HANDBUCH DER MEDIZINISCHEN RADIOLOGIE

ENCYCLOPEDIA OF MEDICAL RADIOLOGY

HERAUSGEGEBEN VON · EDITED BY

L. DIETHELM **O. OLSSON** **F. STRNAD**
MAINZ   LUND   FRANKFURT/M.

H. VIETEN **A. ZUPPINGER**
DÜSSELDORF   BERN

BAND/VOLUME II
TEIL/PART 3

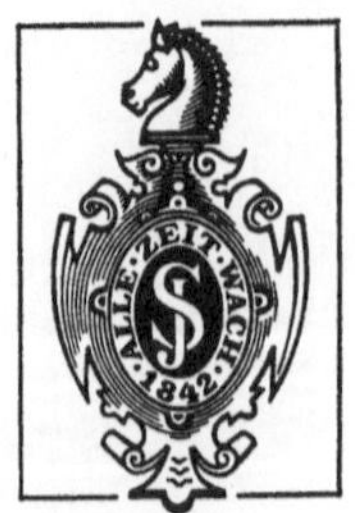

SPRINGER-VERLAG · BERLIN · HEIDELBERG · NEW YORK · 1972

STRAHLENBIOLOGIE
TEIL 3

RADIATION BIOLOGY
PART 3

VON · BY

M. BAUCHINGER · E. P. CRONKITE · T. M. FLIEDNER
FRAU H. FRITZ-NIGGLI · O. HUG · A. M. KELLERER
E. C. LORENZ · E. F. OAKBERG · E. E. POCHIN
K. R. TROTT · FRAU E. ULLRICH-GREVE

REDIGIERT VON · EDITED BY

O. HUG
MÜNCHEN

A. ZUPPINGER
BERN

MIT 186 ABBILDUNGEN
WITH 186 FIGURES

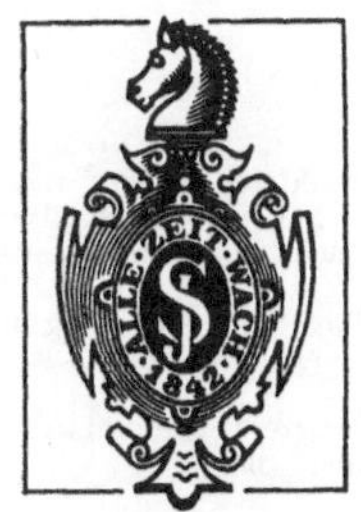

SPRINGER-VERLAG · BERLIN · HEIDELBERG · NEW YORK · 1972

ISBN-13:978-3-642-80711-4   e-ISBN-13:978-3-642-80710-7

DOI: 10.1007/978-3-642-80710-7

Vorwort

Bei der Konzeption des Bandes Strahlenbiologie gingen die Herausgeber von der Annahme aus, daß sich der derzeitige Stand des Faches in zwei Teilbänden befriedigend darstellen lasse. Dabei war Teil 1 den primären chemischen und biochemischen Auswirkungen ionisierender Strahlen auf Zellen und Zellbestandteile, den genetischen Effekten und generellen Faktoren der Strahlenwirkung, wie in der relativen biologischen Wirksamkeit und dem Zeitfaktor zugedacht; Teil 2 sollte die Phänomenologie der Strahlenwirkung auf Einzeller und Vielzeller, insbesondere die Pathomorphologie und -physiologie der Säugetiere einschließlich des Menschen, darstellen.

Spätestens nach Eingang der letzten Manuskripte zeigte sich dann, daß trotz sorgfältiger Planung noch einige erhebliche Lücken offen geblieben waren, die einen dritten Teil notwendig machten. Das ergab sich vor allem aus der rapiden Entwicklung mancher Gebiete der Strahlenbiologie, und zwar gerade solcher, die für die klinische Radiologie wachsende Bedeutung gewonnen haben. Einige Themen sind in der Zwischenzeit sozusagen handbuchwürdig geworden. Besondere Fragestellungen und Ergebnisse, die in den bisherigen Beiträgen oft nur angeschnitten oder unter einem besonderen Aspekt behandelt worden waren, forderten nunmehr eine geschlossene Darstellung.

So war es an der Zeit, eine neue Interpretation der Dosiswirkungsbeziehungen vorzulegen, die zwar von der klassischen Treffertheorie ausging, inzwischen aber zu umfassenderen mathematischen Modellen gelangt ist. Auch stand im deutschen Schrifttum noch immer eine geschlossene Darstellung der Proliferationsstörungen und der Inaktivierung von Säugetierzellen in vitro und in vivo aus — ein Gebiet, das sich im letzten Jahrzehnt eine zentrale Position innerhalb der Strahlenbiologie erobert hat. Gleiches gilt für die Beschreibung und Deutung der Chromosomenaberrationen — nicht nur im Tierexperiment sondern bei den verschiedensten Formen der Strahlenexposition des Menschen. Besondere Bearbeitung verdienten ferner die Strahlenwirkungen auf das Zellplasma und die Keimzellen, die Pathogenese und Klinik der akuten Strahlenkrankheit, die Störungen der Embryonalentwicklung und die Entstehung von Spätschäden, vor allem des Strahlenkrebses. Die einzelnen Beiträge des Teiles 3 hat man sich also als Einfügungen an verschiedenen Stellen im logischen Aufbau der beiden vorhergehenden Teilbände zu denken; im ganzen aber sind sie als eine Art Nachlese auf Grund eines wissenschaftlichen Reifungsprozesses zu betrachten.

München und Bern, Dezember 1972 O. Hug und A. Zuppinger

Preface

In planning the volume on radiobiology, the editors started out with the assumption that the present state of the art could be covered adequately in two subvolumes. The first of these was to deal with the primary chemical and biochemical effects of ionizing radiation on cells and their components, their genetic consequences, and such general aspects of radiation as relative biological efficiency and the time factor. The second subvolume was to cover the phenomenology of radiation effects on single- and multi-cell organisms, with particular reference to the pathomorphology and pathophysiology of mammals, including man.

However, when all the manuscripts were finished, it became clear that, despite careful planning, there were some substantial gaps and that a third subvolume would be required to fill them. This was due for the most part to the rapid advances being made in many fields of radiobiology, not least those which have acquired increasing significance in clinical radiology. Some topics have in the meantime become ripe for inclusion in a handbook. Other problems and results, which the existing contributions had merely touched upon or treated from one particular angle, now demanded a fuller presentation.

For instance, it was time to put forward a new interpretation of dose-effect relationships which, while taking the older hit theory as its basis, had in the meantime evolved more sophisticated mathematical models. Moreover, in the German literature there was still no balanced treatment of proliferative diseases and the inactivation of mammalian cells, both in vitro and in vivo — a subject which over the last decade has moved into a key position in radiobiology. The same is true of the description and interpretation of chromosome aberrations, not in animal experiments alone, but also in a wide variety of forms of radiation exposure of humans. Other themes which required separate treatment comprise: the effects of radiation on cell plasma and germ cells, the pathogenesis and clinical course of acute radiation sickness, defects in embryonic development, and the appearance of late damage, particularly radiation-induced cancer. While the individual contributions to subvolume 3 are to be regarded as interpolations at various places within the logical structure of the two preceding subvolumes, as a whole they are to be seen as a late harvest arising out of the process of scientific maturation.

Munich and Bern, December 1972   O. HUG and A. ZUPPINGER

Inhaltsverzeichnis · Contents

Mitarbeiter von Band II/3 · Contributors to Volume II/3

Priv.-Doz. Dr. M. Bauchinger, Institut für Biologie der Gesellschaft für Strahlen- und Umweltforschung MbH, D-8000 München, Neuherberg und Strahlenbiologisches Institut der Universität München, D-8000 München 15, Bavariaring 19

E. P. Cronkite, M. D. Chairman, Medical, Department, Brookhaven/National Laboratories, Upton/L. I., N. Y. 11973, USA

Prof. Dr. T. M. Fliedner, Med. naturw. Hochschule, Institut für klinische Physiologie, D-7900 Ulm, Parkstr. 10

Frau Prof. Dr. Hedi Fritz-Niggli, Strahlenbiologisches Institut der Universität Zürich, CH-8008 Zürich, August-Forel-Str. 7

Prof. Dr. O. Hug, Vorstand des Strahlenbiologischen Instituts der Universität, D-8000 München 15, Bavariaring 19

Prof. A. Kellerer, M. D., Radiological Research Laboratories, Department for Radiology, Columbia University, New York, N.Y. 10032, USA

Evelyn C. Lorenz, M. D., Biology Division, National Laboratory, Oakridge, Tenn., USA

E. F. Oakberg, M. D., Biology Division, National Laboratory, Oakridge, Tenn., USA

E. E. Pochin, M. D., Medical Research Council Department of Clinical Research, University College Hospital Medical School, University Street, London WCl E 6 JJ, Great Britain

Dr. K.-R. Trott, Gesellschaft für Strahlen- und Umweltforschung, Institut für Biologie, Abt. für Strahlenbiologie und Biophysik, D-8042 Neuherberg, Ingolstädter Landstr. 1

Frau Dr. Etta Ullrich-Greve, D-7806 Ebnet, Rehmattenstr. 4

A. Theory of dose-effect relations*

By

Albrecht M. Kellerer

and

Otto Hug

With 20 figures

I. Introduction

Quantitive dose-effect relations are equally important in the medical application of ionizing radiation and in radiation protection; moreover they are fundamental for an understanding of the mechanisms of radiation action. The practical and theoretical aspect cannot always be clearly separated. Many of the equations and parameters, for example, which are used for the description of dose-effect relations go back to theoretical models which have been used in the past but have now lost relevancy. Stripped of its original meaning the mathematical formalism has often been retained because it permits a suitable representation of typical dose-effect relations, and because it is convenient in many cases to describe a dose-effect relation by a formula or by a few parameters instead of giving it in tabular form or graphical representation. In the following an attempt will be made to distinguish between formal description of dose-effect relations for practical purposes and the mathematical analysis which aims at an understanding of the mechanisms of radiation action. Attention will mainly be given to the dose dependence of cellular radiation actions but the focus will be on general principles which are equally applicable to other levels of radiation action such as molecular systems or multicellular systems. Techniques and arguments applicable to the analysis of dose-response relations are discussed, and no attempt is made to review the experimental techniques, the modifying factors, such as the oxygen effect, or the radiobiological results. Numerical data are used to elucidate the structure of the essential arguments. They are not representative for the great number of dose-effect relations studied in radiation biology and radiology, and neither their experimental accuracy nor their statistical significance will be considered.

II. The concepts of dose and effect

It is useful to clarify the concepts of dose and effect before their quantitative relations are discussed. In the following the word dose always stands for absorbed dose measured in the unit rad. The unit rad corresponds to an energy absorption of 100 erg per gram of the irradiated medium. This special unit has been chosen mainly for historical reasons. For practical application it would be more convenient to use the unit Joule per kilogram which corresponds to 100 rad and is consistent with the International System of Units. The smaller unit rad has however been chosen because it is approximately equivalent to the older unit roentgen.

---

* This work is partly supported by Contract AT-(11-1)-3243 for the United States Atomic Energy Commission and Public Health Service Research Grant No. CA-12536-01 from the National Cancer Institute.

One often uses the comparison with thermal energy to illustrate the unit rad. In this comparison the energy which is transferred by ionizing radiation to the organism seems to be extremely small. An absorbed dose of 1 rad increases the temperature of the irradiated tissue only by roughly $2 \times 10^{-6}\,°C$, and a dose of 500 rad which is lethal for man corresponds to a temperature increase of only $10^{-3}\,°C$. The comparison with thermal energy is however somewhat misleading insofar as heat is energy in its most dissipated form and is thus relatively harmless to the cell. The illustration of the unit rad by its mechanical energy equivalent is therefore more informative. The absorbed dose of 1 rad corresponds approximately to the energy which is necessary to lift the irradiated object by 1 mm in the gravitational field on earth. The dose of 500 rad therefore corresponds to a lifting of the object by 50 cm which is obviously a sizable amount of energy. One also finds that the energy transferred by ionizing radiation to the cell is quite comparable to the energy involved in the action of cell pharmaca which produce the same levels of effect. As a useful rule, applicable on the microscopic and molecular scale, one can state that in a spherical region of diameter $1\,\mu m$ one has on the average one ionization per rad of absorbed dose; in one cubic micron one has roughly 1.8 ionizations. It is thereby postulated that over a wide range of radiation qualities one ionization is produced in the cell per 34 eV of absorbed energy.

In the discussion of cellular or subcellular radiation effects one must be aware that absorbed dose is a statistical concept which merely determines the expectation value of energy deposition in the cell or in the cellular structure. The interaction between a radiation field and matter occurs in discrete and widely varying random events, and the energy imparted to microscopic regions can therefore deviate considerably from the mean value which is determined by absorbed dose. These statistical fluctuations are most expressed for smallest volumes and for densely ionizing radiation; they can be an important and in some cases even the dominant factor which determines the shape of cellular dose-effect relations. In the new formulation of definitions of fundamental quantities in radiation physics (ICRU, 1971) a clear distinction is made between the random variable specific energy z and the non-stochastic quantity absorbed dose D. The specific energy z is defined as the quotient of the energy imparted to the mass of the observed region; the absorbed dose D on the other hand is the expectation value of z. The determination of the probability distributions of z for microscopic regions of different size and for different radiation qualities is object of the so-called microdosimetry. The concepts of microdosimetry and their application to the analysis of dose-effect relations will be discussed in section 7.

The target theory models which are discussed in section 4 treat the complicated patterns of energy deposition in the cell in a greatly simplified manner; they can therefore be of heuristic value but have only limited quantitative validity.

The notion of radiation effect is less clearly defined than that of absorbed dose. Ionizing radiation produces a wide spectrum of alterations in the cell or in the organism. Radiation effects can therefore be measured in various ways. If one deals with effects on the tissue level the scale for measuring the effect must in most cases remain arbitrary. This is for example the case for the production of an erythema or for the induction of lens opacification. The numerical relations between dose and effect have only very indirect meaning in those cases, and it is therefore in general not possible to infer the primary mechanisms of radiation action from such relations. One can, however, avoid this difficulty by studying relative biological effectiveness (RBE) of different radiation qualities as a function of dose; this will be dealt with in section 7.3.

The dose-effect relations which will be discussed in the following are based on so-called quantal effects, i.e. on effects which are not measured in the individual object in a continuous scale but instead are determined merely by the absence or presence of a specified criterion. The most important example are the so-called survival curves. With multicellular organisms one determines the fraction of surviving elements of a population at a specified time after irradiation; if one deals with the inactivation of isolated cells one determines the fraction of cells which produce a colony of a certain minimal size in a specified time after irradiation. One should be aware that the underlying cellular damage can well be continuous and that the experimental endpoint is reduced to an all-or-none criterion merely in order to simplify the experimental technique.

III. The dose-effect relation

For a graphical representation of dose-effect relations one can either plot as a function of dose the fraction of elements which show a specified effect or one can plot the fraction of elements which do not show this effect. The choice between the two different representations depends on the questions asked. If one is interested in the effect of smallest doses, as for example in all considerations concerning radiation protection, one will plot the fraction $E(D)$ of elements which exhibit the effect. $E(D)$ can be called effect probability; it may for example be the probability that the absorbed dose D produces a certain mutation in the cell. If, on the other hand, one is concerned with the doses necessary to inactivate all cells in a tumor then the quantity of interest is the fraction $S(D)$ of survivors in the irradiated cell population, and one can plot $S(D)$ as a function of absorbed dose[1].

The difference between both representations is trivial, because the quantities $E(D)$ and $S(D)$ are complementary:

$$S(D) = 1 - E(D) . \qquad (3.1)$$

It would therefore be sufficient to consider only one of the quantities $E(D)$ or $S(D)$ if one were to use a linear representation of dose-effect curves. The linear representation has, however, the disadvantage that neither the region of very small effect probabilities nor the region of very small survival probabilities are given with sufficient accuracy. For this reason it is convenient to use different representations depending on whether one deals with small or with high levels of dose and effect.

1. Low levels of dose and effect

If one is interested in the dose-effect relation in the range of smallest doses it is convenient to plot the logarithm of $E(D)$ versus the logarithm of dose. As an example the yield of pink mutations in Tradescantia (SPARROW *et al.*, 1972) is plotted in Fig. 1 in linear and in logarithmic representation. The double-logarithmic representation has not only the advantage of increased accuracy but is useful also for the reason that it indicates directly whether in a given case one deals with a linear or with a quadratic dependence of effect on dose. If one assumes that the effect probability is a power function of dose:

$$E(D) = k\, D^n , \qquad (3.2)$$

one obtains the following relations between the logarithms:

$$\ln E(D) = n \ln D + \ln k . \qquad (3.3)$$

Thus, the power function is transformed to a straight line in the double logarithmic representation and the slope of this line is equal to the dose exponent n. A linear relation between absorbed dose and the effect therefore leads to a straight line of slope 1. A quadratic relation between effect and dose, on the other hand, leads to a straight line of slope 2 as in the case of x rays and larger doses in the example of Fig. 1b. The logarithmic repre-

---

1 Here and in the following the term 'survivors within a population' is used to simplify terminology and because survival curves are the most important case of dose-effect relations. The expression can, however, be understood in a general sense and stands for non-occurrence of the test effect.

sentation is therefore of special importance if one deals with the question whether the effect exhibits some kind of threshold in the range of smallest doses or whether it is proportional to dose.

In section 6 the interpretation of the slope of the dose-effect relation in the logarithmic plot will be discussed in some detail. In the present context it is useful to illus-

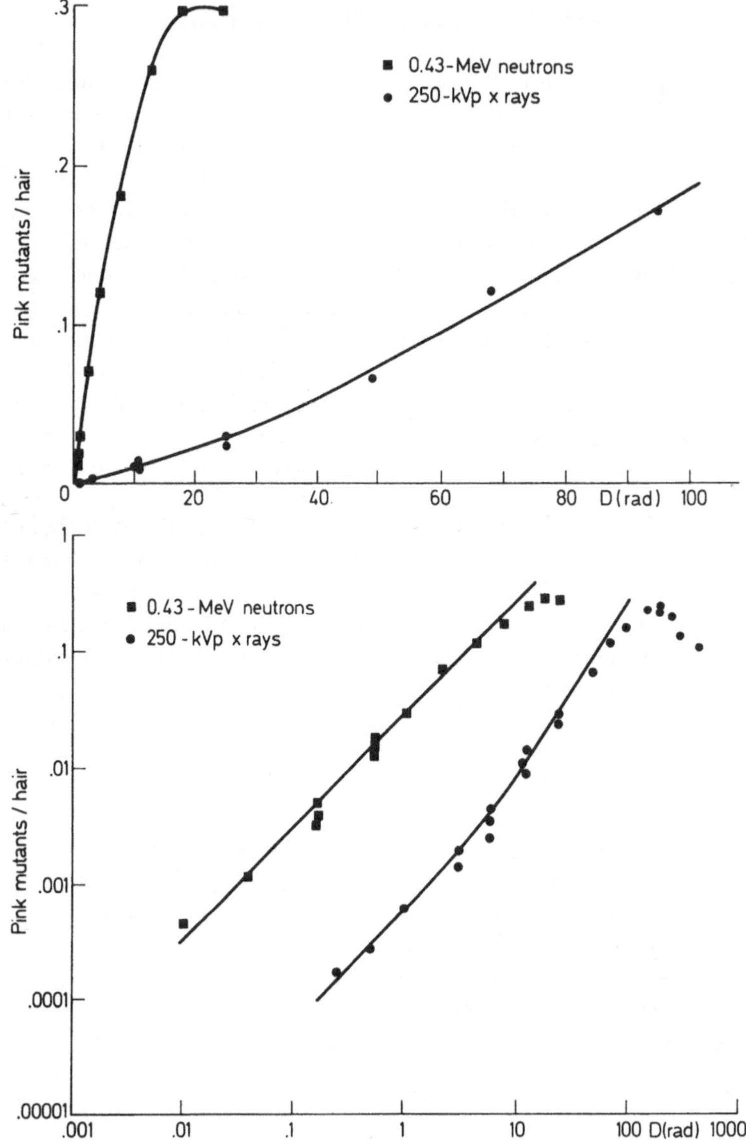

Fig. 1. Linear and logarithmic representation of the dose dependence of the induction of pink mutant cells in the stamen hairs of *Tradescantia* (Sparrow *et al.*, 1972). The spontaneous rate is subtracted. The solid lines in the linear and in the logarithmic plot do not correspond

trate the meaning of the double logarithmic plot by a consideration of dose-effect relations which are commonly used in the analysis of cytogenetic observations (see contribution of Bauchinger to this volume). For densely ionizing radiations and at effect levels which are low enough that one can neglect saturation effects one frequently finds a linear relation between dose and yield of radiation induced chromosome aberrations:

$$E(D) = \alpha D , \tag{3.4}$$

this relation corresponds to a line of slope 1 in the double logarithmic representation. It is essential to subtract the spontaneous rate from the yield; if this were not done the curve would be horizontal at small doses.

For x-rays the situation is more complicated and one frequently observes a quadratic dependence of the yield on dose or more generally a superposition of a linear term and a quadratic term:

$$E(D) = \alpha D + \beta D^2 \, . \tag{3.5}$$

This results in a bent curve in the double logarithmic representation as indicated in Fig. 2. At low doses the curve has the slope 1, at higher doses the slope approaches the value 2. The x-ray data in Fig. 1 agree with eq. (3.5). Cell killing at higher doses and the fact that one can only observe a limited number of aberrations per cell lead to a saturation effect, i.e. to a decrease in slope at higher doses, and in some cases the slope of 2 may not

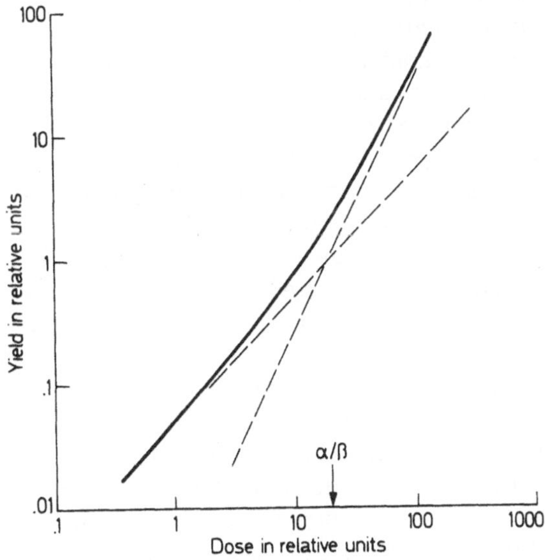

Fig. 2. Dose-effect curves for the linear-quadratic model represented by eq. (3.5)

be reached. This saturation effect which may involve complicated factors and is not always accessible to analysis will not be considered in the present context.

As will be explained in section 7, the linear component in eq. (3.5) represents effects produced by a single particle track, while the quadratic component represents effects due to the interaction of lesions produced by two particles. This interpretation and the possibility to infer the ratio of the linear and the quadratic component on the basis of microdosimetric quantities (see section 7.2) justifies the use of eq. (3.5) at low levels of dose and effect. One must, however, be careful in fitting experimental data to eq. (3.5). If one uses the least squares approximation one has to apply appropriate statistical weights for the different data points. Statistical analysis is not the object of the present discussion, but it has to be pointed out that curve fitting by numerical methods necessitates in general a thorough statistical analysis. Simple eye-ball fitting of a set of data can be useful in cases where such statistical analysis is not feasible, but one must then be careful to use the appropriate scale. The double logarithmic plot should be used instead of the linear plot whenever one deals with low levels of dose and effect.

The double-logarithmic plot has also the advantage that one avoids ill defined statements which are sometimes made when dose relations on a linear scale are fitted to the linear-quadratic model expressed by eq. (3.5). One such statement is that the linear component is large or small as compared to the quadratic component. Strictly speaking, this is meaningless if one does not specify the dose range to which the statement refers. The reason can be understood on the basis of Fig. 2. If one considers the effect relation in the high dose range the slope approaches the value 2 and one has a purely quadratic reaction. If on the other hand one goes to very small doses one reaches a region where the slope of the curve is 1 and where the linear component is completely dominant. In one and the same object and with the same radiation quality one may therefore find a predominantly linear or a predominantly quadratic dose-effect relation depending on whether one works in a range of small or high doses. This simple consideration is especially important for an appraisal of the so-called power law expressed by eq. (3.2) which is sometimes used to fit the dose dependence of radiation induced chromosome aberrations. This relation is used as an alternative to the linear-quadratic model expressed by eq. (3.5) and the dose exponent is taken to indicate the relative importance of the one-track and two-track action. If n is near to 1 the action is mainly linear, if n approaches the value 2 the action is nearly quadratic. The application of eq. (3.2) is an attempt to fit the data by a straight line of intermediate slope in the double logarithmic plot instead of fitting them by the bent curve represented in Fig. 2. Because most experiments cover only a limited dose range such a fit is frequently possible even if the actual dose-effect relation is a superposition of a linear and a quadratic term. However, one can obtain quite different values of the dose exponent n depending on whether the experiments are performed in a range of small doses or in a range of high doses. One may even state that in principle one can always obtain the dose exponent 1 if one goes to sufficiently low doses and that one can approach dose exponents which are considerably larger than 1 if one looks at the effects of higher doses. It is therefore in general not useful to characterize dose-effect relations by merely giving the dose exponent n. Except in those cases where a straight line of intermediate slope actually gives a better fit than the linear-quadratic model expressed by eq. (3.5) this latter model is more meaningful. In order to specify the relative size of the linear and the quadratic component one must give the ratio α/β of the two coefficients in eq. (3.5). This ratio has the dimension of a dose and it is equal to the dose at which the linear and quadratic component are just equal; one can also say that α/β is the dose at which the inflection of the curve in Fig. 2 occurs. Below this dose the linear component is predominant, above this dose the quadratic component is predominant. In certain cases, however, the quadratic component may be hidden by the flattening of the dose effect curve due to saturation of the effect at higher doses. The power law (3.2) may then result in a better fit than the linear-quadratic model (3.5).

2. High levels of dose and effect

Frequently one is not merely interested in the low dose range where only a small fraction of the elements of an irradiated population show the effect. Instead one asks for the overall reaction of the population including the region of high effect probability. In these cases a plot of the logarithm of the effect probability E(D) versus the logarithm of dose is of limited use and it is more meaningful to plot the logarithm of the survival probability S(D) versus dose. This so-called semi-logarithmic representation is of special importance in radiation biology because one deals with the range of smallest survival probabilities whenever one tries to utilize cellular survival curves for radiation therapy. Fig. 3 gives the comparison of a typical inactivation curve in linear and semi-logarithmic plot. Because of its shape in the linear plot such a curve is frequently called sigmoidal; because of its shape in the semi-logarithmic representation one uses the alternative term shoulder curve. Comparison of both plots illustrates the fact that the survival probability at highest doses can be read off the semi-logarithmic but not off the linear representation.

The slope $\frac{d \ln S(D)}{dD}$ of the survival curve in semi-logarithmic plot has a simple meaning. It indicates what fraction of the surviving cells in a population is eliminated by the

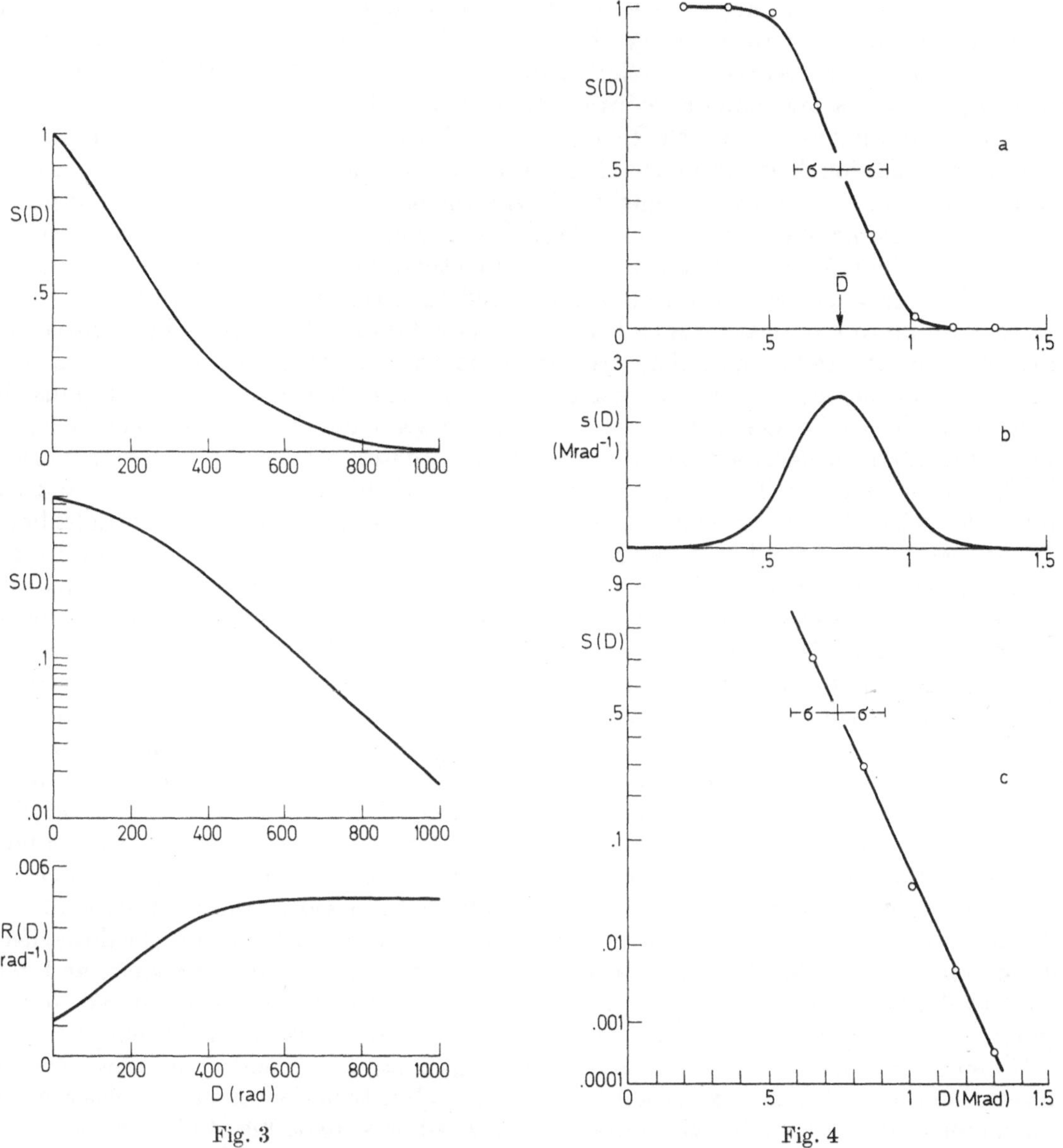

Fig. 3   Fig. 4

Fig. 3. A sigmoidal survival curve in linear and in semi-logarithmic representation, and the dependence of the reactivity, $R(D) = - d \ln S/dD$, on dose

Fig. 4. Survival of *Micrococcus Radiodurans* as function of the x-ray dose (DEAN *et al.*, 1966). Fig. a represents the survival probability S(D), Fig. b its derivative s(D), the differential distribution of the inactivation dose. Fig. c ist the probit plot of the survival probability. $\overline{D}$ is the mean of the inactivation dose, σ its standard deviation

additional application of a unit dose. This fraction can be termed reactivity R(D) (HUG and KELLERER, 1963):

$$R(D) = - \frac{1}{S(D)} \frac{dS(D)}{dD} = - \frac{d \ln S(D)}{dD} \, . \tag{3.6}$$

In the example of Fig. 3 the reactivity increases with dose and reaches a plateau at higher values of dose. One can interpret the increase of reactivity as the accumulation of sublethal damage in the cell. Such sublethal damage could be due to loss of repair mechanisms or the elimination of a compensation mechanism of the cell against the radiation insult.

This interpretation is backed by the observation of dose-rate dependence of the survival curves and especially by the recovery phenomenon found by Elkind (1959). This recovery process consists in a decrease of sublethal damage, i.e. a reversal to the initial value of reactivity, within a few hours after irradiation of the cell.

In the following section which is concerned with the target theoretical models for survival curves additional reasons for the choice of the semi-logarithmic representation will be given. In the present context one might ask why the use of so-called probit plots is not as common in radiobiology as it is in toxicology. The probit plot is based on the postulate of a normal distribution of the dose necessary for inactivation. Such a normal distribution is frequently observed when organisms are exposed to a continuous stimulus which they can tolerate up to a critical threshold. Because the vital objects always exhibit variations in their sensitivity and because they react with some statistical uncertainty even when all cellular parameters are kept equal, a certain washing out of the critical threshold must be observed. If the percentage fluctuations of sensitivity are small then they frequently follow the characteristic bell-shaped distribution which is described by the Gaussian normal distribution. The survival curve is then the integral of this normal distribution, and the probit plot is based on an ordinate scale which transforms these curves into straight lines.

The reaction of the cell to ionizing radiation can in general not be represented by the probit plot because it does not follow a normal distribution. One of the reasons for this fact is that variations of sensitivity within a cell population can be large and also that the process of colony formation is stochastic in nature and subject to considerable random fluctuations. A further reason is that in radiobiological dose-effect relations one deals with a third random factor in addition to biological variability and to the stochastics of the physiological processes; this is the statistical nature of energy deposition in the critical structures of the cell. The latter factor can even be dominant and, as mentioned in section 2, it is most expressed for small sensitive structures and densely ionizing radiation. The relative fluctuations of energy deposition can be extremely large and can deviate far from a normal distribution. As a limiting case one obtains the exponential survival curves which are frequently called single hit curves and which will be discussed in the next section.

There are, however, also cases in which the fluctuations which determine the dose-effect relation are relatively small. In such cases the use of the probit plot is possible, and it is useful to illustrate this by an example because some of the notions encountered in this context are of general applicability and will be used in later sections of this chapter.

If higher organisms are exposed to ionizing radiations one frequently obtains survival curves which to a good approximation follow a normal distribution; a similar observation is made for spores or bacteria which are relatively radioresistant. Fig. 4 gives an example of such a survival curve in linear representation and in the probit plot. If one forms the negative differential quotient $-\frac{dS(D)}{dD}$ of the survival curve one obtains a bell-shaped function which can be considered as the differential distributions of the sensitivity in the population. In the terminology of probability theory one designates the differential curve as probability density while the integral curve, i.e. the original survival curve, is called sum distribution. It is a useful convention to symbolize the probability density by a small letter which corresponds to the capital letter which is used for sum the distribution. In the following the symbol s(D) will be used for the probability density:

$$s(D) = -\frac{dS(D)}{dD} = \frac{dE(D)}{dD} . \tag{3.7}$$

It is obvious from the definition that one could as well choose the symbol e(D) for this function.

S(D) is the probability that a cell randomly selected from the population survives a dose D; one can also express this by the statement that S(D) is the probability that the inactivation dose for a cell is larger than D. The density s(D), on the other hand, gives the probability that the cell will be inactivated at exactly the dose D; this statement is based on the fact that according to eq. (3.7) s(D) dD is the difference of survival rates at dose D and dose D + dD.

In the present example the mean inactivation dose is directly indicated by the center of the bell-shaped probability distribution. The same value is obtained if one reads off the dose for 50 % survival; the reason is that in the special case of a normal distribution the median value of the inactivation dose is equal to the mean value. The variance of the inactivation dose is determined by the width of the bell-shaped distribution. It is also determined by the slope of the straight line in the probit plot. Large slopes correspond to small values of the variance and vice-versa. The more general definition of mean inactivation dose and of the variance of the inactivation dose which is applicable to survival curves of arbitrary shape will be discussed in section 5.3. First, the target theory analysis of dose effect curves will be described.

IV. Target theory analysis of dose-effect relations

1. Exponential dose-effect relations

The historical basis of target theory has been the observation that the inactivation of microbiological objects such as viruses and certain bacteria but also of enzymes depends exponentially on dose. If S(D) is the survival rate in a population then the exponential dependence on dose D is expressed by the following equation:

$$S(D) = e^{-\alpha D} . \tag{4.1}$$

The coefficient α is frequently called inactivation constant; it can be considered as a formal target volume. The exponential dose-effect relation expresses the fact that independent of the dose already applied a certain dose increment dD always eliminates a constant fraction dS/S(D) of the survivors:

$$\frac{dS(D)}{S(D)} = d \ln S(D) = -\alpha \, dD . \tag{4.2}$$

This means that the reactivity, $-d \ln S/dD$, which has been defined in the preceding section is constant and equal to α; the survival curve is accordingly a straight line in the semilogarithmic plot.

In the region of small doses and small effect probabilities which has been discussed in the previous section the exponential relation reduces to a linear dependence between dose and effect:

$$E(D) = \alpha D . \tag{4.3}$$

In analogy to the process of radioactive decay eq. (4.1), i.e. the constant reactivity of the population, can be understood by the assumption that the effect is due not to a continuous or stepwise accumulation of damage but to individual discrete events. Various assumptions have been made concerning the nature of these critical events. DESSAUER (1922) invoked the notion of point heat to characterize the high local energy density generated in molecular cell structures immediately after the absorption of radiation energy. CROWTHER (1924) independently developed the same mathematical formalism to explain the dose effect relations by the statistics of energy absorption but he made more specific assumptions concerning the nature of the hit events and identified them with ionizations in the sensitive structures of the cell.

The coefficient α in the exponential dose-effect relationship can according to eq. (4.2) be considered as the frequency of hits per unit dose and per cell. If in accordance with CROWTHER's postulate one assumes that the critical event is an ionization one can derive a sensitive volume from the value of the constant α. As mentioned in section 2 the mean energy expended per ionization is roughly 34 eV for a wide range of radiation qualities. The hit frequency is then:

$$\alpha = 1.8\ V \tag{4.4}$$

if the volume V is measured in μm^3 and α in rad^{-1}. Accordingly one obtains the following equation for the sensitive volume V:

$$V = 0.55\ \alpha\ . \tag{4.5}$$

It must, however, be noted that the quantity V is a formal sensitive volume and cannot in all cases be interpreted as an actual sensitive volume in a geometrical sense. The sensitive region can be larger than V because individual ionizations may have probabilities less than 1 for being effective. Further limitations of the analysis are due to the fact that the individual ionizations do not occur completely at random in the irradiated medium but are associated in clusters along the tracks of charged ionizing particles. This can result in a saturation effect and also leads to the fact that the value of the sensitive volume V derived according to eq. (4.5) is too small. A detailed analysis of this effect and methods to correct for it in the case of various radiation qualities are described in Lea's monograph (1946).

In spite of the somewhat hypothetical assumptions concerning the nature of the hit events and in spite of the complications of the analysis due to the details of the microscopic distribution of energy deposition there has been some success in the determination of sensitive volumes in enzymes, viruses and bacteria. The method is, however, restricted to structures which do not exceed a size of approximately 100 Å.

Another limiting case which permits a simplified quantitative analysis is the determination of cross sections for cellular inactivation with densely ionizing particles. In this case the critical event is not the occurence of a single ionization in a sensitive structure but the passage of densely ionizing charged particles through the sensitive region. Such studies are in general complicated by the fact that the particle tracks have a halo of secondary electrons (delta rays) and can therefore not be treated as straight lines without radial extension. A heavy charged particle can pass outside the sensitive region and can still inject delta rays into it. If one neglects this factor one obtains values for the cross section of the sensitive region which are too high. Examples for the treatment of these questions are works by Brustad (1962), Powers (1962), and Barendsen (1967). Because the simplified analysis is valid only in certain limiting cases one must in general use exact microdosimetric data. Such data can be obtained experimentally or can be calculated, and the event frequency φ per unit dose is known for various sizes of the reference region and for various radiation qualities. The use of these data for a determination of sensitive volumes in the cell is described in section 7.

2. Multi-hit and multi-target models

Blau and Altenburger (1922) as well as Crowther (1924) went a step beyond the interpretation of exponential dose-effect relations and attempted to explain also nonexponential dose-effect relations by the statistics of energy deposition. As pointed out in the monographs on target theory (Timofeeff-Ressovsky and Zimmer, 1947; Zimmer, 1961) and in recent works concerned with the interpretation of dose-effect relations (Hug and Kellerer, 1966, Dertinger and Jung, 1969) these models are of limited validity. The resulting equations are, however, used frequently in spite of the fact that the original interpretation has been abandoned. For this reason the essential thoughts of the analysis and the main parts of the mathematical formalism will be presented.

If one assumes that the effect is produced not by a single event of energy deposition, but by an accumulation of such events up to a critical number, one obtains curves of the sigmoidal type, such as the one in Fig. 3. In order to derive the equations for the dose-effect relations according to the models employed in target theory, one needs the formula of Poisson. This formula determines the probability $p(\nu)$ for the occurence of exactly ν statistical independent events if the expectation value of the number of events is N:

$$p(\nu) = e^{-N} \frac{N^{\nu}}{\nu!} . \tag{4.6}$$

One may observe that eq. (4.1) is a special case of this Poissonian formula for the case of $\nu = 0$ with $N = \alpha D$.

It should be pointed out that the Poissonian formula is the basis of all the mathematical formalism of target theory. It is, therefore, useful to illustrate this formula by a numerical example. Assume, for instance, that a population of equal cells is exposed to a radiation field in which each cell is on the average traversed by $N = 4$ charged particles. Then the fraction of cells which are traversed by no particle at all is equal to $p(0) = e^{-4} = 0.018$. The fraction of cells which are traversed by exactly one particle is $p(1) = 4\,e^{-4} = 0.072$; and similar expressions are obtained for higher event numbers.

The so-called multi-hit equations result if one assumes that a cell is inactivated if n or more hits occur in its sensitive structure. One then obtains the survival probability as a sum of all Poissonian terms for $\nu < n$:

$$S(D) = \sum_{\nu = 0}^{n-1} e^{-\alpha D} \frac{(\alpha D)^{\nu}}{\nu!} . \tag{4.7}$$

αD is the expectation value of the number of hits in the sensitive structure of the cell.

A different assumption is made in the so-called multi-target model. In this model it is postulated that the cell contains exactly n sensitive targets and that each of these targets must be eliminated by a single event for inactivation of the cell. The probability for each individual target to be eliminated at dose D is given by:

$$p(D) = 1 - e^{-\alpha D} , \tag{4.8}$$

where αD is the mean number of hits per target. The survival probability for the cell is then:

$$S(D) = 1 - p(D)^n = 1 - (1 - e^{-\alpha D})^n . \tag{4.9}$$

In the numerous applications of eqs. (4.7) and (4.9) one has never succeeded to fill the hypothetical hit numbers or the numbers of sensitive targets with concrete biological meaning. This is not surprising because the statistics of energy deposition are not the only factor responsible for the shape of the dose-effect curves. A mathematical approach which neglects this is therefore, at best, an idealization. But even if one restricts the discussion to the statistics of energy deposition, one still finds that the multi-hit model and the multi-target model are arbitrary special cases and that they are therefore void of concrete meaning.

The multi-hit model is based on the assumption of equal, statistically independent hits. Microscopic patterns of energy deposition are, however, characterized by the fact that ionizations and excitations occur in clusters of widely varying size; this is true for all radiation qualities with the possible exception of UV-radiation. Equality of hypothetical hits can, therefore, not be postulated. It is one of the main results of microdosimetric analysis that the spectra of energy deposition in microscopic regions deviate widely from Poisson distributions. The statistical fluctuations exceed the fluctuations, which should result according to Poissonian statistics, by orders of magnitude. Furthermore the hits in individual targets can not be expected to be statistically independent. Statistical independence is, however, required for the validity of eq. (4.9), and this equation is therefore an oversimplification. Similarly, there is little justification to assume that one always deals with equal sensitive targets within the vital object. Finally one would have to consider the general case that it is sufficient for cellular inactivation to damage a limited number out of a larger number of sensitive targets and that the individual targets can have different inactivation kinetics. Such models lead to considerable complexity of the formalism. This, however, is not the main limitation. The various models can be readily solved within the framework of the theory of Markov-processes (see Hug and Kellerer, 1966). A more serious limitation is that the number of free parameters is increased to such a point that it is impossible to distinguish between the various models. Curve fitting by target theory models must therefore remain arbitrary.

The differences in the shape of the survival curves according to eqs. (4.7) and (4.9) are not characteristic for the different models. In both cases the reactivity, i.e. the slope of the curve in the semilogarithmic plot, approximates the value α with increasing dose. The

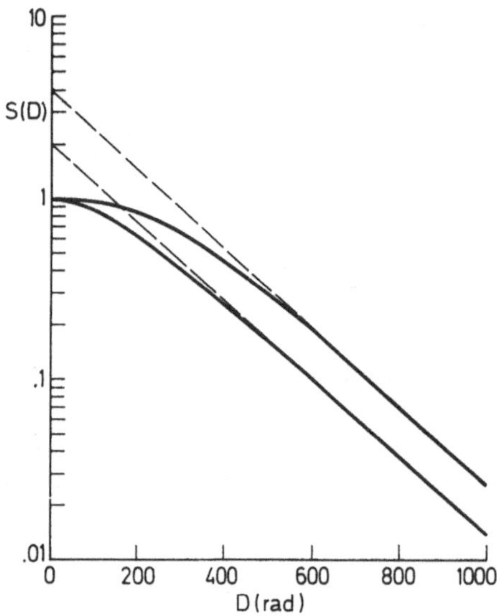

Fig. 5. Survival curves according to the multi-target equation (4.9) with n = 2 and 4

multi-target curves have the additional property that they can be approximated by an exponential function in the range of high doses:

$$S(D) = ne^{-\alpha D} \quad \text{for} \quad D \gg n/\alpha .\tag{4.10}$$

This approximation is symbolized in Fig. 5 by the broken straight line. The intersection of this asymptotic line with the ordinate occurs at the value n, and n has therefore in the past been called the target number. It is, however, merely a formal parameter and the neutral term extrapolation number (Alper, 1960) is now generally preferred. In contrast to eq. (4.9) the curves which correspond to eq. (4.7) do not permit an asymptotic representation by an exponential function. One can, however, show that this property of eq. (4.7) is not characteristic for the multi-hit model. If, for example, one assumes that the probability for further hits is changed after the first hits, or if one takes into account the influence of recombination or recovery processes then one obtains finite extrapolation numbers even in the case of the multi-hit model (Kellerer and Hug, 1963). In summary one can state that the target theory models are merely special cases of a mathematical treatment which describes the energy deposition in the cell and the radiation induced secondary changes as stochastic processes. In spite of the fact that these special cases have in general little quantitative validity they can still be useful as heuristic tools in radiobiology.

Because it is frequently practical to represent experimental survival curves by analytical expressions it is common to use target theory formulae in a purely empirical way without reference to their original interpretation. Frequently eq. (4.9) is used. The reason for this choice is that this equation is more easily evaluated than eq. (4.7); another reason is that it is common use to approximate the experimental data at high doses by an exponential function, i.e. by a straight line in the semi-logarithmic plot. One should however be aware that, as all intra- or extrapolations, the choice of a specific analytic expression always contains a subjective element and that it can lead to a falsification of experimental data.

If one considers only the region of small effect probability then both the n-hit and the n-target model reduce to simple proportionality between the effect and the n-th power of dose. From the multi-hit equation (4.7) one obtains:

$$E(D) = \frac{\alpha^n}{n!}\, D^n \tag{4.11}$$

and from the multi-target equation (4.9):

$$E(D) = \alpha^n\, D^n \,. \tag{4.12}$$

For values n larger than 1 one should therefore have zero initial slope of the dose-effect curve in the semi-logarithmic plot. In general one must however expect that the dose-effect relation has a finite slope at small doses. To account for this it is commonly assumed that in addition to the accumulation of damage up to a critical threshold one deals with a single event mechanism which may, for example, reflect the densely ionizing component of the radiation field. In this case one frequently uses the equation:

$$S(D) = e^{-\alpha D}\left(1 - (1 - e^{-\beta D})^n\right) \,. \tag{4.13}$$

This equation can be considered as a superposition of the multi-target equation with a single event equation, but, strictly speaking, it is nothing but an empirical representation of certain sigmoidal dose-effect curves. In fact one can choose other equations which are equally well suited to fit most of the observed dose-effect curves and which are of somewhat simpler analytical form. An example is the so-called logistic curve:

$$\ln S(D) = -\alpha D - \beta D^2 \tag{4.14}$$

which corresponds to a linear increase of reactivity with dose:

$$R(D) = \alpha + 2\,\beta D \,. \tag{4.15}$$

This relation which has been used by SINCLAIR (1968) to represent cellular survival curves can be modified so that the reactivity approaches a finite value with increasing dose (HAYNES, 1966; HUG and KELLERER, 1963):

$$R(D) = \alpha + \beta\left(1 - e^{-\gamma D}\right) \tag{4.16}$$

and therefore:

$$\ln S(D) = -(\alpha + \beta)\, D + \frac{\beta}{\gamma}\left(1 - e^{-\gamma D}\right) \,. \tag{4.17}$$

An advantage of eqs. (4.14) or (4.17) over the modified multi-target equation (4.13) is that they make it easier to describe the dose-rate dependence of the survival curve. Formulae which account for dose-rate dependence have been derived for the target theory models but they are unnecessarily complicated. If, on the other hand, one choses eqs. (4.14) and (4.17) dose-rate dependent dose-response curves can be readily derived from a differential equation for the reactivity, i.e. the semi-logarithmic slope of the dose-effect curve. The simplest assumption is that the sublethal damage which expresses itself in the increased reactivity recovers exponentially with a time constant λ. For the case of eq. (4.14) one then derives the relation:

$$\frac{dR(D)}{dD} = 2\,\beta - \frac{\lambda}{I}\left(R(D) - \alpha\right), \tag{4.18}$$

where I is the dose rate. In those cases where the dose rate is time dependent one must write the differential equation with time as the independent variable instead of dose:

$$\frac{dR(D)}{dt} = 2\,I\,\beta - \lambda\,(R(D) - \alpha). \tag{4.19}$$

Analogous relations can be obtained for the modified equation (4.17). From the differential equations one readily obtains the solutions for the dose-effect relations determined with constant dose rate, with constant irradiation time, or with split doses. To give explicit solutions in these cases and to discuss complicating factors, such as movement of the cells through the growth cycle, is not the object of the present study; the time factor problem has been treated in detail in a separate article in this handbook (Hug *et al.*, 1966).

V. General description of dose-effect relations

1. Random factors in the response curve

With well synchronized cultures of isolated mammalian cells or with such relatively simple objects as viruses or dried spores one can achieve rather well defined pure populations. But such cases are the exception rather than the rule. And the experimentalist is in general aware of the fact that the dose-effect relation reflects the reaction of a mixed population, and that it must therefore be considered as a superposition of dose-effect relations which belong to the different subpopulations. This can be expressed by the following equation:

$$S(D) = \sum_i p_i\, S_i(D). \tag{5.1}$$

Here S(D) is the survival probability for the total population at dose D and $S_i(D)$ is the survival probability for i-th subpopulations. The factors p_i represent the relative weight of the different subpopulations; the sum of all p_i is equal to unity. The assumption of a finite number of subpopulations is naturally an abstraction. In reality one might deal with a continuous spectrum of different elements and eq. (5.1) should therefore contain an integral instead of a sum. The approximation by a finite number of subpopulations is however in general sufficient; such an approximation corresponds for example to the usual separation of the mitotic cycle of the cell into the discrete states G1, S, G2, and M.

The general result of the superposition of different dose-effect curves is a flattening of the shoulder of the resulting curve. If for example one superimposes different multi-hit curves then the result is always characterized by a hit number which is smaller than the mean hit number of the individual curves. This is illustrated in Fig. 6. The solid line is the

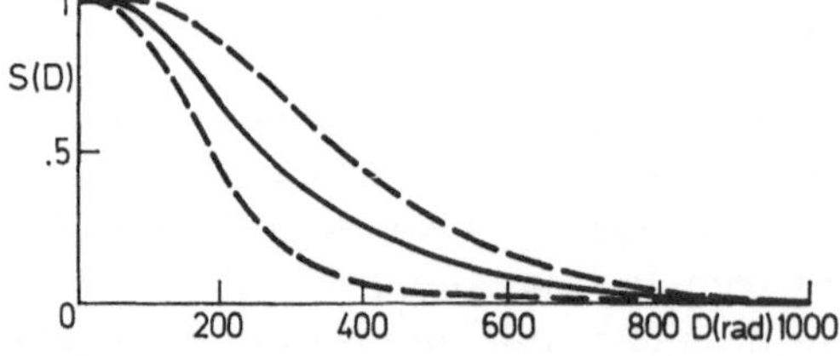

Fig. 6. Superposition of two dose-effect curves. The resulting curve (solid line) deviates more strongly from a step-function than the two component curves (broken lines)

superposition of the two survival curves which are indicated by broken lines. While each of the broken lines could be approximated by a 4-hit curve the resulting curve could more nearly be described by a 2-hit curve. A more rigorous formulation of these statements will be given in the next section. In the present context it is sufficient to state that with increasing biological variability the dose-effect curve loses more and more of its character as a step function. From this fact it follows that the deviations from the simplifying assumptions of the target-theory models do not average out and that therefore the so-called multi-hit or multi-target curves (see eq. [4.7] and [4.9]) have in general only very limited meaning.

A possible exception is the case that the fluctuations of energy deposition are so large that they are the dominant factor in the survival curve and that therefore the biological

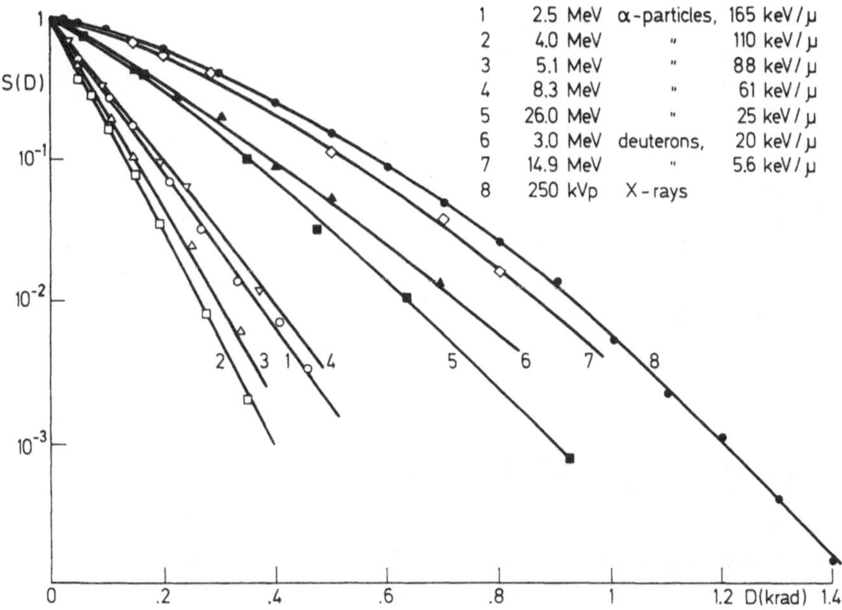

Fig. 7. Survival curves of cultured human cells irradiated with various monoenergetic charged particles (Barendsen, 1967)

variability can be neglected. This can be the case in the inactivation of cells by densely ionizing charged particles. In this case one obtains exponential dose-effect curve which reflect the statistics of charged particle passages:

$$S(D) = e^{-\alpha D} . \tag{5.2}$$

This is confirmed by results which Barendsen (1967) obtained on kidney cells irradiated with heavy charged particles of different ionization density. One can see from Fig. 7 that the survival curve loses its initial shoulder with increasing ionization density. For α-particles one obtains a curve which appears to be exponential and one finds that at the mean inactivation dose (see Section 5.3), $\overline{D} = 1/\alpha$, the nucleus of the cell is, on the average, traversed by only one charged particle. One concludes that the passage of a single α-particle through the nucleus of the cell is sufficient to inactivate the cell. On the other hand, one can show that even in this case the exponential dose-effect relation can only be an approximation.

Hall et al. (1972) find a significant variation of cellular sensitivity against densely ionization radiation in the different phases of the cell cycle. Fig. 8a represents the survival rate after 250 rad of α-irradiation for hamster cells as a function of cell age. If one assumes that the survival curves for synchronized cells are exponential then one must expect that the survival curve for a non-synchronized population deviates from the exponential shape; it must appear as a concave curve from above in a semi-logarithmic plot, i.e. as a curve which bends upwards. Fig. 8b gives the survival curve which should result according to the data represented in Fig. 8a. The curve has indeed a slope which decreases with increasing dose. Because of the limited accuracy of the experimental data it is, however, not possible to observe this deviation from the exponential shape in spite of the fact that the slope, i.e. the reactivity (see eq. [3.6]), changes by nearly a factor of 2 with increasing dose. It is also conceivable that the decrease of reactivity with increasing dose which is due to the biological variability of the cells is compensated by an increase of the reactivity which is due to the accumulation of predamage at higher doses. One can therefore not

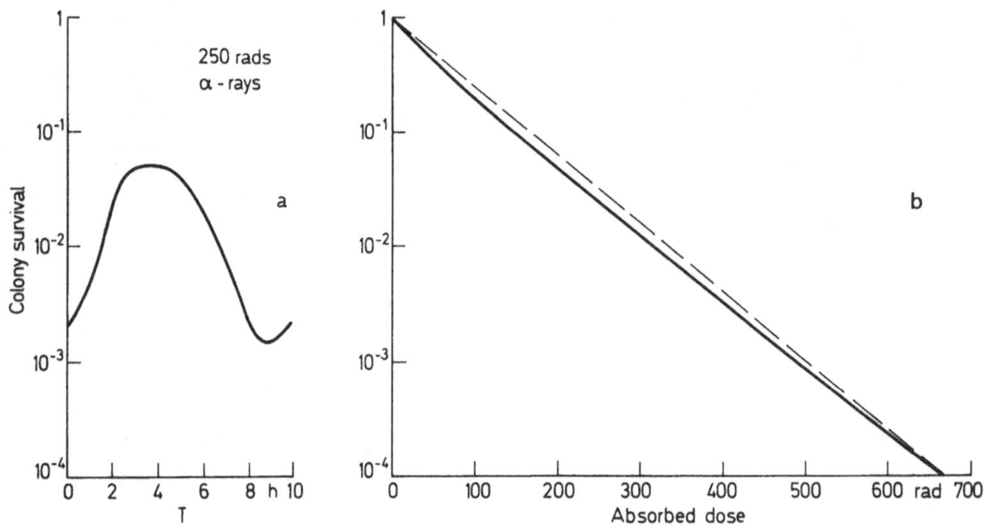

Fig. 8a. Survival of synchronized Chinese hamster cells exposed to 250 rad of 5 MeV α-particles at different times after mitosis

Fig. 8b. Survival curve (solid line) for a non-synchronized population under the assumption that the survival curves for all individual cell ages are exponential. The broken line is inserted to indicate the deviations from an exponential function

with certainty conclude from the apparent exponential shape of the curve that one deals with a pure single-hit mechanism. This case has been discussed in detail because it is a good example for the danger of over-simplification in the interpretation of dose-effect relations. It demonstrates that a detailed analysis is necessary even in the case of seemingly obvious results.

For sigmoid dose effect relations one can state in even greater generality that each of the factors: biological variability, stochastic nature of the physiological processes, and statistics of energy deposition must play its role. Attempts to separate these factors and to determine their individual influence on the dose-effect relations must be based on microdosimetric data, and they necessitate the comparison of dose-effect relations obtained with various radiation qualities.

One must stress — and this will be self-evident for the biologist — that the cell inherently reacts in statistical ways. The random distribution of allele genes to the progeny of the cell is merely one example for this fact. The observation that heating of cells (Dewey et al., 1971) yields survival curves very similar to those obtained with x-rays, demonstrates that it would be pointless to invoke only the statistics of energy deposition in the explanation of survival curves. The random character of colony formation of mammalian cells *in vitro* has in the past years been explicitly studied (see the contribution of TROTT to this volume) and, as alternatives to the target theory analysis, models have been discussed which explain the dose-effect relation by the biological stochastics. In reality these two aspects are not alternatives but they are both equally important to the dose-effect relation which is always influenced by the three factors: statistics of energy deposition, biological variability, and biological stochastics. Any attempt to explain the dose-effect curve by only one of these three aspects must lead to unjustified simplifications.

2. Conventional parameters of the dose-effect relation

As has been mentioned earlier it is common to plot the logarithm of the survival probability S(D) versus dose. The most frequently used parameters for the description of a dose-effect relation are derived from this semi-logarithmic plot.

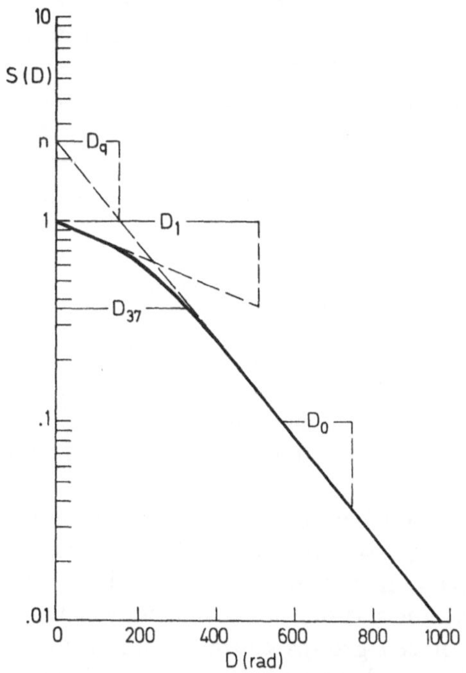

Fig. 9. The conventional parameters of a survival curve

One parameter is the initial slope of the survival curve:

$$s(0) = - \left. \frac{dS(D)}{dD} \right|_0 . \tag{5.3}$$

This quantity which has the dimension rad^{-1} is identical with the initial value R(0) of the reactivity. More frequently one uses the inverse quantity which is occassionally called D_1:

$$\mathbf{D_1} = - \left. \frac{dS(D)}{dD} \right|_0^{-1} . \tag{5.4}$$

D_1 is the dose at which the tangent to the initial point of the dose effect curve in the semi-logarithmic plot intersects the value $S(D) = e^{-1} = 0.37$.

Another parameter is the so-called 37 %-dose (D_{37}) i.e. the dose for which the survival probability is equal to e^{-1}:

$$S(D_{37}) = e^{-1} = 0.37 . \tag{5.5}$$

Finally one frequently uses the so-called extrapolation number n which has already been discussed in section 4.2, and the quantity D_0 which is equal to the inverse of the slope of the dose-effect curve in the region of high doses:

$$D_0 = - \left. \frac{d \ln S(D)}{dD} \right|_{\infty}^{-1} . \tag{5.6}$$

It should be pointed out that there is as yet no established radio-biological terminology. The symbols used for the various quantities may therefore vary; thus the symbol D_{37} is occasionally used for the parameter which has here been defined as D_0.

In the special case of exponential dose-effect relations the three parameters D_1, D_{37}, and D_0 are equal. For the so-called shoulder curves one has the inequation:

$$D_1 > D_{37} > D_0 . \tag{5.7}$$

The parameters D_1 and D_{37} exist for all dose effect relations. The definition of the quantity D_0, on the other hand, is based on the assumption that the slope of the dose effect curve in the semi-logarithmic plot, i.e. the reactivity, converges against a constant value with increasing dose. The definition of the extrapolation number is based on the additional assumption that the dose-effect curve approximates an exponential function at higher doses; this has already been mentioned in section 4.2. The quantity D_0 exists for the multi-hit curves, the multi-target curves, and the curves described by eq. (4.13). It does, however, not exist for the logistic curve (4.14):

$$S(D) = e^{-(\alpha + \beta D)D} , \tag{5.8}$$

which corresponds to a linear increase of the reactivity with dose. If the dose-effect curve is the integral of a normal distribution one also obtains no finite value of D_0. Among the equations which have been discussed for survival curves only the exponential function, the so-called multi-target curves, and the curves described by eq. (4.13) have finite extrapolation numbers.

The initial slope of the dose-effect curves or its inverse D_1 are parameters which are relevant to all considerations pertaining to the effectiveness of smallest doses. The determination of the proliferative ability of mammalian cells is subject to considerable inaccuracies at smallest doses. The fluctuations of the plating efficiency of the cells and the multiplicity, i.e. the existence of cell groups during irradiation, are responsible for the fact that the initial part of the survival curves is in general not very accurately known. A detailed discussion of these factors is given in the monograph of ELKIND and WHITMORE (1967).

It is of great importance for the evaluation of the initial part of cellular inactivation curves whether the irradiation has been performed before or immediately after the plating of the cells or whether the cells have been irradiated several hours after plating. In the latter case it should always be stated whether the experimental data are corrected for multiplicity and, if they are, the details of this correction should be given.

If the survival curve is a superposition of different curves according to eq. (5.1) then the initial slope D_1^{-1} is the arithmetic mean of the corresponding quantities for the subpopulations:

$$D_1^{-1} = \sum_i p_i D_{1,i}^{-1} . \tag{5.9}$$

This additivity of the initial slope of the dose-effect curves simplifies the analysis if one deals with non-synchronized or only partially synchronized cell cultures. If one knows the value of D_1^{-1} for the total population and for certain phases of the cell cycle, one can deduce its value for the remaining part of the cell cycle.

For the quantity D_0 and for the extrapolation number n one does not have additivity of the values of the sub-population. These parameters are exclusively determined by the reaction of the sub-population with the greatest resistance:

$$n = p_r\, n_r\,, \tag{5.10}$$

$$D_0 = D_{0,r}\,.$$

Here p_r is the relative fraction of cells in the most resistant sub-population, for example of the cells which are in the most resistant phase of the cell cycle namely the S phase. n_r and $D_{0,r}$ are the extrapolation number and the D_0 for the resistant sub-population. This is an indication of the rather limited meaning of the quantities D_0 and n.

If one wants to determine the quantities D_0 and n for cells in the more sensitive phases of the cell cycle one must make sure that the population contains no cells at all which belong to the resistant phases. This explains the impossibility to obtain very exact values of D_0 and n for cells in G_1, G_2, and M phase.

Lack of additivity limits the usefulness of the extrapolation number and the quantity D_0, it does, however, not imply that these quantities are inapplicable. The greatest accuracy in the determination of survival probabilities of cell cultures *in vitro* is obtained in the region of smallest survival probabilities. This and the attempts to use the survival data of isolated cells *in vitro* for an understanding of the kinetics of tumor inactivation are the main reasons for the frequent use of the semi-logarithmic plot which stresses the low survival part of the dose-effect relation. In this range of the survival curves the parameter D_0 and the extrapolation number n are useful. One should, however, make it a habit to state explicitly from what dose range or survival range one has derived the estimated values of these quantities. D_0 and n can then be considered as parameters of the tangent to the dose-effect curve in that particular range and need not be considered as absolute characteristics of the dose-effect curve as a whole; this point has been stressed by ELKIND and WHITMORE and is discussed in some detail in their monograph (1967).

An additional parameter which is sometimes used but which is merely a function of D_0 and n is the so-called quasi-threshold dose D_q (ALPER, 1962). It is equal to the dose at which the asymptote to the shoulder curve intersects the abscissa (see Fig. 9). If two large doses D and D', given in quick succession, produce a certain effect then the doses D and $D' + D_q$ are necessary to produce the same effect if separated by a time interval sufficient for recovery of all sublethal damage. D_q can therefore be considered as the dose expended for the production of sublethal damage. The relation between D_q and D_0 and n is:

$$D_q = D_0 \ln n\,. \tag{5.11}$$

One must note that D_q exists only if D_0 and n exist.

The quantity D_{37} is also a parameter which is not additive from the values of the sub-populations. This quantity can not even be calculated if all the values D_{37} are known for the sub-population. One can merely state that D_{37} for the total population must lie between the largest and the smallest value for the sub-populations. Corresponding statements can be made for the so-called median dose D_{50} which is occasionally used.

3. The recommended new parameters and their connection to the conventional quantities

A quantity which is closely related to the parameter D_{37} but which is additive and which is representative for the total population is the mean inactivation dose or mean effect dose $\overline{D}$:

$$\overline{D} = -\int_0^\infty D\,\frac{dS(D)}{dD}\,dD = \int_0^\infty D\,s(D)\,dD\,. \tag{5.12}$$

2*

The survival probability S(D) can, as discussed in section 3, be considered as an integral probability distribution; this is so because S(D) is the probability that a dose larger than D is necessary to inactivate a cell which has been randomly selected from the population. The derivative of S(D) is the corresponding differential probability distribution:

$$s(D) = -\frac{dS(D)}{dD} \, , \tag{5.13}$$

and eq. (5.12) is therefore the common definition of a mean value. By partial integration one can transform eq. (5.12) so that the numerical evaluation is simplified:

$$\overline{D} = \int\limits_0^\infty S(D) \, dD \, . \tag{5.14}$$

This means that the mean inactivation dose is equal to the area under the survival curve in linear representation.

In the case of exponential survival curves the quantities $\overline{D}$ and D_{37} are equal. With increasing shoulder of the survival curve $\overline{D}$ becomes larger than D_{37} and its value approaches that of the median dose D_{50}.

A useful measure of the width of a dose-effect curve or of the degree to which this dose-effect curve deviates from a step function is the variance or mean square deviation of the inactivation dose from its mean value $\overline{D}$:

$$\sigma^2 = \overline{(D - \overline{D})^2} = \overline{D^2} - \overline{D}^2 = \int\limits_0^\infty D^2 \, s(D) \, dD - \overline{D}^2 \, . \tag{5.15}$$

This equation can also be simplified by partial integration and one obtains the following relation:

$$\sigma^2 = 2 \int\limits_0^\infty D \, S(D) \, dD - \overline{D}^2 \, , \tag{5.16}$$

which facilitates numerical evaluation. The functions S(D) and s(D), as well as the parameters $\overline{D}$ and σ^2 are illustrated in Fig. 10.

The quantities $\overline{D}$ and $\overline{D^2}$ are the mean of the inactivation dose and the mean of the square of the inactivation dose; they are frequently called the first moment and the second moment of the distribution. These moments are additive but the variance σ^2 is not. The value of σ^2 for a mixed population is larger than the mean value of the values σ_i^2 for the subpopulations. This is the quantitative formulation of the statement made in section 5.1 that the biological variability always broadens a dose-effect curve. From eq. (5.15) one can obtain the relation between the variance of the total population and the values σ_i^2 for the subpopulations of different sensitivity. If the mean inactivation dose for the subpopulations is designated by $\overline{D}_i$ then one has:

$$\overline{D} = \sum_i p_i \, \overline{D}_i \, ,$$

$$\overline{D^2} = \sum_i p_i \, \overline{D_i^2} \, , \tag{5.17}$$

and therefore:

$$\begin{aligned}
\sigma^2 = \overline{D^2} - \overline{D}^2 &= \sum_i p_i \, \overline{D_i^2} - \overline{D}^2 \\
&= \sum_i p_i \left(\overline{D_i^2} - \overline{D_i}^2 \right) + \sum_i p_i \, \overline{D_i}^2 - D^2 \\
&= \sum_i p_i \, \sigma_i^2 + \sigma_r^2 \, .
\end{aligned} \tag{5.18}$$

The quantity:

$$\sigma_r^2 = \sum p_i \overline{D_i}^2 - \overline{D}^2 = \sum p_i \left(\overline{D_i} - \overline{D}\right)^2 \tag{5.19}$$

is the variance of the mean inactivation dose $\overline{D}_i$ for the different sub-populations. It can also be considered as the variance of radiation resistance throughout the population, because the mean inactivation dose is a measure of the resistance of the cells.

The result expressed by eq. (5.18) is, therefore, that the variance σ^2 of the survival curve exceeds the average of the corresponding values σ_i^2 for the sub-populations by σ_r^2, i.e. by

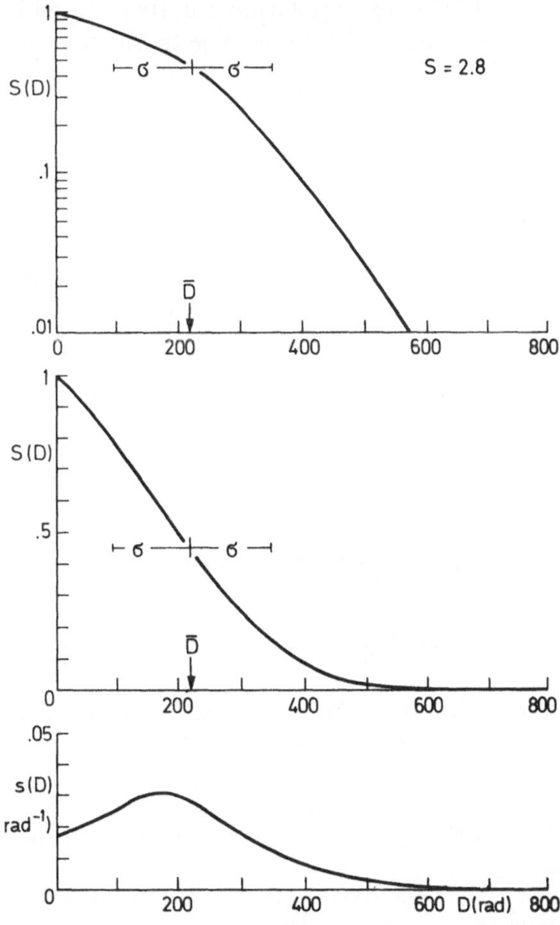

Fig. 10. A survival curve in semi-logarithmic and in linear representation, and its derivative s(D). The values of the mean inactivation dose, $\overline{D}$, and its standard deviation, σ, are indicated

the variance of the resistance in the different sub-populations. The latter term can be considered as the contribution of the biological variability to the width of the survival curve.

It is frequently desirable to measure the width of the survival curve by a parameter which is free of dimensions. In statistics one commonly uses the so-called coefficient of variation $\sigma/\overline{D}$ as a measure for the width of a distribution. In the theory of dose-effect relations it is somewhat more practical to use the square of this quantity, the relative variance:

$$V = \frac{\sigma^2}{\overline{D}^2} = \frac{2 \int\limits_0^\infty D\, S(D)\, dD}{\left(\int\limits_0^\infty S(D)\, dD\right)^2} - 1 . \tag{5.20}$$

Equally useful is the inverse quantity which is called steepness or relative steepness:

$$S = V^{-1} = \overline{D}^2/\sigma^2 \, . \tag{5.21}$$

The possibilities to use these quantities for analysis of the primary mechanisms of radiation action will be discussed in section 7. For exponential survival curves one obtains the value $S = 1$; for shoulder curves the relative steepness is larger than 1. Quite generally one can state that S is a measure of the shoulder of the survival curve: in the mathematical analysis of dose-effect curves this measure takes the place of such simple but poorly defined quantities as hit number or extrapolation number. It will be seen in section 6.2 that S does not represent a number of hits or targets but that it is a lower limit for the

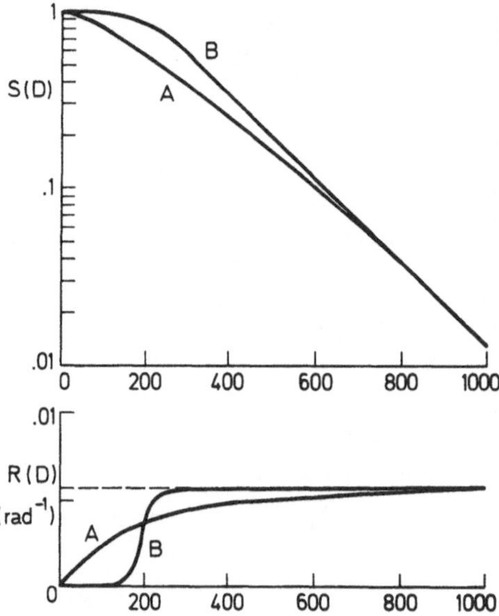

Fig. 11. Two different survival curves with the same parameters n and D_0, and the dose dependence of the reactivity for the two curves

average number of charged particles which must be involved in the mechanism underlying the dose-effect relation.

An example for the fact that the extrapolation number n is not a unique measure for the shoulder of a survival curve is given in Fig. 11. The two curves A and B have the same extrapolation number in spite of the fact that the shoulder of the curve B is much more expressed than the shoulder of the curve A. The steepness S, however, is a realistic measure of the shoulder. It has a value near to 1 for the curve A and a value larger than 3 for the curve B.

The fact that the extrapolation number n is only a poorly defined measure for the shoulder of the survival curve can also be understood in the following way. If one plots the reactivity as a function of dose for the curves A and B then one obtains the curves of Figure 11. In curve A the reactivity, i.e. the sublethal damage in the irradiated population, increases gradually with dose; in the case of the curve B it increases abruptly at a certain threshold value of the dose. In both cases the resulting extrapolation number is the same. The area between the curves and the broken straight line which marks the asymptotic maximum value of reactivity is always equal to the logarithm of the extrapolation number. The survival curve B has a larger shoulder and therefore a higher value of S. One can show in general that for shoulder curves, i.e. for curves in which the reactivity increases with dose, the relative steepness must always lie in the interval given by the following in-equation:

$$1 < S \leq (1 + \ln n)^2 . \tag{5.22}$$

A given value of the extrapolation number is therfore nothing but an upper limit for a possible shoulder in the survival curve. In fact, one can always have a very small shoulder even for large or infinite extrapolation numbers n.

The fact that a survival curve has no finite extrapolation number can be due to the fact that the reactivity keeps increasing with increasing dose. Examples for this are the normal distribution and the so-called logistic curve which has been given in eq. (5.8). On the other hand, it is possible that the reactivity approaches a maximal value $R_0 = D_0^{-1}$ with incrasing dose but in such a way that the area which has been discussed in connection with Fig. 11 is not finite. In other words, there is no finite extrapolation number n if the integral:

$$\ln n = \int_0^\infty \left(R_0 - R(D) \right) dD \tag{5.23}$$

does not converge. This is for example the case with the so-called multi-hit curves (see eq. [4.7]). Experimental data are however always subject to inaccuracies and are limited to a certain dose range. It is, therefore, in general not possible to make definite statements as to the asymptotic behavior of the reactivity. Accordingly one should consider the quantities D_0 and n as parameters of a certain range of the survival curves and not as absolute characteristics of the survival curve.

The preceding considerations are more easily understood if one examines the analogy of the dose dependence of the reactivity with the age dependence of mortality. In this comparison dose corresponds to age, reactivity corresponds to mortality rate, the mean inactivation dose corresponds to the mean lifetime, and the variance σ^2 of the inactivation dose corresponds to the variance of lifetime. A description which fits certain mortality curves is the so-called Gompertz function for the mortality rate as function of age. According to this function the mortality rate (reactivity) is very low for a considerable time but increases exponentially and therefore ultimately reaches extremely high values with increasing age. This leads to a very clearly expressed shoulder in the survival curve as function of age if one plots it in a semi-logarithmic representation. A finite extrapolation number does not exist. The characteristic difference between the mortality curves and the radiobiological survival curves is, therefore, that in the latter the reactivity varies only over a relatively narrow range and that it frequently approaches a more or less constant value at higher doses. One can interpret this by stating that radiation can only induce a certain degree of sublethal damage in the cell. The comparison with the mortality curves illustrates the fact that the analysis of the dose dependence of the reactivity (inactivation rate) permits a fundamental description of the survival curve. As has been seen in section 4.2 this description is particularly useful if one deals with the dose-rate dependence of survival curves which is due to the recovery of sublethal damage.

In many practical cases one desires a simple description of dose-effect relations by a few parameters and it is therefore useful to give some rules which connect the fundamental parameters S and $\overline{D}$ of a survival curve with the commonly used parameters n, D_{37}, and D_0 which are less fundamental but which have the advantage that they can be directly read off the survival curve.

In the special case of the so-called multi-hit curves (see eq. [4.7]) S is equal to the hit number; for the multi-target curves (see eq. [4.9]) S is always smaller than n. The modification of the multi-target model expressed by eq. (4.13) is frequently used to fit survival curves. In this equation n is the extrapolation number, $\alpha = D_1^{-1}$ is the initial slope (reactivity), and $\alpha + \beta = D_0^{-1}$ is the slope at the high dose end. The approximative values of the extrapolation number and the final slope D_0^{-1} can be taken directly from the survival curve, but the initial slope D_1^{-1} can usually not be read off with sufficient accuracy. One may therefore select a different set of three parameters, and a suitable choice is D_{37}, D_0, and n. The curves in Fig. 12 permit the determination of α/β from n and the ratio D_{37}/D_0. The two parameters α and β follow then from their ratio α/β and their sum $\alpha + \beta = D_0^{-1}$. One must, however, be aware of the fact that the resulting α need not be the actual initial slope of the survival curve.

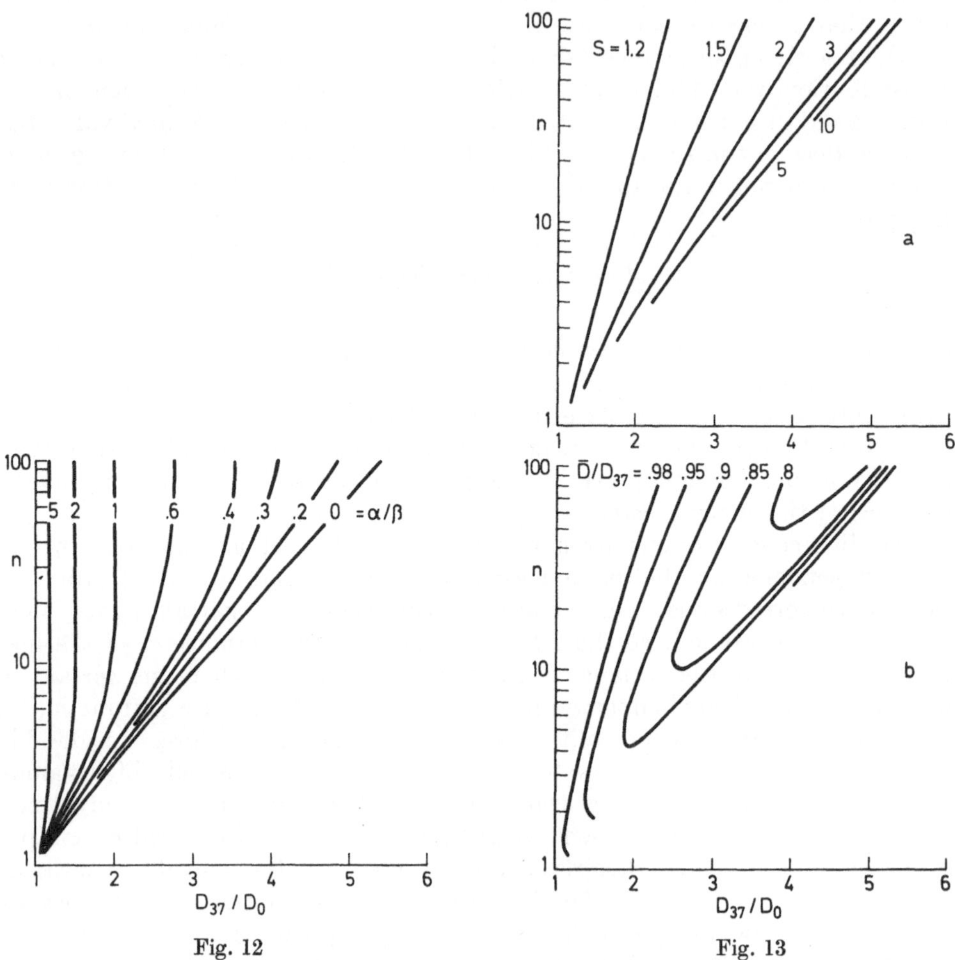

Fig. 12. The ratio of the parameters α and β which have to be chosen if a survival curve with the extrapolation number n and with a given ratio D_{37}/D_0 is to be approximated by the modified multi-target equation (4.13)

Fig. 13a. The steepness S of a survival curve which corresponds to the parameters n and D_{37}/D_0 according to the modified multi-target equation (4.13)

Fig. 13b. The relation of the mean inactivation dose $\overline{D}$ to D_{37} according to the modified multi-target equation (4.13) with the parameters n and D_{37}/D_0

Fig. 13 gives the relative steepness S and the mean inactivation dose $\overline{D}$ as function of the parameters n and D_{37}/D_0. The explicit calculation of S and $\overline{D}$ according to eqs. (5.20) and (5.14) is in general to be preferred because eq. (4.13) may not always appropriately describe a survival curve. For a quick determination of S and $\overline{D}$ the graphs are, however, useful.

As an example for this approximative method for the derivation of the steepness S and the mean inactivation dose $\overline{D}$ one can use the data represented in Fig. 14. These data describe the effect of x-irradiation on mammalian cells *in vitro* in the different phases of

Table 1. *Parameters of survival of Chinese hamster cells exposed to x-rays at different cell-cycle stages* (SINCLAIR, 1968). *The values in brackets are derived from Fig. 13*

	n	D_0 (rad)	D_{37} (rad)	S	$\overline{D}$ (rad)
Mitosis	1	130–135	135	1.02 (1.00)	135 (135)
G 2	1.2 (3.2)	125–130	145	1.09 (1.05)	143 (142)
G 1	1.9	150–155	255	1.42 (1.48)	208 (212)
Early S	2.5	185–190	335	1.77 (1.95)	297 (308)
Late S	10	195–200	550	2.23 (2.2)	477 (485)

the cell cycle. Table I contains the parameters which have been given by SINCLAIR (1968). Next to the values of S and of $\overline{D}$ which have been directly calculated by SINCLAIR the values are given which result according to the graphs of Fig. 13 if one fits the curves by the modified multi-target equation (4.13). There are slight differences between the values but they are insignificant in view of the experimental uncertainties of the dose-effect relations. The approximative method to obtain estimates of the parameters S and $\overline{D}$ is, therefore, quite satisfactory. One should however note that the value n which has been given by SINCLAIR for the G_2-phase does not correspond to the formal definition of the extrapola-

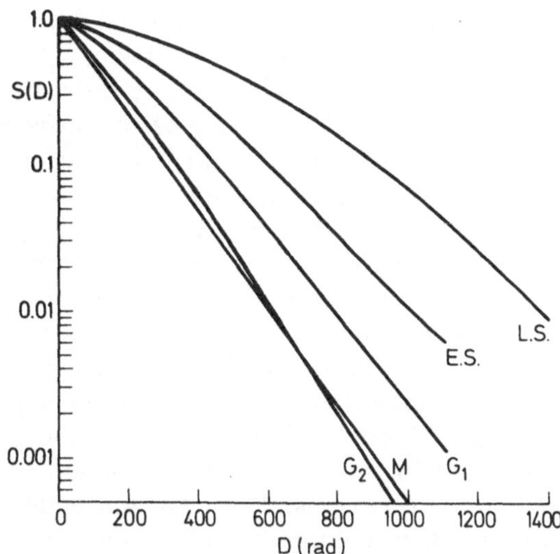

Fig. 14. X-ray survival curves of Chinese hamster cells in different phases of the cell cycle (SINCLAIR, 1968). The parameters of these curves are given in Table 1

tion number as intersection value of the asymptotic tangent of the survival curve with the ordinate; instead, it is apparently chosen to characterize the shoulder of the survival curve. From the survival curve one obtains the value of about 3.2 for the extrapolation number and not 1.2. This confirms that the attempt to use the extrapolation number as a measure for the shoulder of the survival curve is severely restricted and that in general the steepness S must be used. For the approximate determination of the values S and $\overline{D}$ the actual numerical value 3.2 of the extrapolation number has been used, and good agreement with the numerically derived values has been obtained; this would not be the case if one were to use the value 1.2.

In summary one can state that the mean inactivation dose $\overline{D}$ and the variance σ^2 or the steepness S of a survival curve are parameters for the reaction of a cell population over the whole dose range. Contrary to quantities such as the extrapolation number or other parametes which depend only on the reaction of the most resistant part of the population, the values $\overline{D}$, σ^2, and S cannot be derived from a single segment of the dose-effect curve. Due to the limited accuracy of the experimental data in the range of small and intermediate doses it is, therefore, sometimes not possible to give exact values for $\overline{D}$ and S. But, apart from these practical limitations, the mean and the variance of the inactivation dose, and the derived quantity S are fundamental parameters of the survival curve; they are of particular importance because their definition is independent of hypothetical models or equations used to represent the dose-effect relation.

VI. Theorems on dose-effect relations

1. Dose-effect relation and event number

In the following two very general theorems will be discussed which are important for the interpretation of dose-effect relations. These theorems cannot be presented without a certain amount of mathematical formalism and the treatment will, therefore, be less elementary than in the preceding section. The formalism is, however, merely an application of the Poisson statistics which is also the basis of target theory. Both theorems can be understood and applied without knowledge of the mathematical details of their derivation.

First, some general considerations and definitions will be needed. It will be assumed that one deals with a population of cells which do not interact with each other. The cells are not necessarily of equal size or of equal radiation sensitivity. One can, however, associate a region with each cell which is big enough that energy deposition outside this region is irrelevant to the effect. This region can be called *gross sensitive region* (Rossi, 1964). If, for example, one has reason to assume that cellular inactivation is solely determined by energy deposition within the cell nucleus, then the gross sensitive region can be set equal to the nucleus; in the general case, however, the gross sensitive region can be equal to the total volume of the cell and it could even exceed this volume if indirect radiation effects play a role. One must note that the gross sensitive region need not necessarily consist of sensitive structures throughout; the sensitive structures may be dispersed and may occupy only a small fraction of the volume of the gross sensitive region.

In the following a slightly modified concept will be used which is designated by the term *critical region*. This is understood to be a specified region which contains the gross sensitive region; it may be equal to the gross sensitive region or it may be larger. This generalized concept is used for two reasons. First, the statements in section 6.1 and 6.2 apply not only to the gross sensitive volume but also to any larger region containing it. Secondly, the notion of the critical region facilitates the analysis if one deals with mixed cell populations. In such populations, the gross sensitive regions may differ. The critical region can, however, be chosen so that it is of equal size for all cells of the population. This simplifies the mathematical formalism.

Another concept to be used is that of an *energy deposition event* or, for brevity, *event* (see ICRU, 1971). It signifies energy deposition by a charged particle or by a charged particle together with its associated secondary particles. Only if two ionizing particles which pass the region are statistically independent they are counted as separate events. In general, for example in the case of neutron irradiation, one can equate an absorption event with the appearance of a charged particle in the reference region. In the following, the term events in the cell will be used for brevity whenever events in the critical region which belongs to the cell are meant. Smilarly, and in the same way as in the preceding sections, the term survival probability is used in spite of the fact that the considerations refer to any experimental end point and are not restricted to cellular inactivation.

Absorption events are by definition statistically independent. The mean number of events in the cell at dose D is φD. The event frequency, φ, can be derived on the basis of microdosimetric data for microscopic regions of different size and shape and for various radiation qualities.

The actual event number in the cell is a random variable and it fluctuates around its mean value φD. The fluctuations are determined by Poissonian statistics. The probability for exactly ν events in the cell is:

$$p_\nu(D) = e^{-\varphi D}\,\frac{(\varphi D)^\nu}{\nu!}\,. \tag{6.1}$$

This is the same formula which has been discussed in section 4.2.

Instead of the survival probability S(D) as a function of absorbed dose one can consider the survival probability S_ν as function of the event number ν. The relation between these survival probabilities is then:

$$S(D) = \sum_0^\infty S_\nu\, p_\nu(D) = \sum_0^\infty S_\nu\, e^{-\varphi D}\,\frac{(\varphi D)^\nu}{\nu!}\,. \tag{6.2}$$

If instead of the survival probabilities S(D) and S_ν one considers the effect probabilities E(D) and E_ν one obtains the analogous equation:

$$E(D) = \sum_1^\infty E_\nu\, p_\nu(D) = \sum_1^\infty E_\nu\, e^{-\varphi D}\,\frac{(\varphi D)^\nu}{\nu!}\,. \tag{6.3}$$

The results which will be derived in the following are all based on these two equations. It is therfore important to understand the meaning of the quantities S_ν and E_ν and to note that these probabilities depend only on event number and not on dose. This condition is for example not fulfilled if the critical region is chosen too small so that it does not contain all events which may influence the cell. It may equally be violated if the irradiated cells within the population interact. The condition also requires that the dose-effect curve is obtained with constant irradiation time, i.e. with a dose rate proportional to dose. Sensitivity variations of the irradiated population in time could otherwise lead to distortions of the dose-effect relation. In certain practical cases one may, of course, have sufficient reason to assume that the shape of the dose-response curve is identical whether one works with constant dose rate or constant irradiation time.

At a given event frequency φ the probabilities S_ν are unequally determined by the dose-effect relation S(D). This is due to the fact that eq. (6.2) can in principle be inverted. From the experimentally observed survival curve one can, therefore, determine the survival probability as function of the number of charged particles which have traversed the cell or its critical region. This means that one can eliminate the Poisson statistics which are responsible for the fluctuations of the number of charged particles which traverse the cell at a given dose. It is however not the object of the present discussion to deal with a numerical method to do this for a given dose-effect relation. The notions which have been introduced here can be used in a more general way.

2. Relative steepness and minimum number of events

As has been discussed earlier S(D) is the probability distribution, or sum distribution, of the inactivation dose. The derivative of S(D) is the probability density or differential distribution of the inactivation dose:

$$-\frac{dS(D)}{dD} = s(D)\,. \tag{6.4}$$

In analogous way, S_ν can be considered as the probability distribution, or sum distribution, of the number of events necessary for cellular inactivation, and the difference:

$$S_{\nu-1} - S_\nu = s_\nu \tag{6.5}$$

is the probability density of the event number necessary for cellular inactivation. The distinction between S_ν and s_ν compared to $S(D)$ and $s(D)$ is that S_ν and s_ν represent a discrete distribution because the event number ν is a discrete variable. According to eq. (6.5) s_ν is the difference of the survival probability at $\nu-1$ and ν events and it can, therefore, be considered as the probability that a cell selected randomly from the population is eliminated by exactly ν events. The schematic diagram in Fig. 15 illustrates the analogy between the distributions $S(D)$ and S_ν and their corresponding probability densities.

The theorem which will be derived in this section applies only to monotonous survival curves, i.e. to cases where S_ν is always smaller or equal to $S_{\nu-1}$. This condition could be violated if one deals with radiation induced reactivation mechanisms, or if an effect other than cellular inactivation is masked at high doses by cell killing. An example for the latter case is the yield of mutations which declines at higher doses because of the elimination

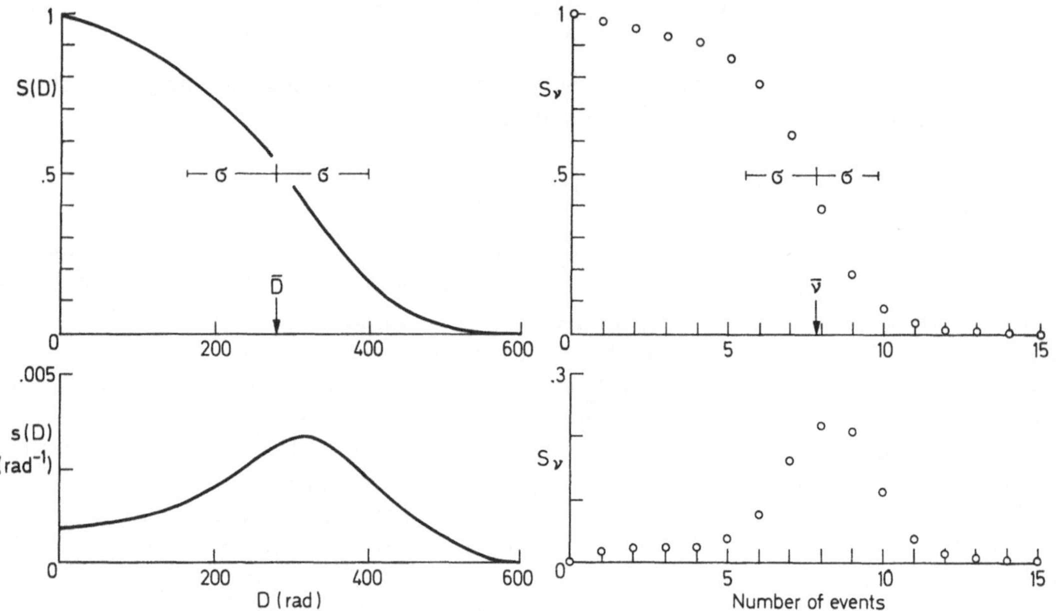

Fig. 15. The survival probability $S(D)$ as a function of dose and its derivative $s(D)$, and the corresponding functions S_ν and s_ν of the number ν of energy deposition events

of the irradiated cells. Only in the case of monotoneous dose-effect relations, i.e. of positive values of $s(D)$ and s_ν, one can talk about probability distributions of the effect dose and the event number.

In analogy to the notions of mean inactivation dose (see eq. [5.12]):

$$\overline{D} = \int\limits_0^\infty D\, s(D)\, dD = \int\limits_0^\infty S(D)\, dD \,, \tag{6.6}$$

and the variance of the inactivation dose (see eq. [5.15]):

$$\sigma^2 = \overline{D^2} - \overline{D}^2 = \int\limits_0^\infty 2\, D\, S(D)\, dD - \overline{D}^2 \tag{6.7}$$

one can use the concept of the mean event number for the induction of the effect:

$$\overline{\nu} = \sum_0^\infty \nu\, s_\nu = \sum_0^\infty S_\nu \tag{6.8}$$

and that of the variance of the number of events necessary for the effect:

$$\sigma_\nu^2 = \overline{\nu^2} - \overline{\nu}^2 = \sum_0^\infty (2\,\nu + 1)\,S_\nu - \overline{\nu}^2\,.$$

(6.9)

The mean values of D and ν and the corresponding values of the variance are symbolized in Fig. 15. In the following it will be shown that the mean event number necessary for the effect is always larger than the relative steepness, $S = \overline{D}^2/\sigma^2$, of the dose-effect relations.

This can be derived from eq. (6.2) and from the definition of $\overline{D}$ and σ^2. One has according to eqs. (6.2) and (6.6):

$$\overline{D} = \int_0^\infty S(D)\,dD = \sum_0^\infty S_\nu \int_0^\infty e^{-\varphi D}\,\frac{(\varphi D)^\nu}{\nu!}\,dD = \sum_0^\infty S_\nu/\varphi = \frac{\overline{\nu}}{\varphi}\,,$$

(6.10)

and according to eqs. (6.2) and (6.7):

$$\overline{D^2} = 2\int_0^\infty D\,S(D)\,dD = 2\sum_0^\infty S_\nu \int_0^\infty D\,e^{-\varphi D}\,\frac{(\varphi D)^\nu}{\nu!}\,dD = 2\sum_0^\infty S_\nu\,\frac{\nu+1}{\varphi^2} = \frac{\overline{\nu^2}+\overline{\nu}}{\varphi^2}\,.$$

(6.11)

Therefore one obtains:

$$\frac{\sigma^2}{\overline{D}^2} = \frac{\overline{D^2}}{\overline{D}^2} - 1 = \frac{\overline{\nu^2}}{\overline{\nu}^2} + \frac{1}{\overline{\nu}} - 1 = \frac{\sigma_\nu^2}{\overline{\nu}^2} + \frac{1}{\overline{\nu}}\,,$$

(6.12)

or:

$$\overline{\nu} = \varphi\overline{D} = \frac{\overline{D}^2}{\sigma^2 - \sigma_r^2/\varphi^2}\,.$$

(6.13)

Because σ_ν^2/φ^2 is always positive, one obtains the inequation:

$$\overline{\nu} \geqq \overline{D}^2/\sigma^2\,,$$

(6.14)

i.e.

$$\overline{\nu} = \varphi\overline{D} \geqq S\,.$$

(6.15)

This means that no model for the explanation of a dose-effect relation of relative steepness S can be valid in which the product $\overline{\nu} = \varphi\overline{D}$ of the event number per unit dose and of the mean inactivation dose is not at least equal to S. If on the average less statistical independent absorption events were needed for the effect then the relative fluctuations of the inactivation dose had to be larger than indicated by the value S. This would be the case even if one were to assume that no other statistical factors except the fluctuations in the number of events were involved in the dose-effect relation.

Equality can occur in relation (6.15) only in the case of a single-hit or a multi-hit model (see eq. [4.7]). In these cases S is equal to the hit number. In other models the mean event number exceeds S. A simple special conclusion from the theorem is, therefore, that superposition of multi-hit curves (see eq. [4.7]) never can lead to a curve which has a higher hit number. For example, it is always possible to simulate an exponential function by the superposition of multi-hit curves, but one never can approximate a multi-hit curve by the superposition of curves of lower hit number. The application to target theoretical models is, however, only a very special example. The importance of the theorem lies in the fact that it is applicable to survival curves without regard to the fact

whether these curves can be represented by a particular equation. Moreover, the importance of the theorem is not restricted to the fact that by determining the relative steepness
of a survival curve one can narrow down the analysis to those models which invoke a
sufficient minimum number of absorption events. The determination of a lower limit of
the number of energy deposition events has general relevance for the determination of
temporal and spatial intervals of interaction between lesions produced by separate charged
particles (see section 7).

3. The meaning of the slope of the dose-effect curve in the logarithmic representation

This section deals with a theorem which is complementary to the one obtained in the
preceding section. The relation between relative steepness of a survival curve and the
minimum number of absorption events refers to the reaction of the total irradiated population and it is applicable whenever the complete dose-effect curve is known. Frequently,
however, the dose-effect curve is only known in a limited dose range, or one is merely
interested in a specific range of doses, for example, when one considers the effects at smallest
level of absorbed dose. Also in such cases one can make theoretical statements concerning
the number of absorption events in the affected and non-affected cells. In the following
such statements will be discussed.

The slope c_E of the dose-effect relation in the double logarithmic representation is:

$$c_E = \frac{d \ln E(D)}{d \ln D} = \frac{D}{E(D)} \frac{dE(D)}{dD} , \qquad (6.16)$$

where $E(D)$ stands for the effect probability at dose D. If one inserts eq. (6.3) into this
expression one obtains:

$$c_E = \frac{D}{E(D)} \sum_{\mu=1}^{\infty} E_\mu \, e^{-\varphi D} \left(\frac{(\varphi D)^{\mu-1}}{(\mu-1)!} \varphi - \varphi \frac{(\varphi D)^\mu}{\mu!} \right)$$

$$= \frac{\displaystyle\sum_{\mu=0}^{\infty} E_\nu \, e^{-\varphi D} \frac{(\varphi D)^\mu}{\mu!} (\mu - \varphi D)}{\displaystyle\sum_{\mu=0}^{\infty} E \, e^{-\varphi D} \frac{(\varphi D)^\mu}{\mu!}} \qquad (6.17)$$

$$= \frac{\displaystyle\sum_{\mu=0}^{\infty} p_\mu \, E_\mu}{\displaystyle\sum_{\mu=0}^{\infty} p_\mu \, E_\mu} - \varphi D .$$

According to the definition of a conditional probability the term:

$$\pi_\mu = \frac{p_\mu \, E_\mu}{\displaystyle\sum_{\mu=0}^{\infty} p_\mu \, E_\mu} \qquad (6.18)$$

is equal to the fraction of cells which have experienced exactly μ absorption events and
which show the effect. This leads to an interesting interpretation of eq. (6.17) if it is written
in the modified form:

$$c_E = \sum_{\mu=0}^{\infty} \pi_\mu \, \mu - \varphi D . \qquad (6.19)$$

φD is equal to the mean number $\bar{\mu}$ of absorption events per cell in the whole population at dose D. The sum $\sum \pi_\mu \, \mu$ is the mean number of events in those cells which show the effect; one can symbolize this mean value by $\bar{\mu}_E$, then eq. (6.19) takes the form:

$$c_E = \bar{\mu}_E - \bar{\mu} \,. \tag{6.20}$$

Thus, one has the very general result that the difference of the mean event numbers in those cells which show the effect and in the cells throughout the total population is equal to the slope of the dose-effect curve in the double-logarithmic representation. An event, as has been stated earlier, is the appearance of an ionizing charged particle and its secondary particles in the cell. The relation remains valid if one chooses a critical region which is larger than the cell. The only condition is that the mean event frequency per unit dose is equal for all critical regions and that energy absorption outside the critical region does not influence the cell.

The theorem is fundamental for the application of microdosimetry to dose effect relations. If for certain values of dose the effect probability E(D) and the slope c_E of the dose-effect curve are known, one can ask how big the sensitive structures must be so that at dose D they are traversed by c_E or more charged particles with a probability E(D). The answer to this question is given by microdosimetric data for various radiation qualities. In this way one can derive lower limits for the dimensions of the sensitive structures in the cell and for the interaction distances of the elementary lesions produced in the cell.

The result obtained in this section can be given by more general form. Eq. (6.19) has been derived from eq. (6.3); an analogous relation can be obtained from eq. (6.2):

$$c_S = \bar{\mu}_S - \bar{\mu} \,. \tag{6.21}$$

In this equation c_S is the slope not of the effect probability but of the survival probability in double logarithmic representation and $\bar{\mu}_S$ is the mean number of absorption events in the fraction of the population that is not subject to the effect while $\bar{\mu}$ is, as before, the mean event number throughout the population. Commonly c_S is negative but the theorem is of general validity and, therefore, also applicable to those dose-effect relations in which the effect reaches a maximum at a certain dose and then decreases with increasing dose.

If one adds eqs. (6.20) and (6.21) one obtains the difference between the mean event numbers in those cells which show the effect and in those cells which do not. One can, therefore, give the following three equations:

$$\bar{\mu}_E - \mu = \frac{d \ln E(D)}{d \ln D} \,, \tag{6.22}$$

$$\bar{\mu} - \bar{\mu}_S = -\frac{d \ln S(D)}{d \ln D} \,, \tag{6.23}$$

$$\bar{\mu}_E - \bar{\mu}_S = \frac{d \ln E(D)}{d \ln D} - \frac{d \ln S(D)}{d \ln D} \,. \tag{6.24}$$

Eq. (6.22) contains as a limiting case a statement which is of particular importance to the analysis of dose-effect curves at smallest doses. The relation implies that in the region of small doses the slope c_E of the effect curve in the double logarithmic plot is equal to the order of the reaction kinetics which determines the effect. In the limiting case when the absorbed dose D approaches 0 this fact may appear obvious. But it is important that eq. (6.22) allows a rigorous statement even in cases where the dose D has a small but finite value. This can be explained by the following special application which has considerable practical implications.

From eq. (6.22) one can derive the fact that a population of non-interacting cells cannot exhibit a dose effect curve with a slope significantly below 1 in a dose range where the mean number of charged particles traversing the cell is much smaller than 1. This is true regardless of the degree of sensitivity variations within the irradiated population. The quantitative formulation of the statement is:

$$c_E \gtrless 1 - \varphi D \, . \tag{6.25}$$

The relation can be derived as follows. φD is the mean number of events per cell at dose D. If one inserts this value for $\overline{\mu}$ in eq. (6.22) one obtains:

$$c_E = \overline{\mu}_E - \varphi D \, . \tag{6.26}$$

The inequation (6.25) follows then directly from the fact that the mean event number $\overline{\mu}_E$ in those cells which show the effects cannot be smaller than 1[1]. The inequation is therefore a special case of relation (6.22).

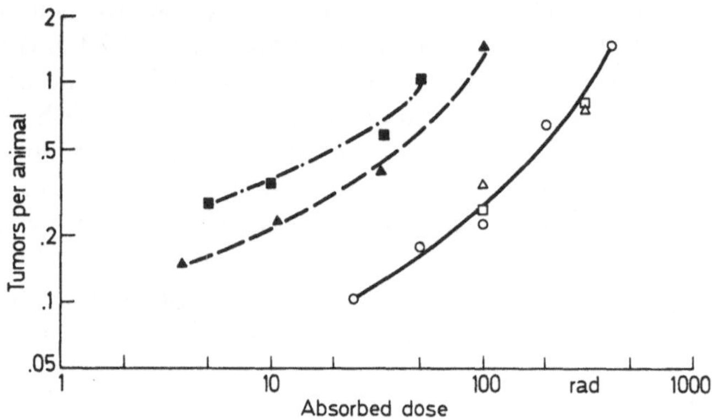

Fig. 16. Mean number of mammary neoplasms induced in the rat by x-rays and neutrons. The spontaneous incidence is subtracted. The data are from a compilation by Rossi and Kellerer (1972)

(X-rays: ○ Bond *et al.*, △ Shellabarger, □ Vogel and Zaldivar; Neutrons: ▲ Shellabarger, ■ Vogel)

As a practical example (Rossi and Kellerer, 1972) one can cite the case of the induction of mammary tumors in the rat by neutrons. The dose-effect relations for this example are given in Fig. 16. Microdosimetric analysis shows that in the case of the neutron irradiations only one out of ten cells is traversed by a charged particle at a dose of 3 rad. The mean value φD of the event number at this dose is, therefore, equal to about 0.1. If the tumor induction were solely the result of radiation action on single cells without interaction between damaged cells, one would have to have, according to eq. (6.25), a slope of at least 0.9 in the dose-effect curve for neutrons. Because the experimentally observed slope of the dose-effect curve is considerably smaller than 0.9 one concludes that the tumor rate is determined by the interaction of damaged cells or by radiation induced disturbances of the hormonal status of the animal.

VII. Dose-effect relations and radiation quality

1. Evaluation of radiation quality

A detailed discussion of radiation quality and its implication to the dose-effect curves exceeds the frame of this article. The detailed and lucid treatment given by Lea (1946) is still of great value, and for the more recent developments one may refer to reviews by Rossi (1967, 1968) who has initiated the new approach to the theory of radiation quality.

---

1 As pointed out in section 3.1 the spontaneous incidence is subtracted in the double-logarithmic representation.

Radiation quality is an important factor in the dose-effect curve. But, as pointed out in the preceding sections, it is only one out of several factors which determine the dose-effect relation. One can therefore in general not explain the dose-effect relation by invoking only this one factor, namely the statistics of energy deposition. Microdosimetric data can however be used in a more general way to derive diameters of the sensitive regions in the cell or to obtain interaction distances of the elementary lesions; such considerations are similar in nature to the arguments applied in section 6.2. Results can be obtained from individual dose-effect relations; they can however be considerably widened if one knows the dose-effect relation for a series of different radiation qualities. The analysis of relative biological effectiveness (RBE) of different radiation qualities will be discussed in section 7.3.

In the following sections some concepts and definitions of the the oryof radiation quality will be needed. An approximative treatment can be based on the concept of linear energy transfer (LET). LET, or stopping power, is the mean energy loss of a charged particle traversing a distance of unit length in the irradiated material. If the value of this quantity is known one can derive the probability that an ionizing particle transfers certain amounts of energy in traversing a microscopic region.

The application of LET if, however, complicated by the fact that a given radiation field always consists of a mixture of particles of different energy and different LET. An exact analysis therefore necessitates consideration of the whole spectrum of LET and not merely a mean value of LET. But even a full spectrum of LET cannot sufficiently characterize a radiation field and its interaction with the irradiated medium; two charged particles can have the same stopping power but different charges and velocities and they will then exhibit different spectra of delta rays, i.e. of the secondary electrons which are liberated in electron collisions. Differences in the delta-ray spectrum lead to different radial distributions of energy deposition around the track core, and particles of the same LET may, therefore, have different effectiveness. In order to account for these differences one frequently uses the so-called restricted LET. This quantity corresponds to LET but its value is determined by excluding all delta electrons which exceed a certain specified maximal energy. Depending on the size of the microscopic regions which are being studied different values of the maximal energy have to be chosen. For this reason one must actually deal with a full set of LET distributions if one wants to characterize a radiation field and its interaction with the irradiated medium. Moreover, LET is an idealized concept, not a directly observable physical quantity; the actual energy deposition in microscopic regions is determined by additional factors such as the curvature and the finite length of the charged particle tracks or the statistics of the electronic collisions. The probability distributions of energy deposition in microscopic regions are therefore not always directly related to the LET distributions and particularly this is the case if one deals with sparsely ionizing radiations or with very small critical regions. The limitations of LET have been dealt with in detail in the literature (ICRU, 1970). These limitations have led to the attempt to measure or compute the probability distributions of energy deposition in microscopic regions directly instead of approximating them on the basis of LET-distributions. The microdosimetric data permit a quantitative analysis in all those cases in which LET theory can only yield an approximative description. In principle, however, one can formulate all arguments either in terms of LET or in terms of microdosimetry. This will not always be pointed out in the following when due to their more general applicability the concepts of microdosimetry are used.

The point of departure in the analysis of the statistics of energy deposition and their influence on cellular radiation effects is the distinction between absorbed dose and the random variable which corresponds to this quantity. The random variable, i.e. the ratio of the energy imparted to a certain region and the mass of that region, is called specific energy z (see ICRU, 1971). One can measure z in the same unit rad which is used for absorbed dose D. For a given absorbed dose the specific energy z can deviate considerably from D. The relative fluctuations are most expressed for smallest regions, for smallest absorbed doses, and for densely ionizing radiation. The mean value of z is equal to D, and the probability distribution of z is designated by f(z; D). The function f(z; D) depends on size and shape of the reference region, on the radiation quality, and on the absorbed dose. f(z; D) dz is the probability that at absorbed dose D the specific energy in the reference volume is between z and z + dz.

In addition to the differential distribution f(z; D) one uses the sum distribution F(z; D). The function F(z; D) is equal to the probability that at absorbed dose D the specific energy is smaller than z:

$$F(z; D) = \int_0^z f(z; D)\, dz\ . \tag{7.1}$$

If the microdosimetric distributions are known for one value of absorbed dose they can be computed for all absorbed doses. Specifically one can compute the distributions for a given dose from the probability distribution of the increments of z produced in individual energy deposition events. This distribution is called the single event spectrum. It is the basic microdosimetric function and the analogue of the LET distribution. The single event spectra are designated by $f_1(z)$ and $F_1(z)$. The function $f_1(z)$ is the differential distribution of the specific energy produced in one event and $F_1(z)$ is the corresponding sum distribution. Accordingly, $f_1(z)$ dz is the probability that a charged particle passing through the region of interest produces a specific energy in this region between z and z + dz. The mean event size is defined as:

$$\bar{z}_F = \int_0^\infty z\, f_1(z)\, dz\ . \tag{7.2}$$

And $\varphi = 1/\bar{z}_F$ is accordingly the mean event number per unit dose. Instead of the specific energy z one frequently uses the related quantity y which is defined as energy deposited in a region in one event divided by the mean chord length of this region (see ICRU, 1971). This quantity has the advantage that it permits a direct comparison with LET, since both quantities have the same dimension. In the following the quantity y will not be used.

In addition to the quantity $\bar{z}_F$ which is averaged over the number of events one uses another mean value of specific energy which is averaged over the energy:

$$\bar{z}_D = \int_0^\infty z^2\, f_1(z)\, dz \Big/ \int_0^\infty z\, f_1(z)\, dz = \int_0^\infty z^2\, f_1(z)\, dz \Big/ \bar{z}_F\ . \tag{7.3}$$

This energy mean $\bar{z}_D$ determines the mean quadratic deviation of the specific energy z from its mean value D:

$$\sigma_z^2 = \overline{(z - D)^2} = \bar{z}_D\, D\ . \tag{7.4}$$

The relevance of $\bar{z}_D$ to the dose-effect relation, particularly its linear component in the range of lowest doses, will be dealt with in the following sections.

The frequency average and the dose average specific energy are analogous to the track average and the dose average of LET. In fact one can approximate these microdosimetric quantities by LET. If one deals with a spherical region of diameter d one has the following approximations:

$$\bar{z}_F = \frac{20.4\, \bar{L}_T}{d^2}\ , \tag{7.5}$$

and:

$$\bar{z}_D = \frac{22.9\, \bar{L}_D}{d^2}\ . \tag{7.6}$$

Here $\bar{L}_T$ and $\bar{L}_D$ are the track average and the dose average of LET (see ICRU, 1970) and the units employed are rad, keV, and μm.

No other relations and definitions will be needed in the following. The principles of microdosimetry and its experimental techniques are described in detail by Rossi (1967,

1968). Rigorous definitions of the microdosimetric quantities and a review of theoretical microdosimetry have been given elsewhere (ICRU, 1971; KELLERER and ROSSI, 1969; KELLERER, 1969).

2. Size of the sensitive regions and interaction distances between absorption events

The most direct application of microdosimetric data is the determination of cross sections or sensitive volumes on the basis of event frequencies. This corresponds to the approach which has been discussed in section 4.1. In the case of an exponential dose-effect relation one can conclude that at the dose D_{37}, i.e. the dose which reduces the survival probability to $e^{-1} = 0.37$, the gross sensitive region of the cell must on the average be subject

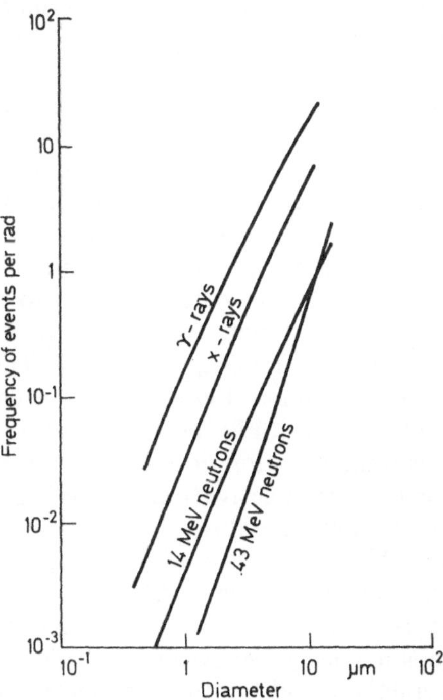

Fig. 17. Event frequency per rad in spherical microscopic tissue regions of diameter d. The curves are based on experimental (ROSSI, 1967) and theoretical (HUG and KELLERER, 1966) data

to at least 1 energy deposition event. If the event frequency per unit dose in the sensitive region is designated by φ one has:

$$D_{37}\, \varphi \geqq 1 \tag{7.7}$$

or:

$$\varphi \geqq 1/D_{37} \, . \tag{7.8}$$

The same consideration applies if one knows only the initial part of the dose-effect relation. Instead of the dose D_{37} one must then use the dose at which the linear extrapolation of the effect relation intercepts the 100 % line.

From the condition that φ is at least $1/D_{37}$, one obtains a lower limit of the diameter of the sensitive region. In Fig. 17 event frequencies for different radiation qualities are plotted as function of the diameter of a spherical region. The concept of an energy deposition event has been defined in section 6.1; in many cases one can identify an event simply as the passage of a charged particle through the critical region. Event frequencies for much smaller regions have been computed by LEA (1946); they are particularly relevant to the study of

3*

radiation effects on bacteria, viruses and enzymes. If one deals with larger objects, such as mammalian cells, the consideration of event frequencies is most relevant for densely ionizing radiations. The reason is that in cellular radiation effects the number of events in the gross sensitive region at the mean effect dose is very large whenever one deals with sparsely ionizing radiation. To inactivate a mammalian cell with x-rays one must have on the average about 1 000 electron traversals through the cell nucleus. With densely ionizing radiations the event frequencies are much smaller and at a LET of about 100 keV/μm one traversal of the nucleus is sufficient for cellular inactivation. From Fig. 7 in section 5.1 one obtains a D_{37} of approximately 70 rad for α-particles of 4 MeV. The sensitive region must have a diameter of about 5 micrometer in order to be traversed on the average by one α-particle at a dose of 70 rad. One concludes that the gross sensitive volume is not significantly smaller than the cell nucleus. There are cases in which one derives an even larger gross sentitive region. This is for example the case in the inactivation of spermatogonia *in vivo*. From results of Bateman *et al.* (1961) on the inactivation of spermatogonia by 430 kV neutrons gross sensitive volumes are obtained which are equal to the total volume of the cell or even somewhat larger (Rossi, 1964). This is consistent with recent observations (see contribution by Oakberg to this volume) on correlated cell death in chains of spermatogonia which are linked by bridges.

From the exponential dose-effect relations for densely ionizing radiations one obtains minimum diameters of the gross sensitive region. This implies that the sensitive structures are dispersed over a region of this minimal size; it does however not exclude the possibility that the individual sensitive structures are much smaller. Next to the determination of the gross sensitive region it is therefore of special interest to determine the distances over which elementary lesions in the cell interact. An answer to this question can be obtained from the dose-effect curves for sparsely ionizing radiations. The mean inactivation dose $\overline{D}$ of a nonsynchronized population of human kidney cells is roughly 350 rad for x-rays; the relative steepness S is larger than 2 (see Fig. 7). According to the theorem in section 6.2 one concludes that at the mean inactivation dose of 350 rad more than two energy deposition events must occur for cellular inactivation. From Fig. 17 one obtains a minimal distance of 0.4 μm for the region in which a dose of 350 rad of x-rays induces on the average at least two absorption events. This indicates a minimal interaction distance of elementary lesions of 0.4 μm. The estimate is-however-conservative and a better estimate is obtained if one considers not only event frequencies but also the actual fluctuations of energy deposition. The statistical variations in energy deposition are considerably greater than the statistical fluctuations in event numbers and they are, therefore, more relevant to the percentage variance of the inactivation dose or to its inverse the relative steepness of the dose response curve.

The microdosimetric analysis of sigmoidal dose-effect relations has been described in detail by Hug and Kellerer (1966). In the present context it is sufficient to present the basic argument in a simplified form. It has been pointed out in section 5 that the variance of the inactivation dose, i.e. the deviation of the dose-response curve from the pure step function, is caused by the combined action of different statistical factors. The observed variance of the dose-effect relation is, therefore, an upper limit of the contribution of each of the factors: statistics of energy deposition, biological variability, and random nature of the physiological processes. The statistics of energy deposition can be the only relevant factor in certain limiting cases. Then the percentage variations of energy deposition in the sensitive region of the cell can be equal to the observed percentage variation of the inactivation dose. In all other cases they must be smaller. From this condition one obtains a more realistic lower limit of the size of the sensitive region in which elementary lesions produced by different particle tracks interact. It is the diameter of the region in which the percentage variations of energy deposition just equal the percentage variation of the inactivation dose. The quantitative formulation of this argument requires the application of microdosimetric functions and leads to somewhat complicated calculations which need not be repeated in the present context. A simplified estimate is sufficient for most applications and will therefore be described[1].

The relative fluctuations of the specific energy z around its mean value D are obtained from eq. (7.4):

$$V_z = \frac{\sigma_z^2}{D^2} = \frac{\bar{z}_D}{D} , \qquad (7.9)$$

at the mean inactivation dose $\overline{D}$ the relative variance V_z in the sensitive region of the cell must be smaller than the relative variance of the inactivation dose found in the survival curve. The relative variance of the inactivation dose is equal to the inverse of the relative steepness S (see section 5.2.2). Accordingly one obtains:

$$\bar{z}_D/\overline{D} \leqq S^{-1} \qquad (7.10)$$

or:

$$\bar{z}_D \leqq \overline{D}/S . \qquad (7.11)$$

This condition for $\bar{z}_D$ determines a lower limit of the site diameter over which the elementary lesions must interact. One may take as an example the data by SINCLAIR (1968) which are represented in Fig. 14 and in Table 1. When the cells are exposed to x-rays during late S phase one obtain a mean inactivation dose of roughly 480 rad and a relative steepness of 2.2 (see Table 1 in section 5.2.2). Thus $\bar{z}_D$ must be less than 215 rad. Fig. 18 gives the value of $\bar{z}_D$ for different radiation qualities as a function of the diameter of the

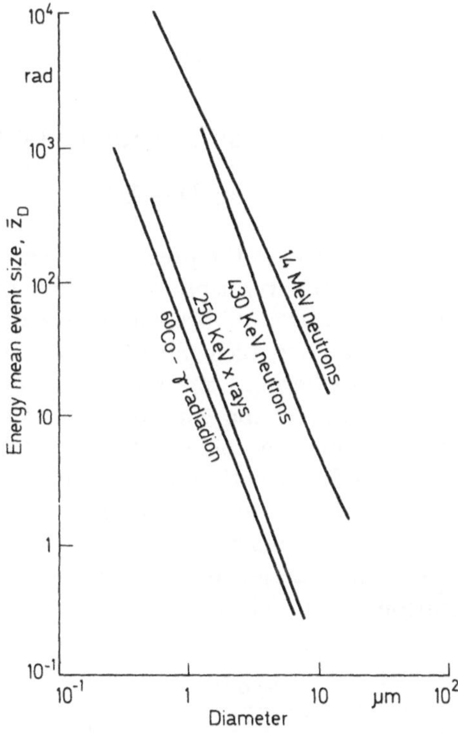

Fig. 18. Energy mean event size, $\bar{z}_D$, in spherical microscopic tissue regions of diameter d. The curves are based on experimental (ROSSI, 1967) and theoretical (HUG and KELLERER, 1966) data

____

1 The simplification consists in substituting the relative variance V_z of z at the mean inactivation dose for the relative variance of the dose necessary to reach a given value of z. For sigmoidal dose-effect relations the difference is not very significant; and the argument applies only to this case.

reference region. From the curve for x-rays one concludes that the sensitive region must be larger than $0.6\,\mu$m and that elementary lesions produced by different charged particle tracks must interact over this distance.

The arguments described above apply to dose-effect relations regardless of the mechanisms of radiation action and the statistical factors which may be involved. The fact that on the basis of a single dose-effect relation one cannot, in general, separate the influence of the various random factors reflects itself in the impossibility to derive actual values whether one deals with the size of the sensitive region, the interaction distance of elementary lesions, or the number of effective events. All results are merely lower limits of the actual values. One can, however, go a step further if one has some detailed knowledge concerning the cellular mechanisms involved in the effect.

Such knowledge is available in the case of the production of chromosome aberrations (see contribution by Bauchinger to this volume). There is evidence that the yield of "single breaks" is more or less independent of radiation quality and that the probability of each individual break to be involved in a structural exchange is determined by the concentration of other breaks within a surrounding region (critical site, or domain of interaction of single breaks).

Quantitatively this can be expressed by the statement that the yield y of chromosome exchanges is proportional to the square of the specific energy z within a certain critical region:

$$y(z) = k\,z^2 \,. \tag{7.12}$$

From this dependence of the yield on specific energy z one obtains the dose dependence of the yield by averaging over the total spectrum $f(z; D)$ of z at a given dose:

$$y(D) = k \int_0^\infty z^2\,f(z; D)\,dz \,, \tag{7.13}$$

this integral can be evaluated (see Kellerer and Rossi, 1971), and one obtains:

$$y(D) = k\,(\bar{z}_D\,D + D^2) \tag{7.14}$$

where $\bar{z}_D$ is the mean event size discussed in the preceding section. This can be understood without detailed reference to its formal derivation. The yield is proportional to the number of breaks times the average concentration of breaks surrounding them. The number of breaks is proportional to dose and the average concentration of neighboring breaks around a break is proportional to $(\bar{z}_D + D)$ where $\bar{z}_D$ represents the concentration of breaks produced by the same particle track and D the contribution of other tracks.

Eq. (7.14) can be used to determine the value of $\bar{z}_D$. This value is equal to the dose for which the linear component in the effect relation is just equal to the quadratic component and it can best be obtained from a double-logarithmic plot of the dose-effect relation (see section 3.1). From the value $\bar{z}_D$ and the curves in Fig. 18 one obtains the diameter of the critical sites or of the domain of interaction of single breaks.

If one uses the approximation of microdosimetric quantities which has been expressed in eq. (7.6) one obtains:

$$y(D) = k \left(\frac{22.9\,\bar{L}_D}{d^2}\,D + D^2 \right) . \tag{7.15}$$

This is the quantitative formulation of arguments which have been variously applied to cytogenetic studies (see Lea, 1946; Wolff et al., 1953; Neary, 1966). Lea obtains typical site diameters of $1\,\mu$m. Wolff et al., on the other hand, conclude that the interaction distances are less than $0.3\,\mu$m, i.e. that the diameter of the critical sites is less than $0.6\,\mu$m. The apparent difference in the results may be due to the fact that Wolff et al.

use a track average of LET for 14 MeV neutrons while according to eq. (7.15) one would have to use the dose average which is considerably larger.

These considerations are simplifications in so far as they do not include the saturation effect, i.e. the waste of energy when particles are too densely ionizing. They also do not account for deviations from the linear-quadratic model which occur if the number of potential sites is limited, or if cell killing and chromosome aberrations are correlated. In the next section a method will be discussed which can eliminate some of these complications and which furthermore makes it possible to widen the applicability of eq. (7.14) to effects other than chromosome exchanges.

3. Analysis of relative biological effectiveness

The inferences from dose-effect relations can be considerably strengthened if dose-response curves for different radiation qualities are known.

BARENDSEN (1967) has determined cellular survival curves for a wide spectrum of radiation qualities (see Section 5.1). From these data he derives the single hit inactivation cross section as function of LET. His results are plotted in Fig. 19. Barendsen combines the arguments of multi-hit theory with accurate analysis of energy loss fluctuations in order to derive the critical number of primary collisions which must occur in a submicroscopic region for cellular inactivation. He concludes that 10 to 15 ionizations must occur within a distance of roughly 100 Å. Similar considerations for other experimental systems have been performed by GRAY (1947) and by HOWARD-FLANDERS (1958).

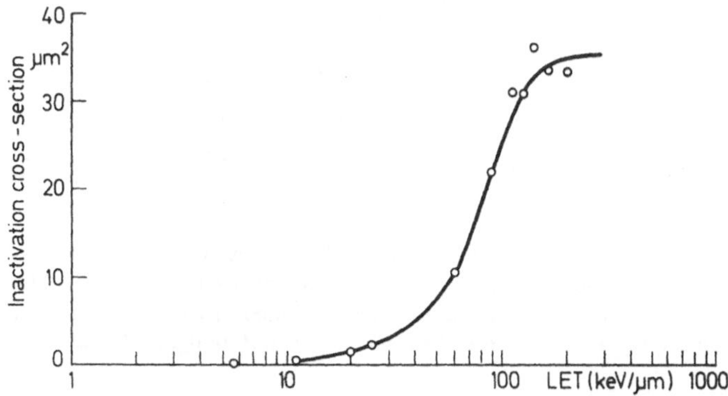

Fig. 19. Inactivation cross sections for human kidney cells exposed to particles of various LET (BARENDSEN, 1967)

This analysis of the relative biological effectiveness is subject to the limitations which have been mentioned in Section 4.2 with reference to the multi-hit theory. The results depend on the assumption of unit effect probability for each ionization or each primary ionization. With intermediate effect probabilities larger interaction distances are obtained. Accordingly the results are valid as lower limits and not as the actual diameter of sensitive sites. The finding that in the action of heavy charged particles on mammalian cells lesions produced at a minimum distance of 100 Å to 150 Å can interact is, therefore, not in conflict with the much larger interaction distances which are inferred from survival curves obtained with sparsely ionizing radiations.

A further restriction lies in the fact that it is not always possible to equate the functional dependence of cellular inactivation cross sections on LET with the LET dependence of the underlying elementary lesions. For microbiological objects such as viruses or bacteria this may be justified. For mammalian cells the situation is complicated by the fact that the cell nucleus contains a large number of sensitive structures and that a densely ionizing particle traversing the gross sensitive volume deposits so much energy that the effect may not merely reflect the action on a single submicroscopic or molecular unit.

A general method for RBE analysis has been introduced by Rossi (1971). It consists in studying RBE as a function of dose instead of dose-effect relations. This has the advantage that the analysis is reduced to the primary steps in the action of radiation. The dose-RBE relation is determined by the microscopic distributions of energy deposition. Processes which take place later in the reaction chain are the same for different radiation qualities and cancel as far as the dose-RBE relation is concerned. RBE is the ratio of doses for equal effect, and both co-ordinates in the plot of RBE versus dose refer therefore directly to physical quantities and the numerical scale of effect is irrelevant. This makes those cases accessible to quantitative analysis where the effect can only be measured in arbitrary scales.

Rossi (1971) finds that for a variety of effects and over a considerable dose range the RBE of neutrons versus x-rays decreases inversely to the square root of the neutron dose.

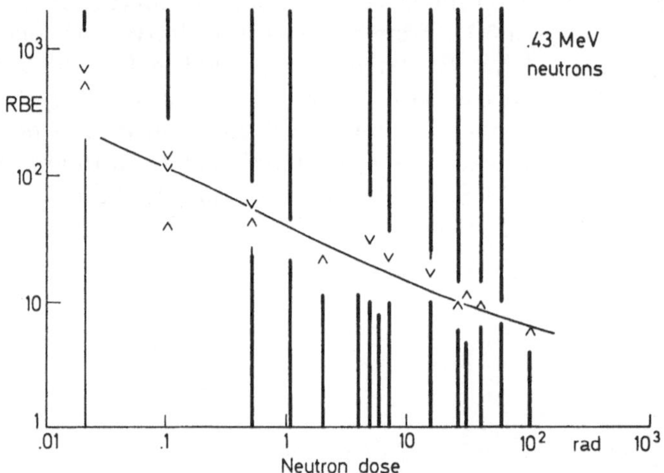

Fig. 20. RBE of 0.43 MeV neutrons relative to x-rays for the induction of lens opacification in the mouse as a function of neutron dose (Bateman et al., 1972). The solid bars indicate the ranges of RBE values which, according to the comparison of x-ray and neutron doses, are excluded. Broad bars: significance exceeding 99%, narrow bars: significance exceeding 95%, arrows: non-significant differences.

In a double logarithmic plot of RBE versus neutron dose one obtains a line of slope $-\,^1/_2$. The observation implies that the elementary lesions underlying the various effects go with the square of the x-ray dose while they are proportional to dose in the case of neutrons.

A theoretical analysis (Kellerer and Rossi, 1971) indicates that the quadratic dependence of elementary lesions on x-ray dose is only an approximation valid in a certain dose range. The more general relation is that the yield of elementary lesions goes with the square of the specific energy z within certain critical sites. This means that eqs. (7.14) and (7.15) which have been related to chromosomal exchange in the preceding section apply to the elementary lesions underlying a wide range of effects. According to these relations one must expect that RBE is inversely proportional to the square root of the neutron dose over a certain range but that it approaches constant values both at very low and very high doses.

From eq. (7.14) one concludes that the RBE at very low doses should be equal to $\bar{z}_{D,n}/\bar{z}_{D,x}$, where $\bar{z}_{D,n}$ is the dose average event size for neutrons and $\bar{z}_{D,x}$ the dose average event size for x-rays. This ratio is nearly independent of the diameter of the region in which the specific energy z is measured; it has a value of approximately 50 for fast neutrons versus x-rays. This limiting value of RBE is indeed found in the experiments of Sparrow et al. (1972) which are represented in Fig. 1 in section 3.1.

Fig. 20 represents a dose-RBE relation which has been established over a particular wide dose range. The biological endpoint is the production of lens opacification in the mouse by 430 keV neutrons (BATEMAN et *al.*, 1972). By direct comparison of the effect of each individual neutron dose with the effect of each individual x-ray dose one can exclude certain ranges of RBE values and thereby obtain a confidence region for the dose-RBE relation. The solid line in the figure and the fact that the limiting RBE may exceed the expected value is discussed by KELLERER and ROSSI (1972).

The part of the dose RBE relation which has the slope $-^1/_2$ is described by the equation:

$$\text{RBE} = \sqrt{\bar{z}_{D,n}/D_n} \, . \tag{7.16}$$

From this equation one concludes that the straight-line extrapolation of this part of the curve intersects the line for which RBE equals 1 at the dose value $\bar{z}_{D,n}$. This is the simplest way to determine the dose average of the event size for neutrons. The dose-RBE relations for various biological effects indicate values of $\bar{z}_{D,n}$ which correspond to site diameters of 1 μm or more (see KELLERER and ROSSI, 1971). The results from the RBE analysis are, therefore, consistent with the findings described in the preceding section.

References

ALPER, T., FOWLER, J. F., MORGAN, R. L., VONBERG, O. O., ELLIS, F., OLIVER, R.: The characterization of the "type C" survival curve. Brit. J. Radiol. **35**, 722–723 (1962).

BARENDSEN, G. W.: Mechanism of Action of Different Ionizing Radiations on the Proliferative Capacity of Mammalian Cells, A. Cole ed., Marcel Dekker (New York). Theoretical and Experimental Biophysics **1**, 167–231 (1967).

BATEMAN, J. L., BOND, V. P.: The effect of Radiations of Different LET on Early Responses in the Mammal. Annals of the New York Academy of Sciences **114** Art. 1, 32–47 (1964).

— ROSSI, H. H., KELLERER, A. M., ROBINSON, C. V., BOND, V. P.: Dose-Dependence of Fast Neutron RBE for Lens Opacification in Mice, Radiat. Res. **51**, 381–390, 1972.

BLAU, M., ALTENBURGER, K.: Über einige Wirkungen von Strahlen. Z. Physik **12**, 315 (1922).

BOND, V. P., CRONKITE, E. P., LIPINCOTT, S. W., SHELLABARGER, C. J.: Studies on Radiation-Induced Mammary Gland Neoplasia in the Rat, Rad. Res. **12**, 276–285 (1960).

BRUSTAD, T.: Heavy Ions and some Aspects of their Use in Molecular and Cellular Radiobiology. Academic Press (New York). Adv. Biol. Med. Phys. **8**, 161 (1962).

CROWTHER, J. A.: Some Considerations Relative to the Action of X-rays on Tissue Cells. Proc. Royal Society (London) **B 96**, 207 (1924).

DEAN, C. J., FELDSCHREIBER, P., LETT, J. T.: Repair of X-Ray Damage to the Deoxyribonucleic Acid in Micrococcus Radiodurans, Nature **209**, 49–52 (1966).

DERTINGER, H., JUNG, H.: Molekulare Strahlenbiologie. Berlin-Heidelberg-New York: Springer 1969.

DESSAUER, F.: Über einige Wirkungen von Strahlen, Z. Physik **12**, 28 (1922).

DEWEY, W. C., WESTRA, A., MILLER, H. H., NAGASAWA, N.: Heat-Induced lethality and Chromosomal Damage in Synchronized Chinese Hamster Cells Treated with 5-Bromodeoxyuridine. Int. J. Radiat. Biol. **20**, 505–520 (1971).

ELKIND, M., SUTTON, H.: X-ray Damage and Recovery in Mammalian Cells in Culture. Nature (London) **184**, 1293–1295 (1959).

— WHITMORE, G.: The Radiobiology of Cultured Mammalian Cells. Gordon and Breach (London) 1967.

GRAY, L. H.: Brit. J. Radiol., Suppl. **1**, 7 (1947).

HALL, E., GROSS, W., DVORAK, R. F., KELLERER, A. M., ROSSI, H. H.: Survival Curves and Age Response Functions for Chinese Hamster Cells Exposed to X rays and High LET alpha-Particles, Radiat. Res. **52**, 88–98, 1972.

HAYNES, R. H.: Molecular Localization of Radiation Damage Relevant to Bacterial Inactivation. Physical Processes in Rad. Biol. 51–78 (1964).

HOWARD-FLANDERS, P.: Physical and Chemical Mechanisms in the Injury of cells by ionizing radiations. Advan. Biol. Med. Phys. **6**, 553–596 (1958).

HUG, O., KELLERER, A. M.: Zur Interpretation der Dosiswirkungsbeziehungen in der Strahlenbiologie. Biophysik **1**, 20–32 (1963).

— — Stochastik der Strahlenwirkung. Berlin-Heidelberg-New York: Springer 1966.

— — ZUPPINGER, A.: Der Zeitfaktor. Handbuch d. medizinischen Radiologie, Bd. II/1, Hrsg. Diethelm, L. et al. Berlin-Heidelberg-New York: Springer 1966, p. 271–354.

ICRU: Linear Energy Transfer, Report-16, International Commission on Radiation Units and Measurements (Washington, D. C.) 1970.

— Radiation Quantities and Units, Report-19, Unternational Commission on Radiation Units and Measurements (Washington, D. C.) 1971.

KELLERER, A. M.: Analysis of Patterns of Energy

— Deposition. Microdosimetry, Euratom, Brussels 107–135 (1969).

— Hug, O.: Zur Kinetik der Strahlenwirkung. Biophysik **1**, 33–50 (1963).

— Rossi, H. H.: Summary of Quantities and Functions Employed in Microdosimetry. „Microdosimetry", 841–853, Euratom, Brussels (1969).

— — RBE and the Primary Mechanism of Radiation Action. Radiat. Res. **47** 15–34 (1971).

— — The Theory of Dual Radiation Action, Current Topics in Radiat. Res., Quarterly **8**, 1972.

Lea, D. E.: Actions of Radiations on Living Cells. Cambridge Univ. Press (Cambridge) 1946.

Neary, G. J.: Chromosome Aberrations and the Theory of RBE, 1. General Considerations. Int. J. Rad. Biol. **9**, 477–502 (1965).

Pollard, E. C., Guild, W. R., Hutchinson, F., Setlow, R. B.: Progr. Biophys. Chem. **5**, 72 (1955).

Powers, E. L.: Considerations of Survival Curves and Target Theory (Seventh Douglas Lea Memorial Lecture). Phys. in Med. Biol. **7**, 1, 3–27 (1962).

Rossi, H. H.: Correlation of Radiation Quality and Biological Effect. Annals of the New York Academy of Sciences, **114**, Art. 1, 4–15 (1964).

— Energy Distribution in the Absorption of Radiation. Adv. in Biol. and Med. Physics **11**, 27–85 (1967).

— Microscopic Energy Distribution in Irradiated Matter. Radiation Dosimetry **1**, p. 43–92, New York: Acad. Press 1968.

— The Effects of Small Doses of Ionizing Radiation. Phys. In Med. and Biology **15**, 255—262 (1970).

Rossi, H. H., Kellerer, A. M.: Carcinogenesis at Low Doses. Science **175**, 200–202 (1972).

Shellabarger, C. J.: unpublished data.

Sinclair, W. K.: The Shape of Radiation Survival Curves of Mammalian Cells Cultured in vitro. Panel on the Biophysical Aspects of Radiation Quality IAEA, Vienna, IAEA, Vienna 1968.

Sparrow, A. H., Underbrink, A. G., Rossi, H. H.: Mutations Induced in Tradescantia by Small Doses of X rays and Neutrons: Analysis of Dose-Response Curves. Science **176**, 916–918, 1972

Timofeeff-Ressovsky, N. M., Zimmer, K. G.: Das Trefferprinzip in der Biologie. Biophysik I, Leipzig: S. Hirzel 1947.

Vogel, H. H.: Mammary Gland Neoplasms after Fission Neutron Irradiation Nature **222**, 1279–1281 (1969).

Vogel, H. H., Zaldivar, R.: Experimental Mammary Neoplasms: A comparison of Effectiveness Between Neutrons, X- and Gamma-Radiation, USAEC Symposium at Oak Ridge, Tenn. **CONF-691106** 207–229 (1969).

Wolff, S., Atwood, K. C., Randolph, M. L., Luippold, H. E.: Factors Limiting the Number of Radiation-Induced Chromosome Exchanges. Journal of Biophysical and Biochemical Cytology **4**, 365–372 (1958).

Zimmer, K. G.: Studies on Quantitative Radiation Biology. London: Oliver and Boyd 1961.

B. Strahlenwirkungen auf die Vermehrung von Säugetierzellen

von

Klaus-Rüdiger Trott

Mit 58 Abbildungen

I. Einleitung

1. Ältere Studien an Gewebekulturen

Die Technik der Gewebekultur, die zu Beginn dieses Jahrhunderts insbesondere durch HARRISON (1907, BURROWS (1910), CARELL (1912) und deren Mitarbeiter entwickelt wurde, eröffnete die Möglichkeit, „die Struktur und das Verhalten lebender Zellen unabhängig von den Einflüssen des Gesamtorganismus zu studieren" (FELL, 1935). Auch die Wirkung von Röngenstrahlen auf Zellen in vitro wurde schon damals untersucht. Mit nahezu unveränderter Technik wurden in den nächsten 40 Jahren vor allem zwei Probleme immer wieder aufgegriffen: zum einen suchte man nach der „tödlichen Dosis für Carcinomzellen" (WOOD u. PRIME, 1922), zum anderen beobachtete man die direkt unter Bestrahlung auftretenden oder unmittelbar folgenden Veränderungen in den kultivierten Zellen, insbesondere die Veränderungen der mitotischen Aktivität.

Die meisten in diesen Arbeiten verwendeten Techniken, z.B. die Plasmakoagulummethode, sind heute vor allem von historischem Interesse. Es soll hier nur insoweit auf sie eingegangen werden, als für das Verständnis der jeweiligen experimentellen Ergebnisse notwendig ist. Im übrigen wird auf die Lehrbücher der Zellkulturtechnik verwiesen (z.B. STRANGEWAYS, 1924; PARKER, 1960; WILLMER, 1965; PAUL, 1970). Umfassendere Übersichten liegen von SPEAR (1935, 1953), CARLSON (1954) und GÄRTNER (1963) vor.

Bei der Suche nach der *tödlichen Dosis für Carcinomzellen* ging man von der Vorstellung aus, daß eine bestimmte Konzentration eines Pharmakons alle Zellen vollständig abtötet. Die damals schon bekannten Vorstellungen über die stochastische Natur der Strahlenwirkung, später zur Treffertheorie ausgebaut, wurden noch kaum auf diese Fragestellung angewendet.

Die ersten eingehenden Versuche zu diesem Problem, abgesehen von Experimenten von WEDD u. RUSS (1912), stammen von WOOD u. PRIME (1921, 1922). Sie bestrahlten kleine Stückchen von transplantablen Tiertumoren in vitro mit Dosen von 1—4 HED (ca. 500—2 000 R). Anschließend wurde die Lebensfähigkeit der Tumorstückchen getestet — indem sie in neue Tiere transplantiert oder in einer Deckglaskultur gezüchtet wurden.

Bei dieser Methode wird ein Gewebestück von ca. 1 mm Kantenlänge in einigen Tropfen Hühnerplasma und Embryonalextrakt auf ein Deckglas explantiert. Das Deckglas wird umgekehrt auf einem Objektträger mit Uhrglasschliff fixiert und bei 37°C inkubiert. Man kann beobachten, wie aus dem Tumorklümpchen nach mehreren Stunden vereinzelt Zellen aussprossen, sich vermehren und innerhalb weniger Tage einen mehr oder weniger breiten Saum von Zellen um das Explantat ausbilden (Abb. 1).

WOOD u. PRIME (1922) stellten fest, daß auch die höchste von ihnen benutzte Dosis (4 HED) nicht in der Lage war, dieses Aussprossen wesentlich zu beeinflussen. Dagegen bewirkte diese Dosis eine Verminderung der Transplantierbarkeit der Tumorstückchen auf die Hälfte. Sie kamen daraufhin zu dem Schluß, daß „der Umfang des Wachstums im Glas kein Anzeichen für die Fähigkeit der Tumorzelle ist, im tierischen Körper weiter zu wachsen. Das Wachstum, welches nach tödlichen Dosen beobachtet wurde, ist offenbar zurückzuführen auf die langsame Wirkung der Strahlen, welche Zellen, die potentiell tot sind, gestattet, in das Medium auszuwandern und einen Teilungsprozeß zu vollenden, bevor ihr Wachstumsmoment endgültig gehemmt wird."

In den folgenden Jahren wurden immer wieder Versuche durchgeführt, um die unterschiedliche Strahlenwirkung auf das Wachstum in vivo und in vitro zu studieren. Opitz (1925) kam zu dem Schluß, daß Bestrahlung des Krebsgewebes außerhalb des Tumorträgers die Krebszelle nicht oder nur dann vernichtet, wenn ein Vielfaches der optimalen Dosis beim lebenden Tier appliziert wird. Roffo (1925) berichtete, daß Strahlendosen, die in vivo als tödlich gelten, das weitere Aussprossen von Zellen aus dem Explantat auch dann nicht hemmen, wenn erst bestrahlt wird, nachdem bereits ein Saum von Zellen

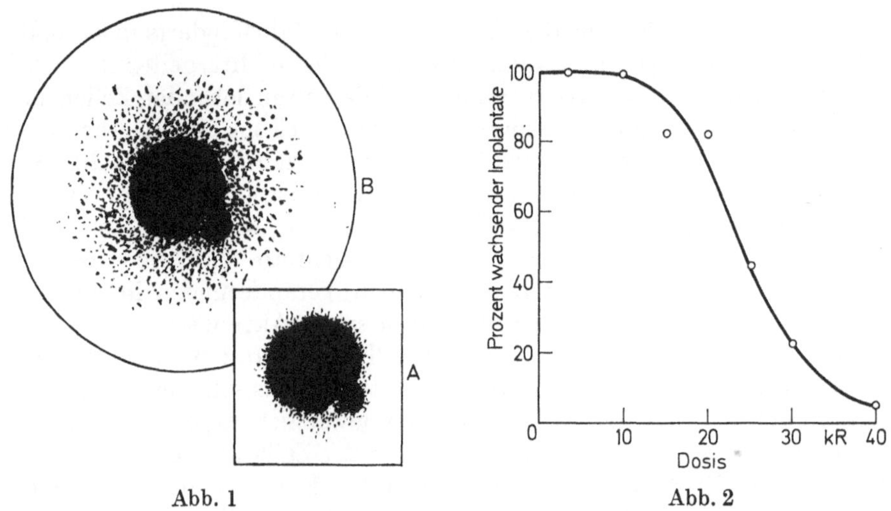

Abb. 1. Das Aussprossen von Fibroblasten aus einer Primärkultur von embryonalem Hühnerherzgewebe nach 12 stündiger (A) bzw. 48 stündiger (B) Inkubation. (Roffo, 1925)

Abb. 2. Die Strahlendosisabhängigkeit des Auswachsens eines Zellsaums von mehr als 20 Zellen nach Bestrahlung eines C3H-Mammacarcinoms in vivo unmittelbar vor der Explantation. (Trott und Hug, unveröffentlicht)

ausgesproßt ist (Abb. 1). Krontowski (1926) fand, daß es keinen Unterschied machte, ob man embryonales Hühnergewebe unmittelbar vor der Explantation im Ei oder nach der Explantation bestrahlt. In beiden Fällen konnte er auch nach 7 HED Röntgenstrahlen noch ein gutes Wachstum beobachten, wobei auch weitere Passagen der Kulturen glückten.

Schubert (1927) beobachtete auch nach 10 HED ein ungehemmtes Aussprossen von Zellen, die jedoch deutliche degenerative Veränderungen, insbesondere Vakuolisierung aufwiesen. Beließ man aber das Gewebe für 3 h nach Bestrahlung im Ei, bevor man es explantierte, war keine Aussprossung mehr zu sehen. Schubert schloß daraus, daß „die Röntgenstrahlung primär die Zellen selbst beeinflußt. Die Abbauprodukte derselben verändern sekundär das Milieu, welches nun seinerseits im Sinne einer Fortführung der Schädigung auch die nicht von den Strahlen getroffenen Zellen alteriert". Zu ähnlichen Ergebnissen kamen auch Strangeways u. Fell (1927).

Mit der von Canti zur Beobachtung des Verhaltens von Gewebekulturen entwickelten Methode der Zeitrafferkinematographie studierten Vollmer u. Rajewski (1937) die unmittelbaren Änderungen der Motilität und Struktur von verschiedenen Gewebekulturen. Nach Dosen von über 960 R fanden sie eindeutige Zeichen der Zellschädigung, vor allem eine Abnahme der amöboiden Bewegungen der Zellen.

Auch wenn bestrahlte Kulturen anfänglich normal wachsen, können sie doch verzögert zugrunde gehen (LASER, 1930). Im Gegensatz zu den Berichten von DOLJANSKI u. Mitarb. (1944) beobachtete SPEAR (1953), daß auch nach Bestrahlung mit 15 000 R nicht selten einige Zellen überleben, sich teilen und die Kultur regenerieren, so daß sie nach einigen Passagen ein normales Aussehen zeigt. Die Dauer der Latenzphase bis zum Auftreten der strahlenbedingten Wachstumshemmung hängt neben der Strahlendosis (nach 15 000 R beträgt die Latenzphase 3 Wochen, nach 20 000 R 2 Wochen [SPEAR, 1953]) auch von der Wachstumsgeschwindigkeit ab, da schneller wachsende Gewebekulturen empfindlicher und schneller reagieren als langsam wachsende. Verschiedene Gewebe weisen also, wenn sie sich in demselben Proliferationszustand befinden, annähernd gleiche Strahlensensibilität auf.

Quantitative Untersuchungen von HALBERSTÄDTER u. Mitarb. (1942) zeigten, daß die D_{50} für die unmittelbare Hemmwirkung auf das Aussprossen von Zellen eines bestrahlten Explantats bei 25 000 R liegt. Das stimmt gut mit eigenen Versuchen überein (TROTT u. HUG unveröffentlicht), (Abb. 2). Wenn man jedoch die unbegrenzte Proliferationsfähigkeit der Gewebekulturen als Überlebenskriterium betrachtet, so sind nach Untersuchungen am gleichen Material schon 2 000—3 000 R in der Lage, diese weitgehend aufzuheben (DOLJANSKI u. Mitarb., 1944). Erst nach Strahlendosen der Größenordnung 100 000 R tritt in einer Fibroblastenkultur sofortiger Tod der ganzen Kultur ein (HOPWOOD u. DONALDSON, 1930; SPEAR, 1930; DOLJANSKI u. Mitarb., 1931).

Die Frage, ob die auch nach hohen Strahlendosen (über 10 000 R) beobachtete Aussprossung nur ein Auswandern steriler Zellen aus dem Gewebsstück darstellt, oder ob wirklich auch Zellen darunter sind, die ihre Fähigkeit zu unbegrenzter Vermehrung bewahrt haben, muß als nicht eindeutig gelöst bezeichnet werden. Eine ganze Reihe von Beobachtungen, z.B. daß gelegentlich Kulturen auch nach 15 000 R weiterwachsen können (SPEAR, 1935), daß auch nach mehreren Wochen in Aussprossungen von mit 10 000 R bestrahlten Tumorstückchen noch DNS-Syntheseaktivität nachweisbar ist (TROTT u. HUG, unveröffentlicht), auch nach extrem hohen Dosen (100 000 R) noch Kernteilungsfiguren gesehen wurden (GOLDFEDER, 1940), und daß gelegentlich implantierte Tumorstückchen auch nach Bestrahlung mit 10 000 R zu neuen Tumoren auswachsen können (THOMLINSON, 1961), weisen darauf hin, daß es in Geweben proliferationsfähige Zellen gibt, die Strahlendosen überleben, die nach unseren heutigen Vorstellungen jede proliferative Aktivität unter den bestrahlten Zellen vernichtet haben sollten. Weitere Versuche zur Erklärung dieser Diskrepanz erscheinen dringend erforderlich.

Seit den Berichten von KIMURA (1919) und STRANGEWAYS (1922) war bekannt, daß auch geringe Strahlendosen in Gewebekulturen die Zellteilung hemmen können. Die Mitosehemmung ist die früheste und empfindlichste Reaktion von tierischen Zellen auf Bestrahlung. Sie wurde in den folgenden Jahrzehnten eingehend untersucht, insbesondere von den Forschern des „Strangeways-Teams" (SPEAR, 1935) in Cambridge: STRANGEWAYS, CANTI, SPEAR, LASNITZKI.

Fibroblastenkulturen, die nahezu ausschließlich für die Untersuchung der Mitosehemmung herangezogen wurden, werden folgendermaßen angelegt: Aus 6–12 Tage lang bebrüteten Hühnereiern wird der Embryo entnommen, die einzelnen Organe werden präpariert und in Stücke von 1 mm Durchmesser geschnitten. Ein Stück wird auf ein Deckglas gebracht, mit 1 Tropfen Nährlösung (meist Embryonalextrakt) und 1 Tropfen Hühnerplasma bedeckt. Das Plasma gerinnt, das Deckglas wird umgekehrt montiert und inkubiert. Nach einigen Tagen wird das Koagulum mit der inzwischen ausgewachsenen Zellschicht geteilt und in einem neuen Koagulum weitergezüchtet. Die meisten Beobachtungen wurden an einem solchen 2. Transplantat von Kulturen aus Sklera- und Chorioideagewebe von Hühnerembryonen gemacht.

STRANGEWAYS u. OAKELEY (1923) fanden, daß schon 20—25 R Röntgenstrahlen deutliche Mitosestörungen auslösen konnten. Die Zahl der pro Kultur beobachteten Mitosen nahm in Abhängigkeit von der Dosis ab, und in den noch vorhandenen Mitosen wurden abnorme Teilungsfiguren beobachtet, insbesondere Verklumpungen von Chromosomen, Kernbrücken, Mikrokerne und multipolare Teilungen. CANTI u. DONALDSON (1926) fanden nach Radiumbestrahlung die gleichen Veränderungen. Bei dauernder Beobachtung bestrahlter Kulturen sahen STRANGEWAYS u. HOPWOOD (1926), daß die Zellen, die sich zum Zeitpunkt der Bestrahlung bereits in den Frühstadien der Mitose befinden, die Teilung ungestört vollenden, und daß die Strahlung somit nicht die Mitose selbst, sondern den Eintritt der Zellen in die Mitose hemmt. Aus diesem Grund ist der maximale Strahleneffekt erst nach ca. 80 Minuten zu beobachten, wenn die zum Zeitpunkt der Bestrahlung in Mitose befindlichen Zellen ihre Kernteilung vollendet haben. Diese Beobachtungen decken sich weitgehend mit den neueren Ergebnissen und Vorstellungen (s. S. 67).

Nachdem der Mitoseindex 80 Minuten nach Bestrahlung auf ein Minimum abgefallen ist, steigt er wieder an, wobei er den Kontrollwert zeitweilig sogar überschreitet (Abb. 3), (CANTI u. SPEAR, 1929). Nach Bestrahlung mit 80 R kompensiert dieser Überschuß gerade den Abfall der Mitoserate unmittelbar nach Bestrahlung. Mit zunehmender

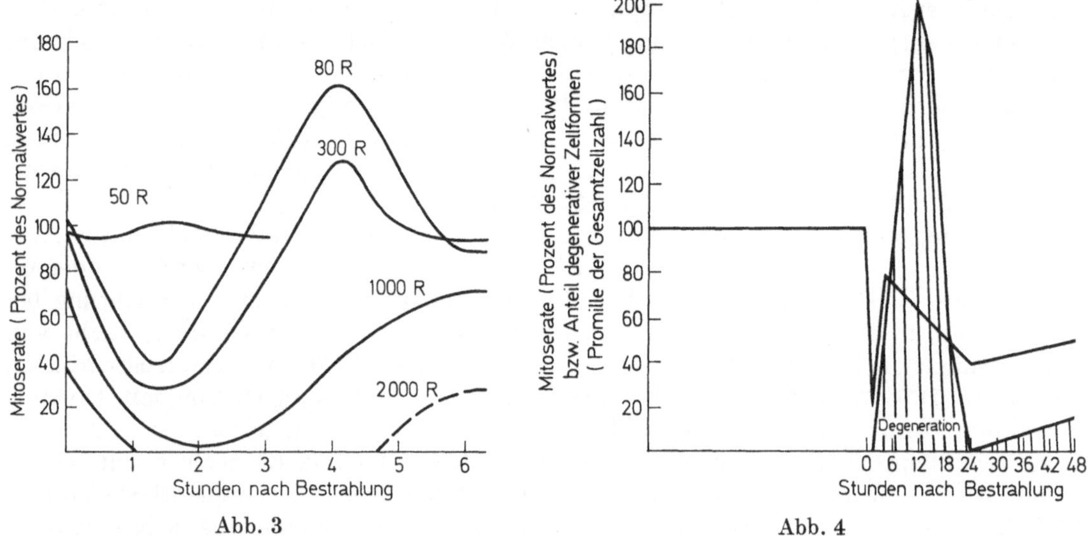

Abb. 3. Die Mitoserate in einer Hühnerfibroblastenkultur im Verlauf der ersten 6 Stunden nach Bestrahlung mit 50–2000 R Gammastrahlen (Ra) einer Dosisleistung von 33 R/min. (CANTI und SPEAR, 1929)

Abb. 4. Mitoserate (ausgezogene Linie) und Anteil degenerativer Zellen (schraffierte Fläche) in einer Hühnerfibroblastenkultur in den ersten 48 Stunden nach einer Bestrahlung mit 96 R. (LASNITZKI, 1940)

Dosis wird der Abfall tiefer und länger und die Erholung der Mitoserate immer geringer.

CANTI u. SPEAR (1927), SPEAR u. GRIMMET (1933) und LASNITZKI (1946) untersuchten die Abhängigkeit der mitosehemmenden Wirkung von Röntgen- und Gammastrahlen von der Dosisleistung und registrierten mit abnehmender Dosisleistung einen immer geringeren Effekt, bis bei Unterschreitung einer Mindestdosisleistung keine Wirkung auf die Mitoserate in der Fibroblastenkultur mehr nachzuweisen war. Dagegen hat eine fraktionierte Bestrahlung, wenn die 2. Dosishälfte zum Zeitpunkt des Mitose-Minimums gegeben wird, eine weitaus stärkere Hemmwirkung als die gleiche Gesamtdosis bei einmaliger Bestrahlung (SPEAR, 1932).

Die relative biologische Wirksamkeit von Röntgen-, Gamma- und Neutronenstrahlen auf die Mitoserate wurde von LASNITZKI u. LEA (1940) und SPEAR u. Mitarb. (1938), die von schnellen Elektronen von GÄRTNER (1953) untersucht.

Von LASNITZKI (1940) stammen die ersten quantitativen Untersuchungen über eine Korrelation des Auftretens von Zelluntergängen zum Wiederanstieg der Mitoserate (Abb. 4). Die Zellen sterben erst, wenn sie eine Zellteilung durchführen wollen, und werden meist am Ende der Prophase zerstört. Zellen, die die Metaphase erreichen, zeigen abnorme

Kernteilungsfiguren und degenerieren später. Bei Dosen bis 1000 R sind außerhalb der Mitose keine Anzeichen einer Zellschädigung zu sehen. Erst bei höheren Dosen (2500—10000 R) tritt der Zelluntergang unabhängig von der Mitose auf und trifft in erster Linie Interphasezellen (LASNITZKI, 1943a).

Von einer Bestrahlung mit 100 R hat sich eine Kultur nach 48 Stunden, von einer Bestrahlung mit 1000 R nach 10 Tagen erholt; d.h. nach diesen Zeiten sind Mitoserate und Verteilung der einzelnen Mitosestadien wieder normal, und es findet sich kein erhöhter Anteil degenerierter Zellen mehr in der Kultur (LASNITZKI, 1943b).

HORNSEY (1953) stellte fest, daß die Zahl der Zelluntergänge nach Bestrahlung von Fibroblastenkulturen entscheidend von der Sauerstoffkonzentration zum Zeitpunkt der Bestrahlung abhängt, wobei anoxische Kulturen etwa doppelt so resistent wie gut mit Sauerstoff versorgte Kulturen sind.

Mit der Gewebekultur, die in den letzten Jahren nur noch vereinzelt bei der Erforschung strahlenbiologischer Probleme angewendet wird, war ein insbesondere für die Strahlentherapie wichtiges Problem nicht zu lösen, nämlich die Abhängigkeit der irreversiblen Schädigung der Vermehrungsfähigkeit von Säugetierzellen von der Strahlendosis. Die Lösung dieses Problems durch die Methode von PUCK u. MARCUS (1956b) brachte eine explosionsartige Erweiterung unserer Kenntnisse über die Strahlenwirkung auf Zellen in Kultur. Die weiteren Abschnitte werden davon handeln.

II. Dosiseffektkurven in vitro

1. Neuere Untersuchungen an Zellkulturen

Die Konstanz der Zellzahl in Mausergeweben und das Wachstum von Tumoren ist wesentlich bedingt durch kontinuierliche Zellteilung von Stammzellen, die eine praktisch unbegrenzte Vermehrungsfähigkeit besitzen. Deshalb war es von entscheidender Bedeutung, daß Methoden entwickelt wurden, die es erlaubten, die Strahlenwirkung auf die „reproduktive Integrität" (GRAY, 1961) der Einzelzelle quantitativ zu erfassen. In der mikrobiologischen Forschung lagen solche Methoden seit Beginn des Jahrhunderts vor: einzelne Bakterien können auf geeigneten Nährböden zu sichtbaren Kolonien auswachsen. Die Wirkungen von Chemotherapeutika, Antibiotika und ionisierenden Strahlen können daran gemessen werden, welcher Prozentsatz der eingesetzten Population noch in der Lage ist, eine Kolonie zu bilden.

Bis 1955 waren Versuche, auch für Säugetierzellen ein Koloniebildungs-Testsystem zu schaffen, erfolglos. Isolierte Zellen wuchsen nur, wenn sie in einer Mindestdichte angesetzt wurden. SANFORD u. Mitarb. (1948) konnten in einer Kapillare zum ersten Mal Klone von Säugetierzellen isolieren. Doch für strahlenbiologische Experimente war dieses Verfahren zu aufwendig.

Es ist das Verdienst von PUCK und seinen Mitarbeitern, eine Methode entwickelt und vervollkommnet zu haben, die es erlaubt, die Strahlenwirkung auf die reproduktive Integrität verschiedener Säugetierzellen über einen weiten Dosisbereich zu studieren. Die Arbeiten der Gruppe um PUCK aus den Jahren 1955—1957 legten den Grundstein zu den heutigen Methoden und Vorstellungen der quantitativen Strahlenbiologie der Säugetierzellen in vitro.

Die meisten Säugetierzellen überziehen den Glasboden von Kulturgefäßen in einer einzigen Zellschicht. Suspensionen von Einzelzellen können leicht mit einer verdünnten Trypsinlösung hergestellt werden. Bei der Inkubation dieser Suspensionen konnte aber nur dann ein Wachstum erreicht werden, wenn in jedem Tropfen Medium mehr als 50 Zellen vorhanden waren (PUCK u. MARCUS, 1955). Auf der Beobachtung, daß zur Unterstützung des Wachstums der Einzelzelle metabolisierende Nachbarzellen notwendig sind, die aber nicht unbedingt vermehrungsfähig sein müssen, bauten PUCK u. MARCUS (1955) ihre „feeder-layer"-Methode auf: In eine Petrischale wurden 300000 Zellen vom Stamm

HeLa pipettiert und über Nacht in den Brutschrank gestellt. Am nächsten Morgen wurden die Zellen mit 5 000—40 000 R bestrahlt. Die so behandelten Zellen waren alle in ihrer Vermehrungsfähigkeit blockiert, doch zeigten sie über mehrere Tage hin eine starke Stoffwechselaktivität. Unter diesen Bedingungen können einzelne, unbestrahlte Zellen, die in solche bestrahlte Kulturen gegeben werden, zu isolierten Kolonien wachsen.

Die Kolonienausbeute (plating efficiency = p.e.) in den ersten Versuchen von Puck u. Marcus (1955) betrug 100 %, d.h. jede morphologisch intakte Zelle aus einer HeLa-Zellkultur war in der Lage, sich bis zur Koloniegröße zu vermehren. Später zeigte sich, daß eine „feeder"-Zellschicht zwar die Zellvermehrung erleichtert, jedoch bei den meisten Zellarten nicht notwendig ist, wenn die Präparation der Einzelzellsuspension in geeigneter Weise vorgenommen wird. Die kritische Stufe ist die Prozedur der Zelldispersion mit Trypsin. Durch eine Modifikation der Präparationstechnik wurde es möglich, mit

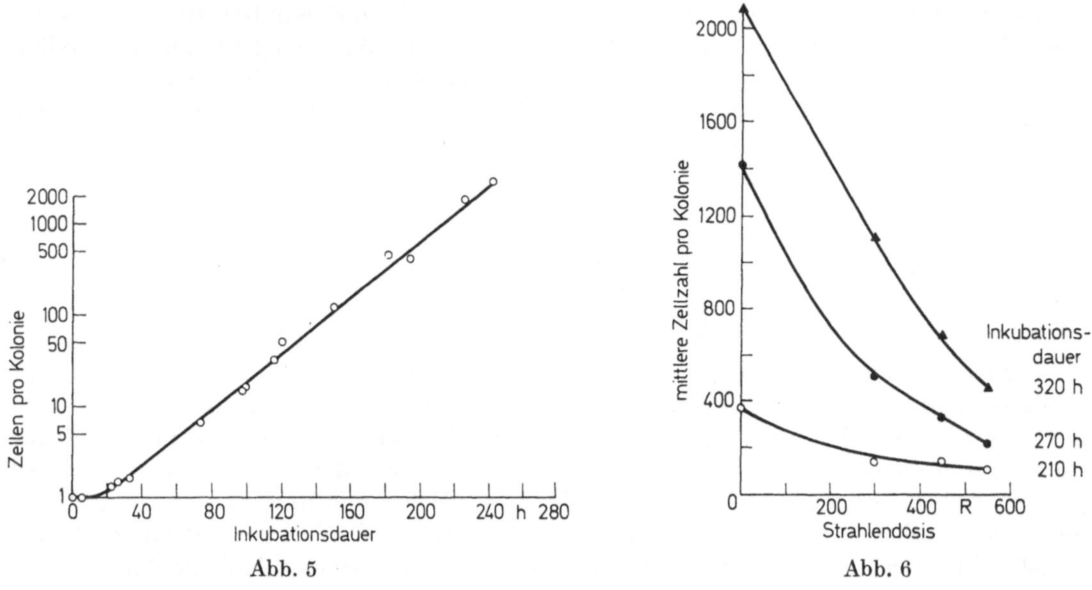

Abb. 5. Die Wachstumskurve von HeLa-Kolonien. (Puck u. Mitarb., 1956)

Abb. 6. Die Abhängigkeit der mittleren Koloniegröße von HeLa-Zellen von der Strahlendosis zu 3 verschiedenen Zeitpunkten nach Bestrahlung mit 230 kV-Röntgenstrahlen. (Puck und Marcus, 1956)

einer Ausbeute von 100 % bestimmte Sublinien von HeLa (z.B. HeLa S-3) ohne „feeder"-Zellschicht zu klonieren. Nach Puck u. Mitarb. (1956) wird das Nährmedium vom Zellrasen der Stammkultur entfernt und 0,25 % Trypsinlösung 1 mm hoch aufpipettiert. Nach 15 minütiger Inkubation bei 37°C wird die Lösung kurz aufgewirbelt, um noch vorhandene Zellklumpen aufzulösen. Dann wird die Suspension mit Medium verdünnt, im Hämozytometer gezählt und mit weiterem Medium auf die gewünschte Konzentration eingestellt.

Für die verschiedenen Zellstämme gibt es unterschiedliche Nährmedien. Sie bestehen in der Regel aus einer isotonischen Lösung von Salzen, Vitaminen und anderen organischen Substanzen und 10—20 % inaktiviertem Serum. Zu weiteren Details der Kulturtechnik wird auf die einschlägige Literatur hingewiesen (z.B. Elkind u. Whitmore, 1967; Paul, 1970).

Zellzählungen in einzelnen Klonen zu verschiedenen Zeiten nach der Inkubation (Abb. 5) ergaben, daß nach einer Verzögerungsphase von etwa 20 Stunden eine exponentielle Vermehrung der Zellzahl bis zu einer Dichte von mehreren tausend Zellen pro Kolonie erfolgte. Danach nahm die Wachstumsgeschwindigkeit ab, wohl weil im Zentrum der Kolonie die Wachstumsbedingungen ungünstiger wurden. Bei Zellen, die das Phänomen der Kontakthemmung zeigen (z.B. 3 T 3), ist sogar von einer Zellzahl von ca. 60 an nur noch eine lineare Zunahme zu beobachten (FISHER u. YEH, 1967). Die Morphologie der einzelnen Kolonien hängt neben der Zellart auch vom Nährmedium, vor allem von der Konzentration und der Art der verwendeten Seren ab.

Mit dieser Methode untersuchten PUCK u. MARCUS die Strahlenwirkung auf das Koloniebildungsvermögen von HeLa-Zellen. Eine definierte Zahl unbestrahlter Zellen wurde ohne feeder-Zellschicht in Petrischalen pipettiert und etwa 5 h lang bei 37° C inkubiert, um den Zellen Zeit zum Festhaften auf dem Glasboden zu geben. Dann wurden sie mit Dosen von 50—1000 R bestrahlt und für weitere 9—17 Tage inkubiert. Unbestrahlte Kontrollen zeigten eine 100%ige Ausbeute an Kolonien. Bei den bestrahlen Zellen wurden 2 Effekte beobachtet:

1. Die Größe der Kolonien nahm in Abhängigkeit von der Strahlendosis ab (Abb. 6).
2. Die Zahl der Kolonien nahm in Abhängigkeit von der Strahlendosis ab.

Nach niedrigen Strahlendosen können sich praktisch alle Zellen noch ein- oder mehrmals teilen, bevor manche weitere Zellteilungen aufgeben und andere mit wechselnder Geschwindigkeit weiterwachsen. So beträgt die mittlere Zellzahl der Kolonien, die später weitere Teilungen eingestellt haben (sog. abortive Kolonien), nach 200 R noch 23 Zellen, nach 400 R 13 und nach 600 R 1,7 Zellen. Da diese abortiven Kolonien in ihrer reproduktiven Integrität geschädigt sind, dürfen sie bei der Bestimmung der Überlebensrate nicht mit berücksichtigt werden. PUCK u. MARCUS (1956) fanden, daß für den von ihnen benutzten Stamm HeLa S-3 eine eindeutige Aussage über die reproduktive Integrität der Zellen nach einer Inkubationsdauer von 11 Tagen gemacht werden kann, wenn man als Mindestzahl für eine Kolonie 50 Zellen annimmt.

Das Kriterium „Kolonienbildung" wurde für die verschiedenen Zellstämme in den einzelnen Labors jeweils anders definiert, wobei sowohl die Inkubationsdauer als auch die Mindestzellzahl variiert wurde. Eine Diskussion der verschiedenen Kriterien findet sich bei NIAS u. FOX (1968).

Die erste Dosiseffektkurve für die Inaktivierung von Säugetierzellen in vitro durch Bestrahlung wurde von PUCK u. MARCUS (1956) veröffentlicht. Im linearen Maßstab ergibt sich eine sigmoide Kurve (Abb. 7a). Die gleiche Kurve präsentiert sich im halblogarithmischen Maßstab als sogenannte Schulterkurve (Abb. 7b): die Reaktivität nimmt mit steigender Dosis zu, um schließlich einen konstanten Wert zu erreichen. An anderer Stelle dieses Bandes (S. 17 ff.) werden die formalen Beschreibungen und die Interpretationen solcher Kurven dargestellt. Die von PUCK u. MARCUS gefundene Dosiseffektkurve läßt sich durch eine mittlere Inaktivierungsdosis von 169 R, eine Varianz der Inaktivierungsdosis von 11 000 R^2 und eine relative Steilheit von 2,5 kennzeichnen. Nach ALPER u. Mitarb. (1960) wird eine Kurve dieser Art durch 2 Bestimmungsgrößen definiert, nämlich die D_0 und die Extrapolationsnummer. Als D_0 wird die Dosis bezeichnet, die im geradlinigen, also exponentiellen Teil der Kurve die Zahl der jeweils noch überlebenden Zellen um den Faktor (1/e) vermindert. Die Extrapolationsnummer ergibt sich, wenn man den geradlinigen Teil der Kurve in der halblogarithmischen Darstellung verlängert, aus dem Schnittpunkt mit der Ordinate. Statt der Extrapolationsnummer kann auch der Schnittpunkt mit der 100 % Überlebensrate angegeben werden; ALPER u. Mitarb. (1962) schlugen vor, diese Größe, die die Einheit Dosis hat, als D_q (Quasi-Schwellendosis) zu bezeichnen.

Aus der von PUCK u. MARCUS (1956) veröffentlichten Kurve (Abb. 7b) kann man folgende Parameter ablesen:

$D_0 = 95$ R; Extrapolationsnummer n = 2,1; $D_q = 70$ R;

mittlere Inaktivierungsdosis $(\overline{D}) = 169$ R; relative Steilheit (S) = 2,5.

Unbeschadet der auf S. 19 ff. dargestellten Überlegungen zur Interpretation von Dosiswirkungsbeziehungen und der Bedenken insbesondere gegen die Definition der Schulter durch die Extrapolationsnummer (n) wird im folgenden stets die Kennzeichnung angegeben, die die zitierten Autoren ihren Kurven gegeben haben, also in der Regel D_0 und n.

Puck u. Mitarb. entwickelten Methoden, um auch andere Zellarten menschlicher Gewebe als Klone wachsen zu lassen. Marcus u. Mitarb. (1956) beschrieben die Kultur von epitheloiden Zellen, die aus der menschlichen Conjunctiva, dem Appendix und der Leber isoliert worden waren und unter optimalen Versuchsbedingungen Kolonieausbeuten von 50—80 % ergaben. Von Puck u. Mitarb. (1957) für diese Zellarten veröffentlichte Dosiseffektkurven waren praktisch deckungsgleich mit der an HeLa S-3 gewonnenen. Die Züchtung von Klonen menschlicher Zellen fibroblastischer Natur bereitete größere Schwierigkeiten. Trotz komplizierterer Nährmedien war die Kolonieausbeute in der Regel niedriger (25—65 %; Puck u. Mitarb., 1957). Die Ergebnisse der Bestrahlungs-

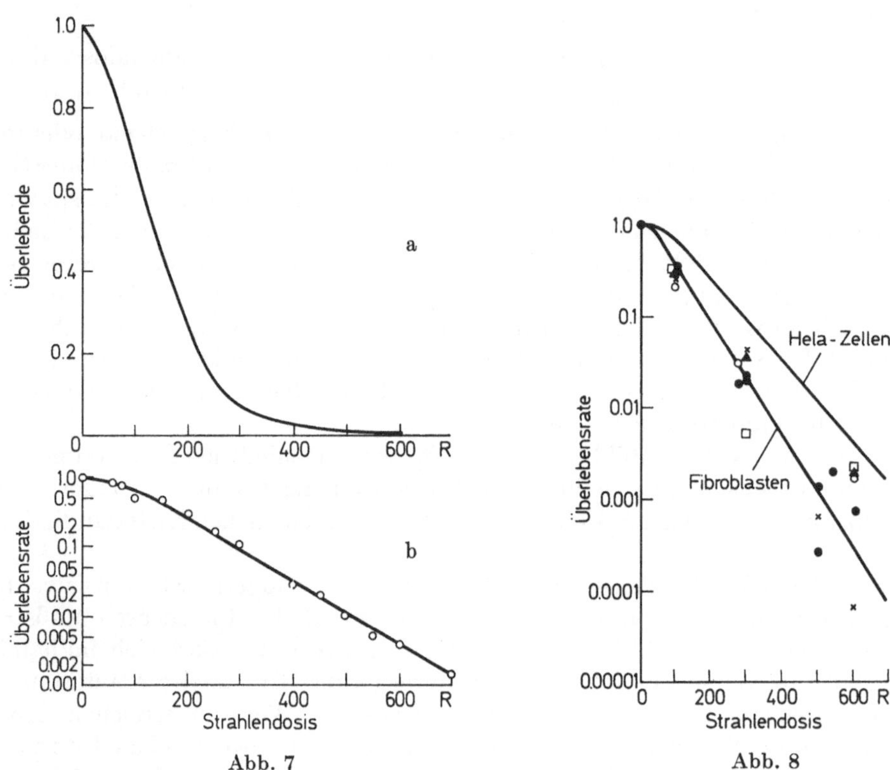

Abb. 7a. Die Überlebensrate von HeLa-Zellen (im linearen Maßstab) in Abhängigkeit von der Strahlendosis. (Werte von Puck und Marcus, 1956)

b. Die Überlebensrate von HeLa-Zellen (im logarithmischen Maßstab) in Abhängigkeit von der Strahlendosis. (Puck und Marcus, 1956)

Abb. 8. Die Überlebensrate von Fibroblasten aus menschlicher Haut, menschlicher Milz und menschlichem Ovar nach Bestrahlung mit 230 kV-Röntgenstrahlen im Vergleich zur Dosiseffektkurve von HeLa-Zellen. (s. Abb. 7b) (Puck u. Mitarb., 1957)

versuche mit Zellen aus 3 verschiedenen Organen (Haut, Milz, Ovar) zeigten größere Streuungen als die mit epitheloiden Zellen durchgeführten (Abb. 8). Die D_0 lag zwischen 50 und 100 R und die Extrapolationsnummer zwischen 1 und 2.

Norris u. Hood (1962) untersuchten eine Reihe direkt von menschlichen Feten explantierter und unterschiedlich lang in vitro weitergezüchteter Zellarten (z.B. Niere, Haut, Lunge) auf ihre Strahlenempfindlichkeit mit der Kolonietestmethode. Im Verlauf der ersten Wochen fand sich eine sehr große Variabilität der Strahlenempfindlichkeit mit Schwankungen der D_0 zwischen 40 und 140 R für die Nachkommen des gleichen Primärexplantats. Häufig hatten Zellen, die eine hohe Kolonieausbeute aufwiesen, auch eine höhere D_0. In allen Fällen blieb im Verlauf der Kultur der ursprüngliche Chromosomensatz erhalten.

Die Arbeiten der Gruppe um PUCK haben die strahlenbiologische Forschung auf völlig neue Grundlagen gestellt, aus denen sich bereits quantitative Aussagen über die Strahlenschädigung von Geweben ableiten ließen (z.B. ELKIND, 1960; MUNRO u. GILBERT, 1961; WILSON, 1961; LAJTHA u. OLIVER, 1961; ELLIS, 1961, 1968; PUCK, 1964; HUG, 1964).

Eine rasch wachsende Zahl von Strahlenbiologen griff die Methode von PUCK auf und wandte sie auf andere Zellstämme tierischen und menschlichen Ursprungs an. Dabei zeigte sich, daß alle Säugetierzellen in vitro nach gleichartigen Dosiswirkungsbeziehungen inaktiviert, d.h. in ihrer reproduktiven Integrität geschädigt werden. Gewisse Variationen der Kurvenform und der numerischen Werte der Bestimmungsgrößen sind teils reell, teils auf die besonderen Versuchsbedingungen in den einzelnen Laboratorien zurückzuführen (s. S. 51 ff.). Besondere Schwierigkeiten bereitet es, die Anfangs- und Endneigung der Dosiswirkungskurve zu bestimmen, weil, wie KELLERER u. HUG auf S. 18 f. ausführen, deren Werte von den jeweils empfindlichsten bzw. resistentesten Zellen der Population abhängen und ihre kleine Zahl zu statistischen Unsicherheiten führt. So ist es in den meisten Fällen nicht definitiv auszumachen, ob die Schulterkurve mit einer endlichen Neigung beginnt und ob die Kurve wirklich in eine Gerade übergeht. Letzteres ist z. B. nicht der Fall in den von BARENDSEN u. Mitarb. (1960) und von BENDER u. GOOCH (1962) veröffentlichten Kurven, die oft als „Mehrtrefferkurven" (s. S. 10 ff.) beschrieben und mathematisch dargestellt werden (z.B. FOWLER, 1966; HUG u. KELLERER, 1966).

Bei dem Studium der Strahlenempfindlichkeit verschiedener Zellarten war man insbesondere bestrebt, Unterschiede zwischen Zellen bösartiger und gutartiger Gewebe zu finden. Bei vergleichenden Untersuchungen von Primärkulturen vor und nach Transformation mit onkogenen Viren fanden WILLIAMS u. TILL (1964) eine Zunahme der D_0 von 175 R auf 200—270 R. Bis auf eine angedeutete Korrelation der Strahlenresistenz mit der klinischen Malignität (gemessen durch die Zahl der Lungentumoren nach i.v. Injektion einer Zellsuspension) fanden sich keine Beziehungen zwischen der Strahlenempfindlichkeit und der Kolonieausbeute, der Wachstumsgeschwindigkeit oder der Chromosomenzahl. Die Zunahme der Strahlenresistenz war vor allem eine Folge der längeren Kultivation in vitro.

Eine erste Zusammenstellung der bei verschiedenen Zellarten gefundenen Extrapolationsnummern stammt von PORTER (1963), die umfassendste Zusammenstellung von Dosiseffektkurvenparametern von WHITMORE u. TILL (1964). Die dort aufgeführten Werte für Mäuse-L-Zellen betragen D_0 = 116—280 rad und n = 2—100 und für Zellen des chinesischen Hamsters D_0 = 117—205 rad und n = 2,5—9,5. Unter Zuhilfenahme dieser Aufstellung wurde die Tabelle 1 für verschiedene Zellarten menschlicher gut- und bösartiger Gewebe angefertigt.

Aus Tabelle 1 geht hervor, daß D_0 und n nicht isoliert betrachtet werden dürfen. Beide Werte schwanken nicht selten von Versuch zu Versuch (LOCKART u. Mitarb., 1961), meist in gegensätzlicher Weise.

Bei der Testung der Strahlenempfindlichkeit von Säugetierzellen mit der PUCKschen Methode fanden sich keine systematischen Abhängigkeiten der Strahlenempfindlichkeit von der Tierspezies, dem Ursprungsorgan (bis auf wenige Ausnahmen), der Malignität des Ausgangsgewebes oder der Chromosomenzahl. Eine ausführliche Diskussion gerade des letztgenannten Problems findet sich bei ELKIND u. WHITMORE (1967).

2. Probleme der Kolonie-Testmethode

Die von verschiedenen Autoren veröffentlichten Dosiseffektkurven der gleichen Zellart weisen nicht selten größere Differenzen auf (s. Tab. 1). Neben Unterschieden, die sich im Lauf der Zeit durch die Züchtung der Zellen in verschiedenen Laboratorien herausge-

Tabelle 1. *Dosiseffektkurvenparameter (D_0 und Extrapolationsnummer n) aus malignen und normalen menschlichen Geweben isolierter Zellstämme nach Bestrahlung mit locker ionisierenden Strahlen und Testung mit der* PUCK*schen Methode. (Zusammengestellt unter Verwendung der Tabelle* WHITMORE *u.* TILL, *1964)*

Gewebe, Zellstamm		Strahlenart	D_0	n	Autoren
Zellen maligner Gewebe					
Cervix-Carcinom	HeLa S-3	230 kV-Röntgenstrahlen	96 R	2	PUCK u. MARCUS (1956)
	HeLa S-3	2,5 MeV-Röntgenstrahlen	150 R	2	BASES (1959)
	HeLa S-3	250 kV-Röntgenstrahlen	130 rad	4	DEERING u. RICE (1962)
	HeLa S-3	76 kV-Röntgenstrahlen	170 R	1,3	HOOD u. NORRIS (1961)
	HeLa S-3-1	55 kV-Röntgenstrahlen	108 rad	2,9	LOCKART u. Mitarb. (1961)
	HeLa S-3-2	55 kV-Röntgenstrahlen	104 rad	4,0	LOCKART u. Mitarb. (1961)
	HeLa S-3-3	55 kV-Röntgenstrahlen	131 rad	1,3	LOCKART u. Mitarb. (1961)
	HeLa S-3-Oxf	75 kV-Röntgenstrahlen	161 rad	1,6	BERRY u. OLIVER (1964)
	HeLa S-3	220 kV-Röntgenstrahlen	125 rad	1,6	TERASIMA u. TOLMACH (1963)
	HeLa S-3	60 Co-Gammastrahlen	181 rad	1,6	BEDFORD u. HALL (1963)
	HeLa S-3	60 Co-Gammastrahlen	140 rad	2	MORKOVIN u. FELDMAN (1960)
Cervix-Carcinom	H. Ep. 1	200 kV-Röntgenstrahlen	130 rad	10	DELIHAS u. Mitarb. (1962)
malignes Melanom		250 kV-Röntgenstrahlen	100 rad	40	BARRANCO u. Mitarb. (1971)
Leukämie (Osgood)		250 kV-Röntgenstrahlen	140 rad	2	MORKOVIN u. FELDMAN (1960)
Burkitt-Lymphom			75 R	1	SATO u. KOJIMA (1971)
Zellen normaler Gewebe					
Leber (Chang)			123 R	5	LITTLE (1971)
embryonale Lunge		230 kV-Röntgenstrahlen	166 R	2	PUCK u. Mitarb. (1957)
embroynale Leber		200 kV-Röntgenstrahlen	119 rad	2	DEWEY (1960)
embryonale Leber		200 kV-Röntgenstrahlen	140 rad	3	DEWEY u. HAWES (1963)
Amnionzellen (AV 2)		250 kV-Röntgenstrahlen	140 rad	2	MORKOVIN u. FELDMAN (1960)
Knochenmark (D-98/AG)		140 kV-Röntgenstrahlen	130 R	10	ERIKSON u. SZYBALSKI (1963)
Lymphoide Zellen (Immunglobulin-produzierend)		250 kV-Röntgenstrahlen	98 rad	6	DREWINKO u. HUMPHREY (1971)
Epitheloide Zellen aus erwachsener Leber, Conjunctiva und Appendix		250 kV-Röntgenstrahlen	140 rad	2	MORKOVIN u. FELDMAN (1960)
Fibroblastische Zellen aus der Haut, der Milz und dem Ovar		250 kV-Röntgenstrahlen	75 R	1,5	PUCK u. Mitarb. (1957)

bildet haben, wobei Sublinien verschiedener Chromosomenzahl, metabolischer Aktivität und Proliferationskinetik entstanden sein können, dürften auch experimentell-technische Faktoren von wesentlichem Einfluß sein.

Zellen können vor und nach dem Platieren bestrahlt werden. Auf jeden Fall muß Sorge getragen werden, daß Temperatur, pH und Sauerstoffpartialdruck (s. u.) konstant sind. Die Unterschiede in der Dosiseffektkurve bei verschiedenen Bestrahlungstemperaturen können beträchtlich sein. Bei 5° C weisen HeLa-Zellen eine um 20 % höhere D_0 auf als bei 37° C (BELLI u. BONTE, 1963). Eine Erniedrigung um wenige Grad über längere Zeit hin hat bei Leukämiezellen in vitro ein deutliches Ansteigen der Überlebensrate zur Folge (BEER u. Mitarb., 1963), (s. S. 103).

Bei Bestrahlung *vor* dem Platieren kann in Suspension bestrahlt werden. Vorteile dieser Methode sind die einfachere Dosimetrie und Herstellung anoxischer Bedingungen. Außerdem wird bei dieser Methode stets die Koloniebildungsfähigkeit einer einzelnen Zelle und nicht einer sich schon entwickelnden Kolonie aus mehreren Zellen (s. u.) getestet. Ein Nachteil könnte darin bestehen, daß die Zellen unmittelbar nach der eingreifenden Methode der Trypsinierung, also in lag-Phase, bestrahlt werden, wodurch nicht immer eine Zufallsverteilung auf die Zellzyklusphasen garantiert ist (s. u.). Außerdem sind manche Synchronisationsmethoden nicht anwendbar (s. S. 91). Auch ist schwierig zu entscheiden, inwieweit die Bestrahlung nicht auch den Vorgang des Festhaftens der Zellen auf dem Boden des Kulturgefäßes beeinflußt (s. BERRY, 1967c).

In den meisten Labors dürfte *nach* dem Platieren bestrahlt werden. Dabei kann das Zeitintervall zwischen Platieren und Bestrahlen die Ergebnisse wesentlich beeinflussen (BENDER u. GOOCH, 1962; TOLMACH u. Mitarb., 1965; BERRY u. Mitarb., 1966), was auf eine vorübergehende, durch das Trypsinieren bewirkte partielle Synchronisation zurückgeführt wird.

Auf der anderen Seite beginnen die Zellen schon wenige Stunden nach dem Platieren mit der ersten Zellteilung, so daß keine Einzelzellen mehr bestrahlt werden, sondern mehrere an der gleichen Stelle liegende Zellen. ELKIND u. Mitarb. (1961) haben gezeigt, daß nach Bestrahlung mit höheren Strahlendosen die Überlebensrate proportional zu der mittleren Zahl der inzwischen aus jeder eingesäten Zelle entstandenen Zellen ansteigt. ELKIND u. WHITMORE (1967) haben ausführlich diskutiert, ob in solchen Fällen die einzelnen Zellen unabhängig voneinander auf Bestrahlung reagieren. Sie kamen zu dem Schluß, daß bei bestimmten Zellarten nachgewiesen sei, daß jede der inzwischen aus der eingesäten Zelle entstandene Zelle unabhängig von der Nachbarzelle inaktiviert wird. Manche früheren Ergebnisse, die als Beweis für eine Interdependenz der Inaktivierung von nahe beieinander liegenden, aus der gleichen Mutterzelle stammenden Zellen eines kleinen Klons angesehen worden waren (PHILLIPS u. TOLMACH, 1964), konnten später als Folge partieller Synchronisation durch den Platierungsvorgang erklärt werden (TOLMACH u. Mitarb., 1965). Die Extrapolationsnummer einer Dosiseffektkurve ist in erster Näherung das Produkt aus der mittleren Zahl der pro eingesetzter Zelle entstandenen Zellen („Multiplizität") zum Zeitpunkt der Bestrahlung und der Extrapolationsnummer, die sich ergeben würde, wenn man wirklich Einzelzellen bestrahlen würde (ELKIND u. Mitarb., 1961). Weil Mikrokolonien im 3—4 Zellstadium eine Gewähr dafür bieten, daß die ausgesäten Zellen asynchron in „log"-Phase wachsen, wird von manchen Untersuchern erst am Tag nach dem Platieren bestrahlt und die Dosiseffektkurve nachträglich korrigiert (s. S. 105). In einem solchen Fall besteht aber keine Möglichkeit mehr, die Form der Dosiswirkungskurve im Schulterbereich zu bestimmen. Gerade der Verlauf der Reaktivität bei Dosen unter 300 R ist aber für die klinische Strahlentherapie bei den heute üblichen Fraktionierungsschemata von ausschlaggebender Bedeutung (s. S. 95).

Für verschiedene Dosiswerte werden in der Regel verschieden große Inokula genommen. In einem typischen Versuch, z.B. von PUCK u. Mitarb. (1957), wurden pro Petrischale für die Kontrollwerte 100 Zellen, für die Bestrahlung mit 100 R auch 100, für 274 R 2000, für 600 R 20000 und für 700 R 200000 Zellen platiert. Aus den verschiedenen Inokula entstanden jeweils 10—50 Kolonien, doch in Anwesenheit von wenigen oder Hunderttausenden von toten Zellen. Die nicht überlebenden Zellen können bei solchen Zellstämmen, die isoliert nur schlecht wachsen und eine niedrige Kolonieausbeute haben, einen Effekt wie „feeder“-Zellen haben (s. S. 47f.), d.h. die Überlebensrate heben. Auf der anderen Seite kann es auch vorkommen, daß die inaktivierten Zellen das Nährmedium verschlechtern, so daß mit zunehmender Strahlendosis und Inokulumgröße zu der direkten Strahlenwirkung noch ein indirekter, nutritiver Schaden kommt, der die Überlebensrate weiter senkt (BENDER u. GOOCH, 1962) — in solchen Fällen kann ein Mediumwechsel einige Tage nach der Bestrahlung von Nutzen sein (BERRY, 1964a). Von verschiedenen Autoren wurde berichtet, daß das bestrahlte Medium selbst eine wachstumshemmende Wirkung entfaltet. Meist waren Dosen von mehreren tausend rad notwendig (z.B. SZUMIEL u. Mitarb., 1971), doch wiesen SCOTT u. Mitarb. (1966) bei L-5178 Y-Zellen schon nach ca. 900 rad eine deutliche Wachstumshemmung nach.

Man sollte, wenn möglich, Erschütterungen der sich entwickelnden Kolonien vermeiden, u.U. kann es zur Versprengung von Zellen aus Kolonien kommen, die an anderer Stelle Satellitenkolonien bilden. So haben wir bei Zellen des chinesischen Hamsters (B-14) nicht selten eine Kolonienausbeute in unbestrahlten Kontrollen von weit über 100% erhalten, was auf Versprengung klonogener Zellen nach den ersten Teilungen zurückzuführen war.

Weitaus häufiger als eine zu hohe Kolonieausbeute ist allerdings eine niedrige „plating efficiency“. Neben der Gefahr, daß bei höheren Inokula ein „feeder“-Effekt die Ergebnisse verfälscht, ist dabei zu bedenken, daß nur die Strahlenreaktion einer Minorität untersucht wird, die nicht unbedingt repräsentativ und identisch mit der in Versuchen am gleichen Zellstamm mit hoher „plating efficiency“ festgestellten Strahlenempfindlichkeit sein muß (ELKIND und WHITMORE, 1967).

3. Dosiseffektkurven von Cytostatika

Mit der gleichen Methode lassen sich auch die Wirkungen anderer Agentien auf die reproduktive Integrität von Säugetierzellen testen. Besonderes Interesse beanspruchen naturgemäß die Cytostatika.

Die Gruppe der alkylierenden Cytostatika inaktiviert Säugetierzellen nach Dosiseffektkurven, die der für Röntgenstrahlen sehr ähnlich sind. Im halblogarithmischen Maßstab

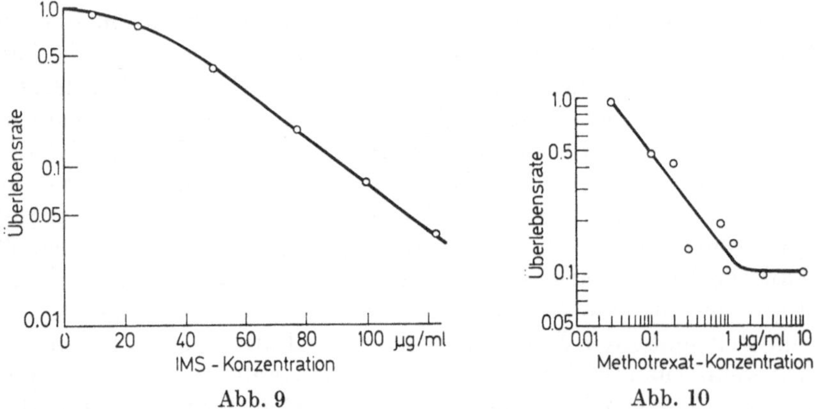

Abb. 9. Die Überlebensrate von HeLa-Zellen nach Behandlung mit verschiedenen Konzentrationen von Isopropylmethansulfonat (Halbwertszeit in Lösung 13 min). (PETROVIC und NIAS, 1967).

Abb. 10. Die Überlebensrate von HeLa-Zellen nach 24stündiger Exposition verschiedener Konzentrationen von Methotrexat. (Man beachte, daß auch die Abszisse im logarithmischen Maßstab aufgetragen ist!). (BERRY, 1968a)

aufgetragen, zeigen sie bei niedrigen Dosen eine Schulter mit endlicher Neigung, die bei zunehmender Dosis steiler wird und schließlich in eine exponentielle Inaktivierungskurve übergeht (Abb. 9). Wendet man den Formalismus von ALPER u. Mitarb. (1960) an, kann man sagen, daß die Dosiseffektkurve von Isopropylmethansulfonat auf HeLa-

Zellen eine D_0 von ca. 25 μg/ml und eine Extrapolationsnummer von 3 hat (Petrovic u. Nias, 1967). Auch Schwefel-Lost (Walker u. Thatcher, 1968; Mauro u. Madoc-Jones, 1970) und Uracil-Lost (Mauro u. Madoc-Jones, 1970) weisen ähnliche Dosiseffektkurven auf. Die Kurven von Berry (1964b) mit Stickstofflost (HN3) haben keine klassische Schulter, sondern eher eine echte Schwelle, während die von Lewis (1963) publizierte Kurve eine typische Schulter zeigt. Noch ausgeprägter ist die Schwellenfunktion bei Thio-TEPA (Berry, 1964b), wo bis zu einer Dosis von 0,3 μg/ml kein Effekt zu sehen war, bis dann die Überlebensrate mit einer D_0 von 1 μg/ml abnahm. Ähnliche Schwellen-Exponentialfunktionen veröffentlichte Berenbaum (1969) mit einer in-vivo-Methode für Anilin-Lost, Cyclophosphamid und Melphalan. Mit einer kombinierten in-vivo-in-vitro-Methode erhielten Brown u. Carbone (1971) an Knochenmarkszellen mit Cyclophosphamid sigmoide Dosiseffektkurven. Eine reine Exponentialfunktion trat nach Zugabe von Epodyl zu HeLa-Zellen auf (Berry, 1964b). Auch bei einigen Versuchen mit Stickstoff-Lost wurden reine Exponentialfunktionen gefunden (Sakamoto u. Elkind, 1969; Mauro u. Madoc-Jones, 1970).

Tabelle 2. *Dosiseffektkurvenparameter (D_0 und Extrapolationsnummer n) für die kurzzeitige Einwirkung verschiedener Pharmaka auf HeLa-Zellen.* (Mod. nach Mauro u. Madoc-Jones, 1970)

Pharmakon	Expositionsdauer	D_0 (μg/ml)	n
Vinblastinsulfat	3 h	0,085	2,4
Vincristinsulfat	3 h	0,028	1,2
Colchizin	3 h	0,02	4,9
Stickstofflost	30 min	0,36	1,6
Senfgas	5 min	0,24	2,7
Uracillost	30 min	1,7	8,0
Actinomycin D	30 min	0,12	1,7
Cycloheximid	3 h	200	2,1
Puromycin	3 h	200	3,1
Hydroxylamin	1 h	110	6,4

Zusammenfassend läßt sich sagen, daß die reproduktive Integrität von Säugetierzellen durch alkylierende Cytostatika nach gleichen oder ähnlichen Dosiseffektkurven zerstört wird wie durch Bestrahlung. Eine bemerkenswerte Ausnahme macht das Degranol, das eine hyperbole Dosiswirkungsbeziehung aufweist (Berry, 1964b), wie sie sonst für Antimetabolite typisch ist (Berenbaum, 1969; Brown u. Carbone, 1971), wie z.B. die von Methotrexat auf HeLa-Zellen (Abb. 10; Berry, 1968a). Die Dosiseffektkurve von Fluorouracil weist den gleichen Typ auf wie die von alkylierenden Cytostatika, wobei jedoch große Empfindlichkeitsunterschiede in den verschiedenen Proliferationsphasen bestehen (Berry, 1964b). Die Kurve von Zellen, die in log-Phase behandelt wurden, ist dreimal steiler als von in Plateauphase behandelten Zellen (Madoc-Jones u. Bruce, 1967). Ähnliche Einflüsse des Proliferationszustandes von Knochenmarkstammzellen auf die Wirkung von alkylierenden Cytostatika fanden van Putten und Lelieveld (1970, 1971).

Mauro u. Madoc-Jones (1970) untersuchten eine Reihe von alkylierenden Cytostatika, Mitosegiften, Mutagenen und Stoffwechselblockern auf die Koloniebildungsfähigkeit von HeLa-Zellen und fanden in allen Fällen (bis auf Hydroxyharnstoff, der bei kurzfristiger Gabe nur Zellen in S-Phase abtötet [Sinclair, 1965; Whitmore u. Mitarb., 1969]), eine typische Dosiseffektkurve wie nach Bestrahlung. Die Ergebnisse sind in Tabelle 2 zusammengefaßt.

Ähnlichkeiten der Dosiswirkungskurven von ionisierenden Strahlen und Chemikalien sind ein Anlaß, Interpretationen der Strahlenwirkung, die sich allzusehr auf hypothetische Mechanismen der Strahlenwirkung bei Mehrtreffer- oder Mehrbereichskurven stützen, die aber bei der Einwirkung von Chemikalien nicht in Frage kommen, kritisch zu beurteilen.

III. Dosiseffektkurven in vivo

Die von Puck und Mitarbeitern 1956 entwickelte Kolonietestmethode ist technisch relativ einfach und erlaubt die Bestimmung der Überlebensrate nach Einwirkung chemischer und physikalischer Agentien über mehrere Dekaden hin mit einer erstaunlichen experimentellen Genauigkeit. Sie konnte für praktisch alle den Strahlentherapeuten interessierenden Zellarten des Menschen angewendet werden. Sie hat der experimentellen Strahlentherapie erst die quantitative Basis gegeben.

Man muß sich jedoch auch ihre Voraussetzungen und Einschränkungen klar machen. Untersucht wird die Fähigkeit einer Zelle, innerhalb einer bestimmten Zeit eine Kolonie von mehr als 30—150 Zellen zu bilden. Das beinhaltet, daß funktionelle Änderungen im weitesten Sinn nicht erfaßt werden, und nur proliferierende oder leicht zur Proliferation anzuregende Zellarten untersucht werden können. Insbesondere beschreibt die Methode nur die Reaktion von Einzelzellen, nicht des organisierten Gewebes. Es konnte jedoch gezeigt werden, daß viele Zellarten in vivo auf Bestrahlung als Einzelzellen reagieren, und ihr Proliferationsverhalten nach Bestrahlung mit der Kategorie der Koloniebildung beschrieben werden kann. In den letzten Jahren sind verschiedene in-vivo-Methoden für normale und maligne Gewebe entwickelt worden, die auf der gleichen theoretischen Basis wie die Pucksche in-vitro-Methode beruhen. Normale Gewebe, an denen solche Untersuchungen durchgeführt wurden, sind

1. die Haut, 2. die Dünndarmschleimhaut, 3. der Knorpel, 4. die Melanozyten der Haarbälge, 5. das Knochenmark.

Da diese Gewebe für den Strahlentherapeuten von besonderem Interesse sind, werden die einzelnen Testsysteme und die Dosiswirkungsbeziehungen auf Bestrahlung hier beschrieben. Auf die Wirkung modifizierender Faktoren wird in den entsprechenden Kapiteln eingegangen.

1. Haut

Die Haut ist ein Mausergewebe. Im stratum basale werden dauernd Zellen gebildet, die die anderen Schichten des Epithels durchwandern und schließlich abgestoßen werden. Die ulzerierende Wirkung hoher Strahlendosen kann u.a. auf die Zerstörung der Teilungsfähigkeit der Basalzellen zurückgeführt werden.

Wenn in einem Hautareal alle Zellen bis auf wenige ihre Proliferationsfähigkeit eingebüßt haben, tritt ein Epitheldefekt auf, in dem die Regeneration von einzelnen überlebenden Zellen in Form von Kolonien sichtbar wird.

Bei Mäusen werden die Haare am Rücken in einem Gebiet von ca. 3 cm Durchmesser ausgezupft. Am nächsten Tag wird eine Fläche von ca. 25 mm Durchmesser mit der Testdosis (1 000—3 000 rad) bestrahlt. Anschließend wird das gleiche Gebiet unter Aussparung der 0,1—285 mm² großen Testareale mit Deuteronen auf 3 000 rad aufgesättigt. Nach etwa 7 Tagen beginnt eine schwere Hautreaktion, die in 15 Tagen bis zur kompletten Ulzeration fortschreitet. Nach 18 Tagen sind in der Regel in dem ulzerierten Gebiet Regenerationsknötchen sichtbar (Abb. 11a). Emery u. Mitarb. (1970) stellten fest, daß eine einzelne überlebende Zelle die Regeneration im Sinne einer klonalen Proliferation bewerkstelligen kann. Das bedeutet, daß in den Testarealen, in denen ein Regenerationsknötchen sichtbar ist, eine oder mehrere Zellen (nach einer Poissonfunktion verteilt) die Bestrahlung überlebt haben. Die Zahl der überlebenden Zellen läßt sich als Funktion der Dosis darstellen (Abb. 11b). Die D_0 dieser Kurven liegt bei 135 rad (Withers, 1967a; Emery u. Mitarb., 1970). Die Schulter dieser Kurve läßt sich direkt nicht bestimmen, weil die Zahl potentiell zur Koloniebildung befähigter (klonogener) Zellen pro mm² Haut nicht bekannt ist. Wenn man den in Fraktionierungsexperimenten gewonnenen Wert $D_2 - D_1$ (s. S. 19) gleich der D_q setzt, ergeben sich Extrapolationsnummern, die höher sind als bei den mei-

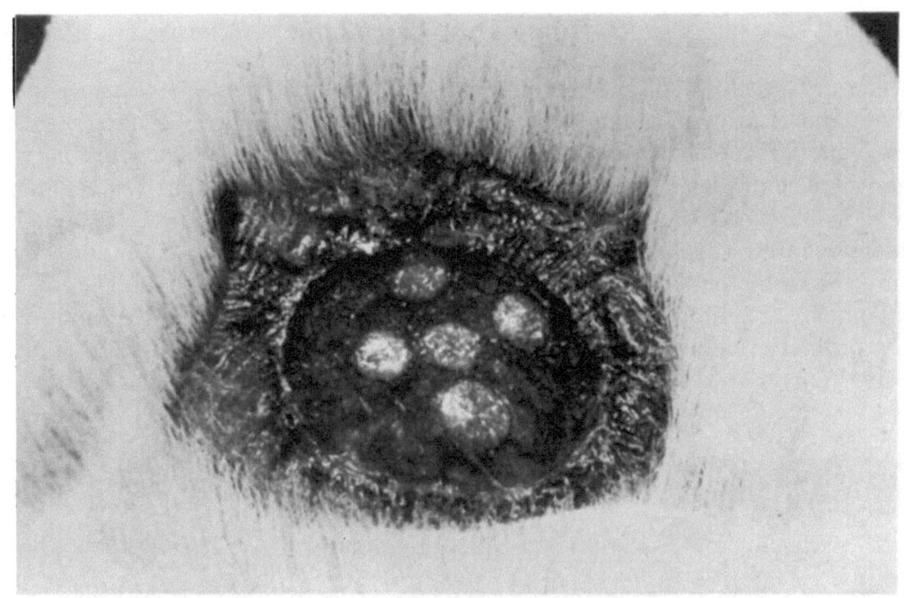

a

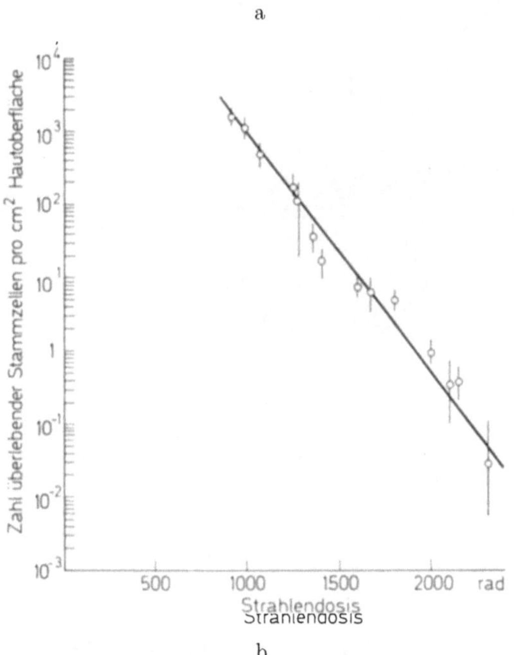

b

Abb. 11a. 5 Regenerationsknötchen (Kolonien) in der ulcerierten Mäusehaut nach Bestrahlung mit der Methode von WITHERS u. Mitarb. (1970). (Freundlicherweise zur Verfügung gestellt von J. DENEKAMP, London)

b. Die Überlebensrate klonogener Hautzellen der Maus nach Bestrahlung mit 150 kV-Röntgenstrahlen. (WITHERS, 1967a)

sten in vivo untersuchten Zellarten: $((D_2 - D_1) = 375$ rad, entspr. n = 16 (WITHERS, 1967b) bzw. $(D_2 - D_1) = 570$ rad, enstpr. n > 60 [EMERY u. Mitarb., 1970]).

LANGE (1970b) berechnete aus den Daten von WITHERS (1967b) eine um den Beitrag der Repopulation korrigierte Extrapolationsnummer von 6.6.

Entsprechend diesen Dosiswirkungskurven müßten nach Bestrahlung 10—20 überlebende Zellen pro cm² Haut in der Lage sein, eine komplette Ulzerierung zu verhindern (unter Nichtbeachtung der subkutanen Veränderungen), indem sie durch Proliferation in 10 Tagen diese Fläche mit funktionsfähigen Zellen bevölkern (WITHERS, 1967a).

2. Dünndarmschleimhaut

WITHERS u. ELKIND (1968) haben eine auf den gleichen Prinzipien basierende Methode beschrieben, die Strahlenwirkung auf die Proliferationsfähigkeit klonogener Kryptenzellen des Dünndarmepithels der Maus zu studieren. Eine Dünndarmschlinge wird eventeriert, und durch eine Dosis von 3000 rad distal und proximal wird ein Testsegment von ca. 2 cm Länge isoliert, das dann mit 1500—2200 rad bestrahlt wird. Nach Reposition wird die Darmschlinge 13 Tage später reseziert. Nach Eröffnung und Reinigung sieht man, eingerahmt von Gebieten totaler Ulzeration auf dem 2 cm langen Darmabschnitt eine mit der Strahlendosis abnehmende Zahl von Regenerationsknötchen, die Kolonien überlebender, aktiv proliferierender Schleimhautepithelzellen entsprechen (Abb. 12a). Bei Dosen dieser Höhe kann man davon ausgehen, daß jede Kolonie eine einzige überlebende klo-

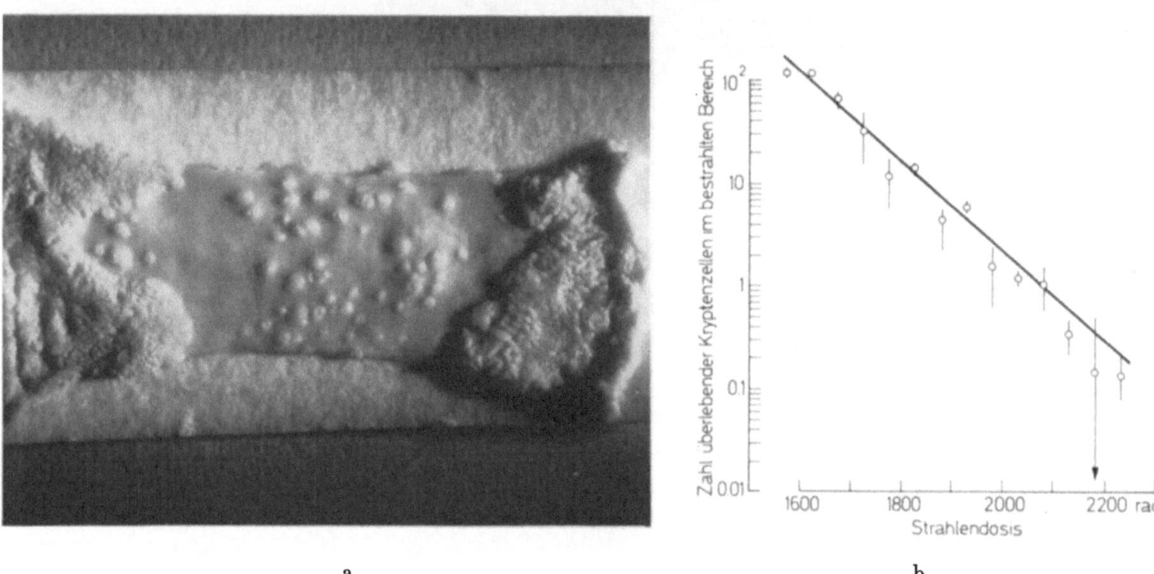

a   b

Abb. 12a. Regenerationsknötchen (Kolonien) in der ulzerierten Darmschleimhaut einer Maus nach Bestrahlung mit der Methode von WITHERS und ELKIND. (Freundlicherweise zur Verfügung gestellt von Dr. H. R. Withers, Houston)

b. Die Überlebensrate von Kryptenzellen des Dünndarms der Maus nach Bestrahlung mit 200 kV-Röntgenstrahlen. (WITHERS und ELKIND, 1969)

nogene Zelle repräsentiert. Die Dosiswirkungsbeziehung (Abb. 12b) weist eine D_0 von 97 rad auf. Eine Abschätzung der Extrapolationsnummer aus Ergebnissen von Fraktionierungsversuchen führt zu Werten zwischen 35 und 160 (WITHERS u. ELKIND, 1969; LANGE, 1970b).

Um die Strahlenempfindlichkeit klonogener Stammzellen der Dünndarmkrypten auch im niedrigen Dosisbereich testen zu können, entwickelten WITHERS u. ELKIND (1970) eine Methode, die auf der mikroskopischen Auszählung regenerierender und degenerierender Krypten im histologischen Querschnitt einer Darmschlinge beruht. Die so gewonnenen Dosiswirkungskurven schließen an die mit der obigen Methode gewonnenen Kurven an und bestätigen im wesentlichen deren Werte ($D_0 = 109$ rad; n = 58).

Wenn man davon ausgeht, daß der „gastrointestinale Strahlentod" durch die Inaktivierung klonogener Dünndarmzellen bewirkt wird, kann man abschätzen, daß bei Mäusen eine Verminderung klonogener Zellen auf weniger als 10000 pro cm Darmlänge in 50% der Tiere tödlich ist (WITHERS u. ELKIND, 1969).

3. Knorpel

1965 beschrieb KEMBER eine Methode, die Strahlenwirkung auf klonogene Knorpelzellen wachsender Epiphysenplatten von Ratten zu studieren. 3—4 Wochen nach einer
Bestrahlung der Hinterbeine von 6 Wochen alten Ratten mit Dosen von 1 700—2 300 R
kann man in histologischen Schnitten der Epiphysenplatte Nester proliferierender Knor-

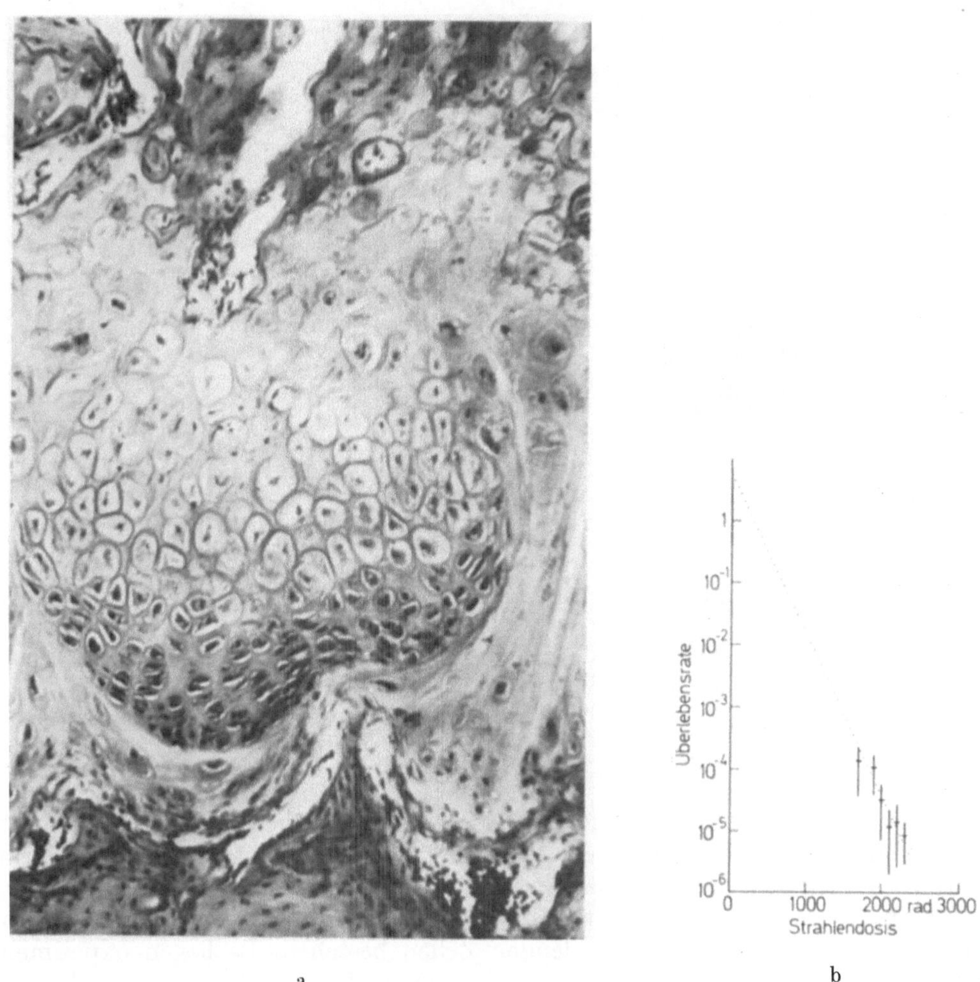

a   b

Abb. 13a. Regenerationsknötchen (Kolonie) im bestrahlten, wachsenden Epiphysenknorpel der Rattentibia.
(Freundlicherweise zur Verfügung gestellt von Dr. N. F. Kember, London)

b. Die Überlebensrate klonogener Knorpelzellen der wachsenden Rattentibia nach Bestrahlung mit 230 kV-
Röntgenstrahlen. (KEMBER, 1965)

pelzellen sehen (Abb. 13a), die aus einzelnen überlebenden Knorpelzellen hervorgegangen
sein könnten. Durch Bestimmung der Zahl der Knorpelzellnester in Serienschnitten konnte
KEMBER eine Dosiswirkungskurve aufstellen (Abb. 13b), die eine D_0 von 190 rad und eine
Extrapolationsnummer von 6 aufweist.

4. Haarbalg

Die Melanozyten in den Haarbälgen entstehen aus Stammzellen, deren reproduktive
Integrität durch Bestrahlung beeinträchtigt wird. POTTEN (1968, 1969) beschrieb eine
Methode, in der die Zahl der Melanozyten pro Haarbalg nach Bestrahlung als Kriterium

der Strahlenschädigung der Stammzellen genommen wird. Nach Auszupfen der Haare wurden Mäuse im Anagen- oder Telogenstadium des Haarwachstums mit Dosen von 250—1 200 rad bestrahlt. In Quetschpräparaten von Follikeln des darauf folgenden Haarzyklus wurde der Prozentsatz der Follikel gezählt, der mehr als 10 Melanozyten enthielt (Abb. 14a). Die dermaßen gewonnenen Dosiswirkungskurven (Abb. 14a) können durch eine D_0 von 180—220 rad und eine Extrapolationsnummer von etwa 6 beschrieben werden.

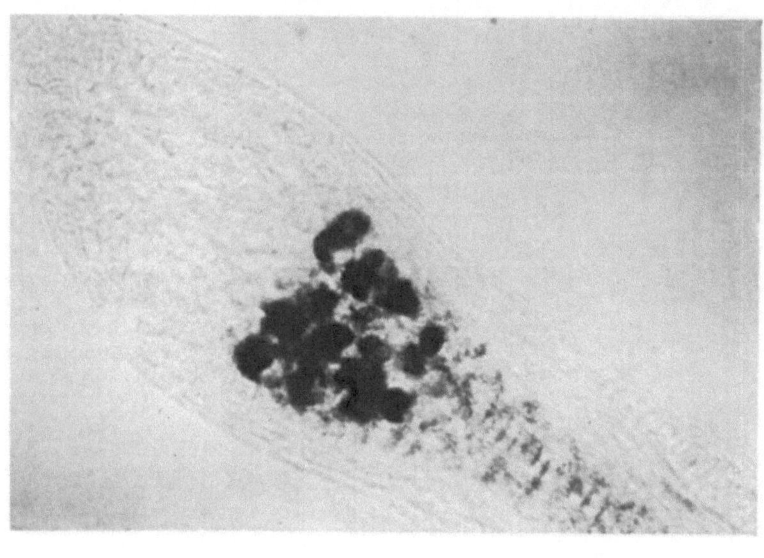
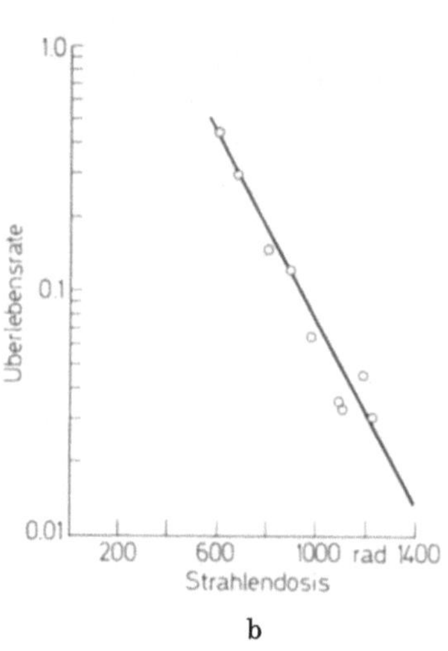

a

b

Abb. 14a. Ein Haarbalg mit einer Melanozytenkolonie von 24 Zellen. (Freundlicherweise zur Verfügung gestellt von Dr. C. S. Potten, Manchester)
b. Die Überlebensrate der melanoblastischen Stammzellen der Haarbälge von Mäusen nach Bestrahlung mit 300 kV-Röntgenstrahlen. (Potten, 1968)

5. Knochenmark

Die älteste in-vivo-Testmethode für normale Zellen ist die von Till u. McCulloch (1961) veröffentlichte Milzkolonietechnik. Sie besteht in der quantitativen Transplantation von Knochenmarkszellen in mit letaler Ganzkörperdosis bestrahlte Mäuse. Die Regeneration der Hämopoese zeigt sich in der Milz in Form von mit bloßem Auge erkennbaren Knötchen (Abb. 15a), die aus blutbildenden Zellen bestehen. Es liegen experimentelle Belege für die Annahme vor, daß jede Kolonie aus einer einzigen klonogenen Zelle entsteht (Becker u. Mitarb., 1963), die mit einem Anteil von etwa 0,01 % unter den Knochenmarkszellen vertreten ist, und die unter besonderen Bedingungen auch in vitro zu Kolonien auswachsen kann (Wu u. Mitarb., 1968; Dicke u. Mitarb., 1971). Die Testmethode besteht in der Präparation einer Suspension von hämopoetischen Zellen aus der Tibia, der Milz oder der foetalen Leber, die intravenös in mit 900—1000 rad vorbestrahlte Empfängertiere injiziert wird. 10 Tage später können in der fixierten Milz die Kolonien, von denen jede etwa 1 Million Zellen enthält, gezählt und als Funktion der Dosis aufgetragen werden. Die von Till u. McCulloch (1961) publizierte Dosiswirkungskurve (Abb. 15b) ist durch eine D_0 von 105 rad und eine Extrapolationsnummer von 2,5 charakterisiert. Aus dieser Dosiswirkungskurve ist zu schließen, daß die mittlere Letaldosis für Mäuse von ca. 700 rad die Zahl von Knochenmarkstammzellen auf weniger als 1% reduziert. Geringere Verluste vermag der Körper noch vor Auftreten allzu schwerer Symptome durch Proliferation der Stammzellen zu kompensieren.

Mit der gleichen Methode lassen sich auch Leukämiezellen in vivo untersuchen (z. B. Bush u. Bruce, 1965).

Die beschriebenen in-vivo-Testmethoden ermöglichen die Untersuchung der reproduktiven Integrität von normalen Körperzellen mit dem gleichen Kriterium, das auch bei der von PUCK entwickelten in-vitro-Methode verwendet wird: der Entwicklung einer Kolonie mit einer Mindestzellzahl innerhalb einer bestimmten Zeit. Auch die Strahlenempfindlichkeit für all diese Zellen in vivo (Tabelle 3) ist praktisch die gleiche wie von denen, die in Zellkultur untersucht wurden.

Das Konzept der Inaktivierung klonogener (Stamm-) Zellen stellt eine brauchbare Basis für die Erklärung mancher Strahlenschäden dar.

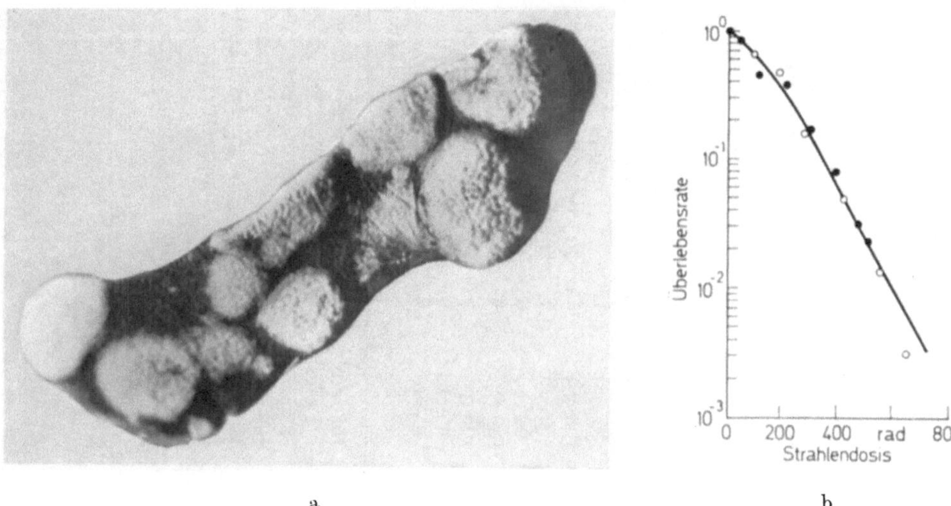

a   b

Abb. 15a. Regenerationsknötchen (Kolonien) in der Milz einer mit 800 rad Ganzkörperdosis bestrahlten Maus 10 Tage nach intravenöser Injektion von 300000 Knochenmarkszellen einer gesunden Maus (eigenes Präparat)

b. Die Überlebensrate von Knochenmarkstammzellen nach Bestrahlung mit ⁶⁰Co-Gammastrahlen und Injektion in letal bestrahlte Mäuse (Werte von 2 Experimenten). (TILL u. McCULLOCH, 1961)

6. Dosiseffektkurven maligner Zellen in vivo

1958 entwickelte HEWITT eine Methode, die reproduktive Integrität von Tumorzellen in vivo mit Hilfe quantitativer Transplantation zu untersuchen.

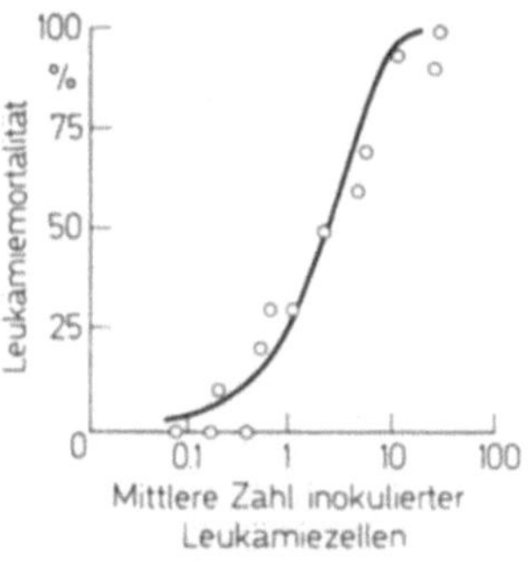

Abb. 16. Die Leukämiemortalität von CBA-Mäusen in Abhängigkeit von der mittleren Anzahl intraperitoneal injizierter Leukämiezellen. (HEWITT, 1958)

HEWITT (1958) isolierte eine in CBA-Mäusen vorkommende lymphozytäre Leukämie, die durch intraperitoneale Injektion einer einzigen Zelle überimpfbar war. Wenn auch bekannt ist, daß Mäuseleukämien durch Viren hervorgerufen werden können, scheint die Erkrankung in diesen Transplantationsversuchen von den übertragenen Leukämiezellen

Tabelle 3. *Dosiseffektkurvenparameter (D_0 und Extrapolationsnummer n) nach Bestrahlung normaler und maligner Mäusegewebe mit locker ionisierenden Strahlen und Testung in vivo*

Gewebe Zellart	Strahlenart	D_0	n	Autoren
Haut, Basalzellen der Epidermis	150 kV-Röntgenstrahlen	135 rad	16	Withers (1967)
	250 kV-Röntgenstrahlen	135 rad	60	Emery u. Mitarb. (1970)
Dünndarm, Kryptenzellen	200 kV-Röntgenstrahlen	97 rad	160	Withers u. Elkind (1968)
	200 kV-Röntgenstrahlen	109 rad	58	Withers u. Elkind (1970)
	1,5 MeV-Elektronen	160 rad	?	Hornsey (1970)
wachsende Epiphyse, Knorpelzellen	230 kV-Röntgenstrahlen	190 rad	6	Kember (1965)
Haar, Melanoblasten des Haarbalgs	300 kV-Röntgenstrahlen	180 rad	6	Potten (1969)
Knochenmark, Stammzellen	^{60}Co-Gammastrahlen	105 rad	2,5	Till u. McCulloch (1961)
	300 kV-Röntgenstrahlen	96 rad	2	Phillips (1968)
	^{137}Cs-Gammastrahlen	85 rad	3,1	Hendry u. Howard (1971)
	300 kV-Röntgenstrahlen	72 rad	2,47	Broerse u. Mitarb. (1971)
Leukämien: CBA-lymphozytäre Leukämie	^{60}Co-Gammastrahlen	162 rad	2	Hewitt u. Wilson (1959)
P-388	3 MeV-Röntgenstrahlen	160 rad	1,6	Berry u. Andrews (1961)
AKR/J-Lymphom	^{60}Co-Gammastrahlen	133 rad	1,9	Bush u. Bruce (1965)
Ehrlich-Aszites-Tumoren, diploid	200 kV-Röntgenstrahlen	109 rad	2,4	Silini u. Hornsey (1962)
tetraploid	200 kV-Röntgenstrahlen	114 rad	10	Hornsey u. Silini (1961)
verschiedene Tumoren von Abb. 19 (ausgezogene Linie)		160 rad	2	Berry (1971a)

und nicht von eventuell mitübertragenen Viren ihren Ausgang zu nehmen, wie ausführlich von ELKIND u. WHITMORE (1967) diskutiert wurde. In Abb. 16 wird die Beziehung zwischen Leukämiemortalität und der Zahl transplantierter, morphologisch intakter Leukämiezellen dargestellt. Die Transplantation von 2 Zellen ruft in 50 % der Empfänger eine Leukämie hervor (die Tumordosis 50 % [TD 50] ist 2).

Zur Bestimmung einer Dosiseffektkurve (HEWITT u. WILSON, 1959) wurden aus den infiltrierten Lebern leukämischer, bestrahlter Spendertiere Einzelzellsuspensionen gewonnen, die Konzentration morphologisch intakter Tumorzellen bestimmt und Serienverdünnungen hergestellt. Verschiedene Verdünnungen wurden je 6—10 Empfängertieren i.p. injiziert und das Auftreten von Leukämie abgewartet. Aus dem Ergebnis dieser Beobach-

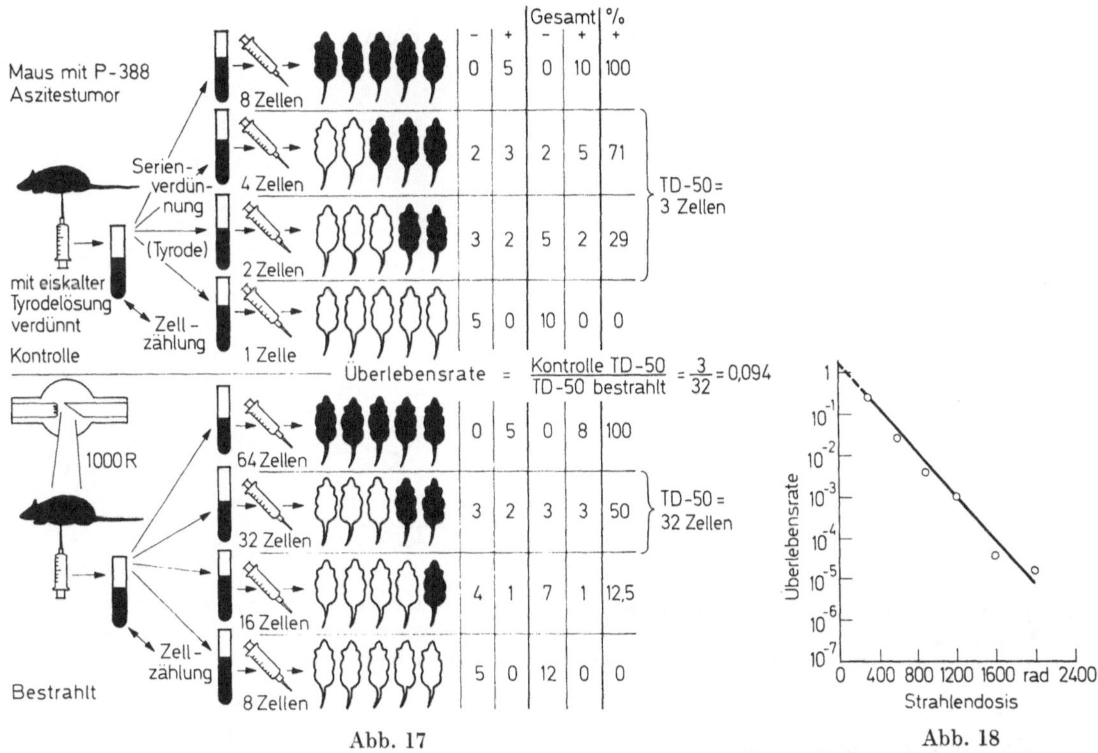

Abb. 17

Abb. 18

Abb. 17. Schematische Darstellung der HEWITTschen Tumortransplantationsmethode zur Bestimmung der Überlebensrate von Tumorzellen in vivo nach der Modifikation von BERRY für die als Aszitestumor wachsende P-388-Leukämie. (BERRY, 1971a)

Abb. 18. Die Überlebensrate von CBA-Leukämiezellen nach Bestrahlung in vivo und Transplantation in unbestrahlte Empfängertiere. (HEWITT u. WILSON, 1959)

tung wurde die Zellzahl berechnet, die in 50 % der Empfänger die Krankheit auslösen kann (TD $50_{\text{bestr.}}$). Die Überlebenskurve der Leukämiezellen läßt sich aufstellen, wenn man die Überlebensrate nach der Gleichung:

$$\text{Überlebensrate} = \frac{\text{TD 50 von Kontrollzellen}}{\text{TD 50 von bestrahlten Zellen}}$$

berechnet (s. Abb. 17). Die von HEWITT u. WILSON (1959) veröffentlichte Kurve ist in Abb. 18 wiedergeben. Sie läßt sich durch eine D_0 von 162 rad und eine Extrapolationsnummer von 2 beschreiben. Besonders bemerkenswert ist, daß mit dieser Methode noch das Überleben einer einzigen Zelle unter 1 Million abgetöteter Zellen exakt zu erfassen ist.

Wenn das Überleben einer einzigen Zelle in Gegenwart einer so großen Überzahl von reproduktiv toten Zellen getestet werden soll, stellt sich dringend die Frage, wie die inaktivierten Zellen die Vermehrung der einzelnen Zellen beeinflussen. Neben nutritiven Problemen besteht die Möglichkeit der Provokation einer immunologischen Reaktion. Dieses Problem wurde eingehend von Scott (1958, 1961) diskutiert. Andererseits wurde von Seelig u. Révész (1960) eine dem „feeder"-Effekt vergleichbare Wachstumsförderung im Ehrlich-Aszites-Tumor beobachtet.

Zusammenfassend kann gesagt werden, daß bei dem von Hewitt u. Wilson (1959) entwickelten System weder nutritive noch immunologische Probleme auftreten. Das gleiche gilt auch für einen anderen Tumor, der von Berry und Andrews (1961) als reiner Aszitestumor propagiert wurde. Da ein Aszitestumor schnell hypoxisch wird, kann man normalerweise nur die Strahlenwirkung auf hypoxische Zellen (s. S. 105) erfassen. Wenn man jedoch für eine gute Sauerstoffversorgung während der Bestrahlung (z.B. durch intraperitoneale Injektion einer geringen Menge von H_2O_2) sorgt, erhält man eine mit der von Hewitt u. Wilson (1959) gut übereinstimmende Kurve.

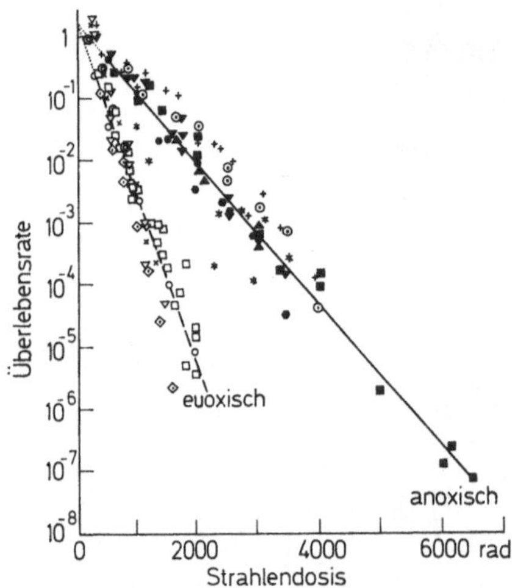

Abb. 19. Die Überlebensrate verschiedener Mäusetumorzellen nach Bestrahlung unter euoxischen und hypoxischen Bedingungen. Eine Zusammenstellung verschiedener, von Berry, Hewitt, Hornsey u. van Putten mit der Tumortransplantationsmethode gewonnener Werte. (Berry, 1971a)

Da als Aszitestumor wachsende Lymphomzellen auch mit der Milzkolonietechnik untersucht werden können, bieten sie sich zu vergleichenden Untersuchungen an. Die mit der Milzkolonietechnik gefundene Dosiseffektkurve ist deutlich steiler ($D_0 = 114$ rad) als die mit der Hewittschen Transplantationsmethode gefundene ($D_0 = 133$ rad), (Bush u. Bruce, 1965).

Auch der Ehrlich-Aszites-Tumor kann unter geeigneten Voraussetzungen durch eine einzige Zelle transplantiert werden. Silini u. Hornsey (1961) fanden, daß bei neugeborenen Mäusen eine einzige Zelle zur erfolgreichen Transplantation genügt, daß aber schon am 2. Tage die TD 50 auf 6 und nach 4 Tagen bereits auf 100 gestiegen ist. Das läßt vermuten, daß sich schnell eine starke Immunreaktion entwickelt. Dennoch lassen sich bei Verwendung von 2 Tagen alten Empfängertieren gute Dosiswirkungskurven gewinnen. Hornsey u. Silini (1961) fanden eine D_0 von 114 rad und eine Extrapolationsnummer von 10—15 bei in vitro-Bestrahlung (und in vivo-Testung) von hypertetraploiden Ehrlich-Aszites-Tumor-Zellen und Silini u. Hornsey (1962) eine D_0 von 109 rad und eine Extrapolationsnummer von 2,4 beim hyperdiploiden Ehrlich-Aszites-Tumor. Scott (1961) erhielt bei Transplantation bestrahlter Ehrlich-Aszites-Tumor-Zellen in ältere Empfängertiere eine Dosiseffektkurve, die mit zunehmender Strahlendosis (und zunehmender Größe des Inokulums) immer steiler wurde (s. S. 53f.), wohl Ausdruck einer Immunreaktion gegen diesen Tumor.

Bei diesem Tumor konnten auch Dosiseffektkurven vom gleichen bestrahlten Zellmaterial in vitro (durch Koloniebildung) und in vivo (durch die Tumorangehrate) bestimmt werden: sie waren praktisch gleich (CULLEN u. HORNSEY, 1966).

In den letzten Jahren wurden auch quantitative Transplantationen solider Tumoren durchgeführt. Dabei liegt in der Regel die TD 50 unbestrahlt deutlich höher. Dennoch konnten auch hier Werte für die Strahlenempfindlichkeit der Einzelzellen bestimmt werden, die im Bereich der in vitro gewonnenen Werte liegen. Eine Zusammenstellung verschiedener Dosiseffektkurven von Mäusetumoren in vivo wurde von BERRY (1971a) veröffentlicht (Abb. 19).

IV. Störungen der Zellvermehrung nach Bestrahlung

1. Die Mitoseverzögerung nach Bestrahlung

Die modernen Techniken der Zellkultur haben es ermöglicht, die Frage der Mitoseverzögerung über die von LASNITZKI erhobenen Befunde (s. S. 46f.) hinaus quantitativ weiter zu studieren, wobei 2 Fragestellungen im Vordergrund standen:

1. Die Dosiswirkungsbeziehung für verschiedene Zellarten und die Abhängigkeit der Mitoseverzögerung vom Zellzyklus.

2. Die Beziehung zwischen Mitoseverzögerung und Verlust der reproduktiven Integrität sowie der Wirkungsmechanismus der Mitoseverzögerung.

Im folgenden sollen neben der eigentlichen Mitoseverzögerung (Verzögerung des Eintritts einer bestrahlten Zellpopulation in die erste Mitose) bzw. Teilungsverzögerung (Verzögerung der ersten Zellteilung einer bestrahlten Zellpopulation) auch reversible Blockierungen in der Progression der Zellen durch den ersten und zweiten Zellzyklus nach der Bestrahlung, insbesondere der Übergänge von einer Zyklusphase in die andere besprochen werden.

1. Der Abfall des Mitoseindex nach Bestrahlung ist völlig gleichartig wie bei primären Hühnerembryofibroblasten auch bei HeLa-Zellen beobachtet worden. Mit der Methode der markierten Mitosen konnten YAMADA u. PUCK (1961) zeigen, daß die Mitoseverzögerung durch eine Verlängerung der G_2-Phase zutande kommt.

Aus dem Verlauf der Wachstumskurven bestrahlter Populationen von chinesischen Hamster-Zellen (V-79) erschlossen ELKIND u. Mitarb. (1963) die Länge der Teilungsverzögerung nach Bestrahlung. Sie erhielten eine lineare Abhängigkeit von der Strahlendosis bis zu Dosen von 1000 rad mit einem Faktor von 0,5 min/rad. Bei L-Zellen beträgt nach WHITMORE (1967) der Faktor 2,4 min/rad, nach WHITFIELD u. RIXON (1959) 1,8 min/rad. TOLMACH fand bei HeLa-Zellen eine Mitoseverzögerung von 1 min/rad (TOLMACH, 1961). In Suspensionskultur wiesen Mäuse-Lymphomzellen (L-5178-Y) wie chinesische Hamsterzellen (CHO) eine gleiche lineare Abhängigkeit von der Strahlendosis (ca. 0,7 min/rad) auf, während HeLa-Zellen entsprechend ihrer längeren Verdoppelungszeit eine doppelt so lange Teilungsverzögerung nach Bestrahlung zeigten (WALTERS u. PETERSEN, 1968). Mitoseverzögerungen dieser Größenordnung wurden auch nach Bestrahlung maligner und normaler Gewebe in Mensch und Tier beobachtet, wobei eine gewisse Korrelation zwischen der mittleren Generationszeit und dem Außmaß der strahleninduzierten Mitoseverzögerung zu bestehen scheint (SEYDEL, 1967).

Der biphasische Verlauf der Kurve des Mitoseindex nach Bestrahlung mit dem über den Kontrollwert ansteigenden Gipfel der Mitoserate erklärt sich daraus, daß Zellen nicht in allen Zyklusphasen gleich stark gehemmt werden, so daß sich eine partielle Synchronisation ergibt. Gegen Ende des Zyklus bestrahlte Zellen werden länger blockiert als in G_1-Phase bestrahlte. Untersuchungen an synchronisierten Zellkulturen haben das im wesentlichen bestätigt. SINCLAIR (1968a) hat in einer Übersichtsarbeit die Abhängigkeit der Mitose- bzw. Teilungsverzögerung von der Zellzyklusphase tabellarisch dargestellt (Tabelle 4).

Tabelle 4. *Mitose- bzw. Teilungsverzögerung von Säugetierzellen in vitro nach Bestrahlung mit locker ionisierenden Strahlen in verschiedenen Zyklusphasen.* (Mod. nach Sinclair, 1968a)

| Zellstamm | Mitose- bzw. Teilungsverzögerung in min/rad nach Bestrahlung in | | | | | | Autoren |
	Mitose	frühe G_1	späte G_1	frühe S	späte S	G_2	
chinesischer Hamster CH 24			0,3	0,2	0,3	0,4	Dewey u. Mitarb. (1966)
chinesischer	0,5	0,44	0,3	0,51	0,71	0,4	Froese (1966)
Hamster V 79	0,3	0,12	0,24	0,31	0,42	0,28	Yu u. Sinclair (1967)
HeLa S-3	0,9		0,3	0,7	1,2	1,3	Terasima u. Tolmach (1963a)
		0,1	0,3	0,64	0,83	0,6	Froese (1966)
menschliche Nieren T			1,0	1,2—1,5		1,5	Bootsma (1967)
L-Zellen							
LP-59			0,5	1,2		1,3	Dewey u. Humphrey (1962)
L 60 T			0,47	0,8	2,3	2,3	Whitmore u. Mitarb. (1967)
LP-59			0,73	2,2		2,6	Thompson u. Suit (1967)

In allen untersuchten Zellstämmen zeigte sich eine Verstärkung der Mitose bzw. Teilungsverzögerung mit Fortschreiten der Zellen im Zellzyklus, wobei in manchen Fällen Zellen in G_2 (z.B. L-Zellen), in den meisten Fällen jedoch in der späten S-Phase (z.B. chinesischer Hamster) am empfindlichsten waren. In Suspensionskultur weisen chinesische Hamsterzellen keine Abhängigkeit der Teilungsverzögerung vom Zellzyklus auf (Walters u. Petersen, 1968).

Untersuchungen von Thompson u. Suit (1969) über die Teilungsverzögerung von L-Zellen (L-59) nach Bestrahlung in verschiedenen Zyklusphasen ergaben z. T. nichtlineare

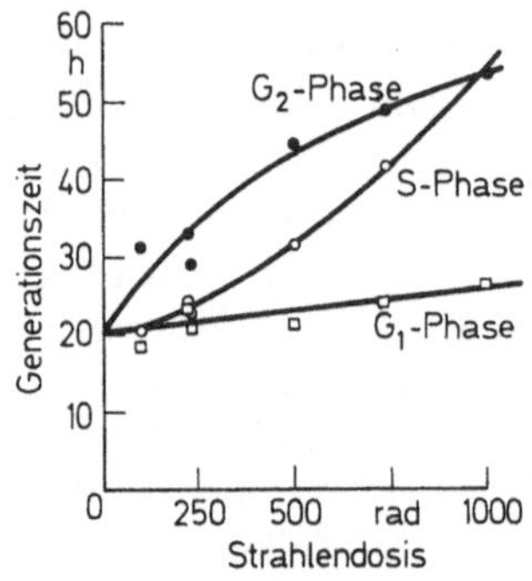

Abb. 20. Die Abhängigkeit des Medianwertes der Dauer der bestrahlten Generation von LP-59-Zellen von der Strahlendosis und der Zellzyklusphase zum Zeitpunkt der Bestrahlung. (Thompson u. Suit, 1969)

Abhängigkeiten von der Strahlendosis (Abb. 20). Auch die Mitoseverzögerung von chinesischen Hamsterzellen zeigte in den verschiedenen Zyklusphasen unterschiedliche Formen der Dosiswirkungsbeziehungen (Yu u. Siclair, 1967). Für asynchron wachsende Populationen wurden mit zunehmender Dosis flacher werdende Dosiswirkungskurven für Teilungs- und Mitoseverzögerung auch von Whitmore u. Mitarb. (1967) gefunden und dahingehend gedeutet, daß die weniger gehemmten Zellen der G_1-Phase bei höheren Strahlendosen die Zellen späterer Zyklusphasen überholen (wie das auch von Bootsma 1965 autoradiographisch nachgewiesen worden war), sich vor ihnen teilen und so die Form der Dosiswirkungskurve im höheren Dosisbereich bestimmen.

Für die verschiedenen Zellarten liegt das Ausmaß der Teilungsverzögerungen nach Bestrahlung relativ nahe beieinander und scheint von der normalen Generationszeit der

Zellen abzuhängen. Die Strahlendosis, die die mittlere Generationszeit von Säugetier-zellen um die Hälfte verlängert, liegt zwischen 300 und 600 rad (SINCLAIR, 1968a).

Am Zustandekommen der Teilungshemmung bei Dosen unter 1000 rad scheinen 3 Prozesse in den einzelnen Zellstämmen in unterschiedlichem Ausmaß beteiligt zu sein:

    a) eine Verlängerung der G_1-Phase,

    b) eine Verlängerung der S-Phase,

    c) ein temporärer Block in G_2.

    a) Bei L-Zellen wurde von MAK u. TILL (1963) nach Bestrahlung in G_1-Phase mit 580 rad eine Verzögerung der Progression von G_1 in S um 50 % beobachtet. Ebenso war bei chinesischen Hamsterzellen (CHO) nach Bestrahlung in G_1-Phase der Beginn der S-Phase (die selbst normale Länge aufwies) um ca. 100 Minuten verzögert (WALTERS u. TOBEY, 1970). Bei sehr langsam proliferierenden Zellen, wie z.B. Primärkulturen von menschlichen Amnionzellen, wird durch Bestrahlung in G_1-Phase der Beginn der DNS-Synthese schon durch eine Dosis von 50 R in der Hälfte aller Zellen tagelang blockiert (LITTLE, 1968, 1970). Ähnliche Effekte wurden bei Bestrahlung von zur Proliferation stimulierten Geweben in vivo beobachtet, jedoch nie in vergleichbarem Maße nach Bestrahlung der üblichen, schnell proliferierenden Zellen in Zellkultur.

    b) Eine deutliche Verlängerung der S-Phase bei gleichzeitiger Verminderung der Syntheseaktivität nach Bestrahlung in der S-Phase wurde von TERASIMA u. TOLMACH (1963) u. BRENT u. Mitarb. (1966) an HeLa-Zellen, von SINCLAIR (1967b) an chinesischen Hamsterzellen, von MAK u. TILL (1963) an L-Zellen, von LITTLE (1970) an Primärkulturen menschlicher Amnionzellen und von KIM u. EVANS (1964) an Ehrlich-Aszites-Tumorzellen in vivo gemessen. 750 rad verlängerten die S-Phase von chinesischen Hamsterzellen um etwa $2^1/_2$ Stunden. Bei HeLa-Zellen war die S-Phase schon nach 300 rad um 3 Stunden verlängert. Mit der Verlängerung der S-Phase ging jeweils eine Verminderung der DNS-Syntheserate einher, die bei L-Zellen besonders gegen Ende der S-Phase ausgeprägt war (HOLFORD, 1966). In allen Fällen wurde aber trotz reduzierter Syntheserate die normale Gesamtmenge an DNS synthetisiert (z.B. WATANABE u. OKADA, 1968). In der G_1-Phase bestrahlte Zellen durchlaufen die S-Phase so schnell wie unbestrahlte Zellen oder schneller. Die Verlängerung der S-Phase bei gleichzeitigem Eindringen weiterer Zellen aus G_1 führt dazu, daß in den ersten Stunden nach Bestrahlung von synchron wachsenden Populationen der Prozentsatz der Zellen in S-Phase beträchtlich, z.T. bis auf das Doppelte ansteigen kann (PAINTER u. ROBERTSON, 1959; KUYPER u. Mitarb., 1962).

    c) Durch in sehr kurzen Abständen vorgenommene Zellzählung in Suspensionskulturen stellten WALTERS u. PETERSEN (1968) fest, daß unabhängig von der Strahlendosis HeLa-Zellen noch 71 Minuten lang, chinesische Hamster-Zellen (CHO) noch 56 Minuten und Mäuselymphomzellen (L-5178 Y) noch 62 Minuten lang sich mit unverminderter Geschwindigkeit vermehrten und erst dann ein dosisabhängiger Block auftrat. Dieser Verlauf muß dahingehend gedeutet werden, daß nicht eine allgemeine, unspezifische Verlängerung der G_2-Phase durch Bestrahlung ausgelöst wird, sondern daß alle Zellen, die vor einem kritischen Punkt im Zellzyklus stehen, weiter wandern bis sie dort angelangt sind und für eine von der Dosis abhängige Zeitspanne aufgehalten werden. Zellen, die zum Zeitpunkt der Bestrahlung diesen Punkt schon passiert haben, beginnen unverzögert mit der Mitose. PUCK u. STEFFEN (1963) lokalisierten diesen Punkt in die Mitte von G_2 und konnten zeigen, daß schon 9 R in der Lage waren, eine meßbare Verlängerung von G_2 zu bewirken.

    Bei Ehrlich-Aszites-Tumorzellen in vivo scheint der Block fast am Ende der G_2-Phase zu liegen (KIM u. EVANS, 1964). Menschliche Nierenzellen in vitro erleiden ihren G_2-Block zu einem Zeitpunkt, in dem die Zelle schon ihre RNS-Synthese in Vorbereitung auf die Mitose eingestellt hat (SCAIFE u. BROHÉE, 1969). CARLSON (1969) beobachtete unter dem Mikroskop, daß H-Ep-2-Zellen, die nach Bestrahlung bis in die späte Prophase gewandert waren, die Mitose normal beenden können, während sie aus der frühen Prophase wieder in die Interphase zurückkehren.

5*

Durch Kombination verschiedener Untersuchungstechniken konnten Doida u. Okada (1969) die blockierenden Wirkungen von ionisierenden Strahlen, Actinomycin D und Puromycin auf L-5178-Y-Zellen exakt auf verschiedene Abschnitte der G_2-Phase lokalisieren. Der Zeitpunkt des Strahlenblocks stimmte mit dem des Puromycinblocks überein; er scheint somit dem Zeitpunkt zu entsprechen, an dem die Zelle die Synthese der zur Zellteilung notwendigen Proteine vornimmt (Walters u. Petersen, 1968). Bacchetti u. Sinclair (1970) wiesen jedoch nach, daß nicht die Hemmung der Proteinsynthese an sich der Faktor ist, der die Mitosehemmung zu diesem Zeitpunkt bewirkt.

Kaufmann (1971) führte diesen Block auf eine strahleninduzierte Störung des Energiestoffwechsels, insbesondere des NAD-Umsatzes zurück.

Durch mehrmalige Bestrahlung mit 25 rad im Abstand von 3 Stunden läßt sich infolge wiederholter Verlängerung der G_2-Phase eine gewisse Synchronisation von L-Zellen in der G_2-Phase erreichen (Linden, 1970; Prévôt, 1971).

Dieser G_2-Block tritt für alle Zellen einer asynchronen Population, gleichgültig zu welchem Zeitpunkt sie bestrahlt werden, im gleichen Phasenpunkt auf. Bei manchen Zellstämmen dürfte auch seine Länge unabhängig vom Zeitpunkt der Bestrahlung sein (Walters u. Petersen, 1968). Dabei könnte der G_2-Block von in G_1-Phase bestrahlten Zellen durch eine Verkürzung der S-Phase (Sinclair, 1967b) soweit kompensiert worden sein, daß für G_1-Zellen eine geringere Mitoseverzögerung resultiert als für Zellen in G_2. Auf Zellen, die eine maximale Verzögerung bei Bestrahlung in G_2 zeigen (wie z.B. L-Zellen) ist diese Erklärung nicht anzuwenden, da eine Bestrahlung in S auf jeden Fall zusätzlich eine Verlängerung der S-Phase zur Folge hat.

2. Welche Beziehung besteht zwischen der strahleninduzierten Teilungsverzögerung und dem Verlust der Reproduktionsintegrität? Zwei Problme sind dabei von besonderem Interesse: a) Haben inaktivierte Zellen, die noch eine oder mehrere (abortive) Teilungen vollführen, die gleiche Teilungsverzögerung wie überlebende Zellen? b) Gibt es Hinweise darauf, daß Teilungsverzögerung und Inaktivierung verschiedene Manifestationen der gleichen primären Schädigung sind?

a) Elkind u. Mitarb. (1963) stellten fest, daß die Teilungshemmung der Zellen, die später zu Kolonien heranwachsen, genau so groß ist wie die der Zellen, die nach einer oder wenigen Teilungen die Proliferation einstellen. Revell (1971) beobachtete bestrahlte Geschwisterzellen unter dem Mikroskop und sah, daß die Verteilung der Generationszeiten in den Fällen, in denen eine der Zellen ihre klonogene Fähigkeit behalten, die andere sie aber verloren hat, für beide Geschwister gleich war. Thompson u. Suit (1967) fanden in Zeitrafferaufnahmen nach 736 rad bei L-Zellen zwar eine relative Verlängerung der mittleren Generationszeit von Zellen abortiver Kolonien in der auf die Bestrahlung folgenden Generation, aber keine signifikant stärkere Vezögerung der ersten Zellteilung nach Bestrahlung. Dagegen registrierten Froese u. Cormack (1968) und Cormack u. Froese (1971) nach Bestrahlung von chinesischen Hamsterzellen (V-79) in der frühen S-Phase eine längere Teilungsverzögerung bei inaktivierten Zellen gegenüber „überlebenden" Zellen.

Außerdem stellten Froese u. Cormack (1968) in Zeitraffer-Untersuchungen fest, daß die Generationszeit einer bestrahlten Zelle wesentlich länger war, wenn eine oder beide Tochterzellen zugrunde gingen, als wenn beide Töchter sich noch mindestens einmal teilten. Hurwitz u. Tolmach (1969a) beobachteten das gleiche Phänomen in verschiedenen Generationen von HeLa-Zellen nach Bestrahlung, Trott (1972) in der ersten Generation nach Bestrahlung von L-Zellen.

b) Die Unterschiede in der Zellzyklusabhängigkeit der Überlebensrate und der Mitoseverzögerung (Sinclair, 1969c) wie auch die Unterschiede der Schutzwirkung von Cysteamin gegenüber Mitoseverzögerung und Inaktivierung (Yu u. Sinclair, 1970) lassen es unwahrscheinlich erscheinen, daß für beide Effekte der gleiche primäre Schaden verantwortlich ist. Für die Mitoseverzögerung scheint die Schädigung der DNS keine große

Rolle zu spielen (SCAIFE, 1970). BACCHETTI u. SINCLAIR (1971) untersuchten den Einfluß verschiedener stoffwechselblockierender Substanzen auf Mitoseverzögerung und Inaktivierung nach Bestrahlung und beobachteten häufig direkt entgegengesetzte Wirkungen. Sie kamen zu dem Schluß, daß „Bedingungen, die für die Zellteilung optimal sind, am ungünstigsten für die Erholung vom potentiell letalen Strahlenschaden" (s. S. 102f.) und damit für die Überlebensrate sind. So wurde z. B. durch eine zeitweilige Blockierung der Proteinsynthese durch Cycloheximid die Teilungshemmung verlängert und die Überlebensrate erhöht.

2. Der 2. Zellzyklus nach Bestrahlung

Der zweite Zellzyklus nach Bestrahlung von HeLa-Zellen mit 500 rad (d. h. die Generation nach der ersten Teilung) weist die gleiche mittlere Dauer auf wie der unbestrahlter Zellen (HURWITZ u. TOLMACH, 1969a). Die folgenden Generationen sind wieder stärker verlängert (Abb. 21). Während bei HeLa-Zellen dieser Ablauf keine Abhängigkeit von der Zyklusphase zum Zeitpunkt der Bestrahlung aufweist, ist bei L-Zellen (L-P 59) ein ähnliches Verhalten der medianen Generationszeit nur für Zellen nachzuweisen, die in den späten Zyklusphasen mit 500 rad bestrahlt worden sind. Bei in G_1-Phase bestrahlten Zellen, bei denen die Verzögerung der ersten Zellteilung relativ am geringsten ist (Abb. 20), ist eine deutlich stärkere Verlängerung des zweiten Zellzyklus nach Bestrahlung zu registrieren (THOMPSON u. SUIT, 1969; TROTT, 1969). Die Zyklusdauer späterer Generatio-

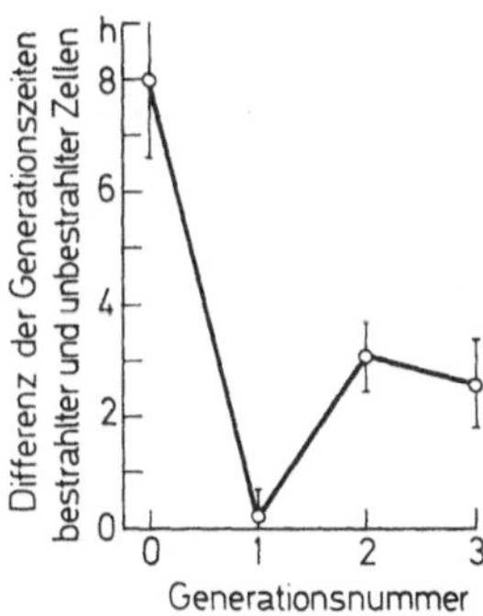

Abb. 21. Mittelwert der Generationszeitverlängerung mit 500 rad bestrahlter HeLa-Zellen bzw. ihrer Nachkommen in 4 aufeinander folgenden Generationen. (HURWITZ u. TOLMACH, 1969)

nen bestrahlter Zellen, die zu Kolonien auswachsen, ist nicht wesentlich verschieden von der unbestrahlter Zellen, während die Generationszeiten in abortiven Klonen wesentlich verlängert sind (THOMPSON u. SUIT, 1969).

In der bestrahlten Generation war nur dann eine deutliche Reduktion in der DNS-Syntheserate zu beobachten, wenn in der S-Phase bestrahlt wurde. In der folgenden Generation von HeLa-Zellen trat in jedem Fall eine Verminderung der DNS-Syntheserate ein unabhängig von der Zyklusphase zum Zeitpunkt der Bestrahlung (BRENT u. Mitarb., 1966). Chinesische Hamsterzellen (DON) wiesen nach einer Dosis, die 90 % der Zellen inaktivierte, zusätzlich zu der Synthesevermindernung noch eine Verzögerung des Eintritts in die S-Phase des 2. Zyklus von ca. 3 h auf (DEWEY u. ROBINETTE, 1969). HOPWOOD u. TOLMACH (1971) stellten fest, daß in G_1-Phase bestrahlte HeLa-Zellen trotz normaler Dauer der G_1- und S-Phasen nur $^2/_3$ der normalen DNS-Menge synthetisierten. Die Gesamtmenge neugebildeter DNS war in den Zellen, die in der folgenden Mitose arretiert wurden, nur etwa ein Drittel der von sich normal teilenden Zellen synthetisierten DNS. HOPWOOD u. TOLMACH (1971) schlossen daraus, daß eine insuffiziente DNS-Synthese eng mit dem Zelltod in Mitose korreliert ist.

3. Die Koloniegrößenverteilung nach Bestrahlung

Schon in Kontrollkulturen sind nicht alle Kolonien gleich groß. Diese Variabilität ist unter den Überlebenden einer Bestrahlung noch vergrößert (Puck u. Marcus, 1956). „Unterschiede in der Größe der Kolonien können dadurch zustande kommen, daß 1. die Generationszeiten der Zellen eine gewisse Schwankungsbreite zeigen, 2. bei jeder Zellteilung ein gewisser Prozentsatz von Zellen entsteht, der sich nicht weiter teilt, 3. eine Korrelation der Generationszeiten zwischen Mutter und Tochterzellen oder zwischen Geschwisterzellen besteht" (Gilbert u. Nias, 1966). Die beobachteten Unterschiede in der Koloniegröße unbehandelter Zellen (Abb. 22) können weitgehend durch die Schwankungsbreite der Generationszeiten und eine gewisse Korrelation verwandter Zellen erklärt werden. Bei ungestörtem Koloniewachstum spielen spontane Zelluntergänge keine entscheidende Rolle für die Größenverteilung der Kolonien.

Sinclair (1964a) maß den Durchmesser von Kolonien chinesischer Hamsterzellen nach Bestrahlung und fand eine Verbreiterung der Verteilungskurve der Koloniedurch-

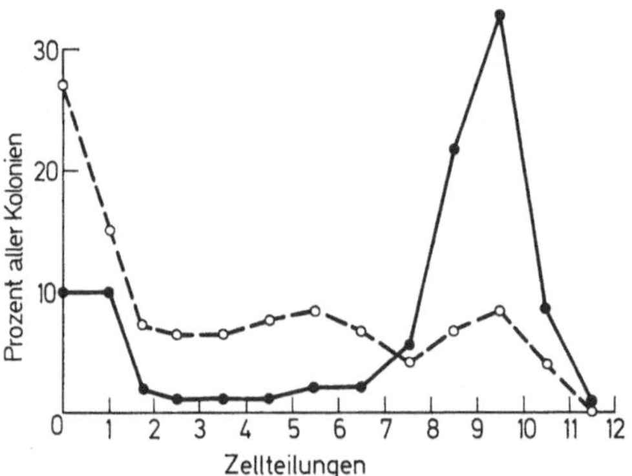

Abb. 22. Die Koloniegrößenverteilung von HeLa-Zellen nach 10 tägiger Inkubation
●————● unbestrahlt
○----------○ nach 300 rad Röntgenstrahlen

Die Koloniegröße ist im logarithmischen Maßstab (2^n) als Anzahl der Zellteilungen, die zu der gezählten Zellzahl geführt haben, angegeben: 0 Teilungen = 1 Zelle; 1 Teilung = 2 Zellen; 2 Teilungen = 3—4 Zellen; 3 Teilungen = 5—8 Zellen; 4 Teilungen = 9—16 Zellen usw. (Nias u. Mitarb. 1965)

messer zu kleineren Werten hin. Bei Dosen von 750 rad waren Kolonien aller Gößenklassen gleich häufig vertreten, bei Dosen über 1 000 rad überwog die Anzahl der kleineren Kolonien mit einem Durchmesser unter 1 mm. Nias u. Mitarb. (1965) zählten die Zellzahl in jeder Kolonie und fanden nach 300 rad bei HeLa-Zellen, daß die gleiche Zahl von Zellen während der Inkubationszeit Zellzahlen erreicht hatte, die 2, 3, 4, 5 usw. bis zu 10 Teilungen entsprechen (Abb. 22). Ähnliche Verteilungen der Koloniegröße hatten Colombo u. Marin (1963) 8 Tage nach Bestrahlung von Meerschweinchen-Nierenzellen mit 450 R gefunden.

In solchen Fällen wird das Kriterium einer bestimmten Mindestzellzahl als Nachweis der ungestörten reproduktiven Integrität fragwürdig. Dagegen machte Berry (1967c) geltend, daß dann, wenn die Zellen (HeLa S-3) vor der Bestrahlung schon platiert und angewachsen sind, die Koloniegrößenverteilung in seinen Experimenten nie die gleichmäßige Verteilung wie bei Nias u. Mitarb. (1965), die in Suspension bestrahlt hatten, aufwiesen. Die Form der Verteilungskurve wurde durch die Bestrahlung nicht prinzipiell verändert. Wenn in den Kontrollen eine eingipfelige Verteilung beobachtet wurde, blieb sie auch nach Bestrahlung mit 1 000 rad bei etwa gleicher Koloniegröße bestehen, ein Hinweis darauf, daß alle Zellen, die sich nicht geteilt hatten oder abortive Kolonien gebildet hatten, sich von der Oberfläche des Kulturgefäßes gelöst hatten.

Die Analyse der Koloniegrößenverteilung ist eine geeignete Methode, um Unterschiede in der Proliferationskinetik der Entwicklung von Kolonien nachzuweisen. Doch zeigte sich, daß nach unterschiedlichsten Behandlungen meist ähnliche Koloniegrößenverteilungen auftraten, wenn nur gleich effektive Dosen verglichen werden, so z.B. nach Isopropylmethansulfonat (Petrovic u. Nias, 1967), aber nicht nach Schwefel-Lost (Mauro u. Mitarb., 1967), nach Alpha-Strahlen (Westra u. Barendsen, 1966), Beta-Strahlen (Nias, 1968), nach Bestrahlung unter Stickstoff (Nias, 1968) und nach Erholung vom potentiell letalen Strahlenschaden (Petrovic u. Nias, 1966), ja sogar nach Hitzeeinwirkung (Westra, 1967) und anderen schädigenden Behandlungen.

Sinclair (1964a) untersuchte das Wachstumsverhalten sogenannter Mikrokolonien von chinesischen Hamsterzellen, d.h. von Kolonien, die nach Bestrahlung und 14tägiger Inkubation aus nur 40—200 Zellen bestanden. Bei fortgesetzter Beobachtung zeigte ein großer Teil dieser Kolonien über längere Zeit hin ein exponentielles Wachstum mit verlängerter Verdoppelungszeit. Diese Verlangsamung der Wachstumsrate war z.T. durch eine Verlängerung der Generationszeiten bedingt, aber auch dadurch, daß etwa 10 % aller Zellen in einer Mikrokolonie sich nicht mehr teilen konnten. Die Zellen dieser Kolonien wiesen eine wesentlich reduzierte Koloniebildungsrate und eine um ein Drittel erhöhte Strahlenempfindlichkeit auf (D_0 etwa 130 rad statt 200 rad in den Zellen der Makrokolonien). Westra u. Barendsen (1966) fanden das gleiche Phänomen bei menschlichen Nierenzellen (T-1) nach Röntgen- und Alpha-Bestrahlung, Todd (1968b) bei T-1-Zellen und einem anderen Stamm chinesischer Hamsterzellen (M 3-1) nach 750 rad Röntgenbestrahlung. Auch bei den Zellen aus den Mikrokolonien bestrahlter T-1-Zellen war die Strahlenempfindlichkeit um ein Drittel größer, und bei den aus bestrahlten M 3-1-Zellen isolierten langsam wachsenden Klonen war die D_0 um ein Drittel bis ein Viertel geringer als in den Kontrollen. In keinem Fall war die Schulter der Dosiseffektkurve wesentlich verändert.

Das anfänglich langsame Wachstum der meisten bestrahlten Zellen ist durch das gehäufte Auftreten steriler Zellen in den ersten Generationen überlebender Zellen nach Bestrahlung bedingt, das in späteren Generationen verschwindet (Miltenburger, 1969b). Aber auch in den Zellen, die nach mehrfachen Passagen ihre langsame Wachstumsgeschwindigkeit beibehalten hatten, nahm diese in der Regel nach längerer Kultivierung, meist nach mehreren Monaten, wieder normale Werte an (Todd, 1968b). Vereinzelt behielten jedoch die Zellen auch nach 4 Jahren ununterbrochener Subkultivation ihren Proliferationsdefekt bei (Stroud u. Resh, 1967).

Auch in Suspensionskulturen von L-5178-Y-Mäuselymphomzellen ist nach Strahlendosen von einigen hundert rad erst nach 8 Wochen wieder die alte Wachstumsgeschwindigkeit erreicht, indem die schnelleren Zellen die langsamer wachsenden überwuchert haben (Beer u. Mitarb., 1968).

Todd (1968b) maß in den aus Mikrokolonien isolierten Zellen einen verminderten Sauerstoffverbrauch. Die Suche nach Unterschieden in der Chromosomenzahl und -form zwischen langsamen und normalen Zellen verlief negativ (Sinclair, 1964a; Todd, 1968b).

In Mikrokolonien treten die verschiedensten degenerativen Zellformen, insbesondere Riesenzellen auf (Colombo u. Marin, 1963). Auch wenn sie häufig während der üblichen Inkubationsdauer die Zellzahl, die das Überlebenskriterium bildet, nicht erreichen, sind sie doch unbegrenzt, wenn auch langsamer proliferationsfähig. Johnson u. Mitarb. (1966) und Berry (1967a) wiesen darauf hin, daß auch in vivo die überlebenden Zellen sich z.T. wesentlich langsamer vermehren als unbestrahlte Zellen und damit ein Wachstumsverhalten wie in Mikrokolonien aufweisen. Ein langsam wachsendes Spätrezidiv eines bestrahlten Mammacarcinoms der C3H-Maus wurde von Suit (1966b) als Mikrokolonieäquivalent gedeutet. Es wies eine deutlich höhere Strahlenempfindlichkeit auf als der Originaltumor.

Mit zunehmender Strahlendosis wird also nicht nur die Zahl der reproduktiv intakten Zellen kleiner, sondern auch die Zahl der von diesen reproduktiv intakten Zellen gebildeten

Nachkommen. Daraus ergibt sich, daß dann, wenn man statt der Zahl klonogener Zellen die Gesamtzellzahl nach bestimmten Inkubations- bzw. Latenzzeiten als Endpunkt nimmt (was für manche Aspekte des Wachstumsverhaltens subletal bestrahlter Tumoren von Bedeutung ist, s. z.B. Thomlinson u. Craddock, 1967), Dosiswirkungskurven resultieren, die nicht in eine Gerade übergehen, sondern mit zunehmender Dosis immer steiler verlaufen (Fowler, 1966). Außerdem erscheint die Strahlenwirkung geringer, wenn 3—4 Tage nach der Bestrahlung die Wachstumshemmung gemessen wird, als wenn erst nach 9—10 Tagen aus der Wachstumshemmung der Strahleneffekt berechnet wird (Dewey u. Mitarb., 1963; Nias u. Fox, 1968).

4. Die direkte Beobachtung des Proliferationsmusters bestrahlter Zellen

Die direkte Beobachtung der Proliferation bestrahlter Zellen durch Zeitrafferkinematographie ist sehr aufwendig und daher nur in wenigen Laboratorien durchgeführt worden. Es wurden insbesondere folgende drei Problemkreise mit dieser Methode untersucht:

1. Wann sterben Zellen, die keine Kolonie mehr bilden können, ab? Wie viele Teilungen können sie noch durchführen? Worin äußert sich der Unterschied zwischen „überlebenden" und „inaktivierten" Zellen?

2. Lassen sich aus dem Proliferationsmuster Schlüsse auf einen Mechanismus der Zellinaktivierung durch Bestrahlung ziehen? Treten die einzelnen Teilungsversager zufällig oder in bestimmten Mustern auf?

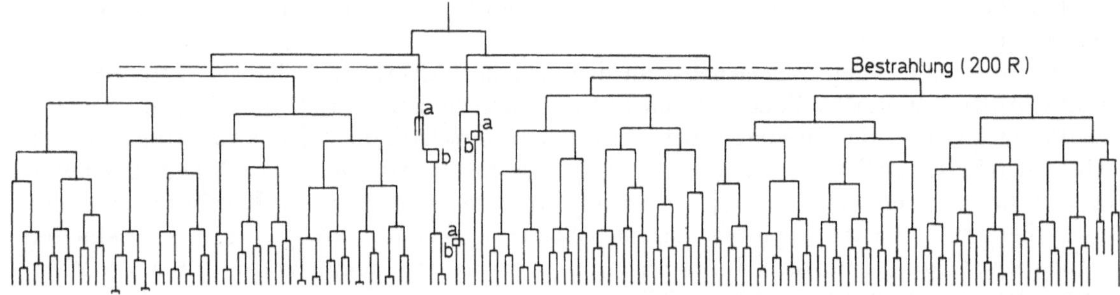

Abb. 23. Diagrammatische Darstellung der Zellvermehrung in Form eines Stammbaums vor und nach Bestrahlung von L-Zellen mit 200 R 45 kV-Röntgenstrahlen (Die Bestrahlung — gestrichelte horizontale Linie — erfolgte im 4-Zellen-Stadium). Die Länge der senkrechten Linien entspricht den Generationszeiten der Zellen. Unter den Nachkommen der 2 zu abortiven Kolonien führenden Zellen erkennt man 3 tripolare Teilungen (a) und 3 Zellfusionen (b). (Trott, 1972)

3. Was geschieht mit den Zellen, die sich nicht weiter teilen? Lassen sich Beziehungen zwischen Mitose und Zelltod, zwischen Generationszeit und Zelltod, zwischen atypischen Zellteilungen und Fusionen und Zelltod herstellen?

Aus Zeitrafferaufnahmen, welche die Proliferation einiger weniger Zellen über 8—14 Tage festhalten, lassen sich Stammbäume einzelner Zellen aufstellen (Abb. 23). Neben der unmittelbaren Anschaulichkeit solcher Darstellungen erlauben sie die Beschreibung der Proliferation auch in quantitativer Hinsicht.

1. Bestrahlte Zellen, die „abortive" Kolonien bilden, können sich noch einige Male teilen, bevor sie ihre Vermehrung einstellen (Puck u. Marcus, 1956). Erst Strahlendosen über 500 R hatten schon in der bestrahlten Generation von L-Zellen eine feststellbare Verminderung der Teilungsrate zur Folge, das Maximum der Inaktivierung trat nach einer oder 2 Teilungen auf (Abb. 24 u. 25), (Trott, 1969). Die hohe Strahlenresistenz der ersten Teilung war schon von Tolmach (1961) festgestellt worden. Nach 400 rad waren noch über

80 % der bestrahlten HeLa-Zellen imstande, sich noch mindestens einmal zu teilen. Bei chinesischen Hamsterzellen (V-79) beobachtete FROESE (1966) erst nach 1000 rad eine deutliche Einschränkung der ersten Teilung. Eine ähnliche Dosisabhängigkeit beschrieben HURWITZ u. TOLMACH (1969a) bei HeLa-Zellen. Die Fähigkeit der bestrahlten Zellen, mindestens noch eine Teilung durchzuführen, hängt von der Zellzyklusphase zum Zeitpunkt der Bestrahlung ab und geht teilweise der mit der Koloniebildungsmethode bestimmten Strahlenempfindlichkeit parallel (THOMPSON u. SUIT, 1969; TROTT, 1969).

Die 2. Teilung ist wesentlich strahlenempfindlicher (FROESE, 1966; THOMPSON u. SUIT, 1967, 1969; HURWITZ u. TOLMACH, 1969a; TROTT, 1969; MILTENBURGER, 1969). Schon bei Dosen von wenigen hundert R ist die Inaktivierungsrate in der auf die Bestrahlung folgenden Generation deutlich erhöht und verstärkt sich z.T. in den folgenden Generationen (Abb. 24). Der Verlust der Koloniebildungsfähigkeit im Dosisbereich unter 500 R kommt also im wesentlichen durch Teilungsversager in späteren Generationen zustande. Nach

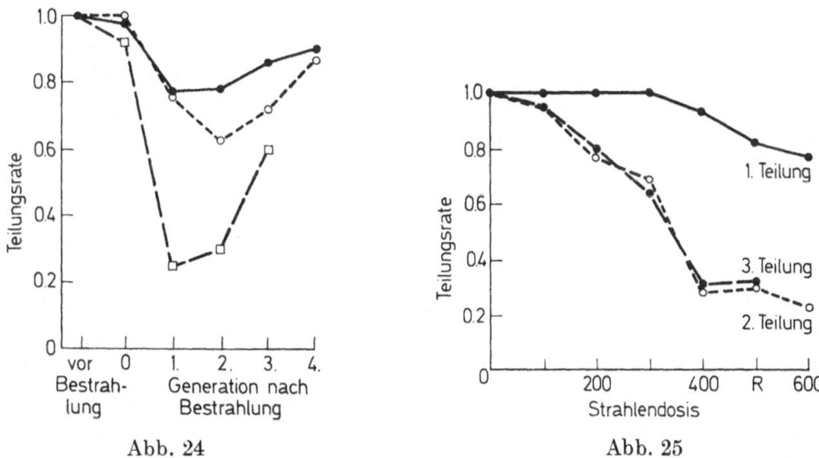

Abb. 24. Die Teilungsraten von L-Zellen vor und in den ersten 5 Generationen nach Bestrahlung in Abhängigkeit von der Strahlendosis

●————● 200 R 45 kV-Röntgenstrahlen in G_1-Phase
○·········○ 300 R 45 kV-Röntgenstrahlen in G_1-Phase
□——□ 400 R 45 kV-Röntgenstrahlen in G_1-Phase
(TROTT u. HUG, 1970)

Abb. 25. Die Erfolgsrate in den ersten 3 Teilungen nach Bestrahlung von L-Zellen in G_1-Phase in Abhängigkeit von der Strahlendosis. (TROTT u. Mitarb., 1970)

Bestrahlung von L-P59-Zellen mit 736 rad waren nur etwa 3 % aller Zellen noch in der Lage, Kolonien zu bilden. Dennoch war praktisch keine Einschränkung der ersten Teilung zu erkennen. Aber weniger als die Hälfte aller Zellen der 2. Generation vollendeten die 3. Teilung und weniger als die Hälfte der 3. Generation die 4. Teilung (THOMPSON u. SUIT, 1967).

Die Teilungsrate ist in der 2.—4. Generation nach Bestrahlung am niedrigsten (THOMPSON u. SUIT, 1969; HURWITZ u. TOLMACH, 1969a). Bei L-Zellen, die mit Dosen von 200—400 R bestrahlt worden waren, trat in der 3. Generation ein Anstieg der Teilungsrate auf (Abb. 24), (TROTT u. HUG, 1970). Er beruht nicht nur darauf, daß Zellen, die die Bestrahlung ohne offensichtliche Beeinträchtigung ihrer Teilungsfähigkeit überstanden hatten, die defekten Zellen überwuchern. Vielmehr zeigte sich auch *innerhalb* von Stammbäumen, bei denen in den ersten 2 Generationen inaktive Zellen aufgetreten sind, in den Folgegenerationen eine Abnahme der Inaktivierungsrate, so daß darauf geschlossen werden kann, daß die Schädigung im Verlauf einiger Zellteilungen aus dem Klon der bestrahlten Zelle heraus selektioniert worden ist.

2. Die experimentellen Untersuchungen über die Frage nach der Verteilung der „Todesfälle" in der Nachkommenschaft bestrahlter Zellen sind insbesondere durch 2 Konzepte stimuliert worden, die als wesentliches Element die Zufälligkeit der Inaktivierungsereignisse ansehen und daher als stochastische Modelle der Zellinaktivierung beschrieben werden. Das Konzept von Whitmore u. Till (1964) geht davon aus, daß eine bestrahlte Zelle und alle ihre Nachkommen eine von der Strahlendosis abhängige reduzierte Teilungswahrscheinlichkeit besitzen und die Entscheidung zwischen Teilung und Versagen zufällig erfolgt. Unter bestimmten experimentellen Bedingungen ist diese Teilungswahrscheinlichkeit konstant vermindert, wie z. B. bei Säugetierzellen in einem BUdR enthaltenden Nährmedium (Pujara u. Whitmore, 1970). Das stochastische Modell der Strahlenwirkung von Hug u. Kellerer (1963, 1966) geht von der weitergehenden Vorstellung aus, daß jede lebende Zelle mit einer gewissen Wahrscheinlichkeit versagt. Dieser Stochastik der Lebensprozesse überlagert sich die Stochastik der Energieabsorption bei Bestrahlung, so daß die Zellen mit einer höheren Wahrscheinlichkeit bei den Zellteilungen versagen. Die bisher vorliegenden Analysen der Daten aus den Stammbaumstudien von Thompson u. Suit, Hurwitz und Tolmach und Trott u. Mitarb. lassen eine Entscheidung über die Gültigkeit des stochastischen Modells in seiner allgemeinen Form nicht zu.

Nur über das Verhalten von Geschwisterzellen lassen sich z. Z. Angaben machen. Bei ungestörter Proliferation weisen Geschwisterzellen eine weitaus geringere Schwankungsbreite in ihren Generationszeiten auf als entfernt verwandte Zellen (Froese, 1964). Diese Korrelation wird durch Bestrahlung gestört (Froese, 1966; Marin u. Bender, 1966). Dagegen zeigten Geschwisterzellen in der Nachkommenschaft bestrahlter Zellen in allen Generationen eine engere Korrelation in bezug auf den Zelluntergang als nicht so nah verwandte Zellen (Froese, 1966; Thompson u. Suit, 1967, 1969; Hurwitz u. Tolmach, 1969a; Trott, 1969). Nur Miltenburger (1969) fand keine überzufällig erhöhte Inaktivierungsrate in verwandten Zellen ersten Grades.

Thompson u. Suit (1969) hatten darüber hinaus den Eindruck, daß besonders in Stammbäumen von mit 200 rad bestrahlten Zellen Versager in einzelnen Ästen des Stammbaumes massiv gehäuft auftraten. Eine besonders charakteristische Form solch überzufälliger Häufung wird als Letalsektor beschrieben, in dem die eine Tochterzelle die unbegrenzte Proliferationsfähigkeit behält und schließlich mehr als 50 Zellen bildet, während die Nachkommenschaft der anderen Tochter ausstirbt. Solche Letalsektoren sind bei Hefezellen und Bakterien bekannt (Haefner, 1965; Haefner u. Striebeck, 1967; James u. Werner, 1966). Thompson u. Suit (1969) fanden sie in 18 % aller „überlebenden", d. h. am Versuchsende mehr als 50 Zellen enthaltenden Klone nach 230 rad.

3. Der reproduktive Zelltod manifestiert sich morphologisch im Auftreten von Riesenzellen, Zellpyknosen, Desintegration von in der Mitose blockierten Zellen und insbesondere in Zellfusionen und multipolaren Zellteilungen. Keine der genannten Zelluntergangsformen ist auf bestrahlte Zellen beschränkt, tritt aber nach Bestrahlung weitaus häufiger auf als in unbestrahlten Populationen (Marin u. Bender, 1966).

Multipolare Teilungen treten in Kulturen menschlicher Carcinomzellen (KB) spontan in etwa 3—4 % aller Mitosen auf (Fetner u. Porter, 1965). Nach Bestrahlung steigt die Häufigkeit multipolarer Teilungen an und erreicht ein Maximum nach mehreren Tagen. Zu späteren Zeitpunkten nimmt die relative Häufigkeit von tetrapolaren gegenüber tripolaren Mitosen zu (Levis u. Marin, 1963). Die Häufigkeit multipolarer Mitosen hängt von der Strahlendosis ab, eine Dosis von 300 rad verzehnfacht in KB-Zellen den in der unbestrahlten Kultur beobachteten Wert (Fetner u. Porter, 1965).

In Zeitrafferfilmen von bestrahlten Zellen lassen sich häufig Zellen beobachten, die über lange Zeit hin, oft das 5—10fache der normalen Generationszeit, ohne Teilung und ohne offensichtliche Desintegrationszeichen liegen bleiben. Meist nehmen sie unterdessen an Größe zu: die von der Zelle bedeckte Fläche wird größer, die Kern-Plasma-Relation nimmt ab (Pomerat u. Mitarb., 1959). Tolmach u. Marcus (1960) und Tolmach (1961) maßen bei mit 1 250 rad bestrahlten HeLa-Zellen eine exponentielle Zunahme der Zellgröße über mehrere Tage hin bis zum 9fachen des Ausgangswertes. Riesenzellen sind jedoch nicht selten die Folge von Zellfusionen, vor allem bei HeLa-Zellen (HURWITZ u. TOLMACH, 1969b).

Die am häufigsten beobachtete Form des Zelltodes in der Nachkommenschaft bestrahlter L-Zellen und L-P59-Zellen bestand in Pyknosen, die keine Beziehungen zu Mitoseversuchen zeigten (THOMPSON u. SUIT, 1969), während bei HeLa-Zellen 75 % aller Zelluntergänge von einem erfolglosen Teilungsversuch eingeleitet wurden (HURWITZ u. TOLMACH, 1969a).

Zellfusionen sind eine besonders eindrucksvolle Störung der normalen Zellproliferation. HURWITZ u. TOLMACH (1969b) bestimmten ihr Vorkommen in normalen HeLa-Zellen in vitro mit 0,9 %. Nach Bestrahlung mit 500 rad folgte etwa einem Viertel aller Zellteilungen eine Zellfusion (MARIN u. BENDER, 1966; HURWITZ u. TOLMACH, 1969b). In der überwiegenden Mehrzahl sind es Schwesterzellen, die sich, meist innerhalb einiger Stunden, wiedervereinigen, doch sind auch Fusionen zwischen anderen Verwandten beobachtet worden, z.B. zwischen Cousinen oder auch zwischen Zellen des gleichen Stammbaumes, die verschiedenen Generationen angehören (HURWITZ u. TOLMACH, 1969b). In vielen Fällen blieb nach der Teilung zwischen den Geschwisterzellen eine Plasmabrücke bestehen, die die Fusion erleichterte.

Zellfusionen traten in einzelnen Klonen überzufällig häufig auf (HURWITZ u. TOLMACH, 1969b). In der Mehrzahl der Fälle fand nach der Zellfusion eine Desintegration der Riesenzelle statt. Eine weitere häufige Folge von Zellfusionen waren multipolare Teilungen (MARIN u. BENDER, 1966; HURWITZ, 1969b), doch führten auch multipolare Teilungen häufig zu Fusionen. In über der Hälfte aller tripolaren Teilungen bestrahlter HeLa-Zellen vereinigten sich 2 der 3 Tochterzellen, in 30 % sogar alle 3 Tochterzellen wieder (HURWITZ u. TOLMACH, 1969b).

V. Die Abhängigkeit der Strahlenwirkung von der Strahlenqualität

Untersuchungen über die unterschiedliche Wirksamkeit von ionisierenden Strahlen verschiedener Qualität wurden schon mit der Gewebekulturmethode durchgeführt (s. S. 46). So testeten LASNITZKI u. LEA (1940) die Unterschiede in der mitosehemmenden

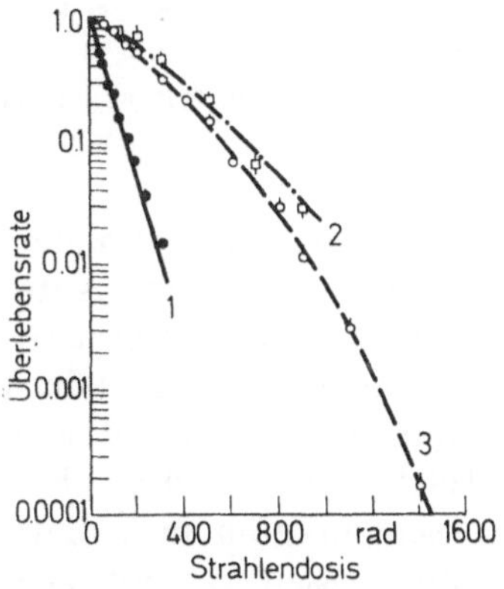

Abb. 26. Dosiseffektkurven menschlicher Nierenzellen (T-1) bei Bestrahlung mit ^{210}Po-Alpha-Teilchen (1), ^{90}SR/^{90}Y-Beta-Strahlen (2) und 250 kV-Röntgenstrahlen (3). (Nach BARENDSEN u. Mitarb., 1960)

Wirkung von Röntgenstrahlen verschiedener Härte und SPEAR u. Mitarb. (1938) die von Gammastrahlen und 2,4 MeV-Neutronen.

Die ersten Versuche, mit der Kolonietestmethode die Wirkung von Strahlung höherer LETs zu untersuchen, stammen von BARENDSEN u. Mitarb. (1960). Menschliche Nierenzellen

(T-1) wurden in speziellen Petrischalen, deren Böden aus einer 6 μ dicken Polyäthylen-terphthalatfolie bestanden, platiert und mit Alphastrahlen einer ^{210}Po-Quelle von unten bestrahlt. Mit einem ^{90}Sr/^{90}Y-Präparat wurde eine Betabestrahlung durchgeführt. Nach Inkubation und Auswertung in üblicher Weise wurden die in Abb. 26 dargestellten Dosiseffektkurven gefunden. Die Kurve 3 ist das Ergebnis der Röntgenbestrahlung: auf-fallend ist die kontinuierliche Zunahme der Reaktivität auch noch bei Überlebensraten unter 1 % (Über die Bedeutung solcher Kurven s. S. 51). Die Kurve für Betastrahlen verläuft deutlich flacher, während die Dosiswirkungskurve nach Alphabestrahlung eine Exponentialfunktion mit einer D_0 von 65 rad ist. In der Proliferationskinetik nach Be-strahlung fanden sich keine wesentlichen Unterschiede gegenüber der nach Röntgen-

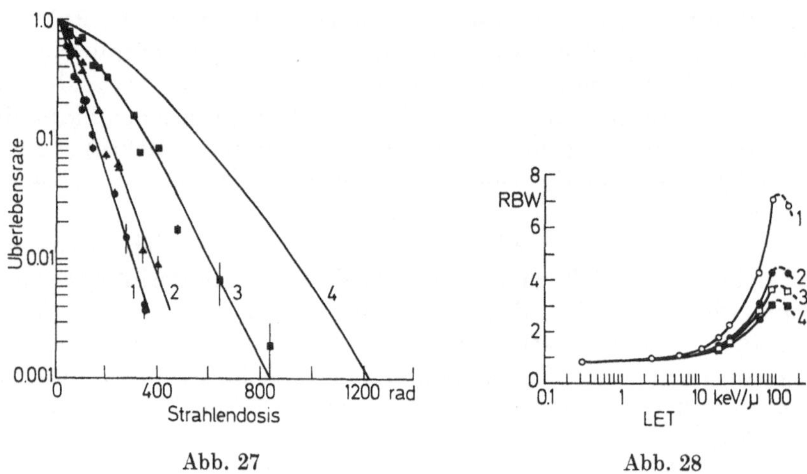

Abb. 27   Abb. 28

Abb. 27. Dosiseffektkurven menschlicher Nierenzellen (T-1) bei Bestrahlung mit Alpha-Teilchen verschie-dener Energie

Kurve 1: LET = 85 keV/μ Kurve 3: LET = 24,6 keV/μ
Kurve 2: LET = 60,8 keV/μ Kurve 4: 250 kV-Röntgenstrahlen

(Barendsen u. Mitarb., 1963)

Abb. 28. Die Abhängigkeit der RBW von Alpha-Teilchen vom LET bei verschiedenen Überlebensraten (bzw. Strahlendosen)

Kurve 1 = Überlebensrate 80 %   Kurve 3 = Überlebensrate 5 %
Kurve 2 = Überlebensrate 20 %   Kurve 4 = Überlebensrate 0,5 %

(Barendsen u. Mitarb., 1963)

bestrahlung. Die Koloniegrößenverteilung ist die gleiche wie nach Röntgenbestrahlung (Westra u. Barendsen, 1966), doch scheint der Anteil der inaktivierten Zellen, die schon vor der ersten Zellteilung ihre weitere Proliferation einstellen, größer zu sein als nach Bestrahlung mit locker ionisierenden Strahlen (Trott u. Mitarb., 1970).

Erste vergleichende Untersuchungen über die Wirkung von beschleunigten Teilchen stammen von Deering u. Rice (1962), die Sauerstoff-, Kohlenstoff-, Lithium- und Helium-Kerne im Linearbeschleuniger beschleunigten und damit HeLa-Zellen bestrahlten. Die Ergebnisse lassen sich so zusammenfassen: 1. mit zunehmendem LET (bis zu einem Wert von 200 keV/μ) nimmt die Wirksamkeit der Strahlung zu; 2. von einem LET von 100 keV/μ an weisen die Dosiseffektkurven keine Schulter mehr auf; 3. bei Zunahme des LET über 200 keV/μ hinaus nimmt die Neigung der Dosiseffektkurve, die weiterhin rein exponentiell ist, wieder ab.

Todd (1967) fand nach Bestrahlung von T-1-Zellen mit Bor-Kernen (LET = 165 keV/μ) noch eine Schulterkurve, mit Kohlenstoff- (LET = 220 keV/μ), Sauerstoff- (LET = 385 keV/μ) und Neon-Ionen (LET = 570 keV/μ) jedoch rein exponentielle Dosiswirkungskurven, die mit zunehmendem LET wieder flacher verliefen. Ähnliche Versuche an chinesischen Hamsterzellen von Skarsgard u. Mitarb. (1967) führten zu ähnlichen Ergebnissen (Tabelle 5). In beiden Fällen ergab sich eine maximale Wirkung bei Bestrahlung mit beschleunigten Kohlenstoffkernen eines LET von 190 bzw. 220 keV/μ.

Beschleunigte Deuteronen und Alpha-Teilchen verschiedener LET wurden von Barendsen u. Mitarb. (1963) und Barendsen (1964) zur Bestrahlung von T-1-Zellen verwendet und Dosiseffektkurven bestimmt (Abb. 27). Mit zunehmendem LET wurde die Schulter immer geringer und ging bei einem LET über 60 keV/μ verloren. Die steilste Dosiswirkungskurve wurde bei Bestrahlung mit 4 MeV-Alpha-Teilchen eines LET von 110 keV/μ gefunden. Bei dieser Kurvenschar läßt sich besonders deutlich erkennen, wie

Tabelle 5. *Dosiseffektkurvenparameter (D_0 und Extrapolationsnummer n) nach Bestrahlung von Säugetierzellen mit beschleunigten Kernen unterschiedlicher Energie*

Deering u. Rice (1962) HeLa S-3				Skarsgard u. Mitarb. (1967) chinesische Hamsterzellen (CH2B$_2$)				Barendsen u. Mitarb. (1968) menschliche Nierenzellen (T-1)			Berry u. Mitarb. (1970) Leukämie P-388 in vivo			
LET keV/μ	Partikel	D_0 (rad)	n	LET keV/μ	Partikel	D_0 rad	n	LET keV/μ	Partikel	D_0 rad	LET keV/μ	Partikel	D_0 rad	n
	Rö	130	4		Rö	170	5		Rö	180		Rö	160	2
								5,6	Deuteronen	160	6	Deuteronen	123	13,7
											14	,,	118	7,9
19	4 He	90	4	19	4 He	165	2,6	20	4 He	145				
								26	,,	120	26	4 H	138	1,6
43	6 Li	70	3	44	6 Li	143	1,9				45	,,	93	2,1
								61	,,	84	62	,,	121	0,9
				72	6 Li	106	1,8							
								88	,,	70	86	,,	80	1,9
				126	11 B	107	1,3	110	,,	57				
								140	,,	64				
								166		79				
190	12 C	55	1	189	12 C	100	1,6							
350	16 O	105	1	351	16 O	142	0,9							
				561	20 Ne	202	1,1							
				1950	40 A	500	1,1							

sehr die Relative Biologische Wirksamkeit der verschiedenen Strahlenarten von der Form der Dosiseffektkurven abhängt und für verschiedene Dosisbereiche bzw. Überlebensraten verschieden ist (Abb. 28), (s. S. 39 ff.).

Einen weiteren Bereich der Strahlenqualität umfassen die Versuche, die von Barendsen u. Mitarb. (1966) am gleichen Zellmaterial durchgeführt wurden und deren Ergebnisse in Tabelle 5 zusammengestellt sind (Abb. 7, S. 15).

Untersuchungen über die Veränderungen der RBW mit der Tiefe in einem Phantom bei Bestrahlung von T-1-Zellen mit 910 MeV-Helium-Kernen wurden von Raju u. Mitarb. (1971) veröffentlicht.

Auch bei in vivo Systemen lassen sich vergleichbare Dosiseffektkurven nach Bestrahlung mit beschleunigten Alpha-Teilchen und Deuteronen demonstrieren. Die Bestrahlung der Mäusehaut mit 28 MeV-Alpha-Teilchen ergab eine D_0 von 95 rad (d.h. eine RBW$_{D_0}$ von 1,4), (Leith u. Mitarb., 1971). Die Ergebnisse der Versuche von Berry (1970) mit in-vivo getesteten P-388-Leukämiezellen sind in Tabelle 5 aufgeführt.

Zunehmendes Interesse haben Experimente mit schnellen Neutronen gefunden, da diese auch von therapeutischer Bedeutung sein könnten. Erste Untersuchungen mit der HEWITTschen Tumortransplantationsmethode zeigten, daß nach Bestrahlung eines tetraploiden Ehrlich-Aszites-Tumors mit Neutronen einer mittleren Energie von 6 MeV eine D_0 von 55 rad gegenüber einer D_0 von 114 rad nach Röntgenbestrahlung auftrat, ohne daß die Extrapolationsnummer sich änderte (HORNSEY u. SILINI, 1961). Dagegen verlief die Dosiseffektkurve nach Bestrahlung von P-388-Leukämiezellen mit Spaltneutronen exponentiell mit einer D_0 von 85 rad (ANDREWS u. BERRY, 1962). Die RBW_{D_0}, das Verhältnis der exponentiellen Endneigungen der Dosiswirkungskurven, war in beiden Fällen etwa 2. Bei Bestrahlung der gleichen P-388-Leukämiezellen wie in den Versuchen von ANDREWS u. BERRY mit den 6 MeV-Neutronen des gleichen Zyklotrons wie in den Versuchen von HORNSEY u. SILINI fanden BERRY u. Mitarb. (1965) eine Verminderung der Extrapolationsnummer von 3,9 auf 1,6 und eine RBW_{D_0} von 2,1.

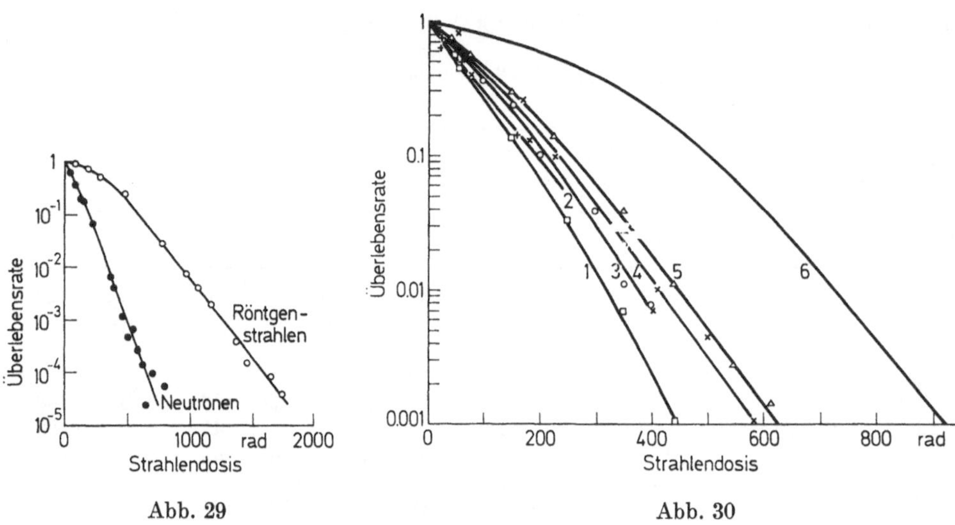

Abb. 29   Abb. 30

Abb. 29. Dosiseffektkurven von chinesischen Hamsterzellen (H 1) nach Bestrahlung mit 6 MeV-Neutronen und 280 kV-Röntgenstrahlen. (SCHNEIDER u. WHITMORE, 1963)

Abb. 30. Dosiseffektkurven von menschlichen Nierenzellen (T-1) bei Bestrahlung mit Neutronen verschiedener Energie

Kurve 1: Spaltneutronen
Kurve 2: 3 MeV-Neutronen
Kurve 3: Neutronen nach Beschuß eines Be-Targets mit 20 MeV-^{3}He-Teilchen (mittl. Energie 10 MeV)
Kurve 4: Neutronen nach Beschuß eines Be-Targets mit 16 MeV-Deuteronen (mittl. Energie 6 MeV)
Kurve 5: D-T-Neutronen (15 MeV)
Kurve 6: 250 kV-Röntgenstrahlen

(BROERSE u. Mitarb., 1968)

Die ersten Versuche, die Wirkung von 6 MeV-Neutronen auf das Koloniebildungsvermögen in vitro zu testen, wurden von SCHNEIDER u. WHITMORE (1963) an zwei Stämmen chinesischer Hamsterzellen und an L-Zellen durchgeführt. Die Zellen wurden in Suspension bestrahlt und dann platiert (Abb. 29). Alle von SCHNEIDER u. WHITMORE (1963) publizierten Neutronen-Dosiswirkungskurven verlaufen steiler als die nach Röntgenbestrahlung mit D_0-Werten von etwa 65 rad und RBW_{D_0}-Werten von 2,2—2,5, und alle weisen eine Schulter auf, die aber kleiner ist als die nach Röntgenbestrahlung. Nur Knochenmarkzellen, in der gleichen Versuchsserie mit der Milzkolonietechnik getestet, wurden nach einer rein exponentiellen Dosiswirkungskurve mit einer D_0 von 41 rad inaktiviert.

14-MeV-Neutronen der D-T-Reaktion inaktivieren HeLa-Zellen nach einer Dosiswirkungskurve, deren D_0 und Extrapolationsnummer jeweils etwa halb so groß sind wie nach Röntgenbestrahlung (NIAS u. Mitarb., 1967). Bei P-388-F-Zellen in vitro fanden die gleichen Autoren keine sichere Verkleinerung der Schulter bei 14 MeV-Neutronenbestrahlung. Vergleichende Untersuchungen über die Wirkung von Neutronen verschiedener Energiespektren auf Zellen in vitro wurden von BROERSE u. Mitarb. (1968) und auf Zellen in vivo von BERRY (1971b) durchgeführt. BROERSE u. Mitarb. (1968) fanden in allen Fällen nach Neutronenbestrahlung von menschlichen Nierenzellen in vitro (T-1) eine geringere Schulter als nach Röntgenbestrahlung (Abb. 30) und mit abnehmender mittlerer Neutronenenergie einen steileren Verlauf der Dosiseffektkurve. Die Unterschiede in den Energiespektren von 6 MeV-Neutronen in verschiedenen Tiefen eines gewebeäquivalenten Materials führten in den Versuchen von EVANS u. Mitarb. (1971) zu unterschiedlichen Dosiseffektkurven in verschiedenen Phantomtiefen, während McNALLY u. BEWLEY (1969)

Tabelle 6. *Dosiseffektkurvenparameter (D_0 und Extrapolationsnummer n) für euoxische und hypoxische Mäuselymphomzellen (P-388), in vitro mit Neutronen verschiedener Energie an der Oberfläche und in 10 cm Tiefe eines gewebeäquivalenten Phantoms bestrahlt und mit der HEWITTschen Tumortransplantationsmethode in vivo getestet.* (Nach BERRY, 1971b)

Neutronenquelle	mittlere Energie MeV	an der Oberfläche des Phantoms D_0 (rad) euoxisch	hypoxisch	OER	n	in 10 cm Tiefe des Phantoms D_0 (rad) euoxisch	hypoxisch	OER	n
Spaltneutronen TRIGA	1	91	102	1,1	0,9	96	119	1,2	2,8
Zyklotron Hammersmith	6	77	125	1,6	1,9	99	127	1,3	0,8
D-T-Reaktion									
(Lawrence Lab.)	14	87	153	1,8	3,1	115	146	1,3	1,2
(Aldermaston)	14	76	139	1,8	0,8	73	113	1,5	1,0
Zyklotron Texas A & M									
30 MeV-Beryllium	15	94	168	1,8	2,2	139	154	1,1	0,8
50 MeV-Beryllium	25	102	201	2,0	2,4	112	181	1,6	3,5

bei Bestrahlung von Ehrlich-Aszites-Tumorzellen mit 6 MeV-Neutronen und NIAS u. Mitarb. (1971) bei Bestrahlung von HeLa-ZELLEN mit 14 MeV-Neutronen keinen Einfluß der Phantomtiefe auf die Parameter der Dosiswirkungskurven fanden.

Auch BERRY (1971b) sah nach Bestrahlung von P-388-Leukämiezellen mit Neutronen 6 verschiedener Spektren in vitro und Testung ihrer reproduktiven Integrität in vivo neben der Abhängigkeit von Schulter und Endneigung der Dosiseffektkurven von der Neutronenenergie ausgeprägte Unterschiede je nach Lage im Phantom. Die Ergebnisse von BERRY (1971b) sind in Tabelle 6 zusammengefaßt. Neben den Parametern der Dosiseffektkurven für euoxische Zellen sind auch die für hypoxische Zellen und der Sauerstoffverstärkungsfaktor angegeben. (Auf diese Werte wird auf S. 107 eingegangen.)

Unterschiede im Proliferationsverhalten neutronenbestrahlter Zellen gegenüber röntgenbestrahlten wurden nicht gefunden (BERRY, 1967a; NIAS, 1968).

Die Wirkung von 14 MeV-Neutronen auf die reproduktive Integrität von Zellen normaler Gewebe in vivo wurde von WITHERS u. Mitarb. (1970) an Darmschleimhautzellen untersucht, wo im Vergleich zur Röntgenbestrahlung die Reduktion der Extrapolationsnummer von 40 auf 8 der hervorstechende Effekt war, während sich die Steilheit der Kurve nur unwesentlich änderte, von DENEKAMP u. Mitarb. (1971) an klonogenen Hautzellen, wo die Schulter der Dosiseffektkurve auf ein Drittel vermindert war, während die D_0 nur von 135 rad auf 109 rad abnahm, und von BROERSE u. Mitarb. (1971) und HENDRY u. HOWARD (1971) an Knochenmarkzellen, wo ebenfalls die Reduktion der Extrapolationsnummer auf Werte von 1,34 (BROERSE) bzw. 1,7 (HENDRY) deutlicher war als die Veränderung der D_0.

In der Arbeit von Broerse u. Mitarb. (1971), die über ein gemeinsames Projekt mehrerer Gruppen berichtet, fällt auf, daß bei gleichen Versuchsbedingungen die D_0 der 14 MeV-Neutronenkurven in den zwei zusammenarbeitenden Zentren einmal 62,5 rad, im anderen Fall 78,3 rad betrug.

Ähnliche Unterschiede fand Berry (1971b) zwischen seinen beiden 14 MeV-Neutronenquellen.

Kember (1969) beobachtete bei Bestrahlung klonogener Knorpelzellen mit 6 MeV-Neutronen eine geringere D_0 und Extrapolationsnummer im Vergleich zur Röntgenbestrahlung.

Die Relative Biologische Wirksamkeit von Neutronen hängt entscheidend von ihrer Energie und ihrer Dosis ab (Abb. 31), (Barendsen, 1971; vgl. Beitrag Kellerer u. Hug, S. 39ff.). Auf die unterschiedliche Wirkung von Neutronenbestrahlung auf Zellen verschiedener Zellzyklusphasen und Sauerstoffversorgung wird auf S. 89 u. 106 f. eingegangen.

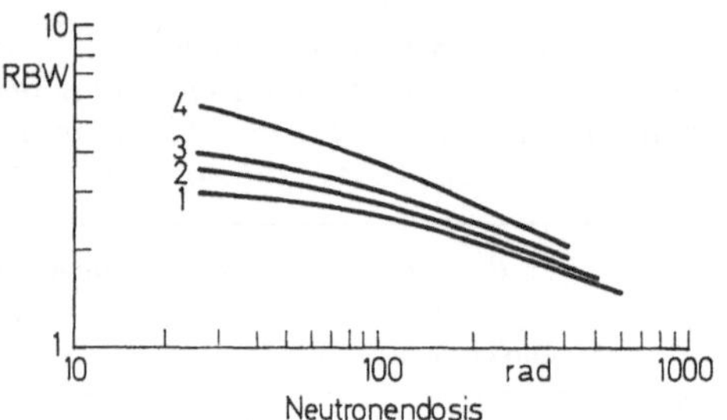

Abb. 31. Die Abhängigkeit der RBW von Neutronen unterschiedlicher Energie von der Neutronendosis bei Bestrahlung von menschlichen Nierenzellen (T-1) in vitro
Kurve 1: Neutronen der D-T-Reaktion (15 MeV)
Kurve 2: Neutronen nach Beschuß eines Be-Targets mit 16 MeV-Deuteronen (mittl. Energie 7 MeV)
Kurve 3: Neutronen nach Beschuß eines Be-Targets mit 20 MeV-^{3}He-Teilchen (mittl. Energie 10 MeV)
Kurve 4: Neutronen aus dem Zerfall von ^{235}U
(Barendsen, 1971)

Die Probleme, die die Untersuchungen mit Strahlung unterschiedlicher Qualität an Zellkulturen für Fragen des Mechanismus der zellulären Inaktivierungsvorgänge und mikrodosimetrische Überlegungen aufwerfen, können hier nicht angesprochen werden. Es wird dazu auf den Beitrag von Kellerer u. Hug in diesem Band (S. 32ff.) sowie auf die Diskussionen von Elkind (1970, 1971), Bewley (1968), Barendsen (1968) und Kellerer u. Rossi (1971) verwiesen.

VI. Die Abhängigkeit der Strahlenwirkung von der Dosisleistung

Die oben beschriebenen Versuche über die Strahlenwirkung auf die Vermehrungsfähigkeit von Säugetierzellen wurden alle bei Dosisleistungen von einigen rad bis zu einigen hundert rad pro Minute durchgeführt.

1. Sehr hohe Dosisleistung

Town (1967) beobachtete, daß eine Erhöhung der Dosisleistung auf $3,5 \times 10^9$ rad/sec eine biphasische Dosiseffektkurve zur Folge hatte: bei niedrigen Dosen zeigte sich eine normale Schulterkurve, bei Dosen über 900 rad nahm die Neigung der Kurve ab und verlief wesentlich flacher weiter. Da solche Kurven von Bestrahlungsversuchen an Bakterien mit ähnlich hoher Dosisleistung her bekannt (Dewey u. Boag, 1959) und als Ausdruck eines radiogenen Sauerstoffentzugs erklärt waren, nahm Town (1967) an, daß auch bei Säugetierzellen die Bestrahlung mit extrem hoher Dosisleistung zu einer Sauerstoffverarmung im strahlenempfindlichen Bereich führt. Da eine Nachdiffusion von Sauerstoff in der kurzen Bestrahlungszeit nicht erfolgen kann, trifft der Rest einer höheren Strahlendosis hypoxische und damit resistente Zellen. TODD u. Mitarb. (1968) fanden keinen Knick in der Dosiseffektkurve bei Dosen unter 1000 rad, während PHILIPS u. WORNSOP (1968), KANNON u. Mitarb. (1968), GRIEM u. Mitarb. (1969) und BERRY u. Mitarb. (1969) bei Dosisleistungen über 10^{10} rad/sec alle den typischen Knick im Dosisbereich von etwa 1000 rad sahen. NIAS u. Mitarb. (1969) konnten nur dann eine biphasische Dosiseffektkurve bei Bestrahlung mit Pulsen von 1 μsec Dauer beobachten, wenn der Sauerstoffgehalt des Mediums vorher schon auf 0,35 % reduziert worden war. Auch bei Verkürzung der Pulsdauer auf 10 nsec konnten NIAS u. Mitarb. (1970) bis zu Dosen von 1600 rad (DL = 10^{11} rad/sec) keinen Knick in der Kurve entdecken. Bei Überprüfung der eigenen Versuche konnten auch BERRY u. STEDEFORD (1971) die alten Ergebnisse nicht verifizieren. Es muß angenommen werden, daß technische Artefakte — z.B. eine ungleiche Dosisverteilung bei den höchsten Dosen, d.h. dem geringsten Abstand vom Target, oder eine primär verminderte Sauerstoffkonzentration in den Bestrahlungsgefäßen — für den Knick in der Dosiseffektkurve verantwortlich waren. Somit ist anzunehmen, daß die Strahlenempfindlichkeit von Säugetierzellen in vitro bei Dosisleistungen im Bereich von $1-10^{11}$ rad/sec praktisch gleich bleibt.

2. Sehr kleine Dosisleistungen

Bei niedrigen Dosisleistungen ist eine Änderung in der Dosiswirkungskurve zu erwarten, denn „ist die Schädigung auf irgend einer Stufe der zum Endeffekt führenden Ursachenkette reversibel, so verringert sich die Wirkung einer Strahlendosis mit Verlängerung der Bestrahlungszeit" (HUG u. Mitarb., 1966). Die theoretischen Grundlagen des Zeitfaktors werden an anderer Stelle dieses Werkes (HUG u. Mitarb., 1966) erläutert. Es soll hier nur darauf hingewiesen werden, daß bei zunehmendem Einfluß rückläufiger Prozesse die Dosiswirkungskurve immer flacher wird und schließlich in eine exponentielle Funktion mit der Neigung der Anfangsreaktivität übergeht. Bei Dosisleistungen um 5 rad/h dürften ausschließlich die auf die irreversible Komponente zurückzuführenden Strahlenwirkungen zum Zug kommen und den Verlauf der Dosiswirkungskurve bestimmen (HUG u. KELLERER, 1965).

BEDFORD u. HALL (1963) und HALL u. BEDFORD (1964) bestrahlten Einzelzellen eines HeLa-Stammes mit Dosisleistungen zwischen 44,9 rad/min und 9,5 rad/h Gammastrahlen bei optimalen Wachstumsbedingungen. Die Bestrahlungsdauer betrug bis zu 50 Stunden. Anschließend wurden die Kulturen in normaler Weise weiterinkubiert und die Überlebensrate durch Auszählen der entstandenen Kolonien bestimmt. Die so gewonnenen Dosiswirkungskurven stimmten mit der von LAJTHA u. OLIVER (1961) vorausgesagten Form weitgehend überein: die Kurve wurde bei Bestrahlung mit niedrigerer Dosisleistung immer flacher (die D_0 nahm von 181 rad bei 44,9 rad/min über 205 rad bei 16,9 rad/min und 259 rad bei 2,37 rad/min auf 320 rad bei 9,5 rad/h zu), und die Extrapolationsnummer wurde schließlich 1. Es muß bei der Bewertung dieser Versuche berücksichtigt werden, daß die höchsten Dosen über zwei Generationszeiten (ohne Berücksichtigung einer strahleninduzierten Generationszeitverlängerung) verteilt waren und durch die Bestrahlung Unterschiede in der Phasenverteilung induziert worden sein könnten. So fand HALL (1969c) bei Bestrahlung von HeLa-Zellen mit einer Dosisleistung von 30 rad/h eine biphasische Dosiswirkungskurve, was er auf eine Akkumulation der Zellen in einer strahlenresistenten Zyklusphase im Verlauf der Bestrahlung (d.h. eine partielle Synchronisation) zurückführte. Von FOX u. NIAS (1970) wurde eine Dosiseffektkurve veröffentlicht, bei der durch Erniedrigung der Temperatur auf 20° C die Proliferation ausgeschaltet war, ohne daß andere Zelleigenschaften, insbesondere die Koloniebildungsfähigkeit und der Fraktionierungseffekt, sich wesentlich verändert hatten (Abb. 32). Die Kurve bei Bestrahlung mit einer Dosisleistung von 25 rad/h verlief exponentiell mit einer D_0

von 625 rad, während die Kurvenparameter bei akuter Bestrahlung $D_0 = 200$ rad und
$n = 3$ waren. Lajtha u. Oliver (1961), Hug u. Kellerer (1965) und Porter (1965)
hatten unter der Annahme, daß die Schulter der Dosiseffektkurve mit Halbwertszeiten von
1,5—3 Stunden restituiert wird (s. S. 93f.), berechnet, daß bei einer Dosisleistung von
5—10 rad/h die Dosiswirkungskurve eine Gerade mit der Neigung der Anfangsreaktivität ist.

Die Dosisleistungsabhängigkeit der Wirkung locker ionisierender Strahlen auf Zellen
in vitro ist am ausgeprägtesten im Bereich von 1—100 rad/min (Hall, 1969b).

Dünndarmepithelzellen zeigen der großen Schulter entsprechend einen besonders ausgeprägten Einfluß der Dosisleistung auf die Neigung der Dosiseffektkurve: so steigt bei
einer Dosisleistung von 160 rad/h Radium-Gammastrahlen die D_0 von 100 rad auf 390 rad
an (Withers u. Mitarb., 1971).

Bei in-vivo-Bestrahlung von Aszitestumoren mit einer Dosisleistung von 20 rad/h
Gammastrahlen verläuft die Dosiswirkungskurve flacher und nach einer Exponentialfunktion, während bei 40 rad/h noch eine Extrapolationsnummer von 1,5 (gegenüber 3 bei
akuter Bestrahlung) zu finden ist (Berry u. Cohen, 1962; Berry, 1968b).

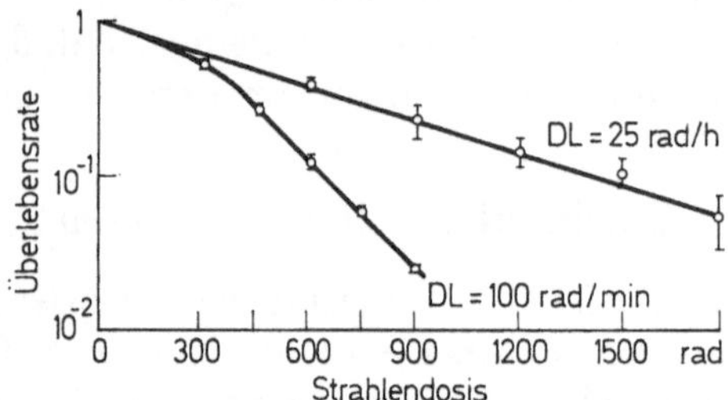

Abb. 32. Dosiseffektkurven von chinesischen Hamsterzellen (CHO) bei Bestrahlung mit einer Dosisleistung
von 100 rad/min bzw. 25 rad/h bei 20°C. (Fox u. Nias, 1970)

Die mit abnehmender Dosisleistung flacher werdende Dosiswirkungskurve geht mit
einer Verminderung des Sauerstoffeffektes einher, so daß bei niedrigsten Dosisleistungen
die aerobe Dosiswirkungskurve sich der anoxischen Kurve annähert (Oliver, 1967; s. S. 110).

Bei Bestrahlung von Aszitestumorzellen in vivo mit 6 MeV Neutronen einer Dosisleistung zwischen 15 und 300 rad/min tritt keine Abhängigkeit von der Dosisleistung auf
(Berry u. Mitarb., 1965). Seit kurzem steht dem Strahlentherapeuten ^{252}Cf, das neben
Gammastrahlen (ca. 37 % der Dosis) vor allem Neutronen emittiert, zur intracavitären
Therapie mit niedriger Dosisleistung zur Verfügung. Fairchild u. Mitarb. (1970) fanden
unter Bestrahlung von HeLa-Zellen mit einem Californium-252-Präparat auch bei
einer Dosisleistung von 6 rad/h kein Abflachen der Dosiswirkungskurve. Das bedeutet, daß
die RBW von Neutronen stark von der Dosisleistung abhängt. Aus Wachstumskurven mit
Radium bzw. Californium bestrahlter chinesischer Hamsterzellen (CHL-F) bestimmten
Hall u. Mitarb. (1971) die Abhängigkeit der RBW von Californiumneutronen von der
Dosisleistung. Sie nahm von einem Wert von 5 bei 5 rad/h auf einen Wert von 12
bei 1 rad/h zu.

Bei Bestrahlung von HeLa-Zellen bei $-196°$ C ist eine Dosisleistung von 100 rad/d
Gammastrahlen genau so wirksam wie eine akute Bestrahlung (Nias u. Ebert, 1969).

Bei Bestrahlung mit Dosisleistungen von wenigen rad/h, wie sie von Bedford, Hall
und Fairchild beschrieben wurden, tritt das Problem der Zellproliferation unter der
Bestrahlung als experimentelles Hindernis auf. Es ist jedoch auch von praktischer Bedeutung, inwieweit Zellen unter dauernder Strahleneinwirkung proliferieren können.

Die Wachstumsgeschwindigkeit einer in Suspension kultivierten Population von
L-M-Mäusezellen nimmt unter Dauerbestrahlung in linearer Abhängigkeit von der Dosisleistung im Bereich einiger rad/h ab (Hellmann u. Merchant, 1963a). Diese Verlangsamung wird durch Erniedrigung der Temperatur noch relativ verstärkt (Hellmann u.

Merchant, 1963 b), wahrscheinlich eine Folge der verlängerten Generationszeit der Zellen bei niedrigen Temperaturen, wodurch die Einzelzellen eine höhere Strahlendosis erhalten. Bei Bohnenkeimlingen konnten Hall u. Cavanagh (1967) nachweisen, daß „die pro Zellzyklus erhaltene Strahlendosis das Ausmaß des Schadens einer Population proliferierender Zellen bestimmt, die einer Dauerbestrahlung exponiert ist".

Werden Zellen dauernd mit Dosisleistungen von einigen rad/h bestrahlt, nehmen allmählich die Zellzahl sowie der Anteil klonogener Zellen an der Gesamtzellzahl konstante Werte in Abhängigkeit von der Dosisleistung an (Nias u. Lajtha, 1964; Nias u. Fox, 1969).

Eine Population von Mäuselymphomzellen, die unbestrahlt in Suspensionskultur mit einer Verdoppelungszeit von 10 h wächst, kann bei einer Bestrahlung mit 6 rad/h ihre Zellzahl

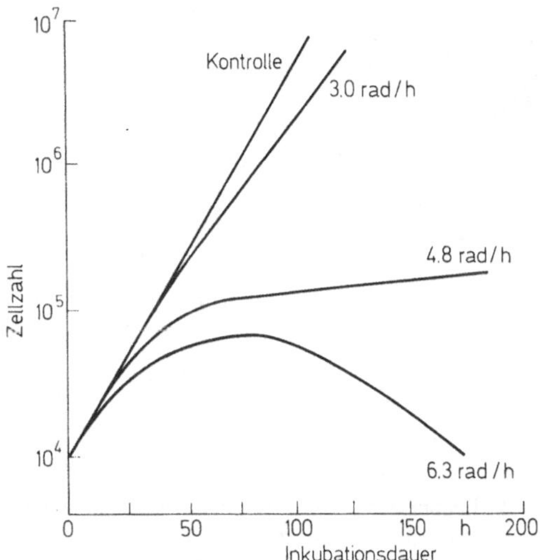

Abb. 33. Die Zunahme der Zahl morphologisch intakter L 5178 Y-Zellen in Suspensionskultur unter Dauerbestrahlung mit Tritium-Wasser bei Dosisleistungen von 3,0, 4,8 und 6,3 rad/h. (Nach Daten von Courtenay, 1965 und 1969)

nach anfänglichem Wachstum nicht mehr aufrecht erhalten und geht allmählich ein (Courtenay, 1965), (Abb. 33). Die Grenzdosisleistung, bei der gerade noch eine Zunahme der Zellzahl, wenn auch mit auf das Zehnfache verlängerter Verdoppelungszeit erfolgt, liegt bei 4,8 rad/h (Courtenay, 1969). Die Verringerung der Wachstumsgeschwindigkeit ist vor allem Folge einer erhöhten Absterberate und nur zum geringen Teil durch eine Verlängerung der Generationszeit bedingt. In einem verwandten Zellstamm haben Fox u. Gilbert (1966) und Fox u. Nias (1970) die Proliferationsparameter für verschiedene Dosisleistungen bestimmt. Aus der Tabelle 7, in der diese Daten zusammengefaßt sind, ist zu entnehmen, daß eine von der Dosisleistung abhängige Zellzyklusverlängerung auftritt, daß der Anteil

Tabelle 7. *Proliferationskinetische Parameter von Leukämiezellen in vitro (P-388-F) unter Dauerbestrahlung mit verschiedener Dosisleistung im Gleichgewichtszustand.* (Mod. nach Fox u. Gilbert, 1966, und Fox u. Nias, 1970)

Dosisleistung rad/d	Verdoppelungszeit h	Generationszeit h	Generationsdosis rad	% tote Zellen	% begrenzt teilungsfähige Zellen	% klonogene Zellen	% inaktivierte Zellen pro Zellzyklus
0	12,9	12	0	9	1	90	
60	14,4	12,5	31,5	16	24	60	8
90	15,8	13,3	50	22	28	50	11
120	17,3	14,1	71	23	37	40	12
150	21,2	14,2	89	39	39	22	20
210	27,5	18	157	42	44	14	50

klonogener Zellen in der Population mit der Dosisleistung abnimmt und daß der Anteil der toten wie auch der nur begrenzt lebensfähigen Zellen mit der Dosisleistung zunimmt. Aus diesen Daten bestimmten Fox u. Nias (1970) den pro Zellzyklus inaktivierten Prozentsatz an Zellen für die verschiedenen Generationsdosen (Tabelle 7). Auch aus Wachstumskurven von auf dem Glasboden der Kulturgefäße haftenden Zellen lassen sich solche Dosiswirkungsbeziehungen berechnen (Abb. 34).

Die in vitro gewonnenen Befunde lassen sich auch bei den in-vivo-Systemen bestätigen. So stellt sich die Zahl der klonogenen Knochenmarkszellen auf ein Gleichgewicht ein, das

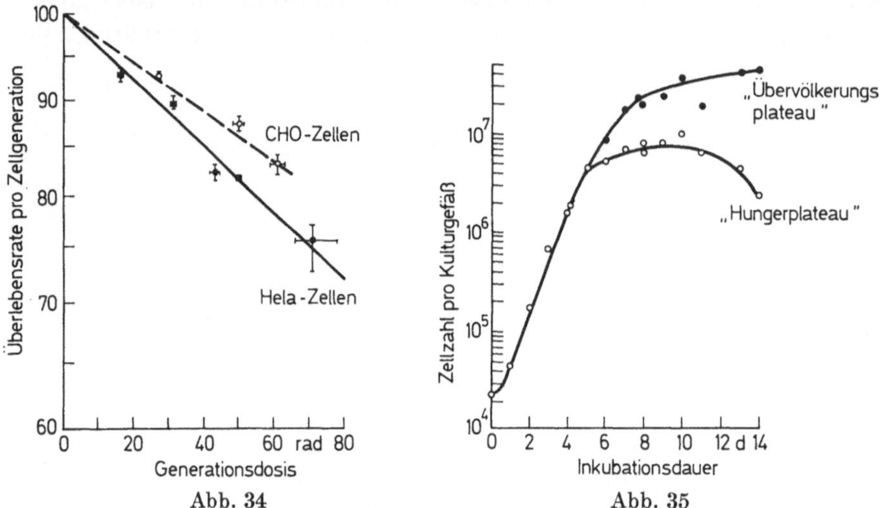

Abb. 34. Die Überlebensrate pro Zellgeneration von chinesischen Hamsterzellen (CHO) bzw. HeLa-Zellen in Abhängigkeit von der Generationsdosis unter einer Dauerbestrahlung. (Fox u. Nias, 1970)

Abb. 35. Wachstumskurven von chinesischen Hamsterzellen (HAZ) mit (ausgefüllte Punkte) und ohne (Kreise) täglichem Mediumwechsel. (Hahn u. Mitarb., 1968)

unter 24 rad/d bei 40 % (Drasil, 1966) und unter 50 rad/d bei 10 % (Lamerton, 1966) liegt, während die Darmepithelien offensichtlich durch Dauerbestrahlung dieser Größenordnung weniger betroffen werden, wohl auch Folge der wesentlich kürzeren Generationszeit und somit der relativ geringeren Generationsdosis (Lamerton, 1966).

Unter Dauerbestrahlung können gelegentlich auch strahlenresistente Mutanten auftreten und durch ihren Selektionsvorteil die Überhand gewinnen. Diese Strahlenresistenz, die nicht mit einer Veränderung der Chromosomenzahl verbunden ist, zeigt sich auch in den Dosiswirkungskurven bei akuter Bestrahlung (Courtenay, 1969).

VII. Die Strahlenwirkung auf Säugetierzellen in vitro in verschiedenen Wachstums- und Zellzyklusphasen

1. Die Strahlenempfindlichkeit von Zellen in Plateau-Phase

Zellen in vitro können sich nicht unbegrenzt vermehren. Man unterscheidet in Zellkulturen drei Wachstumsphasen: eine meist nur wenige Stunden dauernde „lag"-Phase im Anschluß an Trypsinierung und Passagieren der Zellen (über die Strahlenempfindlichkeit dieser Phase s. S. 53), gefolgt von der Phase der exponentiellen Zellvermehrung. Bei Erreichen einer kritischen Zelldichte verlangsamt sich die Zunahme der Zellzahl und erreicht schließlich ein Plateau. Bei L-Zellen in Suspensionskultur liegt die Plateau-Zelldichte bei etwa 2 000 000 Zellen/ml (Eidam u. Merchant, 1965). Auch Kulturen, in denen die Zellen auf der Glasoberfläche ausgebreitet wachsen, zeigen die drei Wachstumsphasen

Abb. 35). Die Proliferationskinetik von Plateauphasezellen wurde insbesondere von HAHN u. Mitarb. (1968) an chinesischen Hamsterzellen (HAZ) untersucht. Wenn in den Petrischalen das Medium täglich gewechselt wird, bildet sich bei einer Zelldichte von 10^6 Zellen/cm^2 Oberfläche ein lange dauerndes Plateau aus. Da kein nutritiver Mangelzustand für die Wachstumshemmung verantwortlich sein kann, beschrieb HAHN (1969) diesen Zustand als Übervölkerungseffekt. Die reproduktive Integrität der Zellen in übervölkerten Kulturen nimmt um etwa 15 % pro Tag ab. Etwa 90 % der Zellen befinden sich in einer Art Ruhephase (wohl einer stark verlängerten G_1- oder G_0- Phase), nur 10 % der Population wachsen mit einer stark verlängerten Generationszeit weiter. Ganz andere Verhältnisse liegen vor, wenn das Plateau durch einen nutritiven Mangelzustand (d.h. durch Belassen des gleichen Mediums für die Dauer des Versuchs) bewirkt wird. In solchen „hungernden" Kulturen wird das Plateau bei etwa 10^5 Zellen/cm^2 Oberfläche erreicht. Weniger als 1 % der Zellen proliferiert mit praktisch normaler Generationszeit, alle anderen Zellen sind in einem Ruhezustand, in dem sie ohne wesentliche Beeinträchtigung ihrer reproduktiven Integrität verbleiben.

Da Plateauphase-Zellen vielleicht den Eigenschaften von Zellen in soliden Tumoren näher kommen als die üblichen exponentiell wachsenden Zellkulturen (HAHN, 1969), sind Veränderungen der Strahlenempfindlichkeit mit dem Wachstumszyklus von besonderem Interesse. In den beiden oben beschriebenen unterschiedlichen Plateau-Zuständen von chinesischen Hamsterzellen ergaben sich folgende Dosiseffektkurven: die D_0, die in exponentiell wachsenden Kulturen 142 rad betrug, nahm in übervölkerten Kulturen auf 135 rad, in den „hungernden" Kulturen auf 127 rad ab. Die Extrapolationsnummer änderte sich bei „hungernden" Zellen kaum, in den übervölkerten Kulturen war die Schulter aber völlig verschwunden, so daß eine rein exponentielle Dosiseffektkurve resultierte (STEWART u. Mitarb., 1968; HAHN, 1969). Auch RÉVÉSZ u. LITTBRAND (1969b) fanden bei chinesischen Hamsterzellen eines anderen Stammes (V-79) eine ausgeprägte Verkleinerung der Schulter mit einer Abnahme der Extrapolationsnummer von 10 auf 2, ohne daß eine Änderung der D_0 auftrat.

LUDOVICI u. Mitarb. (1961) bestimmten die D_{50} von HeLa-Zellen in verschiedenen Wachstumsphasen und beobachteten einen Anstieg von 107 R auf 130 R im stationären Zustand. MADOC-JONES (1964) fand, daß die Dosiseffektkurve von Rattensarkomzellen in vitro mit zunehmendem Alter der Kultur bei gleichzeitigem Anwachsen der Schulter immer steiler wurde, wie auch LITTLE (1969) an Chang-Leberzellen eine Abnahme der D_0 von 152 rad auf 123 rad und einen Anstieg der Extrapolationsnummer von 2,2 auf 3,7 beobachtete.

HAHN (1969) und BERRY u. Mitarb. (1970) stellten fest, daß die Strahlenwirkung auf Zellen in Plateauphase stark von der Art des Mediums, in dem die Zellen wachsen, abhängt. Die deutlich höhere Strahlenempfindlichkeit von HeLa-Zellen bei Bestrahlung in Plateauphase in einem nukleotidarmen Nährmedium (die D_0 nahm von 201 rad auf 135 rad ab [BERRY u. Mitarb., 1970]) läßt sich durch eine Akkumulation der Zellen am Übergang von G_1- in S-Phase erklären.

Werden chinesische Hamsterzellen (V-79) aus der Plateauphase in neue Kulturgefäße umgesetzt, durchlaufen sie den ersten Zellzyklus fast synchron, wobei allerdings die G_1-Phase deutlich verlängert ist. Entsprechend dieser teilsynchronen Progression ändert sich die Strahlenempfindlichkeit der Zellen in den ersten 25 Stunden nach der Subkultivierung (CHAPMAN u. Mitarb., 1970; s. a. BERRY u. Mitarb., 1966).

Die Erforschung der Strahlenbiologie von Säugetierzellen in stationären Kulturen ist noch nicht abgeschlossen. Soweit die vorliegenden Ergebnisse überhaupt eine zusammenfassende Darstellung erlauben, ist zu sagen, daß Zellen in Plateauphase in der Regel strahlenempfindlicher sind als entsprechende Zellen in der exponentiellen Wachstumsphase. Das äußert sich z.T. in einer Verkleinerung der Schulter, z.T. in einer Abnahme der D_0 der Dosiswirkungskurve. Die höhere Strahlenempfindlichkeit von Zellen in Plateauphase dürfte vor allem in der Akkumulation von Zellen in einer relativ strahlenempfindlichen Zellzyklusphase, d.h. einer partiellen Synchronisation ihre Ursache haben.

2. Die Abhängigkeit der Strahlenwirkung vom Zellzyklus

Bei direkter Beobachtung proliferierender Zellen kann man nur zwischen zwei Zuständen der Zelle unterscheiden: der Mitose und der intermitotischen Phase. Während des exponentiellen Wachstums der Population sind die Generationszeiten der Zellen, d.i. die Zeitspanne zwischen zwei Teilungen, relativ festgelegt und schwanken nur wenig um einen Mittelwert (Abb. 36), der für die meisten Zellarten in vitro zwischen 8 und 30 Stunden liegt.

In der Zeit zwischen den Teilungen, bereitet sich die Zelle durch Verdoppelung ihres DNS-Gehaltes auf die nächste Mitose vor. Howard u. Pelc (1953) stellten fest, daß diese DNS-Neusynthese nicht kontinuierlich während der ganzen intermitotischen Phase erfolgt, sondern nur in einer auf deren Mitte beschränkten Zeitspanne. Sie bezeichneten die damit abgrenzbaren Zyklusphasen als präsynthetisches Intervall (G_1), Synthesephase (S), postsynthetisches Intervall (G_2) und Mitose (M). Es muß ausdrücklich betont werden, daß diese Bezeichnungen sich nur auf die DNS-Synthese und die Mitose beziehen, und daß die Phasen des DNS-Zyklus in sich nicht homogen sind und auch nicht unbedingt für andere

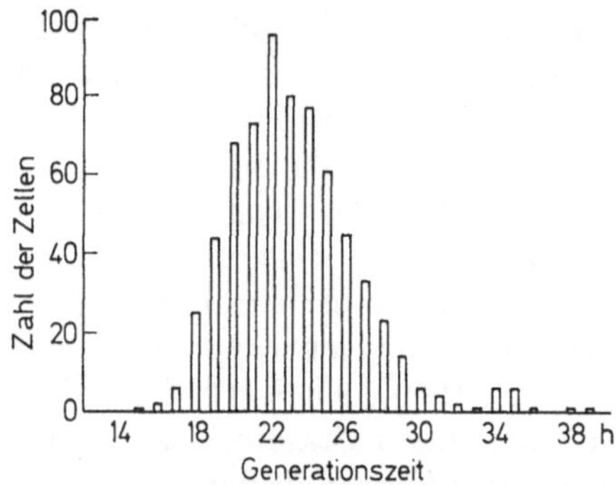

Abb. 36. Verteilung der Generationszeiten unbestrahlter L-Zellen (Die Werte wurden durch Auswertung von Zeitrafferfilmen an 650 Zellen eines Klons gewonnen). (Trott, unveröffentlicht)

zyklisch verlaufende Zellprozesse den Zeitmaßstab setzen. Da die Phasen des DNS-Zyklus am einfachsten feststellbar und bei nahezu allen proliferierenden Zellarten vorhanden sind, werden sie allgemein zur Markierung bestimmter Abschnitte innerhalb der Generationszeit der Zellen verwendet.

Zellen weisen in verschiedenen Zellzyklusphasen unterschiedliche Strahlenempfindlichkeiten auf. Versuche zur Testung dieser Unterschiede werden in der Regel an synchronisierten Zellkulturen durchgeführt. Auf die verschiedenen Methoden der Synchronisation wird auf Seite 91 f. kurz eingegangen.

Die ersten Versuche mit synchronisierten Säugetierzellen in vitro stammen von Terasima u. Tolmach (1961). HeLa-Zellen wurden in Mitosephase synchronisiert und zu verschiedenen Zeitpunkten nach der Synchronisation mit 300 rad bestrahlt. Die Überlebensraten waren je nach Intervall zwischen Synchronisation und Bestrahlung verschieden hoch (Abb. 37).

Wenn zwischen Synchronisation und Bestrahlung 2—3 Stunden vergangen waren, überlebten fast 8 mal so viele Zellen, als wenn die gleiche Dosis sofort nach der Synchronisation gegeben wurde, d.h. die frühe G_1-Phase war ausgesprochen strahlenresistent. Diesem Gipfel der Strahlenresistenz folgte eine Phase zunehmender Strahlenempfindlichkeit. Aus der in Abb. 37 im gleichen Zeitmaßstab hinzugefügten Kurve der nach ³HTdR-Zugabe markierten, d.h. in S-Phase befindlichen Zellen, kann man ersehen, daß das 2. Maximum der Strahlenempfindlichkeit (= Minimum der Kurve) mit dem Beginn der DNS-Synthese zusammenfiel. Es folgte eine zweite Steigerung der Strahlenresistenz bis zu einem Maximum etwa am Ende der DNS-Synthesephase.

Mit zunehmendem Zeitabstand von der Synchronisation wird die Auflösung der Kurve schlechter, weil die Population sich entsprechend den statistischen Schwankungen der Generationszeiten (Abb. 36) unterschiedlich schnell durch den Zyklus bewegt. Aus diesem Grund ist insbesondere eine Bestimmung der Strahlenempfindlichkeit der Zellen der G_2-Phase problematisch (s. S. 88).

In späteren Versuchen bestimmten TERASIMA u. TOLMACH (1963a und b) Dosiseffektkurven synchronisierter HeLa-Zellen (Abb. 38). Man muß beachten, daß nur die Dosiseffektkurve zum Zeitpunkt 0 die einer Einzelzelle ist, während die anderen alle von den beiden Tochterzellen der in Mitose synchronisierten Mutterzelle ausgehen. Wenn man die Kurven entsprechend korrigiert, haben alle eine Extrapolationsnummer von 1—2, aber unterschiedliche Neigungen. Den empfindlichen Zyklusphasen entsprechen D_0-Werte von

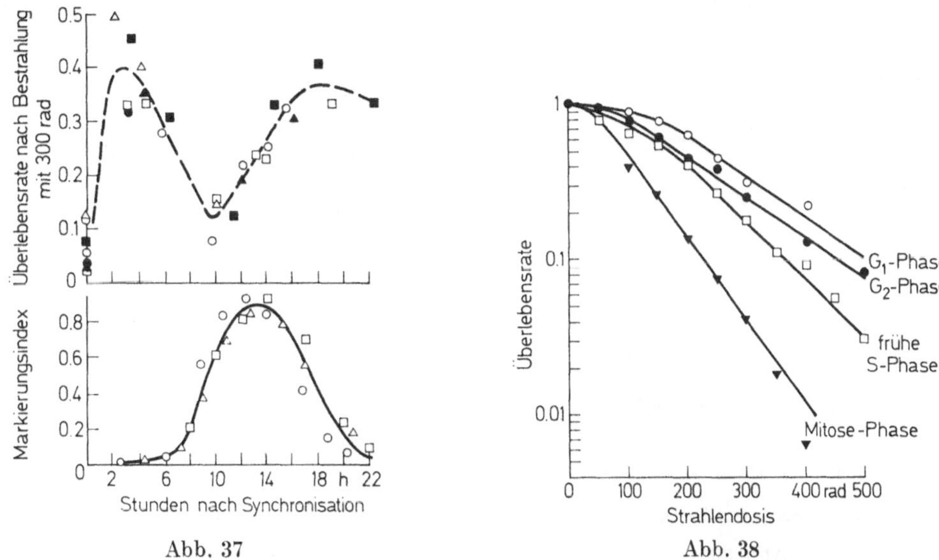

Abb. 37. Überlebensrate von synchronisierten HeLa-Zellen nach 300 rad Röntgenstrahlen zu verschiedenen Zeiten nach Synchronisation in Mitose (obere Kurve) sowie der Markierungsindex (Anteil der in S-Phase befindlichen Zellen) zu verschiedenen Zeiten nach der Synchronisation (untere Kurve). (TERASIMA u. TOLMACH, 1963a)

Abb. 38. Dosiseffektkurven von HeLa-Zellen bei Bestrahlung 4 Stunden (G_1-Phase), 13 Stunden (frühe S-Phase), 19 Stunden (G_2-Phase) und unmittelbar nach Synchronisation in Mitose mit 220 kV-Röntgenstrahlen. (TERASIMA u. TOLMACH, 1963a)

82 rad (Mitosephase) und 121 rad (G_1-S-Übergang), den resistenten Phasen D_0-Werte von 164 rad (frühe G_1-Phase) und 170 rad (späte S-Phase).

Die ausführlichsten Arbeiten über die Abhängigkeit der Strahlenwirkung vom Zellzyklus stammen von SINCLAIR und verschiedenen Mitarbeitern (1963ff.). Er arbeitete vor allem mit dem Stamm V-79 chinesischer Hamsterzellen, für die eine besonders kurze Generationszeit von 10 Stunden typisch ist (SINCLAIR u. MORTON, 1964). Diese ist vor allem durch eine sehr kurze G_1-Phase bedingt. Im Gegensatz zu der zweigipfeligen Kurve der Strahlenempfindlichkeit von HeLa-Zellen weisen V-79-Zellen nur ein einziges Resistenzmaximum auf, das in der S-Phase gelegen ist (SINCLAIR u. MORTON, 1963). Spätere, detailliertere Untersuchungen ergaben, daß der Gipfel gegen Ende der S-Phase auftritt (Abb. 39), (SINCLAIR, u. MORTON, 1966). Eine bessere Auflösung der verschiedenen Zeitpunkte war durch eine „Nachsynchronisation" zu Beginn der S-Phase möglich. Dabei wurden die Zellen, die schon mit der DNS-Synthese begonnen hatten, während die meisten Zellen noch in G_1-Phase waren, durch ein S-Phasen-spezifisches Agens (hier ³HTdR hoher Aktivität) zerstört. Nach Anwendung dieser „Nachreinigung" konnte auch der ursprüngliche Befund, daß die Dosiseffektkurven der Zellen in verschiedenen Zyklusphasen alle die gleiche D_0 besitzen und nur in ihrer Extrapolationsnummer verschieden sind (Sinclair u. Morton, 1965) nicht aufrecht erhalten werden. Bei Betrachtung der verschiedenen Kurven (Abb. 40) fällt auf, daß die Zellen in Mitose eine rein exponentielle Dosiswirkungskurve zeigen, während mit zunehmendem Alter der Zelle sowohl die Schulter als auch die D_0 größer werden.

Unterschiede in der Strahlenempfindlichkeit werden meist als Dosismodifikationsfaktor angegeben (DMF), d.h. als Quotient der Strahlendosen, die benötigt werden, um die Überlebensrate auf den gleichen Wert zu drücken. Aus den Versuchen von Terasima u. Tolmach (Abb. 38) ergibt sich ein maximaler DMF von über 2 zwischen den empfindlichsten und den resistentesten Zyklusphasen, aus den Daten von Sinclair und Morton (Abb. 40) ergeben sich sogar noch höhere Werte. Somit sind die Schwankungen der Strahlenempfindlichkeit mit dem Zellzyklus in ihrer Größenordnung durchaus mit den durch unterschiedliche Sauerstoffversorgung bedingten Empfindlichkeitsschwankungen (s. S. 105) vergleichbar.

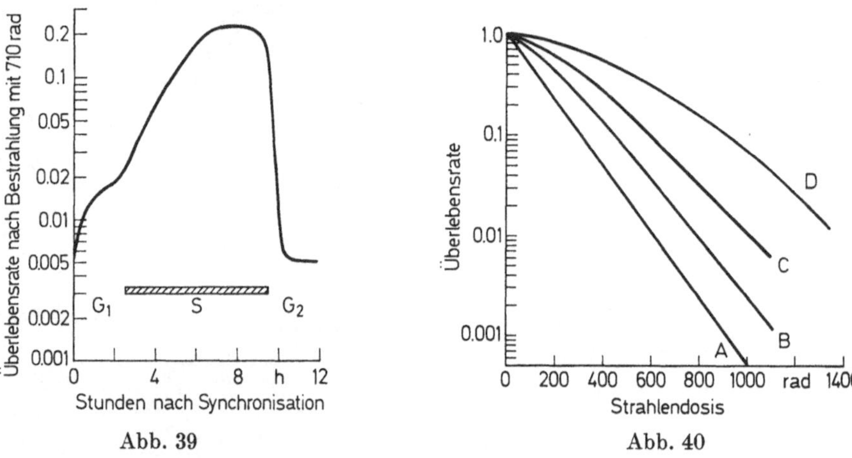

Abb. 39. Überlebensrate von synchronisierten chinesischen Hamsterzellen (V-79) nach Bestrahlung mit 710 rad Röntgenstrahlen zu verschiedenen Zeiten nach Synchronisation in Mitose (Nachsynchronisation mit ^{3}H-TdR). (Nach Sinclair, 1968a)

Abb. 40. Dosiseffektkurven von chinesischen Hamsterzellen (V-79) bei Bestrahlung in Mitose (A), G_1-Phase (B), früher S-Phase (C) und später S-Phase (D) mit 250 kV-Röntgenstrahlen. (Nach Sinclair, 1968a)

Es kann nicht Aufgabe dieser Arbeit sein, die Schwankungen der Strahlenempfindlichkeit für die verschiedenen untersuchten Zellarten aufzuzählen. Es wird daher auf die Übersichtsarbeit von Sinclair (1968a) zu diesem Thema verwiesen. Es sollen nur einige wichtig erscheinende spezielle Probleme herausgegriffen werden.

Die Bestimmung der Strahlenempfindlichkeit von Zellen in G_2-Phase ist praktisch nur durch die kombinierte Anwendung mehrerer Synchronisationsverfahren möglich. Sinclair u. Morton (1966) und Djordjevic u. Tolmach (1967) verwendeten zur „Nachsynchronisation", in diesem Fall zur Elimination „verspäteter" Zellen, ^{3}HTdR hoher spezifischer Aktivität. Eine Dreifachbehandlung wandten Thompson u. Humphrey (1969) bei L-Zellen an: Als die Mehrzahl der in Mitose synchronisierten Zellen in G_2-Phase erwartet wurde, wurde die Kultur mit Colcemid und ^{3}HTdR versetzt. Während ^{3}HTdR alle Zellen, die noch in S-Phase waren, abtötete, blockierte Colcemid alle Zellen, die eine Mitose versuchten. Übrig blieben ausschließlich G_2-Zellen. Elkind u. Kano (1971) synchronisierten chinesische Hamsterzellen, die nur eine extrem kurze G_1-Phase haben (V-79-661), in G_2-Phase, indem sie durch gleichzeitige Zugabe von Hydroxyharnstoff und des Proteinsynthesehemmers Cycloheximid die Zellen der S-Phase abtöteten und die der G_2-Phase blockierten. In allen Fällen, in denen besondere Mühe darauf verwendet worden war, reine G_2-Populationen zu erhalten, zeigte sich, daß die G_2-Phase zu den strahlenempfindlichsten Phasen des Zellzyklus gehört, daß diese hohe Strahlenempfindlichkeit aber dann, wenn sich beträchtliche Anteile der Population in den „benachbarten", besonders strahlenresistenten Phasen (z.T. Anfang G_1 und besonders Ende S) befinden, maskiert wird (s. Abb. 37), (vgl. S. 19).

Es besteht Übereinstimmung darüber, daß Zellen in der späten S-Phase besonders strahlenresistent sind. Dagegen gibt es widersprüchliche Angaben über die Strahlenempfindlichkeit der Zellen in G_1. Von verschiedenen Beobachtern wurde immer wieder bestätigt, daß die frühe G_1-Phase bei HeLa-Zellen zu den resistentesten Phasen gehört (TERASIMA u. TOLMACH, 1961; TOLMACH u. Mitarb., 1965; PETROVIC u. NIAS, 1967; DJORDJEVIC u. TOLMACH, 1969). In L-Zellen, die eine ähnlich lange Generationszeit wie HeLa-Zellen besitzen, ist die G_1-Phase die strahlenresistenteste Phase (WHITMORE u. Mitarb., 1965). Dagegen war die G_1-Phase in chinesischen Hamsterzellen besonders strahlenempfindlich (Abb. 39, 40). Eine Lösung brachten die Versuche von HAHN u. BAGSHAW (1966), die bei chinesischen Hamsterzellen mit einer kurzen G_1-Phase diese Phase künstlich verlängern konnten, ohne daß die anderen Phasen beeinflußt worden wären. Dabei fanden sie, daß die G_1-Phase um so strahlenresistenter wurde, je länger sie dauerte, so daß bei den längsten erreichbaren G_1-Phasendauern (12—15 Stunden) die G_1-Phase zur strahlenresistentesten Phase des Zellzyklus geworden war. Ebenso trat bei chinesischen Hamsterzellen (V-79), die aus der frühen Plateauphase passagiert wurden, eine Verlängerung der G_1-Phase mit deutlicher Erhöhung der Strahlenresistenz auf (CHAPMAN u. Mitarb., 1970).

Diese und weitere Untersuchungen über die Zyklusabhängigkeit der Strahlenempfindlichkeit zusammenfassend kam SINCLAIR (1968a) zu folgenden Schlußfolgerungen:

"1. Generell sind Zellen in Mitose am empfindlichsten.

2. Wenn G_1 relativ lang ist, findet man meist am Anfang eine resistente Periode, gefolgt von einem Abfall der Überlebensrate, wenn die Zellen sich der S-Phase nähern. Das Ende der G_1-Phase dürfte so empfindlich sein wie die Mitose.

3. In den meisten Zellarten steigt die Strahlenresistenz während der S-Phase bis zu einem Maximum am Ende von S. Das ist in der Regel der resistenteste Teil des Zellzyklus.

4. In den meisten Zellarten ist die G_2-Phase strahlenempfindlich, vielleicht so empfindlich wie die Mitose" (SINCLAIR, 1968a).

Untersuchungen über die Zyklusabhängigkeit der Wirkung ionisierender Strahlen hohen LETs liegen kaum vor. ARLETT (1969) und BIRD u. BURKI (1971) fanden bei synchronisierten chinesischen Hamsterzellen (F bzw. V-79) keine Unterschiede in der Wirkung von Alphastrahlen bzw. beschleunigten Teilchen eines LET von 190 keV$/\mu$ in den verschiedenen Zyklusphasen. Die Strahlenempfindlichkeit der verschiedenen Zellzyklusphasen gegenüber Neutronen weist das gleiche Muster auf wie nach Röntgenbestrahlung, die Schwankungen sind jedoch deutlich geringer (SINCLAIR, 1968b bei Spaltneutronen; HALL, 1969a und MASUDA, 1971 bei D-T-Neutronen [14 MeV]). Während sich die Extrapolationsnummer bei Bestrahlung von chinesischen Hamsterzellen mit Spaltneutronen nicht mit dem Zellzyklus änderte, stieg die D_0 in der S-Phase auf 80 rad, während sie in G_1 und G_2 60 rad betrug (SINCLAIR, 1969c).

Die meisten Zellen sind in der S-Phase nicht zu dem Zeitpunkt der maximalen DNS-Syntheseaktivität am resistentesten, sondern erst dann, wenn $^2/_3$ der DNS schon synthetisiert sind (SINCLAIR, 1969c). Auch dann, wenn die DNS-Synthese blockiert wird, weisen die Zellen mit nur geringer Verzögerung eine phasentypische Steigerung der Strahlenresistenz auf (VOS u. Mitarb., 1966; SINCLAIR, 1967a). Es muß also eine Stoffwechselsituation, die typisch für die S-Phase ist, aber nicht direkt mit der DNS-Synthese gekoppelt ist, für die Resistenzsteigerung verantwortlich sein. Die Entkoppelung läßt sich auch durch Bestrahlung von chinesischen Hamsterzellen am Übergang von G_1- in S-Phase erreichen: zwar wird die DNS-Synthese dabei nicht gehemmt, aber der Anstieg der Strahlenresistenz wesentlich gebremst (Elkind u. Kano, 1971). Hinweise auf die Ursache dieser Strahlenempfindlichkeitsschwankungen boten Untersuchungen über die Zyklusabhängigkeit der Strahlenschutzwirkung von Cysteamin (Sinclair, 1969a). Je größer die Empfindlichkeit der Zellen bestimmter Zyklusphasen war, desto größer war die Schutzwirkung von Cysteamin, so daß nach Cysteaminzugabe die Dosiswirkungskurven der verschiedenen Zyklusphasen dichter beieinander verliefen. Auch bei HeLa-Zellen wurden besonders die empfindlichen Zyklusphasen durch Cysteamin geschützt: In M und am Übergang von G_1 in S-Phase nahm die D_0 von 71 bzw. 66 rad auf 109 bzw. 116 rad (also um den Faktor 1,5—1,75) zu, während in der frühen G_1-Phase nur eine Zunahme von 186 rad auf 203 rad (also um 1,09) zu erreichen war (Mauro, unveröff. zit. n. Tolmach, 1969). Sinclair (1969c) zog daraus den Schluß, daß die Veränderungen der Strahlenempfindlichkeit mit dem Zellzyklus zumindest teilweise Ausdruck unterschiedlicher intrazellulärer Konzentrationen nicht proteingebundener Sulfhydrylgruppen sind. Ohara u. Terasima (1969) fanden tatsächlich bei synchronisierten HeLa-Zellen eine lineare Korrelation von nicht proteingebundenen Sulfhydrylgruppen zur Überlebensrate nach Bestrahlung. Mauro u. Mitarb. (1969) stellten eine ausgeprägte Zyklusabhängigkeit der Konzentrationen von Disulfiden, proteingebundenen Sulfhydrylgruppen und nicht proteingebundenen Sulfhydrylgruppen bei HeLa-Zellen fest; eine enge Korrelation zur Strahlenempfindlichkeit zeigten auch hier die nicht proteingebundenen Sulfhydrylgruppen. Sogar Unterschiede zwischen Zellstämmen verschiedener Strahlenempfindlichkeit konnten auf Unterschiede im SH-Geahlt zurückgeführt werden (Parkhomenco u. Mitarb., 1970).

3. Die Abhängigkeit der Zytostatikawirkung vom Zellzyklus

Viele Zytostatika zeigen ausgeprägte Schwankungen ihrer Wirksamkeit während des Zellzyklus. Die Wirkung alkylierender Zytostatika weist bei L-Zellen (Walker u. Helleiner, 1963), HeLa-Zellen (Mauro u. Madoc-Jones, 1970) und chinesischen Hamsterzellen (Mauro u. Elkind, 1968; Elkind u. Sakamoto, 1969) meist eine ähnliche Abhängigkeit vom Zellzyklus auf wie die von Röntgenstrahlen, während Petrovic u. Nias (1967) eine ganz unterschiedliche Zyklusabhängigkeit von Röntgenstrahlen und Isopropylmethansulfonat fanden.

Mitosegifte, wie Colchizin und Vinca-alkaloide, sind am wirksamsten in der S-Phase des Zellzyklus von chinesischen Hamster- und HeLa-Zellen (Mauro u. Madoc-Jones, 1970). Auffallend ist die relativ hohe Resistenz von Zellen in der Mitosephase gegenüber einer 10 Minuten dauernden Exposition dieser Zytostatika.

Besonderes Interesse gewann die zytotoxische Wirkung von Actinomycin D, weil es die Erholung vom subletalen Strahlenschaden blockiert. Untersuchungen an chinesischen Hamsterzellen (Elkind u. Mitarb., 1968; Elkind u. Sakamoto, 1969; Elkind u. Mitarb., 1969) und an HeLa-Zellen (Djordjevic u. Kim, 1968) zeigten eine maximale Wirkung in der frühen S-Phase und eine maximale Resistenz in der G_2-Phase an, während nach Mauro u. Madoc-Jones (1970) und Bacchetti u. Whitmore (1967) eine enge Parallelität der Zyklusabhängigkeit von Actinomycin D mit der der Strahlenwirkung besteht.

Stoffwechselgifte, welche die Proteinsynthese hemmen, wie z.B. Cycloheximid, sind am wirksamsten am Ende der G_1-Phase von HeLa-Zellen (Mauro u. Madoc-Jones, 1970).

Die Stoffwechselgifte, die direkt die DNS-Synthese blockieren, wie z.B. Hydroxyharnstoff, sind nur während der DNS-Synthesephase wirksam (Sinclair, 1965; Mauro u. Madoc-Jones, 1970). Die DNS-Synthesehemmung scheint nicht direkt für den Zelltod verantwortlich zu sein. Eher dürfte er Folge des durch die Hydroxyharnstoffzugabe induzierten unbalancierten Wachstums sein (Bacchetti u. Whitmore, 1969). Die zytotoxische Wirkung von Fluordesoxyuridin hängt nicht vom Zellzyklus der chinesischen Hamsterzellen ab (Lozzio, 1969).

4. Synchronisation

Die Untersuchungen über die Zyklusabhängigkeit der Strahlenwirkung erfordern die Verwendung synchronisierter Zellpopulationen. Während man manchen primitiven Organismen (z.B. Tetrahymena) durch periodische Reize ein synchrones oder teilsynchrones Wachstum von außen aufprägen kann, sind solche Versuche bei Säugetierzellen in vitro bisher nicht geglückt. In vivo ist jedoch in vielen Geweben eine spontane rhythmische, d.h. teilsynchrone Aktivität der Zellproliferation zu beobachten.

Die Methoden, Zellen einer asynchronen Population zu synchronisieren, beruhen im wesentlichen auf 2 Prinzipien: entweder wird ein Proliferationsblock durch Zugabe eines Stoffwechselgiftes gesetzt, nach dessen Entfernung die Zellen, die auf den Block aufgelaufen sind, synchron weiterwachsen, oder es werden aus einer asynchronen Population Zellen, die sich alle in der gleichen Zyklusphase befinden, entnommen, indem man entweder alle anderen Zellen abtötet oder die gewünschte Population isoliert.

Letzteres Prinzip ist das in der Zellkultur am längsten verwendete und für viele Zellstämme und Fragestellungen am besten geeignete, da es die geringste Alteration der iso-

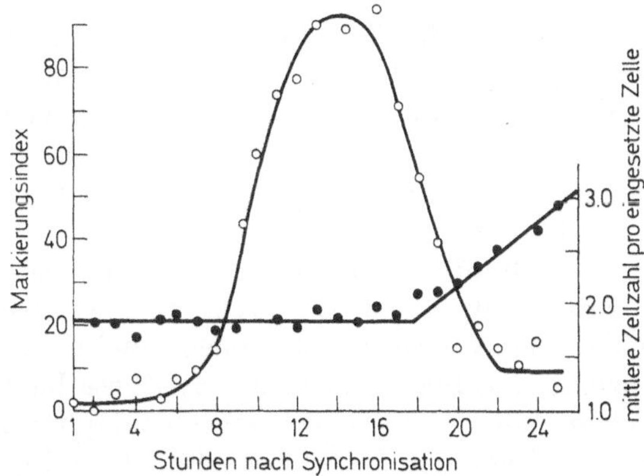

Abb. 41. Markierungsindex (Kreise und linke Ordinate) und mittlere Zellzahl pro eingesetzte Zelle (Punkte und rechte Ordinate) in synchronisierten HeLa-Zellen nach Markierung mit Tritium-Thymidin zu verschiedenen Stunden nach Synchronisation in Mitose. (PETROVIC u. NIAS, 1967)

lierten Zellen garantiert. TERASIMA u. TOLMACH (1961) nutzten die Tatsache aus, daß Zellen, die während der intermitotischen Zeitspanne breitflächig auf dem Glasboden des Kulturgefäßes sitzen, für die Zeit der Mitose eine Kugelform annehmen und dadurch weniger fest haften. Durch vorsichtiges Schütteln der Kultur lassen sich diese Zellen ablösen und isolieren. Nach erneuter Inkubation vollenden die Zellen den Teilungsprozeß innerhalb kurzer Zeit und wachsen synchron weiter. Die Ausbeute an synchronen Zellen ist nicht sehr groß, da die Mitose nur einen kleinen Bruchteil des Zellzyklus ausmacht, dafür ist die Synchronisationsschärfe um so besser. Die Ausbeute kann durch Vorinkubation mit Colcemid für einige Stunden wesentlich verbessert werden (STUBBLEFIELD u. KLEVECZ, 1965).

Die Synchronisationsschärfe nimmt mit der Zeit wieder ab. Ein Beispiel für die fortschreitende Desynchronisation bietet Abb. 41 (PETROVIC u. NIAS, 1967). In einer in Mitosephase synchronisierten Population von HeLa-Zellen wurden in kurzen Abständen die Zahl der Zellen in S-Phase und die Zahl der geteilten Zellen bestimmt. Gleich nach der Synchronisation waren aus 90% der Zellen zwei Zellen entstanden (mittlere Zellzahl pro eingesetzte Zelle = 1,8). Wenn die Population synchron weiterwachsen würde, müßte die Zahl der S-Phase-Zellen nach Ende der G_1-Phase ebenso schlagartig auf über 90 % steigen und am Ende der S-Phase ebenso plötzlich wieder auf 0 absinken. Die Zellzahl pro Mikrokolonie dürfte auch erst einige Zeit nach dem Abfall des Markierungsindex ansteigen. Die zunehmende Verschleifung dieser Kurven ist ein Maß für die Desynchronisation, so wie sie sich auch in der Verteilungskurve der Generationszeiten (Abb. 36) ausdrückt. Eine Desynchronisation tritt nach allen Synchronisationsmethoden auf.

Eine andere Methode der Isolierung von Zellen einer Zyklusphase nutzt die Größenunterschiede der Zellen während des Zellzyklus aus. Durch Sedimentation in Sucrose-Gradienten kann man G_1-Zellen in der oberen Fraktion anreichern (SINCLAIR u. BISHOP, 1965). Verschiedene Gruppen haben sich um die Verbesserung der Methode bemüht, doch ist die Synchronisationsschärfe noch unbefriedigend (NIAS u. FOX, 1971).

Auch die selektive Abtötung von Zellen bestimmter Zyklusphasen kann zur Synchronisation verwendet werden. Wenn die geeignete toxische Substanz für längere Zeit gegeben wird und dabei keine Störungen in der Progression der nicht betroffenen Zellen auftreten, wandern immer mehr Zellen in die Phase, in der sie abgetötet werden. Nach Auswaschen der toxischen Substanz bleibt ein „Fenster" gleich alter, lebensfähiger Zellen, das beliebig schmal gemacht werden kann (WHITMORE u. Mitarb., 1965). Die für diese Methode am besten geeignete Substanz ist ^{3}HTdR hoher spezifischer Aktivität: Zellen in S-Phase inkorporieren die aktive Substanz in letalen Mengen („Radioaktiver Selbstmord"), Mit dieser Methode, die allgemein anwendbar ist, läßt sich eine gute Synchronisation am Ende der G_1-Phase erreichen.

Die Progression der Zellen durch den Zellzyklus läßt sich mit FUdR blockieren (EIDINOFF u. RICH, 1959). Nach Zugabe von Thymidin oder Auswaschen des FUdR beginnen die Zellen synchron mit der DNS-Synthese. Es muß darauf hingewiesen werden, daß durch die Blockierung der DNS-Synthese die anderen zyklischen Wachstumsvorgänge nicht notwendigerweise auch blockiert werden. Die sonst aufeinander abgestimmten Stoffwechselprozesse werden entkoppelt, und es tritt ein pathologischer Zustand auf, der als „unbalanciertes Wachstum" (RUECKERT u. MUELLER, 1960) bezeichnet wird. Eine Blockierung an gleicher Stelle läßt sich durch hohe Konzentrationen von Thymidin erreichen (XEROS, 1962). Hydroxyharnstoff kann chinesische Hamsterzellen synchronisieren, indem es S-Phase-Zellen abtötet und gleichzeitig den Beginn der DNS-Synthese blockiert (SINCLAIR, 1965).

Auf Grund der zyklischen Unterschiede in der Strahlenempfindlichkeit wirkt auch eine Bestrahlung synchronisierend. Nach den Daten der Abb. 40 sind nach einer Strahlendosis von mehreren hundert rad etwa 90 % der überlebenden chinesischen Hamsterzellen einer asynchronen Population in der strahlenresistenten S-Phase. Das hat natürlich Folgen für die Wirkung einer fraktionierten Bestrahlung (s. S. 97). Die Zyklusabhängigkeit der mitosehemmenden Wirkung einer Bestrahlung kann zur Synchronisation in G_2-Phase ausgenützt werden (LINDEN u. Mitarb., 1970; PRÉVÔT u. Mitarb., 1971).

Diese unvollständige Übersicht über die verschiedenen Synchronisationsmethoden (ausführlichere kritische Darstellungen liegen von SINCLAIR, 1969b und NIAS u. FOX, 1971 vor) sollte die Wirkungsprinzipien der wichtigsten Synchronisationsmethoden aufzeigen. Die Synchronisationsschärfe und die Ausbeute wechseln von Methode zu Methode und von Zellstamm zu Zellstamm. Durch Kombination verschiedener Methoden (s. S. 88) lassen sich Desynchronisationseffekte teilweise kompensieren.

VIII. Erholungsprozesse nach Bestrahlung

1. Fraktionierungseffekt

a) Der Fraktionierungseffekt bei locker ionisierenden Strahlen

Die Reaktivität von Säugetierzellen — graphisch gesehen die Neigung der halblogarithmischen Dosiswirkungskurve — nimmt in der Regel mit zunehmender Dosis zu, bis sie bei Dosen über 300—500 rad einen konstanten Wert erreicht hat (s. S. 6f.). Werden Zellen, die eine erste Strahlendosis von einigen hundert rad überleben, unmittelbar im Anschluß an diese erste Bestrahlung einer 2. Bestrahlung ausgesetzt, werden sie entsprechend ihrer durch die Vorbestrahlung erhöhten Reaktivität inaktiviert. Vergeht jedoch zwischen der ersten und der zweiten Strahlendosis einige Zeit, so haben die Überlebenden der ersten Dosisfraktion ihre ursprüngliche Reaktivität wieder gewonnen und werden nach einer Schulterkurve inaktiviert, so wie Zellen, die nie vorher bestrahlt worden waren (Abb. 42). Diese Restitution der ursprünglichen Reaktivität nach einer ersten Strahlendosis wird nach ELKIND allgemein als *Erholung vom subletalen Strahlenschaden* (recovery of sublethal damage) bezeichnet. Sie führt dazu, daß eine fraktionierte Bestrahlung weniger wirksam ist als eine Einzeitbestrahlung gleicher Gesamtdosis (=*Fraktionierungseffekt*, nach ALPER u. Mitarb. [1969]: sparing effect of fractionation). Der Fraktionierungseffekt wird meist quantifiziert als die Änderung der absoluten Überlebensraten der fraktioniert bestrahlten gegenüber der einzeitig bestrahlten Population oder als der Quotient dieser Überlebensraten (= *Fraktionierungsfaktor*). Mit Blick auf die strahlentherapeutische Bedeutung (s. S. 97) wird häufig auch die Differenz gleich wirksamer Dosen (Gesamtdosis bei fraktionierter Bestrahlung — Dosis bei Einschlagbestrahlung = $D_2 - D_1$) als Maß des Fraktionierungseffektes angegeben.

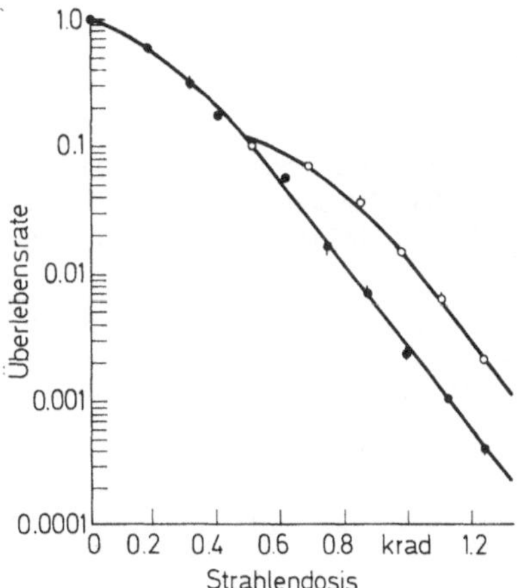

Abb. 42. Dosiswirkungskurven von chinesischen Hamsterzellen (V-79) bei einmaliger Bestrahlung (Punkte) und bei fraktionierter Bestrahlung nach einer ersten Dosis von 505 rad und einem Fraktionierungsintervall von 18 Stunden (Kreise). (Nach ELKIND u. SUTTON, 1960)

Seit 1959 hat sich vor allem ELKIND mit dem Problem der Wirkung fraktionierter Strahlendosen auf Säugetierzellen in vitro befaßt. Ein typisches Experiment zeigt Abb. 42. Die ausgefüllten Punkte geben die Dosiswirkungskurve bei Einzeitbestrahlung an — eine typische Schulterkurve. Wird eine Dosis von 505 rad appliziert und dann 18 Stunden lang die Kultur bei 37° C inkubiert, so reagiert die Restpopulation auf die 2. Bestrahlung wie die ursprüngliche Population: die Dosiswirkungskurve hat die gleiche Schulter und die gleiche Endneigung. Den zeitlichen Verlauf der Wiederherstellung der Schulter zeigt Abb. 43 (ELKIND u. SUTTON, 1960) bei der gleichen Zellinie nach einer ersten Dosis von 505 rad und einer 2. Dosis von 487 rad. Werden beide Dosen ohne Intervall appliziert, ist die Überlebensrate wie nach 992 rad Einzeitdosis 0,186 %. Schon ein bestrahlungsfreies Intervall von 30 Minuten läßt die Gesamtüberlebensrate auf etwa das Doppelte ansteigen. Einem sehr raschen Anstieg und ersten Maximum bei einem Intervall von 2 Stunden folgt ein Absinken auf ein Minimum bei 4—6 Stunden, worauf sich ein erneuter Anstieg auf ein Plateau anschließt. Schematisch dargestellt als Schwankungen der Extrapolationsnummer der 2. Dosiseffektkurve nach einer ersten Dosis von 433 rad läßt sich für chinesische Hamsterzellen (V-79) folgender Verlauf erkennen (Abb. 44): Das erste Maximum, etwa dem halben Wert der Extrapolationsnummer der Ursprungspopulation entsprechend, ist nach ca. 2,5 h erreicht. Das Minimum, hier ein völliges Verschwinden der Schulter, liegt bei 5,5 Stunden. Der Wiederanstieg auf das Plateau fällt mit dem Ende der Mitosehemmung zeitlich zusammen. Das Plateau bleibt bestehen, bis durch weitere Zellteilungen die Zellzahl ansteigt und allein aus diesem Grund die Extrapolationsnummer weiter ansteigt (s. S. 53). Dieser oszillierende Verlauf des Fraktionierungseffektes ist durch das 1961 zum ersten Mal formulierte Restitutions-Progressions-Modell erklärt (ELKIND u. Mitarb., 1961) (s. S. 97).

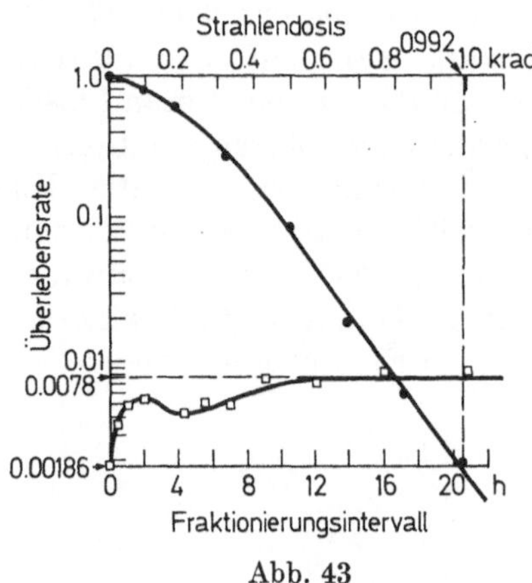
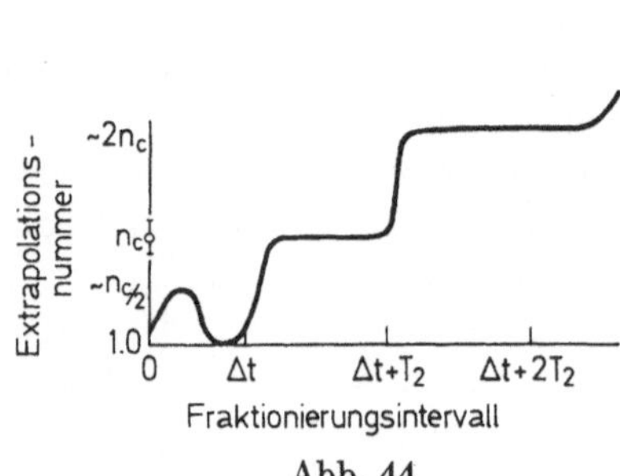

Abb. 43   Abb. 44

Abb. 43. Dosiseffektkurve von chinesischen Hamsterzellen (V-79) bei Röntgenbestrahlung —●—●— (Strahlendosis in der oberen Abszisse) sowie die Überlebensrate nach einer Gesamtdosis von 992 rad bei fraktionierter Bestrahlung (1. Dosis = 505 rad, 2. Dosis = 487 rad) mit zunehmendem Fraktionierungsintervall —□—□— (untere Abszisse). (Nach ELKIND u. SUTTON, 1960)

Abb. 44: Schematische Darstellung der zeitlichen Schwankungen der Extrapolationsnummer einer Zweitbestrahlung nach einer konditionierenden Strahlendosis von 433 rad. n_c = Extrapolationsnummer der ursprünglichen Population; Δt = Zeitdauer der Mitoseverzögerung; T_2 = Generationszeit der Zellen. (Nach ELKIND u. Mitarb., 1961)

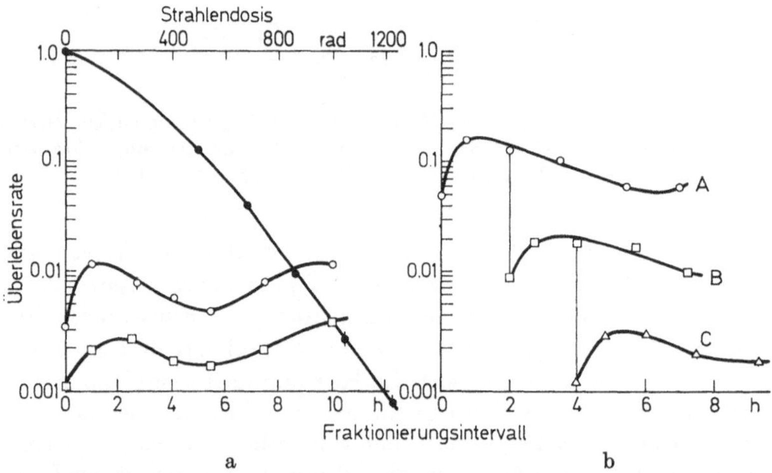

a   b

Abb. 45a. Verlauf des ersten und zweiten Fraktionierungszyklus bei Bestrahlung von chinesischen Hamsterzellen (V-79) mit 2 bzw. 3 Dosen von 505 rad (Erläuterung im Text). (Nach ELKIND u. SUTTON, 1960)

b. Die Überlebensrate von chinesischen Hamsterzellen (V-79) bei mehrfach fraktionierter Bestrahlung:
Kurve A: 433 rad — zunehmendes Fraktionierungsintervall — 433 rad
Kurve B: 433 rad — nach 2 h wieder 433 rad — zunehmendes Fraktionierungsintervall — 433 rad
Kurve C: 433 rad — nach 2 h wieder 433 rad — nach weiteren 2 h wieder 433 rad — zunehmendes Fraktionierungsintervall — 433 rad. (Nach ELKIND u. SINCLAIR, 1965)

Bei mehrfacher Fraktionierung kann sich jedesmal der gleiche Vorgang wiederholen (Abb. 45a), (ELKIND u. SUTTON, 1960). Die Kreise zeigen den Verlauf der Überlebensrate nach 2 Dosen von 505 rad mit zunehmendem Intervall. Die untere, durch Quadrate markierte Kurve gibt den Verlauf der Überlebensrate nach 3 Dosen von 505 rad an, wobei zwischen erster und zweiter Dosis ein bestrahlungsfreies Intervall von 23 Stunden liegt.

Den Anfangsverlauf der Erholungskurve bei 2—4 Fraktionen mit Intervallen von 2 Stunden zeigt Abb. 45b. Hier wird noch deutlicher, wie nach jeder Dosisfraktion die überlebende Population von neuem die zyklischen Schwankungen der Schultergröße durchläuft.

Idealisiert kann man sich den Verlauf der Dosiswirkungskurve für mehrfach fraktionierte Bestrahlung mit bestrahlungsfreien Intervallen, die lang genug sind, um einen maximalen Fraktionierungseffekt zu gestatten, wie in Abb. 46a vorstellen (ELKIND u. SUTTON, 1960): jede neue Dosisfraktion bildet eine neue, gleichgroße Schulter aus. Die resultierende Dosiswirkungskurve für fraktionierte Bestrahlung ergibt in ihrem mittleren Verlauf eine Exponentialfunktion, deren Neigung um so flacher ist, je kleiner die Dosis der Einzelfraktionen ist. Diese idealisierte Dosiswirkungskurve wurde von ELKIND u. SUTTON auch experimentell bestätigt (Abb. 46b). Neben der Dosiswirkungskurve für Einzeitbestrahlung sind die Überlebensraten nach Bestrahlung in 1, 2, 3, 4 und 5 Fraktionen von 505 rad, jeweils mit 22stündigem bestrahlungsfreien Intervall angegeben. Sie liegen auf einer Geraden, die der theoretisch angenommenen Exponentialfunktion entspricht.

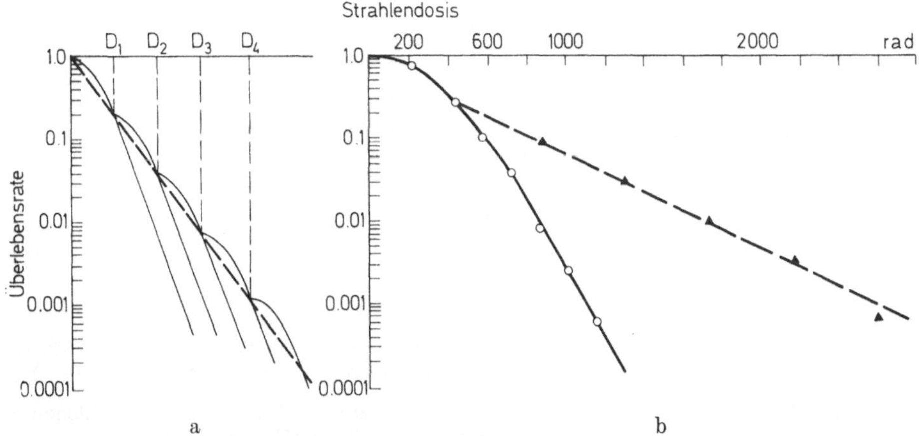

Abb. 46a. Schema der wiederholten Restitution der Schulter bei mehrfach fraktionierter Bestrahlung mit der Einzeldosis D. (ELKIND u. SUTTON, 1960)
b. Überlebensraten von chinesischen Hamsterzellen nach einmaliger Bestrahlung (Kreise) sowie nach mehrmaliger Bestrahlung mit 433 rad bei Bestrahlungsintervallen von je 22 h. (Nach ELKIND u. SUTTON, 1960)

Die Überlebensrate nach 2600 rad, in 5 solchen Fraktionen gegeben, ist 1600 mal höher, als wenn die gleiche Dosis auf einmal gegeben wurde.

Für nahezu alle untersuchten Zelltypen in vivo wie in vitro wurden ähnliche Kurven gefunden, wobei je nach Zellart und Einzeldosen die Höhe des ersten Maximums, der Zeitpunkt und das Ausmaß der vorübergehenden Senke und der spätere Verlauf variierten.

HeLa-Zellen weisen eine vorübergehende Senke in der Erholungskurve bei etwa 5 Stunden auf (LOCKART u. Mitarb., 1961). Je höher die erste Strahlendosis ist, desto weniger ausgeprägt ist die Senke nach dem ersten Anstieg der Erholungskurve (größere Störungen in der Progression der Zellen durch den Zellzyklus anzeigend). Dagegen ist bei kleineren Erst-Dosen, die noch im Bereich der Schulter der Dosiswirkungskurve liegen, die Höhe des ersten Anstiegs geringer. Bei Einzeldosen unter 100 rad fand BARENDSEN (1968) an menschlichen Nierenzellen (T-1g) keinen Fraktionierungseffekt. MALONE u. Mitarb. (1971) variierten in Versuchen an HeLa-Zellen systematisch die Höhe der ersten Dosis bei gleichbleibender zweiter Dosis von 420 rad sowie die Höhe der 2. Dosis bei gleichbleibender erster Dosis von 420 rad. Der Fraktionierungfaktor zeigte in beiden Fällen eine sehr ähnlich verlaufende Zunahme mit der Strahlendosis bis zu einem Maximum bei den Dosen, wo die Dosiseffektkurve ihre Endneigung erreicht (Abb. 47a und b). Ähnliche Befunde hatte auch BERRY (1967b) schon an HeLa-Zellen erhoben und außerdem festgestellt, daß sich neben der Schulter der Dosiswirkungskurve der zweiten Bestrahlung auch deren D_0 deutlich verändern kann: Bei einem Fraktionierungsintervall von 6 Stunden nach einer Erst-Dosis von 500 rad ist die D_0 um ein Drittel höher als die der ursprünglichen Population.

Auch bei anderen Zellen menschlichen Ursprungs in vitro wurden ähnliche Fraktionierungseffekte beobachtet, z.B. bei Nierenzellen (T-1), (Barendsen, 1962), bei lymphoiden Zellen (Drewinko u. Humphrey, 1971) oder bei menschlichen Melanomzellen in vitro (Barranco u. Mitarb., 1971), desgleichen bei verschiedenen Zellstämmen, die aus Mäusegeweben isoliert wurden, wie z.B. bei L-Zellen (Han u. Mitarb., 1964). Eine Besonderheit weisen Zellen einer Mäuseleukämie in vitro auf, die schon bei Einzeitbestrahlung durch eine besonders hohe Strahlenempfindlichkeit ausgezeichnet sind (D_0 = 62 rad). Die Kurve des Fraktionierungseffektes steigt nach einer konditionierenden Dosis von 100 rad erst an, obwohl die Einzeitdosiseffektkurve keine Schulter aufweist, der Fraktionierungseffekt also auch nicht als Restitution einer Schulter interpretiert werden kann, und sinkt dann weit unter den Ausgangswert ab. Das bedeutet,

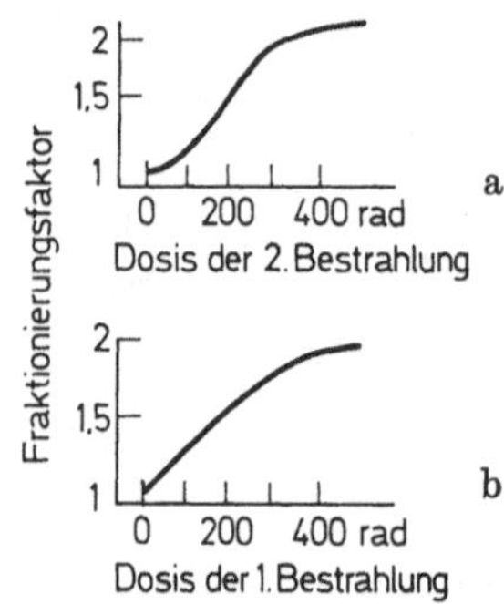

Abb. 47a. Die Abhängigkeit des Fraktionierungsfaktors von der Höhe der 2. Strahlendosis nach einer konditionierenden Dosis von 420 rad bei HeLa-Zellen. Fraktionierungsintervall 2 h. (Malone u. Mitarb., 1971)

b. Die Abhängigkeit des Fraktionierungsfaktors von der Höhe der konditionierenden Strahlendosis bei einer 2. Strahlendosis von 420 rad. Fraktionierungsintervall 2 h. (Malone u. Mitarb., 1971)

daß bei diesen Zellen eine geeignet fraktionierte Bestrahlung wirksamer sein kann als eine Einzeitbestrahlung gleicher Gesamtdosis (Caldwell u. Mitarb., 1965). Über interessante Unterschiede in den zeitlichen Schwankungen des Fraktionierungsfaktors Bei 2 Stämmen des Ehrlich-Aszites-Tumors in vitro berichteten Bhaskaran u. Dittrich (1969): Bei gleicher Einzeitdosiseffektkurve (D_0 = 130 R; n = 2,8) zeigte der eine Stamm einen typischen, oszillierenden Verlauf der Überlebensrate nach 2×350 R, während sie beim anderen Zellstamm innerhalb eines Zeitraums von 3 Stunden auf den Maximalwert anstieg und sich nicht weiter veränderte. Dittrich u. Göhde (1970) zeigten, daß ein unterschiedliches Proliferationsverhalten im Intervall für die Differenzen im Verlauf des Fraktionierungseffektes verantwortlich war.

Auch bei fraktionierter Bestrahlung mit locker ionisierenden Strahlen in vivo tritt der Fraktionierungseffekt mit einem ähnlichen zyklischen Verlauf auf. Dieser ist besonders ausgeprägt bei den klonogenen Zellen der Epidermis, wo 2 Minima (nach 6 und 12 Stunden) auftreten (Withers, 1967b; Emery u. Mitarb., 1970). Auch bei klonogenen Dünndarmepithelien tritt neben einem ausgeprägten Minimum nach etwa 12 h ein 2. Minimum nach etwa 2 Tagen auf (Withers u. Elkind, 1969). Bei der Bestrahlung klonogener Knochenmarkszellen scheinen Höhe des ersten Anstiegs und Ausprägung des passagären Minimums neben der Strahlendosis wesentlich vom Proliferationszustand der Zellen abzuhängen. Stimulierte Knochenmarkszellen zeigen einen Fraktionierungsfaktor von 1,6 (Phillips u. Hank, 1968) bis 2 (Till u. McCulloch, 1963) nach 4—5 Stunden, mit einer ausgeprägten Senke bei einem 10 Stunden-Intervall. Wenn aber ruhende (also in G_0-Phase befindliche) klonogene Knochenmarkszellen bestrahlt werden, tritt diese Senke nicht auf. Das Ausmaß der Schulter der 2. Kurve ist deutlich größer (n = 2,8) und die D_0 steigt von 85 rad auf 105 rad (HENDRY u. HOWARD, 1971).

Auch bei in vivo untersuchten Tumorzellen ist ein Fraktionierungseffekt verschiedentlich beschrieben worden, so z. B. von BELLI u. Mitarb. (1966). Eine ausführliche Darstellung des Fraktionierungseffektes bei Zellen normaler und maligner Gewebe in vivo findet sich bei WITHERS (1969). FOWLER u. STERN (1963) wiesen nach, daß die Erholung vom subletalen Strahlenschaden die in der klinischen Strahlentherapie gefundenen Fraktionierungseffekte, wie z. B. die Strandquist-Gerade, weitgehend erklärt.

Das komplizierte Verhalten des Fraktionierungseffektes wurde zum ersten Mal 1961 von ELKIND u. Mitarb. dahingehend gedeutet, daß neben der Restitution der Schulter auch Veränderungen in der Zusammensetzung der Zellpopulation auftreten. KALLMAN stellte 1963 ein Modell auf, das auf folgenden Annahmen beruht:

1. Die erste Strahlendosis hinterläßt eine partiell synchronisierte Population von resistenten Zellen (s. S. 92).

2. Die überlebenden Zellen erfahren eine Verzögerung in ihrer Progression durch die verschiedenen Zyklusphasen, die von der Dosis und der Zyklusphase zum Zeitpunkt der Bestrahlung abhängt. Das führt dazu, daß weitere Zellen vorübergehend in einer resistenten Phase auflaufen.

3. Die mittlere Strahlenempfindlichkeit der Population überlebender Zellen verändert sich entsprechend dem teilsynchronen Durchgang der Zellen durch die folgenden Zellzyklusphasen unterschiedlicher Strahlenempfindlichkeit.

Dieses Modell wurde von HAHN u. Mitarb. (1965) und HAHN u. KALLMAN (1967) durchgerechnet. Obwohl sehr grob verallgemeinernde Annahmen gemacht werden mußten (z. B. wurde der Zellzyklus in 4 starre, homogene Kompartimente aufgeteilt), ergaben die Kalkulationen doch eine Abhängigkeit des Fraktionierungseffektes vom Bestrahlungsintervall, die dem allgemein beobachteten Verlauf des Fraktionierungseffektes nahe kam. Ein wesentlich differenzierteres Modell von YOUNG u. FOWLER (1969), das 10 variable Kompartimente benutzte und mit den von SINCLAIR (1968a) gewonnenen Daten für die Altersabhängigkeit von Dosiseffektkurven, Mitoseverzögerung und einer Verteilung von Generationszeiten arbeitete, konnte den zeitlichen Verlauf vom 1. Maximum, Minimum und 2. Maximum sehr genau simulieren. Insbesondere die Dosisabhängigkeit des ersten Maximums, die Veränderungen in den Dosiseffektkurvenparametern für die 2. Dosis in Abhängigkeit vom Bestrahlungsintervall und die Größe des Fraktionierungseffektes in Abhängigkeit von der Höhe der Einzeldosen ließen sich danach berechnen und die beobachteten Phänomene reproduzieren.

(Mit einer ultraschnellen Methode der Fluoreszens-Impuls-Cytophotometrie konnten DITTRICH und GÖHDE (1970) an Ehrlich-Aszites-Tumorzellen in vitro diese Veränderungen der Zusammensetzung der Zellpopulation in den ersten Stunden nach einer Strahlendosis von 500 R direkt demonstrieren.)

Das Modell ging von der Voraussetzung aus, daß auch die 2. Dosis die Überlebenden der ersten Dosis nach den Dosiseffektkurven der entsprechenden Zellzyklusphase inaktiviert. Daher errechneten sich für die kurzen Zeitintervalle zu hohe Überlebensraten, die von YOUNG u. FOWLER (1969) dahingehend gedeutet wurden, daß die Erholung vom subletalen Strahlenschaden noch nicht abgeschlossen war. Offensichtlich spielen für den zeitlichen Ablauf des Fraktionierungseffektes 2 Prozesse eine Rolle: die Restitution der Schulter und die Progression der partiell synchronisierten Population überlebender Zellen durch die Zyklusphasen verschiedener Strahlenempfindlichkeit. Dieses *„Repair-Progression-Model"* wurde zum ersten Mal konsequent von ELKIND (1967b) vorgestellt und experimentell belegt. Computerberechnungen der oben genannten Art, die sowohl die Erholung vom subletalen Strahlenschaden als auch die Progression berücksichtigen, liegen von PASKIN u. Mitarb. (1968) vor.

In einem vorhergehenden Kapitel (s. S. 88) wurde gezeigt, daß sowohl die Extrapolationsnummer als auch die Endneigung der Dosiseffektkurve sich mit der Zellzyklusphase verändern. Daher wird verständlich, daß Dosiswirkungskurven zu verschiedenen Zeiten nach einer konditionierenden Dosis unterschiedliche Neigungen aufweisen, die nicht mit der der ursprünglichen Population übereinstimmen (z. B. Lockart u. Mitarb. [1961] und Berry [1967b] an HeLa-Zellen in vitro; Frindel u. Mitarb. [1966] und Hendry u. Howard [1971] an Knochenmarkszellen in vivo).

In der Plateauphase des Wachstums trat bei chinesischen Hamsterzellen kein Fraktionierungseffekt auf (Hahn, 1968), was auf Grund der für diese Wachstumsphase typischen Form der Dosiseffektkurve auch zu erwarten war.

Sinclair (1964) und Sinclair u. Morton (1964) hatten gezeigt, daß bei synchronisierten chinesischen Hamsterzellen besonders dann ein erheblicher Anstieg der Überlebens-

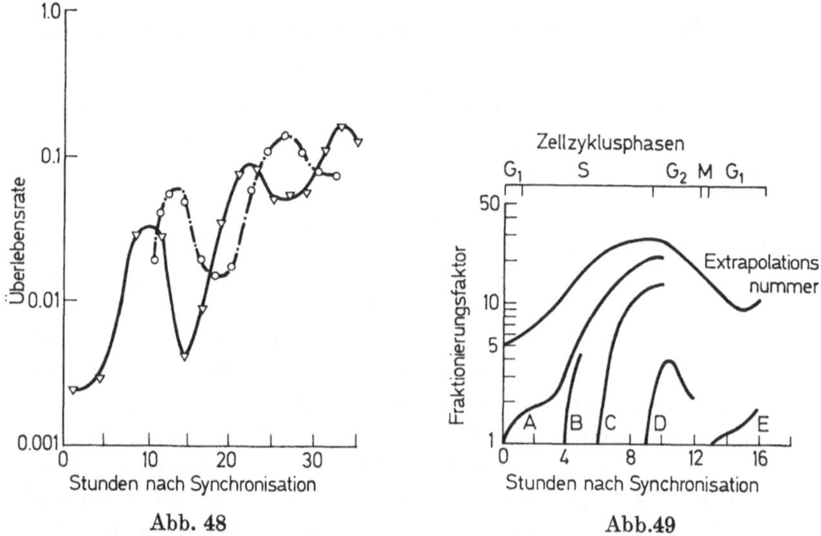

<table>
<tr><td style="text-align:center">Abb. 48</td><td style="text-align:center">Abb.49</td></tr>
</table>

Abb. 48. Überlebensraten synchronisierter chinesischer Hamsterzellen (V-79) nach Bestrahlung mit 1320 rad zu verschiedenen Zeiten nach Synchronisation in Mitose (Dreiecke) sowie nach fraktionierter Bestrahlung, wobei die erste Dosis von 660 rad in der S-Phase (10,6 h nach Synchronisation) und die 2. Dosis von 660 rad nach unterschiedlichem Intervall gegeben wurde (Kreise). (Sinclair, 1964)

Abb. 49. Die Schwankungen der Extrapolationsnummer von synchronisierten L-Zellen während des Zellzyklus (obere Kurve) sowie der Verlauf des Fraktionierungsfaktors während des Zellzyklus (untere Kurven). Die konditionierende Dosis von 700 rad wurde am Ende der G_1-Phase (A), in der S-Phase (B, C), in G_2-Phase (D) und zu Beginn der G_1-Phase (E) gegeben, die 2. Dosis von 500 rad nach verschiedenen Intervallen. Die Synchronisation erfolgte mit der „Fenster-Technik" am Übergang von G_1- in die S-Phase (s. S. 92). (Withmore u. Mitarb., 1965)

rate zu erreichen ist, wenn die erste Dosis gegen Ende der S-Phase gegeben wurde (Abb. 48). Bei den Zellen, die zu anderen Zeitpunkten des Zellzyklus bestrahlt wurden, war der Fraktionierungseffekt vor allem vom Einfluß der Progression der Zellen in Zellzyklusphasen anderer Strahlenempfindlichkeit bestimmt. Elkind u. Kano (1971) konnten bei der gleichen Zellart auch nach einer in G_2-Phase gegebenen Erst-Dosis eine deutliche Erholung vom subletalen Strahlenschaden nachweisen. Auch bei synchronisierten L-Zellen war der Fraktionierungsfaktor am größten, wenn die erste Dosis in der S-Phase gegeben wurde (Whitmore u. Mitarb., 1965). In der Abb. 49 sind die zeitlichen Schwankungen des Fraktionierungsfaktors für synchronisierte L-Zellen zusammen mit den zyklusspezifischen Veränderungen der Extrapolationsnummer aufgetragen. Daraus zogen Whitmore u. Mitarb. (1965) den Schluß, daß „unmittelbar nach einer konditionierenden Dosis die überlebenden Zellen ihre Extrapolationsnummer zumindest teilweise restituieren".

Von da an verläuft ihre Extrapolationsnummer parallel zu den Veränderungen, die man in einer Population erwarten würde, die nie zuvor bestrahlt worden war".

LANGE (1970) untersuchte den Einfluß der Erholung vom subletalen Strahlenschaden und der Progression durch den Zellzyklus auf die Überlebensrate von synchronisierten HeLa-Zellen nach fraktionierter Bestrahlung mit 2×200 rad. Unter diesen Bedingungen fand er, daß die Veränderungen der Überlebensrate nach einer 2. Bestrahlung weitgehend auf die Progression der Überlebenden durch den Zellzyklus zurückzuführen waren. Eine sofortige Restitution über die zyklusspezifischen Änderungen hinaus erfolgte nur dann in signifikantem Ausmaß, wenn die 2. Dosis in der frühen und mittleren G_1- und insbesondere der späten S-Phase appliziert wurde. Wird die konditionierende Dosis einer fraktionierten Bestrahlung chinesischer Hamsterzellen (V-79) in der Phase des Übergangs von der G_1-Phase in die S-Phase gegeben, verzögert sie die mit der Progression in die S-Phase normalerweise verbundene Ausprägung einer größeren Schulter (ELKIND u. KANO, 1971). Die Reaktivität der Zellen auf eine 4 Stunden später gegebene 2. Strahlendosis ist so, als hätten die Zellen gerade erst die 1. Dosis erhalten. Die Überlebensrate der nach diesem Fraktionierungsschema bestrahlten Zellen ist somit deutlich geringer als wenn die Gesamtdosis auf einmal zum Zeitpunkt der Zweitbestrahlung gegeben worden wäre. Wird außerdem noch die Progression der im Übergang von G_1-Phase in S-Phase bestrahlten Zellen durch Cycloheximid blockiert, tritt auch nach stundenlangem Intervall kein Fraktionierungseffekt auf (ELKIND u. KANO, 1971).

Bei einem anderen Stamm von chinesischen Hamsterzellen (CHO) stellte MUNRO (1971) fest, daß die Erholung vom subletalen Strahlenschaden nur für relativ kurze Zeit, etwa bis zum Auftreten des ersten Minimums der Überlebensrate nachzuweisen ist. Der dann folgende Anstieg der Überlebensrate ist vollständig durch den Anstieg der Zellzahl erklärbar.

Es muß also zum jetzigen Zeitpunkt noch als offen gelten, in welchem Ausmaß Restitution der Schulter und Progression bzw. Multiplikation der Zellen bei den verschiedenen Zellarten zu dem zeitlichen Ablauf des Fraktionierungseffekts beitragen.

b) Abhängigkeit des Fraktionierungseffektes von der Strahlenart

Bei dem Zustandekommen des Fraktionierungseffektes spielen die Restitution der Schulter der ursprünglichen Dosiswirkungskurve und die unterschiedliche Strahlenempfindlichkeit der verschiedenen Zellzyklusphasen zusammen. Man kann daher erwarten, daß bei fraktionierter Bestrahlung mit Strahlen hohen LETs, wie z. B. Alpha-Strahlen, bei denen eine exponentielle Dosiseffektkurve gefunden wird (s. S. 76) und bei denen keine Abhängigkeit der Strahlenwirkung vom Zellzyklus besteht (s. S. 89), auch kein Fraktionierungseffekt auftritt. An menschlichen Nierenzellen (T-1) fand BARENDSEN (1962, 1968) keinen Fraktionierungseffekt bei fraktionierter Alpha-Bestrahlung. Ebensowenig trat er auf bei fraktionierter Bestrahlung von chinesischen Hamsterzellen mit schnellen Teilchen von einem LET über 126 keV/μ (SKARSGARD u. Mitarb., 1967) und bei Bestrahlung von menschlichen Nierenzellen (T-1) bei einem LET von 220 keV/μ oder höher (TODD, 1968b). Die RBW dicht ionisierender Strahlen nimmt also mit zunehmender Fraktionierung zu. Wenn aber eine endliche Anfangsneigung für Dosiseffektkurven nach Einzeitbestrahlung besteht (D_1) und wenn mit abnehmender Höhe der Einzeldosis bei fraktionierter Bestrahlung eine Dosiswirkungskurve erreicht wird, deren Neigung dieser D_1 entspricht, dann kann die RBW mit zunehmender Fraktionierung nicht beliebig groß werden, sondern strebt einem Endwert zu, was auch experimentell nachzuweisen war (BARENDSEN, 1968).

Wenn eine der beiden Fraktionen einer fraktionierten Bestrahlung aus Strahlung niedrigen LETs, die andere aus Strahlung hohen LETs (z. B. Alpha-Teilchen) besteht, wird keine gegenseitige Beeinflussung der Dosiswirkungskurven gefunden. Nach einer ersten Alpha-Strahlendosis tritt die Inaktivierung durch eine unmittelbar folgende 2. Dosis

7*

(250 kV-Röntgenstrahlen) nach einer typischen Schulterkurve auf, während nach einer ersten Röntgen- oder Gammastrahlendosis auch bei längerem Intervall die 2. Dosis (Alpha-Teilchen) die Zellen nach der bekannten Exponentialfunktion inaktiviert (Barendsen, 1968; Arlett, 1969), (Abb. 50).

Von derzeit besonderem klinischen Interesse ist der Fraktionierungseffekt bei Neutronenbestrahlung. Dieses Problem wurde 1970 von Elkind umfassend diskutiert, so daß auf diese Darstellung verwiesen werden kann. Entsprechend der unterschiedlichen Form der Dosiswirkungskurven verschiedener Zellstämme in Abhängigkeit von verschiedenen Neutronenenergien (s. S. 78 f.) fanden sich Fraktionierungseffekte unterschiedlichen Ausmaßes. So trat kein Fraktionierungseffekt auf bei Bestrahlung von Mäuseleukämiezellen in vivo mit Spalt-Neutronen (Andrews u. Berry, 1962), von Hamsterfibroblasten in

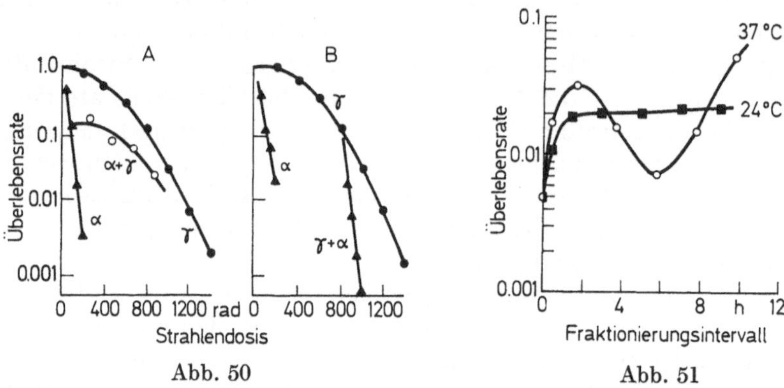

Abb. 50   Abb. 51

Abb. 50. Dosiseffektkurven chinesischer Hamsterzellen (Klon F) bei Bestrahlung mit Alpha-Teilchen eines ^{241}Am-Präparates oder ^{60}Co-Gammastrahlen. Außerdem ist in A die Dosiswirkungskurve bei fraktionierter Bestrahlung mit Alpha-Teilchen und unmittelbar folgender Gamma-Bestrahlung (Kreise: $\alpha + \gamma$) und in B die Dosiswirkungskurve bei fraktionierter Bestrahlung mit Gammastrahlen und später folgender Alpha-Bestrahlung eingezeichnet ($\gamma + \alpha$). (Arlett, 1969)

Abb. 51. Die Überlebensrate chinesischer Hamsterzellen (V-79) nach fraktionierter Bestrahlung bei unterschiedlicher Temperatur im Fraktionierungsintervall:
37° C = erste Dosis 747 rad, 2. Dosis 804 rad, Temperatur im Intervall 37° C,
24° C = erste Dosis 763 rad, 2. Dosis 795 rad, Temperatur im Intervall 24° C.
(Nach Elkind u. Mitarb., 1965 a)

vitro mit 6 MeV-Neutronen (Schneider u. Whitmore, 1963) und Knochenmarkszellen in vivo (Hendry u. Howard, 1971) sowie HeLa-Zellen in vitro (Nias u. Mitarb., 1971) mit 14 MeV-Neutronen. In anderen Fällen wurde ein geringer, meist etwa halb so großer Fraktionierungseffekt im Vergleich zur Bestrahlung mit locker ionisierenden Strahlen nachgewiesen, z.B. in vitro von Broerse u. Barendsen (1969) und in vivo von Withers u. Mitarb. (1970 a), Kember (1969), Broerse u. Roelse (1971) und Denekamp u. Mitarb. (1971).

Man kann verallgemeinernd sagen, daß, wenn sich bei Einzeitbestrahlung sigmoide Dosiseffektkurven ergaben, *meist* auch ein Fraktionierungseffekt gefunden wurde und *immer*, wenn eine exponentielle Dosiswirkungsbeziehung bestand, kein Fraktionierungseffekt eintrat (Todd, 1968 b; Elkind, 1970).

c) Untersuchungen zum Wirkungsmechanismus des Fraktionierungseffektes

α) *Temperaturabhängigkeit*

Die Abhängigkeit des Fraktionierungseffektes von der Temperatur im bestrahlungsfreien Intervall wurde verschiedentlich untersucht. Berry u. Oliver (1964) fanden bei Inkubation von HeLa-Zellen bei 20° C eine ausgeprägte Verzögerung im ersten Maximum, das statt nach 2 Stunden erst nach 8 Stunden erreicht war, in seiner Höhe aber nicht wesentlich vermindert war. Der weitere Verlauf mit Minimum und 2. Maximum war nicht wesentlich verändert. LANGE (1970) sah bei synchronisierten HeLa-Zellen bei 20° C keine signifikante Erholung vom subletalen Strahlenschaden, aber eine langsame Progression der Zellen bis zu einem Block in der Mitte der G_1-Phase.

Chinesische Hamsterzellen (CHO) und P-388-F-Mäuseleukämiezellen zeigten auch bei 20° C einen normalen Fraktionierungseffekt (Fox u. NIAS, 1970). Bei Inkubation von chinesischen Hamsterzellen des Stammes V-79 im Intervall bei 24° C nahm die Überlebensrate etwas langsamer zu und erreicht nicht ganz die Höhe wie bei 37° C, blieb aber auf dieser Höhe stehen und zeigte nicht die üblichen Fluktuationen (Abb. 51), (ELKIND u. Mitarb., 1965a).

Selbst bei 3° C war bei V-79-Zellen noch ein geringer Fraktionierungseffekt zu sehen (ELKIND u. Mitarb., 1965a). TERASIMA (1969) fand jedoch an L-Zellen bei dieser Temperatur keinen Fraktionierungseffekt.

Bei fraktionierter Bestrahlung von HeLa-Zellen im tiefgefrorenen Zustand trat keinerlei Fraktionierungseffekt mehr auf, obwohl nach Einzeitbestrahlung eine sigmoide Dosiseffektkurve gefunden wurde (NIAS u. Mitarb., 1969).

Die Form der Fraktionierungseffektkurve bei 24° C stützt nach ELKIND (1967) wesentlich das Restitutions-Progressions-Modell des Fraktionierungseffektes. Wenn Zellen bei 24° C sich nicht vermehren und wenn keine wesentlichen Verschiebungen in der Verteilung auf die einzelnen Zyklusphasen vorkommen, stellt der Anstieg den reinen Restitutionsvorgang, isoliert von dem Einfluß der Progression durch den Zellzyklus, dar.

β) *Die Stoffwechselabhängigkeit des Fraktionierungseffektes*

Die Abhängigkeit des Fraktionierungseffektes von der Funktion verschiedener Stoffwechselprozesse wurde häufig untersucht. Es sollen nur die wichtigsten Ergebnisse zusammengestellt werden:

Nach Unterbrechung des Energiestoffwechsels durch Dinitrophenol wurde ein eher größerer Fraktionierungseffekt gefunden (BERRY, 1966a; DALRYMPLE u. Mitarb., 1969). Selbst wenn man die Zellen im Intervall in einer reinen Salzlösung ohne wichtige Stoffwechselmetabolite hält, tritt ein typischer Fraktionierungseffekt auf (ASHBY u. BONTE, 1968). Nur mit Fluorid ließ sich der Fraktionierungseffekt unter bestimmten Bedingungen ausschalten (ASHBY u. BONTE, 1968). Über den Einfluß des Sauerstoffmangels auf den Fraktionierungseffekt wird auf S. 109 f. berichtet.

Eine Blockierung des Proteinstoffwechsels durch Zugabe von Cycloheximid oder Puromycin beeinflußt den Verlauf des Fraktionierungseffektes in den ersten Stunden nicht, bis später die toxischen Wirkungen der beiden Substanzen vorherrschen (BERRY, 1966a; ELKIND u. Mitarb., 1967a; KIM u. Mitarb., 1966; TERASIMA, 1969).

Eine Hemmung des DNS-Stoffwechsels durch Fluoruracil, Fluordesoxyuridin oder Thymidin in hoher Konzentration hemmt den Fraktionierungseffekt nicht (BERRY, 1966a; ELKIND u. Mitarb., 1967a; KIM u. Mitarb., 1964; TERASIMA, 1969). Wird den Kulturen für längere Zeit Methotrexat zugefügt, weisen die Zellen eine exponentielle Dosiseffektkurve auf, so daß auch kein Fraktionierungseffekt auftreten kann. 24 Stunden nach Entfernen des Methotrexat ist jedoch mit der dann sigmoiden Dosiseffektkurve auch wieder ein Fraktionierungseffekt nachzuweisen (BERRY, 1966a, 1968a).

Actinomycin D, das die Bildung der m-RNS hemmt, blockiert den Fraktionierungseffekt bei chinesischen Hamsterzellen (ELKIND u. Mitarb., 1964b; 1967a; ELKIND, 1967). Da jedoch manche Substanzen, die keinen Einfluß auf den Fraktionierungseffekt ausüben, die RNS-Synthese weitaus stärker blockieren als Actinomycin, stellte ELKIND 1967 die Theorie auf, daß die Erholung vom subletalen Strahlenschaden nicht eine intakte RNS-Synthese zur Bedingung habe, sondern ein nicht-enzymatischer Prozeß sei, ,,der eine bestimmte stereochemische Beziehung der DNS zu ihrer molekularen Umgebung voraussetzt" (ELKIND, 1967). TERASIMA (1969) fand zwar bei L-Zellen keine Hemmung der Erholung vom subletalen Strahlenschaden durch Actinomycin D, jedoch durch andere Stoffe, die sich wie Actinomycin D an die DNS anlagern, z.B. Proflavin und Phleomycin.

Eine Reihe von Ergebnissen legen nahe, den molekularen Mechanismus der Erholung vom subletalen Strahlenschaden in der Wiedervereinigung von Einstrangbrüchen des DNS-Moleküls zu suchen. Es soll hier jedoch nicht auf diese Problematik, die inzwischen ein eigenes, umfangreiches Forschungsgebiet geworden ist, eingegangen werden. Eine neuere Übersicht findet sich bei PAINTER (1970).

d) Fraktionierungseffekt bei Cytostatika

Die enge Korrelation zwischen der Erholung vom subletalen Strahlenschaden und einer sigmoiden Einzeitdosiseffektkurve besteht nicht bei der fraktionierten Zufuhr von Cytostatika. Bei phasenspezifisch wirkenden Cytostatika, wie z.B. Actinomycin D, kann durch Progression und Akkumulation in resistenten Phasen ein Fraktionierungseffekt gefunden werden (ELKIND u. KANO, 1970). Bei den meisten alkylierenden Zytostatika, wie z.B. Stickstoff-Lost, deren Dosiswirkungskurven ausgeprägte Schultern aufweisen, ist dennoch keinerlei Fraktionierungseffekt festzustellen (WALKER u. THATCHER, 1968; SAKAMOTO u. ELKIND, 1969). Ähnliche Befunde liegen für andere alkylierende Cytostatika vor, z.B. Isopropylmethansulfonat (Fox u. Mitarb., 1970b) und Methylmethansulfonat (Fox u. NIAS, 1968). Um so auffallender ist der Befund einer sehr schnell vollendeten Restitution der Schulter bei fraktionierter Gabe von Schwefel-Lost, die von MAURO u. ELKIND (1968b) an chinesischen Hamsterzellen nachgewiesen wurde, während an L-Zellen bei fraktionierter Gabe dieses Cytostatikums kein Fraktionierungseffekt auftrat (WALKER u. THATCHER, 1968).

MARIN u. LEVIS (1964) untersuchten die Frage, wie sich Bestrahlung und Stickstoff-Lost gegenseitig beeinflussen. Beide Agentien inaktivieren aus Meerschweinchenherzen isolierte Zellen (RCP) nach sigmoiden Dosiseffektkurven. Eine Vorbestrahlung mit 300 rad bewirkte, daß die Dosiseffektkurve der die konditionierende Stahlendosis überlebenden Zellen nach Gabe des Cytostatikums einer schulterlosen Exponentialfunktion folgte. Eine Vorbehandlung der Zellen mit Stickstoff-Lost beeinflußte dagegen die Strahlenwirkung nicht, und es fand sich eine typische Schulterkurve.

e) Fraktionierungseffekt und Dosisleistungseffekt

An anderer Stelle wurde ausgeführt (s. S. 81), daß ein Zeitfaktor auftreten muß, wenn an irgendeiner Stufe der Wirkungskette ein rückläufiger Prozeß auftritt. LAJTHA u. OLIVER (1961) hatten den Fraktionierungseffekt als Abnahme einer durch die erste Strahlendosis induzierten Vorschädigung angesehen, die mit einer Halbwertzeit von $1^1/_2$ Stunden vonstatten geht. Auf dieser Basis kamen sie zu der Voraussage, daß mit abnehmender Dosisleistung auch die Dosiseffektkurve immer flacher verlaufen müßte. Allgemeiner gefaßt wurde die Verbindung von Fraktionierungseffekt und Dosisleistung von HUG u. KELLERER (1965) diskutiert, die den Schluß zogen, daß sich bei abnehmender Dosisleistung (im Bereich weniger rad/h) die Steilheit der Dosiswirkungskurve allmählich der Anfangsneigung der Dosiswirkungskurve D_1 bei akuter Bestrahlung annähern dürfte. Besonders mit Blick auf strahlentherapeutische Probleme wurde diese Frage von LIVERSAGE (1969) diskutiert. Von Fox u. NIAS (1970) wurden die experimentellen Belege dieser Beziehung von Fraktionierungseffekt und Dosisleistungseffekt zusammenfassend dargestellt.

2. Erholung vom potentiell letalen Strahlenschaden

In den letzten Jahren wurde neben dem Fraktionierungseffekt ein weiterer rückläufiger Prozeß beschrieben, der meist als Erholung vom potentiell letalen Strahlenschaden bezeichnet wird.

Durch verschiedene *nach der Bestrahlung zugeführte* Agentien kann die Überlebensrate nach einer einmaligen akuten Strahlendosis gesteigert werden. Blockierung der Proteinsynthese durch Cycloheximid erhöht die Überlebensrate von HeLa-Zellen, die in S-Phase mit 500 rad bestrahlt wurden, um den Faktor 3 (PHILLIPS u. TOLMACH, 1966).

Eine Blockierung der Energieversorung der Zellen durch Dinitrophenol für 2 Stunden nach einer Bestrahlung hat eine Abflachung der Dosiswirkungskurve von L-Zellen um 15 % zur Folge (DALRYMPLE u. Mitarb., 1967). Während Dinitrophenol auf die Zellen in allen Zyklusphasen resistenzsteigernd wirkt, wird durch Zugabe von Arsen nach Bestrahlung vor allem die Überlebensrate der in der frühen S-Phase bestrahlten Zellen erhöht (BAKER u. Mitarb., 1970). Auch eine Verminderung der Temperatur während und unmittelbar nach der Bestrahlung erhöht die Überlebensrate von HeLa-Zellen (BELLI u. BONTE, 1963), L-Zellen (WHITMORE u. Mitarb., 1969), chinesischen Hamsterzellen (Don) (DEWEY u. MILLER, 1970) und Mäuseleukämiezellen in vitro (BEER u. Mitarb., 1963), zum Teil um das Mehrfache. Durch das Aufbewahren der Zellen in einer isotonischen Salzlösung für mehrere Stunden kann die Überlebensrate von in G_1- und G_2-Phase mit 900 R bestrahlten chinesischen Hamsterzellen (V-79) auf das 3—4fache erhöht werden (BELLI u. SHELTON, 1969). Auch eine Zufuhr von isologer DNS (MILETIC u. Mitarb., 1964) und DNS-Bausteinen kann die Überlebensrate von HeLa-Zellen und L-Zellen, insbesondere nach Bestrahlung in der S-Phase, um den Faktor 4—5 ansteigen lassen (PETROVIC u. NIAS, 1966; PETROVIC, 1968; PETROVIC u. FERLE-VIDOVIC, 1968).

Werden Plateauphasenzellen (s. S. 84 f.) nach Bestrahlung noch für 6 Stunden in Plateau-Phase gelassen, bevor sie trypsiniert und platiert werden, zeigen sie eine etwa doppelt so hohe Überlebensrate als wenn sie unmittelbar nach Bestrahlung platiert werden (HAHN, 1969), was eine Erholung vom potentiell letalen Strahlenschaden bedeutet, während unter den gleichen Wachstumsbedingungen keine Erholung vom subletalen Stralenschaden auftreten kann (HAHN, 1968a).

Die Erholung vom potentiell letalen Strahlenschaden tritt nur dann auf, wenn die Plateauphasezellen im alten Medium belassen werden. Wird dagegen unmittelbar nach Bestrahlung das Medium gewechselt, ergibt sich die gleiche Dosiseffektkurve wie nach unmittelbar auf die Bestrahlung folgender Platierung (LITTLE, 1971). Das läßt darauf schließen, daß im Medium von Plateauphasekulturen eine Substanz vorhanden ist, die für die Erholung vom potentiell letalen Strahlenschaden verantwortlich ist. LITTLE (1971) konnte zeigen, daß die Zugabe von Medium aus stationären Kulturen für 6 Stunden nach Bestrahlung eine Erhöhung der Überlebensrate in exponentiell sich vermehrenden Kulturen bewirkte, wobei die D_0 von ca. 150 R auf 175 R zunahm. In menschlichen Leberzellen (CHANG) in Plateauphase wies LITTLE (1969) sowohl einen Fraktionierungseffekt mit einem Fraktionierungsfaktor von 3 wie auch eine Erholung vom potentiell letalen Strahlenschaden um den Faktor 2 bei Belassung der Zellen für 2—6 Stunden in der übervölkerten Kultur nach.

Diese Untersuchungen können vielleicht auch die Beobachtung von LUND u. ROSENGREN (1966) erklären, daß selbst nach Bestrahlung von HeLa-Zellen in Plateauphase mit 20000 rad nach 6—8 Wochen vereinzelt Kolonien auftraten.

ELKIND u. Mitarb. (1967 b) fanden, daß Actinomycin D nicht nur den Fraktionierungseffekt hemmt, sondern auch, nach der Bestrahlung gegeben, die Schulter der Dosiseffektkurve verkleinert: ein Zeichen für die Hemmung der Reparatur potenziell letaler Schäden. Ob die beiden reparativen Prozesse unabhängig sind, verschiedene Stoffwechselprozesse benötigen und unter unterschiedlichen Bedingungen ablaufen oder äquivalente Ausdrucksformen des gleichen Vorgangs, zum einen in letal geschädigten, zum anderen in überlebenden Zellen sind, wie ELKIND u. Mitarb. (1967 b) und WHITMORE u. Mitarb. (1969) vermutet haben, kann zur Zeit nicht entschieden werden. Die Erholung vom potenziell letalen Schaden scheint eine Proliferationshemmung zur Voraussetzung zu haben, die es den Zellen ermöglicht, den Reparationsprozeß durchzuführen, bevor sie weiter proliferieren (s. S. 69).

IX. Die Abhängigkeit der Strahlenwirkung von der Sauerstoffkonzentration

1. Der Sauerstoffverstärkungsfaktor bei Bestrahlung mit locker ionisierenden Strahlen

Vereinzelte Mitteilungen von Strahlentherapeuten und Strahlenbiologen (z. B. Schwarz, 1909; Holthusen, 1921; Mottram, 1936) hatten vermuten lassen, daß in anoxischem Gewebe die Strahlenwirkung wesentlich geringer ist als bei guter Durchblutung. Nachdem an Pflanzenzellen der Einfluß des Sauerstoffs auf die Strahlenempfindlichkeit von Read (1952) in umfassenden Versuchen nachgewiesen worden war, klärte Gray mit seinen Mitarbeitern (1953) die Bedeutung des Sauerstoffeffektes für tierische Zellen. Sie fanden, daß das gleiche Ausmaß der Strahlenwirkung, wie Chromosomenaberrationen in Ehrlich-Aszites-Tumorzellen, Zelluntergänge in einer Gewebekultur (s. S. 47) und Wachstumshemmung eines soliden Tumors, unter anoxischen Bedingungen eine doppelt bis dreimal so hohe Strahlendosis erforderte wie unter euoxischen Bedingungen. Entscheidend für die Wirkungsunterschiede war die Konzentration des im Gewebe gelösten Sauerstoffs zum Zeitpunkt der Bestrahlung. Schon Read (1952) hatte festgestellt, daß der Sauerstoff als Verstärkungsfaktor für die Strahlendosis wirkt (OER = oxygen enhancement ratio). Dieser Verstärkungsfaktor wurde zuerst von Alper u. Howard-Flanders (1956) an Bakterien quantitativ untersucht und eine Gleichung zu seiner Bestimmung angegeben:

$$S = S_N \cdot \frac{m(O) + k}{(O) + k}$$

S = die Strahlenempfindlichkeit bei der Sauerstoffkonzentration (O),
S_N = die Strahlenempfindlichkeit in Stickstoff,
m = Verhältnis der Strahlenempfindlichkeiten von optimal mit Sauerstoff versorgten Zellen zu maximal anoxischen Zellen (= maximale OER).
k = Sauerstoffkonzentration für den halbmaximalen Sauerstoffeffekt).

Die Sauerstoffkonstante k beträgt bei Bakterien 7,2 μM/l (Alper u. Howard-Flanders, 1956). Die ersten Versuche, den Sauerstoffeffekt auf die strahleninduzierte Hemmung der reproduktiven Integrität von Säugetierzellen quantitativ zu erfassen, stammen von Dewey (1960). Menschliche Leberzellen wurden in Suspension mit Gasen verschiedenen Sauerstoffpartialdrucks equilibriert, bestrahlt und auf ihre reproduktive Integrität getestet. Die gewonnenen Dosiswirkungskurven zeigt Abb. 52. Die Neigung der Kurven nimmt mit abnehmendem Sauerstoffgehalt ab, die D_0 von 118 rad in Luft auf 263 rad in Stickstoff zu. Das Verhältnis der Strahlenempfindlichkeiten ist 2,2. Aus der Gleichung von Alper u. Howard-Flanders und den experimentellen Werten berechnete Dewey (1960) eine für halbmaximalen Sauerstoffeffekt notwendige Sauerstoffkonzentration von 8,5 μM/l. Elkind u. Mitarb. (1965b) untersuchten die Abhängigkeit des Sauerstoffverstärkungsfaktors (OER) über einen besonders weiten Bereich an Sauerstoffkonzentrationen (Abb. 53) und fanden eine maximale OER von 3,1 und eine Sauerstoffkonzentration für halbmaximalen Effekt von 8 μM/l. Untersuchungen von Barendsen (1961) ergaben einen k-Wert von 7 μM/l.

Der maximale Sauerstoffverstärkungsfaktor wurde an den verschiedensten Zellstämmen in vitro bestimmt; die Werte liegen in der Regel zwischen 2,3 und 3,0, z. B. für HeLa-Zellen bei 2,4 (Hall u. Mitarb., 1966a; Nias u. Mitarb., 1967) und für chinesische Hamsterzellen bei 2,6 (Hall, 1969a) bzw. bei 3,0 (Berry u. Mitarb., 1970), bzw. 3,1 (Elkind u. Mitarb., 1965b; Belli u. Roach, 1968).

Bei in vitro-Versuchen ist die Herstellung wirklich anoxischer Bedingungen schwer, vor allem wenn bestrahlt wird, nachdem die Zellen platiert und angewachsen sind. Wenn das Medium über den Zellen nicht abgezogen wird, ist eine maximale Anoxie auch nach stundenlanger Begasung nicht zu erreichen (Baker und Town, 1966). Auf der anderen Seite besteht die Gefahr der Austrocknung, wenn man nach Entfernen des Mediums

Stickstoff über die Zellen leitet, um den Rest Sauerstoff zu entfernen (Belli und Roach, 1968). Komplizierend kommt hinzu, daß in Polystyren, aus dem die gebräuchlichen Plastikkulturgefäße gefertigt sind, Sauerstoff in beträchtlicher Menge löslich ist. Wird der Sauerstoff aus dem Nährmedium entfernt, so diffundiert er aus der Wandung nach und verhindert die Einstellung wirklich anoxischer Verhältnisse (Chapman u. Mitarb., 1968; Davies und Baker, 1970). Dementsprechend ist der Sauerstoffverstärkungsfaktor in Plastikgefäßen kleiner, als wenn die Versuche in Glasgefäßen durchgeführt werden (Chapman u. Mitarb., 1969). Diese Schwierigkeiten lassen sich umgehen, wenn man die Zellen in Suspension bestrahlt, insbesondere, wenn man sehr hohe Zellkonzentrationen verwendet (z.B. 6×10^6 Zellen/ml). Bei dieser Zelldichte vermindert die Zellatmung die Sauerstoffkonzentration in wenigen Minuten auf sehr niedrige Werte (Nias u. Mitarb., 1970).

Auch in vivo lassen sich anoxische Bedingungen erreichen. Entweder kann durch Abtöten des Tieres oder durch Abklemmung des Versuchsorgans (z.B. einer Extremität) in kurzer Zeit auf Grund des Sauerstoffverbrauchs der Zellen ein Sauerstoffmangel hergestellt werden. Die so bestimmten Sauerstoffverstärkungsfaktoren liegen im gleichen Be-

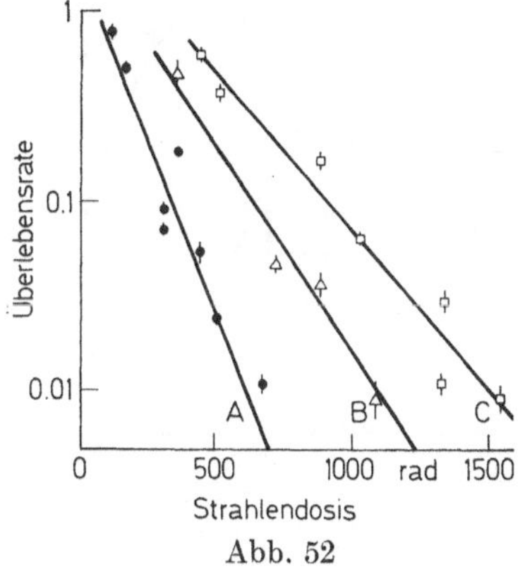
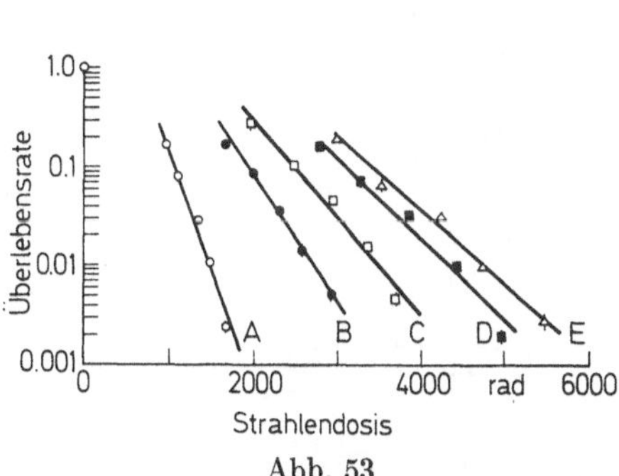

Abb. 52   Abb. 53

Abb. 52. Dosiswirkungskurven bei Bestrahlung menschlicher Leberzellen in vitro in Luft (A), in 0,275% Sauerstoff (B) und in Stickstoff (C) mit 200 kV-Röntgenstrahlen. (Dewey, 1960)

Abb. 53. Dosiswirkungskurven chinesischer Hamsterzellen (V-79) nach Bestrahlung bei verschiedenen Sauerstoffkonzentrationen:

Kurve A: in Luft: $D_0 = 187$ rad

Kurve B: in 2,5 μM/l Sauerstoff: $D_0 = 343$ rad

Kurve C: in 0,4 μM/l Sauerstoff: $D_0 = 443$ rad

Kurve D: in 0,1 μM/l Sauerstoff: $D_0 = 538$ rad

Kurve E: in 0,01 μM/l Sauerstoff: $D_0 = 589$ rad

(N.B.: Die Zellen wurden lange nach dem Platieren bei einer mittleren „Multiplizität" (s. S. 53) von 10 bestrahlt. Daher erklären sich die um den Faktor 10 zu hohen Überlebensraten im Vergleich zu anderen Versuchen). (Nach Elkind u. Mitarb., 1965b)

reich wie die in vitro gewonnenen (s. Abb. 19). Bei Aszitestumoren sind die meisten Zellen hypoxisch (Deschner u. Gray, 1959), so daß die Herstellung euoxischer Bedingungen das größere Problem aufwirft. Nach Injektion von subtoxischen Konzentrationen von H_2O_2 in den Aszites wird durch Katalase Sauerstoff freigesetzt, der für einige Minuten eine normale Sauerstoffkonzentration erzeugt, so daß der typische Sauerstoffeffekt mit einem Verstärkungsfaktor von 2,3—2,5 beobachtet wird (Berry u. Andrews, 1961; Berry u. Mitarb., 1965).

Zellen normaler Gewebe in vivo zeigen einen ähnlichen Sauerstoffeffekt, wenn die Strahlenwirkung mit einer Klon-Testmethode geprüft wird: klonogene Hautzellen OER = 2,6 (Withers, 1967c), klonogene Dünndarmzellen OER = 2,6 (Hornsey, 1970a), klonogene Knorpelzellen OER = 2,1 (Kember, 1967), Melanozyten OER = 2,75 (Potten u. Howard, 1969), Knochenmark OER = 2,32 (Phillips, 1968).

Die Bedeutung des Sauerstoffeffektes für die Strahlentherapie von Tumoren, die auf Grund ihrer unzureichenden Gefäßarchitektur Bereiche enthalten, in denen hypoxische, lebensfähige (klonogene) Zellen liegen (Thomlinson u. Gray, 1956), wurde von Gray (1953, 1961, 1965), Wilson (1961), Munro (1967) u.v.a. betont.

2. Die Abhängigkeit des Sauerstoffverstärkungsfaktors von der Strahlenqualität

Die oben mitgeteilten Werte des Sauerstoffverstärkungsfaktors zwischen 2 und 3 wurden mit locker ionisierenden Strahlen gewonnen. Mit zunehmendem LET der Strahlung nimmt der Sauerstoffeffekt ab. Für Alphastrahlen beträgt z. B. die OER nur 1,15 gegenüber 2,7 bei 250 kV-Röntgenstrahlen (BARENDSEN, 1962). ALPER u. MOORE (1967) schlugen vor, das Verhältnis der OER von locker ionisierenden Strahlen zur OER von Strahlung höheren LETs als „therapeutischen Gewinnfaktor" (therapeutic gain factor) zu bezeichnen, da es ein Maß sei für die effektivere Inaktivierung anoxischer Zellen durch die jeweilige Strahlenart.

Die Abhängigkeit des Sauerstoffverstärkungsfaktors von der Strahlenqualität (LET) wurde u. a. von BARENDSEN u. Mitarb. (1966), TODD (1967), FEOLA u. Mitarb. (1969) und

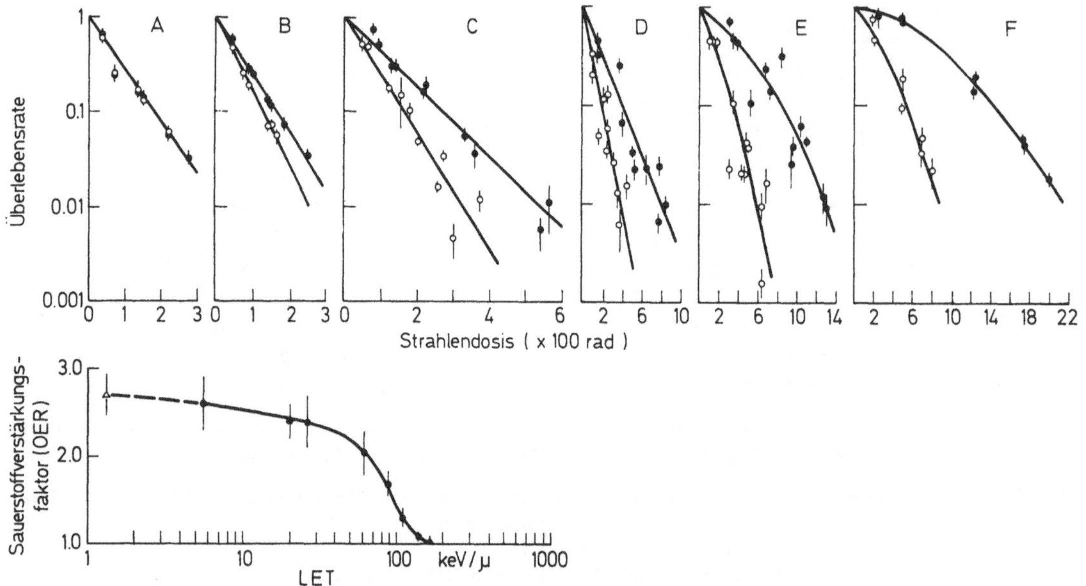

Abb. 54. Dosiseffektkurven menschlicher Nierenzellen (T-1) nach Bestrahlung unter euoxischen (Kreise) und hypoxischen (Punkte) Bedingungen mit verschiedenen Stahlenarten (obere Kurven)

Kurve A: 2,5 MeV-Apha-Teilchen (LET = 166 keV/μ)
Kurven B: 4 MeV-Alpha-Teilchen (LET = 110 keV/μ)
Kurven C: 5,1 MeV-Alpha-Teilchen (LET = 88 keV/μ)
Kurven D: 8,3 MeV-Alpha-Teilchen (LET = 61 keV/μ)
Kurven E: 25 MeV-Alpha-Teilchen (LET = 26 keV/μ)
Kurven F: 14,9 MeV-Deuteronen (LET = 5,6 keV/μ)

Untere Kurve: Die Abhängigkeit des Sauerstoffverstärkungsfaktors vom LET beschleunigter Teilchen. (BARENDSEN u. Mitarb., 1966)

BERRY (1970) untersucht. Die Ergebnisse von BARENDSEN (1966) sind in Abb. 54 graphisch dargestellt. Bei Strahlung mit einem LET über 150 keV/μ ist mit einem Sauerstoffeffekt nicht mehr zu rechnen.

Da für die Therapie mit Strahlen hohen LETs insbesondere Neutronen in Frage kommen, wurde der Sauerstoffverstärkungsfaktor für Neutronen mehrfach untersucht. Für HeLa-Zellen in vitro ergab sich eine OER von 1,5 mit 14 MeV-Neutronen (NIAS u. Mitarb., 1967), ebenso für chinesische Hamsterzellen mit 14 MeV-Neutronen 1,5 (HALL, 1969a), für chinesische Hamsterzellen mit 6 MeV-Neutronen 1,3 (SCHNEIDER u. WHITMORE, 1963). Bei Bestrahlung von Aszitestumoren (P-388) in vivo ergab sich bei 6 MeV-Neutronen eine OER von 1,69 (BERRY u. Mitarb., 1965), bei Bestrahlung eines anderen Aszitestumors (Ehrlich-) in vitro mit dem gleichen Gerät eine OER von 1,8 (HORNSEY u. SILINI, 1961).

Zwei Untersuchungen, bei denen an dem gleichen Zellmaterial verschiedene Neutronen-quellen mit Energien von 1—15 MeV getestet wurden, sind von besonderem Interesse. Während BROERSE u. Mitarb. (1968) bei Neutronen von 1—15 MeV stets den gleichen Sauer-stoffverstärkungsfaktor (1,5—1,6) bei menschlichen Nierenzellen (T-1) fanden, sah BERRY (1971b) eine deutliche Abnahme des Verstärkungsfaktors von 1,74 mit 14 MeV-Neutronen auf 1,2 mit Spalt-Neutronen (1 MeV) bei Untersuchungen an P-388-Leukämiezellen in vivo (s. Tabelle 6).

Zusammenfassend ist zu sagen, daß Neutronenbestrahlung das Problem, das anoxische Zellen für die Strahlentherapie vielleicht darstellen, verringern könnte (BARENDSEN, 1971), wobei ein therapeutischer Gewinnfaktor von 1,5—1,7 zu erwarten wäre.

Der Sauerstoffeffekt wurde bisher nur unter dem Gesichtspunkt betrachtet, inwieweit er ein dosismodifizierender Faktor ist. Es bestehen keine Zweifel, daß Sauerstoff im we-sentlichen einen Dosisverstärkungsfaktor darstellt, der auf radiochemische Reaktionen zurückzuführen ist.

Das legen auch Versuche nahe, die zeigten, daß keine Abhängigkeit des Verstärkungs-faktors vom Zellzyklus besteht (KRUUV u. SINCLAIR, 1968; LEGRYS u. HALL, 1969). Doch muß damit gerechnet werden, daß Sauerstoffmangel auch tiefgreifende Veränderungen im Stoffwechsel der Zellen verursacht, die ihrerseits die Strahlenwirkung modifizieren können.

3. Die Form der Dosiseffektkurve bei Bestrahlung hypoxischer Zellen

Wenn der Sauerstoff einen bloßen Verstärkungsfaktor darstellen würde, müßten die Dosiswirkungskurven in Luft und Stickstoff die gleiche Form haben, d.h. z.B. die gleiche Extrapolationsnummer aufweisen. Das ist aber durchaus nicht immer der Fall. Mit dieser Problematik hat sich vor allem die Gruppe um RÉVÉSZ befaßt.

Während in einer Reihe von Untersuchungen, in denen unzweifelhaft ein beträchtliches Ausmaß an Hypoxie erreicht wurde (z.B. ELKIND u. Mitarb., 1965a), die Extrapolations-nummer sich kaum änderte, fanden andere Untersucher bei Bestrahlung unter starker Hypoxie eine deutliche Verkleinerung der Extrapolationsnummer (z.B. HUMPHREY u. Mitarb., (1963) von 12 auf 3; VAN PUTTEN u. KALLMAN (1968) von 10,9 auf 2,7). In vivo erhielt PHILLIPS (1968) bei Bestrahlung von klonogenen Knochenmarkszellen unter Anoxie eine rein exponentielle Dosiseffektkurve.

RÉVÉSZ u. LITTBRAND konnten an verschiedenen Zellstämmen immer wieder zeigen, daß, wenn besondere Sorgfalt auf das Erreichen einer wirklich maximalen Anoxie gelegt wurde (d.h. wenn Glasgefäße benutzt, das Medium bis auf kleine Reste entfernt und die Begasung mit besonders sauerstofffreiem Argon durchgeführt wurde, wobei alle Gaslei-tungen aus sauerstoffdichtem Metall waren), unter solchen extrem sauerstoffarmen Be-dingungen die Dosiswirkungskurven immer einer reinen Exponentialfunktion folgten.

Während die meisten Untersucher eine Dosiswirkungskurve in einem Versuchsansatz mit möglichst vielen Punkten festzulegen versuchen, bestimmen LITTBRAND (1970a) und RÉVÉSZ stets nur drei Punkte im exponentiellen Teil der Schulterkurve mit möglichst vie-len unabhängigen Versuchsansätzen. Dadurch ist eine bessere statistische Behandlung der Daten möglich. Andere Untersucher stehen dieser Methode jedoch kritisch gegenüber (z.B. ELKIND u. WHITMORE, 1967).

RÉVÉSZ u. LITTBRAND fanden eine exponentielle Inaktivierungskurve bei Ehrlich-Aszites-Tumorzellen (1964) und bei chinesischen Hamsterzellen (1967).

Die Abnahme der Extrapolationsnummer tritt erst bei sehr geringen Sauerstoffkonzen-trationen auf, die weit unter den oben genannten k-Werten liegen (s. S. 106). Schon bei 0,14 μM/l, d.h. der Sauerstoffkonzentration, bei der die Zellen nur noch 50% ihres norma-len Sauerstoffverbrauches aufweisen (FROESE, 1962, 1968), tritt eine Schulter auf (RÉVÉSZ u. LITTBRAND, 1966). Der Sauerstoffverbrauch der Zellen und der Anstieg der Extrapola-tionsnummer lassen sich gut korrelieren (Abb. 55), (LITTBRAND u. RÉVÉSZ, 1969).

Der exponentielle Verlauf der Dosiseffektkurve erklärt die Beobachtung, daß kein Fraktionierungseffekt auftritt, wenn die erste Bestrahlung unter Bedingungen kompletter Anoxie durchgeführt wurde (Révész u. Littbrand, 1967). In Abb. 55 ist zu sehen, wie Extrapolationsnummer, Zellatmung und Fraktionierungseffekt in gleicher Weise mit der Sauerstoffkonzentration ansteigen. Analoge Beobachtungen machten Phillips u. Hank (1968) nach Bestrahlung von Knochenmarkszellen in vivo unter Anoxie. Andererseits beobachteten Elkind u. Mitarb. (1965) entsprechend der Schulterkurve bei Einzeitbestrahlung auch einen Fraktionierungseffekt bei ca. 0,02 μM/l Sauerstoff, bei dem gleichen Zellstamm übrigens, den auch Littbrand u. Révész (1969) verwendeten.

Wenn unter anoxischen Bedingungen die Dosiswirkungskurve exponentiell verläuft, hängt der Sauerstoffverstärkungsfaktor von der Strahlendosis ab, wobei im Bereich kleiner Dosen anoxische Zellen mindestens so strahlenempfindlich sein dürften wie euoxische Zellen (Cohen, 1967). Nach Strahlendosen zwischen 100 und 200 rad ist die Überlebensrate

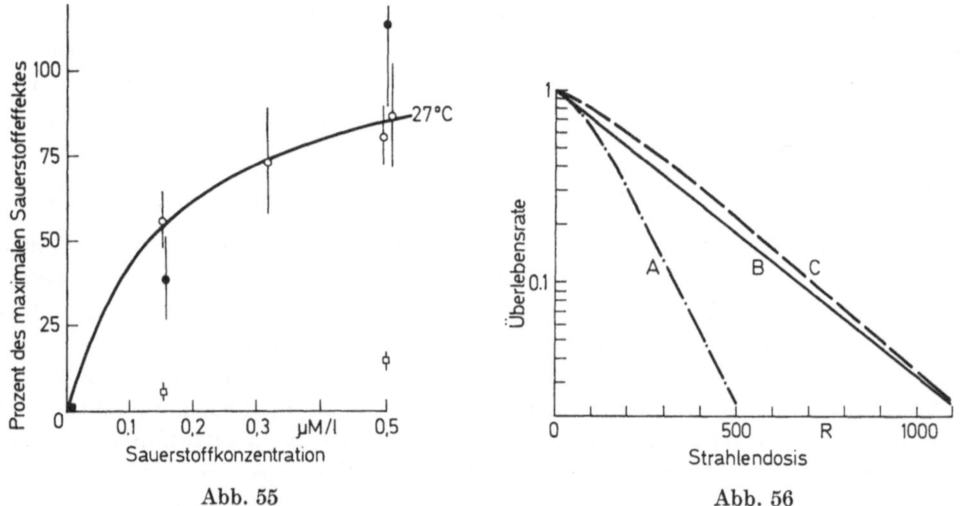

Abb. 55   Abb. 56

Abb. 55. Die Abhängigkeit der Endneigung der Dosiseffektkurve (□), der Extrapolationsnummer (●), des Fraktionierungseffektes (○) und der Atmungskonstanten (Q_{O_2}) bei 27° C (—27°) von der Sauerstoffkonzentration. (Nach Littbrand u. Révész, 1969)

Abb. 56. Idealisierte Dosiseffektkurven von Säugetierzellen bei Bestrahlung in Luft (A), in absoluter Anoxie ($<$ 0,002 μM/l Sauerstoff) (B) und in 0,15 μM/l Sauerstoff (C). (Littbrand u. Révész, 1969)

von anoxischen Zellen in Plateauphase nicht größer als die von mit Luft equilibrierten Zellen der log-Phase (Révész, 1971, unveröffentlicht), während Berry u. Mitarb. (1970) sogar bis zu Dosen von 600 rad eine bevorzugte Inaktivierung von Zellen in hypoxischer stationärer Phase fanden. Aber auch bei Zellen gleicher Wachstumsphase ist bis zu einer Dosis von 150 rad keine größere Resistenz von anoxischen gegenüber euoxischen Zellen (Littbrand, 1970a) festzustellen.

Bei Dosen zwischen 150 R und 450 R ist bei einer Sauerstoffkonzentration von 0,15 μM/l die Überlebensrate um ca. 10 % höher als bei 0,002 μM/l (Révész u. Littbrand, 1969a). Sauerstoff hat also einen ambivalenten Einfluß auf die Strahlenwirkung: Je nach Konzentration und Strahlendosis kann er radioprotektiv oder sensibilisierend wirken. Littbrand u. Révész (1969) veröffentlichten folgende (idealisierte) Dosiswirkungskurven für Bestrahlung in Luft, in kompletter Anoxie und bei 0,15 μM/l Sauerstoff (Abb. 56). Bei Sauerstoffkonzentrationen, die eine Atmung der Zellen noch ermöglichen, ist die Inaktivierungsrate geringer als in Anoxie. Dieser Strahlenschutzeffekt geringer Mengen

Sauerstoff könnte die Folge einer Erholung vom potentiell letalen Strahlenschaden (s. S. 102f.) sein, der in weniger als einer halben Minute nach Bestrahlungsende schon fixiert ist (LITTBRAND u. RÉVÉSZ, 1969). Außerdem wird unter diesen Bedingungen (0,15 μM/l Sauerstoff) ein subletaler Strahlenschaden induziert, der sich in Fraktionierungsversuchen nachweisen läßt. Wenn die Zellen während des Intervalls in Luft gehalten werden, so tritt auch bei der 2. Bestrahlung unter 0,15 μM/l Sauerstoff die gleiche Schulterkurve auf. Unter kompletter Anoxie ist jedoch kein subletaler Strahlenschaden induzierbar.

Es treten also unter Stickstoff und Sauerstoff nicht nur quantitative Unterschiede in der Strahlenwirkung auf (READ, 1952) sondern auch qualitative Unterschiede. Neben der Überlebensrate wurde in einigen Untersuchungen auch die Proliferationsfähigkeit in Anoxie bestrahlter Zellen verändert gefunden: Die von überlebenden chinesischen Hamsterzellen gebildeten Kolonien hatten einen größeren mittleren Durchmesser (SIRACKA u. Mitarb., 1969), wogegen NIAS (1968) keine Änderung in der Koloniegrößenverteilung von HeLa-Zellen feststellte. Auch die Wachstumshemmung von Ehrlich-Aszites-Tumorzellen nach hohen Strahlendosen in Anoxie ist wesentlich geringer als bei in Luft bestrahlten überlebenden Zellen (LITTBRAND, 1970b). Dem stehen Ergebnisse von ELKIND u. Mitarb. (1965a) gegenüber, die nach Bestrahlung unter 0,01 μM/l Sauerstoff gleiche Teilungshemmung und gleiches Proliferationsverhalten fanden wie nach Bestrahlung mit der entsprechenden Strahlendosis in Luft.

Die Restitution der Schulter in der Dosiswirkungskurve von längere Zeit in Hypoxie gehaltenen Zellen nach plötzlicher Zufuhr von Sauerstoff erfolgt nicht sofort und ist erst nach ca. 3—5 Stunden komplett (FOSTER u. Mitarb., 1971). Die Form und die Temperaturabhängigkeit dieser Restitution der Schulter zeigen auffallende Ähnlichkeit mit dem ELKINDschen Fraktionierungseffekt (s. S. 93 ff.).

4. Der Fraktionierungseffekt bei hypoxischen Zellen

Anoxie hat noch einen weiteren Einfluß auf den Fraktionierungseffekt. Bei Bohnenkeimlingen (HALL u. CAVANAGH, 1967) ebenso wie bei Algenzellen (HOWARD, 1968) ist bei 0,01 μM/l Sauerstoffkonzentration im Bestrahlungsintervall keine Erholung vom subletalen Strahlenschaden zu bemerken. Bei HeLa-Zellen ist die Überlebensrate bei zweistündigem Intervall in 0,01 μM/l Sauerstoff nur um den Faktor 1,44 höher als bei Einzeitbestrahlung, während der Fraktionierungseffekt unter gleichen Bestrahlungsbedingungen, aber mit Sauerstoffzufuhr im Intervall, den Faktor 2,52 ausmacht (FOX u. NIAS, 1970). Unterschiede im Fraktionierungseffekt sind hier, im Gegensatz z.B. zu den Versuchen von LITTBRAND u. RÉVÉSZ (1969), nicht Ausdruck unterschiedlicher Schultergrößen der Dosiseffektkurven der konditionierenden Bestrahlung, da in beiden Fällen die erste Dosis in Hypoxie gegeben wurde und dabei eine normal große Schulter auftrat.

Das gleiche Ergebnis erhielt KEMBER (1968) bei der fraktionierten Bestrahlung klonogener Knorpelzellen der Rattentibia; wenn die Extremität zwischen beiden Dosisfraktionen dauernd abgebunden war, war kein Fraktionierungseffekt zu beobachten, eine Öffnung des Blutstromes nach 2 Stunden für weitere 2 Stunden und anschließende Bestrahlung machte jedoch einen typischen Fraktionierungseffekt möglich. Diese Ergebnisse sprechen dafür, daß bei extremer Hypoxie keine Erholung vom subletalen Strahlenschaden auftritt. Dem stehen Ergebnisse von ELKIND u. Mitarb. (1964, 1965c) gegenüber, die bei bis auf 0,01 μM/l reduziertem Sauerstoffdruck nicht nur keine Reduktion der Schulter sondern auch vollständige Erholung im bestrahlungsfreien Intervall trotz unveränderter Hypoxie gefunden hatten. Die Überlebensrate stieg unter 0,4 μM/l Sauerstoff so schnell an wie bei besser mit Sauerstoff versorgten Zellen. Bei längeren Intervallen aber zeigte sich eine relativ höhere Überlebensrate von im Intervall hypoxischen Zellen (also umgekehrt wie erwartet). Nachdem das Absinken der Überlebensrate nach dem ersten Anstieg auf einer Progression der partiell synchronisierten Population in empfindliche Zyklusphasen beruht, kann aus dem Fehlen eines Minimums nach dem ersten Gipfel des

Fraktionierungseffektes auf eine Retardierung oder gar Blockierung der Progression der überlebenden Zellen im Zellzyklus geschlossen werden.

An synchronisierten chinesischen Hamsterzellen (V–79) fanden Koch u. Kruuv (1971) bei Sauerstoffkonzentrationen unter 0,1 μM/l noch eine normale Progression der Zellen durch den Zyklus, aber ein völliges Fehlen einer Erholung vom subletalen Strahlenschaden.

Auch der Oxygenierungsstatus der Zellen in der Zeit vor der fraktionierten Bestrahlung beeinflußt das Ausmaß des Fraktionierungseffektes, wahrscheinlich über eine partielle Synchronisation der chronisch hypoxischen Zellpopulation (s. S. 111), (Hall, 1969c).

Informationen über das Ausmaß der Erholung vom subletalen Strahlenschaden lassen sich auch aus den Bestrahlungsversuchen mit niedriger Dosisleistung gewinnen, die von Bedford u. Hall (1966), Hall u. Mitarb. (1966a) und Berry (1968b) durchgeführt wurden. Die Bestrahlung von HeLa-Zellen unter 0,4 μM/l Sauerstoff hatte eine Verminderung der Dosisleistung von 103 rad/min auf 30 rad/h, aber keine signifikante Veränderung der Dosiswirkungskurve zur Folge (D_0 akut = 435 rad, D_0 protrahiert = 405 rad). Bei Bestrahlung in Luft nahm die D_0 dagegen von 180 rad auf 260 rad zu (Bedford u. Hall, 1966). Bei noch niedrigerem Sauerstoffdruck (0,02 μM/l für 6 Stunden) wurden ähnliche Ergebnisse gefunden (Hall u. Mitarb., 1966a). Dagegen zeigte sich bei protrahierter Bestrahlung (40 rad/h) von P-388-Leukämiezellen unter hypoxischen Bedingungen in vivo oder in vitro ein ausgeprägter Dosisleistungseffekt (D_0 akut = 291 rad; D_0 protrahiert = 592 rad).

Bei Bestrahlung von HeLa-Zellen mit Neutronen einer Californiumquelle bei einer Dosisleistung von 16 rad/h fanden Fairchild u. Mitarb. (1970b) einen Sauerstoffverstärkungsfaktor von 1,3.

Wenn also mit abnehmender Sauerstoffkonzentration Fraktionierungseffekt und Dosisleistungseffekt immer kleiner werden, dann wird auch mit abnehmender Dosisleistung und zunehmender Fraktionierung der Sauerstoffverstärkungsfaktor abnehmen. Oliver (1967) postulierte, daß bei extrem niedrigen Dosisleistungen schließlich die Dosiseffektkurven anoxisch und euoxisch bestrahlter Zellen identisch sind.

5. Proliferationskinetik hypoxischer Zellen

Um die Strahlenwirkung auf hypoxische Zellen in Tumoren abschätzen zu können, ist es nicht nur erforderlich, die Dosiswirkungsbeziehungen hyp- und anoxischer Zellen sowie den Fraktionierungseffekt und die Erholung vom potentiell letalen Strahlenschaden zu kennen, sondern es ist auch wichtig zu wissen, ob Zellen unter an- bzw. hypoxischen Bedingungen längere Zeit überleben und proliferieren können, und ob dabei Umverteilungen in der relativen Dauer der einzelnen Zyklusphasen auftreten.

Untersuchungen zur Frage der Proliferationsfähigkeit unter Sauerstoffmangel leiden unter dem technischen Problem, definierte niedrige Sauerstoffkonzentrationen zu erzeugen und aufrecht zu erhalten. Das wird besonders deutlich, wenn man sieht, daß allein der im Polystyren der Kulturgefäße gelöste Sauerstoff ausreicht, für mehrere Tage kaum gestörte Zellvermehrung zu ermöglichen (Born u. Hug, 1970). Normales Wachstum unter hypoxischen Bedingungen fanden Brosemer u. Rutter (1961) an HeLa-Zellen, Harris (1956) an Primärkulturen von Rattenherzen, Pace u. Mitarb. (1962) an L-, Mäuseleber- und HeLa-Zellen. Eine Reduktion der Wachstumsgeschwindigkeit beobachteten Dales (1960) bei L-Zellen und Rueckert u. Mueller (1970b) bei HeLa-Zellen. Clark (1969) sah bei Mäusefibroblasten keinerlei Wachstum und Gifford (1963) fand, daß nach kurzem Wachstum HeLa-Zellen unter Anoxie abstarben. Ehrlich-Aszites-Tumorzellen, HeLa-Zellen und chinesische Hamsterzellen verlieren unter Anoxie ihre reproduktive Integrität (Littbrand u. Révész, 1968; Hall u. Mitarb., 1966; Born u. Trott, 1971). Die Abnahme der Koloniebildungsfähigkeit ist neben der Sauerstoffkonzentration vor allem von der Dauer der Hypoxie abhängig — es wurden Schulterkurven (Hall u. Mitarb., 1966; Bedford, 1970; Abb. 57) und hyperbole Dosiswirkungskurven (Littbrand u. Révész; Born

u. Trott) gefunden. 36 Stunden Aufenthalt in 0,08 μM/l Sauerstoff zerstörte die reproduktive Integrität von 90 % aller Zellen (chinesische Hamsterzellen, CHL-F), während nach der gleichen Zeit in 0,8 μM/l Sauerstoff noch über die Hälfte der Zellen überlebten. Die in der Abb. 57 dargestellten Sauerstoffkonzentrationen liegen alle, und das muß ausdrücklich betont werden, um eine bis zwei Größenordnungen unter der Sauerstoffkonzentration, bei der schon ein halbmaximaler „Sauerstoffeffekt" auftritt. Dabei wird der Verlust der reproduktiven Integrität bei 0,8 μM/l Sauerstoff zumindest zeitweilig mehr als ausgeglichen durch Zellproliferation, die, wenn auch mit größerer Verdoppelungszeit, weitergeht.

Über das Problem der Zellproliferation unter Sauerstoffmangel in vitro liegen nur spärliche Daten vor. Auch nach längerer Hypoxie nimmt der Markierungsindex nach

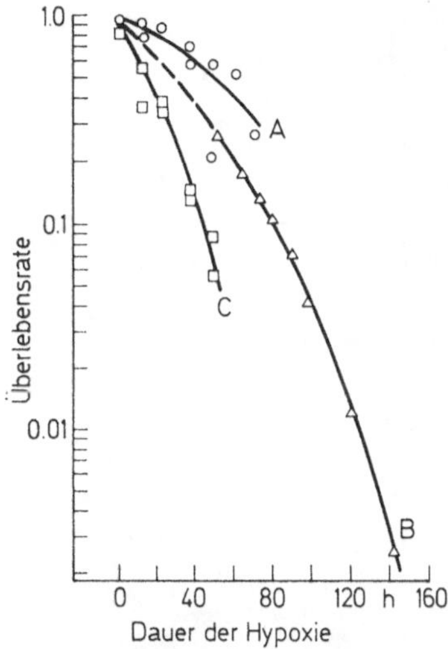

Abb. 57. Die Überlebensrate von chinesischen Hamsterzellen (CHL-F) in vitro unter Sauerstoffmangel unterschiedlicher Dauer und Schwere:
Kurve A: Sauerstoffkonzentration 0,8 μM/l
Kurve B: Sauerstoffkonzentration 0,15 μM/l
Kurve C: Sauerstoffkonzentration 0,08 μM/l
(Bedford, 1970)

[3]HTdR-Zugabe nicht wesentlich ab, obwohl die Verdoppelungszeit der Zellpopulation stark ansteigt (Bedford, 1970; Born u. Trott, 1971), was auf eine entsprechende Verlängerung der S-Phase hinweist. Proliferationskinetische Untersuchungen haben aber auch Hinweise auf einen Block in der G_1-Phase ergeben (Bedford, 1970; Born u. Trott, 1971). Die flacher verlaufende Dosiseffektkurve nach Bestrahlung von längere Zeit unter Sauerstoffmangel stehenden Zellen könnte auf einer partiellen Synchronisation beruhen (Bedford, 1970).

In Aszitestumoren, die mit zunehmendem Alter immer hypoxischer werden (Del Monte, 1967; Frindel u. Mitarb., 1969b), findet man eine zunehmende Akkumulation von Zellen in G_1- und G_2-Phase (Frindel u. Mitarb., 1969a).

6. Die Bedeutung des Sauerstoffeffektes für die Strahlentherapie

Für den Strahlentherapeuten stellt sich die Frage, inwieweit hyp- und anoxische Zellen im Tumor den Erfolg einer Strahlentherapie beeinflussen können. Bei einem Tumor, der ca. 1 % hypoxische klonogene Zellen enthält, wird die Form der Dosiseffektkurve bei Dosen über 1 000 rad ausschließlich von der Empfindlichkeit der durch ihre Hypoxie resistenten Zellen bestimmt. Berechnungen der Dosiswirkungskurven gemischter Populationen aus euoxischen und hypoxischen Zellen sind wiederholt durchgeführt worden und haben entmutigend hohe Strahlendosen ergeben, die zur Inaktivierung aller Zellen eines Tumors notwendig wären (Wilson, 1961; Suit, 1966a; Munro, 1967).

Eine besondere Zellkulturtechnik ermöglicht das Kultivieren sphärischer Klone in vitro, die wie Tumorläppchen aus zentraler Nekrose und proliferierender äußerer Zellschicht bestehen (Abb. 58a), (Sutherland u. Mitarb., 1970, 1971; Dalen u. Burki, 1971; Trott, 1971). Die Dosiswirkungskurve nach Bestrahlung solcher sphärischer Klone gleicht der Dosiseffektkurve von in vivo bestrahlten Tumoren (Powers u. Tolmach, 1964;

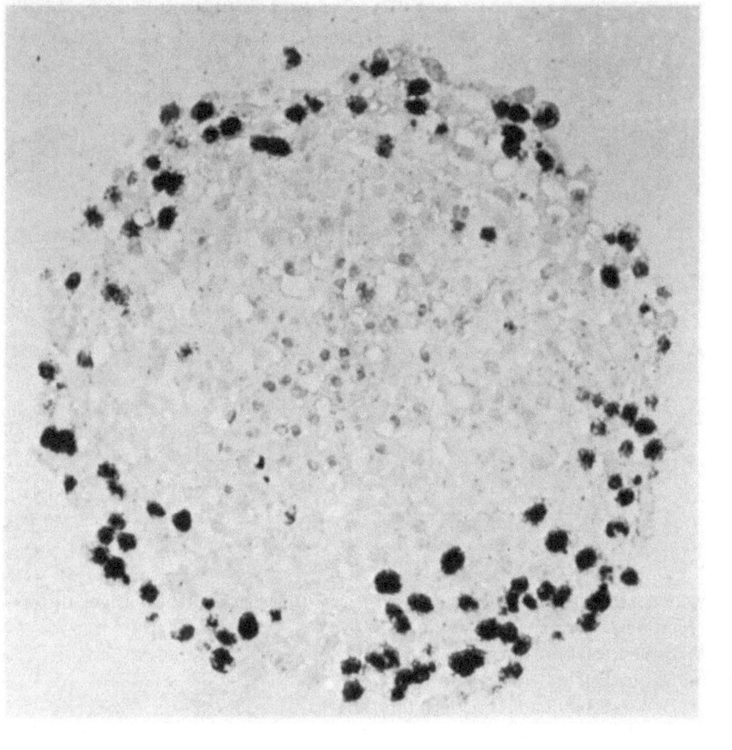
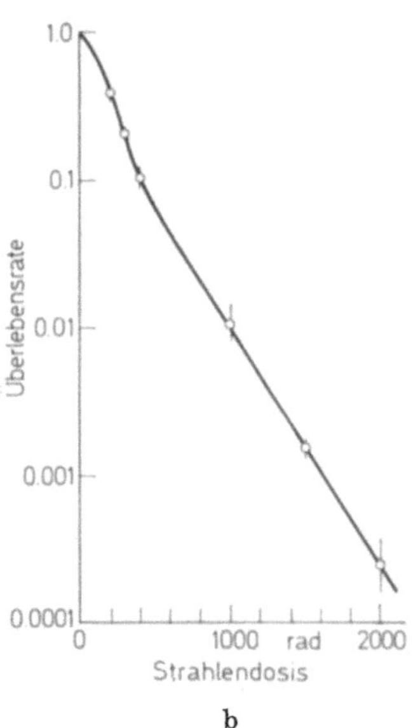

a   b

Abb. 58a. Autoradiographisches Bild der Zellproliferation in einem sphärischen Klon chinesischer Hamsterzellen (Durchmesser ca. 0,3 mm) nach 18 h dauernder Markierung mit Tritium-Thymidin. Man erkennt, daß die Inkorporation des Tritium-Thymidins auf die peripheren Zellen beschränkt ist und sich im Zentrum eine Nekrose ausbildet. (Trott u. Mitarb., unveröffentlicht)
b. Die Überlebensrate von HeLa-Zellen nach Bestrahlung sphärischer Klone von je 5000 Zellen. (Trott u. Mitarb., unveröffentlicht)

Barendsen u. Broerse, 1969), indem sie wie diese eine resistente Fraktion aufweisen, die mit zunehmender Größe des Klons größer wird (Sutherland u. Mitarb., 1970; Trott, 1971), (Abb. 58b).

Wenn auch in Tumoren hypoxische Zellen vorkommen, die eine wesentlich höhere Strahlenresistenz aufweisen und ihre volle reproduktive Integrität bewahren können, so ist es doch möglich, daß auf Grund der verminderten Erholungsfähigkeit hypoxischer Populationen (Hall u. Mitarb., 1966b), von Reoxygenierung (Thomlinson, 1967), von Gefäßveränderungen (Reinhold, 1971) und von anderen geweblichen Reaktionen im Verlauf einer sich über Wochen hinziehenden Strahlentherapie hypoxische Zellen ihre Bedeutung für die Kurabilität des Tumors verlieren. Durch Sauerstoffüberdruckbehandlung, Abbinden tumortragender Extremitäten und Verwendung von Strahlung höheren LETs wird derzeit versucht, dem Problem hypoxischer Zellen im Tumor beizukommen (Diskussion z.B. bei FOWLER, 1966). Durch Hypoxie bedingte Veränderungen des Zellmetabolismus und der Proliferationskinetik können aber bei geeigneter Behandlungsplanung dazu beitragen, die durch die Hypoxie bedingte Strahlenresistenz zu kompensieren. In einer sich über viele Hefte des British Journal of Radiology hinziehenden Diskussion (z.B. HALL u. Mitarb., 1966 b; OLIVER, 1967; HALL, 1967 a; LIVERSAGE, 1967) kam HALL (1967 b) zu dem Schluß: ,,We suggest that the oxygen effect is unimportant in clinical radiotherapy and has been, in fact, something of a red herring".

Gerade bei der Betrachtung des Sauerstoffeffektes kommen die Möglichkeiten der zellulären Strahlenbiologie für die Strahlentherapie, aber auch ihre Grenzen zum Ausdruck, was ALPER (1967) zu der Bemerkung veranlaßte: ,,There is moreto the cure of tumours than cell survival curves", was nur eine Feststellung von OPITZ aus der Pionierzeit der experimentellen Strahlentherapie wiederholt: ,,So lange wir nur die Epithelzellen des Krebses beachten, ist ein Fortschritt in der Strahlenbehandlung des Krebses nicht zu erwarten" (1925).

Literatur

ALPER, T., HOWARD-FLANDERS, P.: Role of oxygen in modifying the radiosensitivity of E. coli B. Nature **178**, 978–979 (1956).

— GILLIES, N. E., ELKIND, M. M.: The sigmoid survival curve in radiobiology. Nature **186**, 1062–1063 (1960).

— FOWLER, J. F., MORGAN, R. L., VONBERG, O. O., ELLIS, F., OLIVER, R.: The characterization of the "type C" survival curve. Brit. J. Radiol. **35**, 722—723 (1962).

— Applications of radiobiology in radiotherapeutic developments. Modern trends in radiotherapy 1, ed. by T. J. Deeley and C. A. P. Wood, London: Butterworths 1967.

— MOORE, J. L.: The interdependence of oxygen enhancement ratios for 250 kVp X-rays and fast neutrons. Brit. J. Radiol. **40**, 843–848 (1967).

— HOWARD, A., KIEFER, J.: Radiobiological terminology. Nature **224**, 625–626 (1969).

ANDREWS, J. R., BERRY, R. J.: Fast neutron irradiation and the relationship of radiation dose and mammalian tumor cell reproductive capacity. Radiat. Res. **16**, 76–81 (1962).

ARLETT, C. F.: The response of Chinese hamster cells to alpha particle irradiation. studia biophysica **18**, 99–106 (1969).

ASHBY, R. R., BONTE, F. J.: The metabolic requirements for repair of sublethal damage (Abstr.). Radiat. Res. **35**, 512–513 (1968).

BACCHETTI, S., WHITMORE, G. F.: Actinomycin D and X-ray sensitivity in synchronized mouse L-cells. Radiat. Res. **31**, 577–578 (1967).

— — The action of hydroxyurea on mouse L-cells. Cell Tissue Kinet. **2**, 193–211 (1969).

— SINCLAIR, W. K.: The relation of protein synthesis to radiation-induced division delay in Chinese hamster cells. Radiat. Res. **44**, 788–806 (1970).

— — The effects of X-rays on the synthesis of DNA, RNA, and proteins in synchronized Chinese hamster cells. Radiat. Res. **45**, 598–612 (1971).

BAKER, D. J., TOWN, C. D.: "Anoxia" in radiobiology. Brit. J. Radiol. **39**, 706–707 (1966).

BAKER, M. L., DALRYMPLE, G. V., SANDERS, J. L., Moss, A. J.: Effects of radiation on asynchronous and synchronized L-cells under energy deprivation. Radiat. Res. **42**, 320–330 (1970).

BARENDSEN, G. W., BEUSKER, T. L. J., VERGROESEN, A. J., BUDKE, L.: Effects of different ionizing radiations on human cells in tissue culture. II. Biological experiments. Radiat. Res. **13**, 841–849 (1960).

— Damage to the reproductive capacity of human cells in tissue culture by ionizing radiations of different linear energy transfer. The initial effects of ionizing radiations, ed. by R. J. C. Harris. New York: Academic Press 1961.

— Dose-survival curves of human cells in tissue culture irradiated with α, β, 20-kV X- and 200-kV X-radiation. Nature **193**, 1153–1155 (1962).

— WALTER, H. M. D., FOWLER, J. F., BEWLEY, D. K.: Effects of different ionizing radiations on human cells in tissue culture. III. Experiments with cyclotron-accelerated alpha-particles and deuterons. Radiat. Res. **18**, 106–119 (1963).

— Impairment of the proliferative capacity of human cells in culture by α-particles with different linear-energy transfer. Int. J. Rad. Biol. **8**, 453–466 (1964).

— WALTER, H. M. D.: Effects of different ionizing radiations on human cells in tissue culture. IV. Modification of radiation damage. Radiat. Res. **21**, 314–329 (1964).

— The influence of oxygen on damage to the proliferative capacity of cultured human cells produced by radiations of different LET. Cellular Radiation Biology, Baltimore: Williams & Wilkins 1965.

— KOOT, C. J., VAN KERSEN, G. R., BEWLEY, D. K., FIELD, S. B., PARNELL, C. J.: The effect of oxygen on impairment of the proliferative capacity of human cells in culture by ionizing radiations of different LET. Int. J. Rad. Biol. **10**, 317–327 (1966).

— Responses of cultured cells, tumours and normal tissues to radiations of different linear energy transfer. Current topics in radiation research **IV**, 293–356 (1968).

— BROERSE J. J.: Experimental radiotherapy of a rat rhabdomyosarcoma with 15 MeV neutrons and 300 kV-rays. II. Effects of single exposures. Europ. J. Cancer 5, 373–391 (1969).

Barendsen, G. W.: Cellular responses determining the effectiveness of fast neutrons relative to X-rays for effects on experimental tumours. Europ. J. Cancer 7, 181–190 (1971).

Barranco, S. C., Romsdahl, M. M., Humphrey, R. M.: The radiation response of human malignant melanoma cells grown in vitro. Cancer Res. 31, 830–833 (1971).

Bases, R. E.: Some applications of tissue culture methods to radiation research. Cancer Res. 19, 311–315 (1959).

Becker, A. J., McCulloch, E. A., Till, J. E.: Cytological demonstration of the clonal nature of spleen colonies derived from transplanted mouse marrow cells. Nature 197, 452–454 (1963).

Bedford, J. S., Hall, E. J.: Survival of HeLa cells cultured in vitro and exposed to protracted gamma-irradiation. Int. J. Rad. Biol. 7, 377–383 (1963).

— — Threshold hypoxia: its effect on the survival of mammalian cells irradiated at high and low dose-rates. Brit. J. Radiol. 39, 896–900 (1966).

— The effect of prolonged hypoxia on the radiation response of mammalian cells. IVe congrès international de radiobiologie et de physico-chimie des rayonnements, Evian (unveröffentlichtes Manuskript) 1970.

Beer, J. Z., Lett, J. T., Alexander, P.: Influence of temperature and medium on the X-ray sensitivities of leukaemia cells in vitro. Nature 199. 193–194 (1963).

— Rosiek, O., Sablinski, J. M., Ziemba-Zak, B.: Radiation-induced heritable lesions in cultures of murine leukaemic cells L 5178 Y. studia biophysica 6, 103–111 (1968).

Belli, J. A., Bonte, F. J.: Influence of temperature on the radiation response of mammalian cells in tissue culture. Radiat. Res. 18, 272–276 (1963).

— — Rose, M. S.: Radiation recovery response of mammalian tumour cells in vivo. Nature 211, 662–663 (1966).

— Roach, A.: "Anoxic" radiation response in cultured mammalian cells. Brit. J. Radiol. 41, 390–391 (1968).

— Shelton, M.: Potentially lethal radiation damage: repair by mammalian cells in culture. Science 165, 490–492 (1969).

Bender, M. A., Gooch, P. C.: The kinetics of X-ray survival of mammalian cells in vitro. Int. J. Rad. Biol. 5, 133–145 (1962).

Berenbaum, M. C.: Dose-response curves for agents that impair cell reproductive integrity. A fundamental difference between dose-response curves of antimetabolites and those for radiation and alkylating agents. Brit. J. Cancer 23, 426–433 (1969).

Berry, R. J., Andrews, J. R.: Quantitative relationships between radiation dose and the reproductive capacity of tumor cells in a mammalian system in vivo. Radiology 77, 824–830 (1961).

— Cohen, A. B.: Some observations on the reproductive capacity of mammalian tumour cells exposed in vivo to Gamma radiation at low dose-rates. Brit. J. Radiol. 35, 489–491 (1962).

— Oliver, R.: Effect of post-irradiation incubation conditions on recovery between fractionated doses of X-rays. Nature 201, 94–96 (1964).

Berry, R. J.: On the shape of X-ray dose-response curves for the reproductive survival of mammalian cells. Brit. J. Radiol. 37, 948–951 (1964a).

— A comparison of effects of some chemotherapeutic agents and those of X-rays on the reproductive capacity of mammalian cells. Nature 203, 1150–1153 (1964b).

— Bewley, D. K., Parnell, C. J.: Reproductive capacity of mammalian tumour cells irradiated in vivo with cyclotron-produced fast neutrons. Brit. J. Radiol. 38, 613–617 (1965).

— Effects of some metabolic inhibitors on X-ray dose-response curves for the survival of mammalian cells in vitro, and on early recovery between fractionated X-ray doses. Brit. J. Radiol. 39, 458–463 (1966a).

— Distribution of clone-sizes in surviving and non-surviving HeLa-S-3 cells in vitro: possible evidence for radiation-induced synchrony. Int. J. Rad. Biol. 11, 301–304 (1966b).

— Evans, H. J., Robinson, D. M.: Perturbations in X-ray dose response in vitro with time after plating: a pitfall in the comparison of results obtained by different laboratories using asynchronous cell systems. Exp. Cell Res. 42, 512–522 (1966).

— "Small clones" in irradiated tumour cells in vivo. Kinetics of re-growth of murine leukaemia cells surviving irradiation with X-rays, fast neutrons and accelerated charged particles. Brit. J. Radiol. 40, 285–291 (1967a).

— Effects of small and large first X-ray doses on the two-dose recovery pattern in HeLa S-3 cells in vitro. Radiat. Res. 32, 13–20 (1967b).

— On the use of an arbitrary minimum clone size to define survival of cell reproductive capacity. Radiat. Res. 30, 237–247 (1967c).

— Some observations on the combined effects of X-rays and methotrexate on human tumor cells in vitro with possible relevance to their most useful combination in radiotherapy. Am. J. Roentgen. 102, 509–518 (1968a).

— Hypoxic protection and recovery in tumour cells irradiated at low dose-rates and assessed in vivo. Brit. J. Radiol. 41, 921–926 (1968b).

— Hall, E. J., Forster, D. W., Storr, T. H., Goodman, M. J.: Survival of mammalian cells exposed to X-rays at ultra-high dose-rates. Brit. J. Radiol. 42, 102–107 (1969).

— Survival of murine leukaemia cells in vivo after irradiation in vitro under aerobic and hypoxic conditions with monoenergetic accelerated charged particles. Radiat. Res. 44, 237–247 (1970).

— Hall, E. J., Cavanagh, J.: Radiosensitivity and the oxygen effect for mammalian cells cultured in vitro in stationary phase. Brit. J. Radiol. 43, 81–90 (1970).

— Zelluläre Faktoren der Strahlenempfindlichkeit. Präoperative Tumorbestrahlung. Hrsg. O. Hug. München: Urban & Schwarzenberg 1971a.

— Hypoxic protection against fast neutrons of different energies – a review. Europ. J. Cancer 7, 145–152 (1971b).

— Stedeford, J. B. H.: Brit. J. Radiol. (1971) (in Druck).

BEWLEY, D. K.: A comparison of the response of mammalian cells to fast neutrons and charged particle beams. Radiat. Res. **34**, 446–458 (1968).

BHASKARAN, S., DITTRICH, W.: Radiosensitivity of different Ehrlich-ascites-tumour mutants in vivo and in tissue culture. Atomkernenergie **14**, 51–55 (1969).

BIRD, R., BURKI, J.: Inactivation of mammalian cells at different stages of the cell cycle as a function of radiation linear energy transfer. Physical Aspects of Radiation Quality, IAEA – SM – 145/26, 241–250. Wien, 1971.

BOOTSMA, D.: Changes induced in the first post-irradiation generation cycle of human cells studied by double labeling. Exp. Cell Res. **38**, 429–431 (1965).

— Mitotic delay of human cells in tissue culture irradiated at different phases of the generation cycle. Progress in radiology, ed. by L. Turano, A. Ratti and C. Biagini. Amsterdam: Excerpta Medica Found. 1967.

BORN, R., HUG, O.: Cell growth on plastic and glass surfaces under anoxia. Brit. J. Radiol. **43**, 430 (1970).

— TROTT, K.-R.: Proliferation kinetics of Chinese hamster cells under prolonged hypoxia. 8th annual meeting Europ. Soc. Radiat. Biol. Basko Polje (unveröffentlichtes Manuskript) 1971.

BRENT, T. P., BUTLER, J. A. V., CRATHORN, A. R.: Effects of irradiation on synthesis of deoxyribonucleic acid and mitosis in synchronous cultures of HeLa cells. Nature **210**, 393–395 (1966).

BROERSE, J. J., BARENDSEN, G. W., VAN KERSEN, G. R.: Survival of cultured human cells after irradiation with fast neutrons of different energies in hypoxic and oxygenated conditions. Int. J. Rad. Biol. **13**, 559–572 (1968).

— — Recovery of cultured cells after fast neutron irradiation. Int. J. Rad. Biol. **15**, 335–339 (1969).

— ROELSE, H.: Survival of intestinal crypt cells after fractionated exposure to X-rays and 15 MeV neutrons. Int. J. Rad. Biol. 20, 391–395 (1971).

— ENGELS, A. C., LELIEVIELD, P., VAN PUTTEN, L. M., DUNCAN, W., GREENE, D., MASSEY, J. B., GILBERT, C. W., HENDRY, J. H., HOWARD, A.: The survival of colony-forming units in mouse bone-marrow after in vivo irradiation with D–T neutrons, X- and Gamma-radiation. Int. J. Rad. Biol. **19**, 101–110 (1971).

BROSEMER, R. W., RUTTER, W. J.: The effect of oxygen tension on the growth and metabolism of a mammalian cell. Exp. Cell Res. **25**, 101–113 (1961).

BROWN III, C. H., CARBONE, P.P.: Effects of chemotherapeutic agents on normal mouse bone marrow grown in vitro. Cancer Res. **31**, 185–190 (1971).

BURROWS, M. T.: The cultivation of tissues of the chick embryo outside the body. J. Am. med. Ass. **55**, 2057 (1910).

BUSH, R. S., BRUCE, W. R.: The radiation sensitivity of a transplanted murine lymphoma as determined by two different assay methods. Radiat. Res. **25**, 503–513 (1965).

CALDWELL, W. L., LAMERTON, L. F., BEWLEY, D. K.: Increased sensitivity of in vitro murine leukaemia cells to fractionated X-rays and fast neutrons. Nature **208**, 168–170 (1965).

CANTI, R. G., DONALDSON, M.: The effect of radium on mitosis in vitro. Proc. Roy. Soc. Lond. B **100**, 413–419 (1926).

— SPEAR, F. G.: The effect of Gamma irradiation on cell division in tissue culture in vitro. Proc. Roy. Soc. Lond. B **102**, 92–101 (1927).

— — The effect of Gamma irradiation on cell division in tissue culture in vitro. Proc. Roy. Soc. Lond. B. **105**, 93–98 (1929).

CARLSON, J. G.: Immediate effects on division, morphology, and viability of the cell. Radiation Biology, ed. by A. Holländer. Vol. I/2, 763–824. New York: McCraw-Hill 1954.

— X-ray-induced prophase delay and reversion of selected cells in certain avian and mammalian tissues in culture. Radiat. Res. **37**, 15–30 (1969).

CARREL, A.: The permanent life of tissue outside the organism. J. exp. med. **15**, 516 (1912).

CHAPMAN, J. D., STURROCK, J., BOAG, J. M., CROOKALL, J. O.: Anoxia in radiobiology. Brit. J. Radiol. **41**, 951–952 (1968).

— — — — The oxygen tension around mammalian cells growing on plastic petri dishes and its effect on cell survival curves. Brit. J. Radiol. **42**, 399 (1969).

— TODD, P., STURROCK, J.: X-ray survival of cultured Chinese hamster cells resuming growth after plateau phase. Radiat. Res. **42**, 590–600 (1970).

CLARK, M. E.: Growth and morphology of adult mouse fibroblasts under anaerobic conditions and at limited oxygen tensions. Exp. Cell Res. **36**, 548–560 (1964).

COHEN, L.: A critical "dose-per-fraction" factor. Brit. J. Radiol. **40**, 154 (1967).

COLOMBO, G., MARIN, G.: Cytological analysis of colonies developed from mammalian cells irradiated in vitro with X-rays. Exp. Cell Res. **29**, 268–277 (1963).

CORMACK, D. V., FROESE, G.: A correlation between division delay and loss of colony-forming ability in cultured Chinese hamster cells. Physical Aspects of Radiation Quality, IAEA-SM-145/26, 251–259. Wien, 1971.

COURTENAY, V. D.: The response to continuous irradiation of the mouse lymphoma L 5178Y grown in vitro. Int. J. Radiat. Biol. **9**, 581–592 (1965).

— Radioresistant mutants of L 5178 Y cells. Radiat. Res. **38**, 186–203 (1969).

CULLEN, B., HORNSEY, S.: A comparison of X-ray survival curves obtained from cells cultured in vitro with those of the parent strain assayed in vivo. Int. J. Rad. Biol. **11**, 35–41 (1966).

DALEN, H., BURKI, H. J.: Some observations on the three-dimensional growth of L 5178 Y cell colonies in soft agar culture. Exp. Cell Res. **65**, 433–438 (1971).

DALES, S.: Effects of anaerobiosis on the rates of multiplication of mammalian cells cultured in vitro. Can. J. Biochem. Physiol. **38**, 871–878 (1960).

DALRYMPLE, G. V., SANDERS, J. L., BAKER, M. L.: Dinitrophenol decreases the radiation sensitivity of L-cells. Nature **216**, 708–709 (1967).

— — WILKINSON, K. P.: The role of energy metabolism in the rapair of radiation injury by L-cells (Abstr.). Radiat. Res. **39**, 515 (1969).

Davies, R. W., Baker, D. J.: Anoxia in radiobiology. Oxygen in polystyrene dishes – a further experiment. Brit. J. Radiol. **43**, 496–497 (1970).

Deering, R. A., Rice, R.: Heavy ion irradiation of HeLa cells. Radiat. Res. **17**, 774–786 (1962).

Delihas, N., Rich, M. A., Eidinoff, M. L.: Radiosensitization of a mammalian cell line with 5-bromodeoxyuridine. Radiat. Res. **17**, 471–491 (1962).

del Monte, U.: Changes in oxygen tension in Yoshida ascites hepatoma during growth. Proc. Soc. Exp. Biol. Med. **125**, 853–856 (1967).

Denekamp, J., Emery, E. W., Field, S. B.: Response of mouse epidermal cells to single and divided doses of fast neutrons. Radiat. Res. **45**, 80–84 (1971).

Deschner, E. E., Gray, L. H.: Influence of oxygen tension on X-ray induced chromosomal damage in Ehrlich ascites tumor cells irradiated in vitro and in vivo. Radiat. Res. **11**, 115–146 (1959).

Dewey, D. L., Boag, J. W.: Modification of the oxygen effect when bacteria are given large pulses of radiation. Nature **183**, 1450–1451 (1959).

— Effect of oxygen and nitric oxide on the radiosensitivity of human cells in tissue culture. Nature **186**, 780–782 (1960).

Dewey, W. C., Humphrey, R. M.: Relative radiosensitivity of different phases in the life cycle of L-P 59 mouse fibroblasts and ascites tumor cells. Radiat. Res. **16**, 503–530 (1962).

Dewey, D. L., Hawes, C.: 6-Aminonicotinamide and the radiosensitivity of human liver cells in culture. Nature **200**, 1176–1178 (1963).

Dewey, W. C., Humphrey, R. M., Cork, A.: Comparison of cell-multiplication and colony formation as criteria for radiation damage in cells grown in vitro. Int. J. Rad. Biol. **6**, 463–471 (1963).

— — Sedita, B. A.: Cell cycle kinetics and radiation-induced chromosomal aberrations studied with C-14 and H-3 labels. Biophys. J. **6**, 247–260 (1966).

— Robinette, S. M.: Progression of viable and non-viable synchronized Chinese hamster cells into the S-phase after X-irradiation in mitosis or the S-phase. Int. J. Rad. Biol. **16**, 495–500 (1969).

— Miller, H. H.: Effect of temperature on X-ray-induced cell lethality and chromosomal aberrations. Int. J. Rad. Biol. **18**, 91–93 (1970).

Dicke, K. A., Platenburg, M. G. C., van Bekkum, D. W.: Colony formation in agar: in vitro assay for haemopoietic stem cells. Cell Tissue Kinet. **4**, 463–477 (1971).

Dittrich, W., Göhde, W.: Phase progression in two dose response of Ehrlich ascites tumor cells. Atomkernenergie **15**, 174–176 (1970).

Djordjevic, B., Tolmach, L. J.: X-ray sensitivity of HeLa S 3 cells in the G_2 phase. Comparison of two methods of synchronization. Biophys. J. **7**, 77–94 (1967).

— Kim, J. H.: Different lethal effects of mitomycin C and actinomycin D during the division cycle of HeLa cells. J. Cell Biol. **38**, 477 (1968).

— — Modification of radiation response in synchronized HeLa cells by metabolic inhibitors: effects of inhibitors of DNA and protein synthesis. Radiat. Res. **37**, 435–450 (1969).

Doida, Y., Okada, S.: Radiation-induced mitotic delay in cultured mammalian cells (L 5178 Y). Radiat. Res. **38**, 513–529 (1969).

Doljanski, L., Trillat, J.-J., du Noüy, P. L., Rogozinski, A.: L'action des rayons X sur les cultures de tissu in vitro. C. R. Acad. Sci. **192**, 304–306 (1931).

— Goldhaber, G., Halberstädter, L.: Comparative studies on the radiosensitivity of normal and malignant cells in culture. II. The delayed lethal effect. Cancer Res. **4**, 106–109 (1944).

Drasil, V., Juraskova, V., Koukalova, B.: The influence of continuous irradiation on the colony-forming activity of mouse bone-marrow. Int. J. Rad. Biol. **11**, 613–614 (1966).

Drewinko, B., Humphrey, R. M.: Repair mechanisms in human lymphoid cells. Int. J. Rad. Biol. **20**, 169–171 (1971).

Eidam, C. R., Merchant, D. J.: The plateau phase of growth of the L-M strain mouse cell in a protein-free medium. Patterns of protein and nucleic acid synthesis and turnover. Exp. Cell Res. **37**, 132–139 (1965).

Eidinoff, M. L., Rich, M. A.: Growth inhibition of human tumor cell strain by 5-Fluoro-2'-deoxyuridine: time parameters for subsequent reversal by thymidine. Cancer Res. **19**, 521–526 (1959).

Elkind, M. M.: Cellular aspects of tumor therapy. Radiology **74**, 529–540 (1960).

— Sutton, H.: Radiation response of mammalian cells grown in culture. I. Repair of X-ray damage in surviving Chinese hamster cells. Radiat. Res. **13**, 556–593 (1960).

— — Moses, W. E.: Postirradiation survival kinetics of mammalian cells grown in culture. J. Cell. Comp. Physiol. **58** suppl. 1, 113–134 (1961).

— Han, A., Volz, K. W.: Radiation response of mammalian cells grown in culture. IV. Dose dependence of division delay and post-irradiation growth of surviving and non-surviving Chinese hamster cells. J. Natl. Cancer Inst. **30**, 705–721 (1963).

— Alescio, T., Swain, R. W., Moses, W. B., Sutton, H.: Recovery of hypoxic mammalian cells from sublethal X-ray damage. Nature **202**, 1190–1193 (1964a).

— Whitmore, G. F., Alescio, T.: Actionmycin D: suppression of recovery in X-irradiated mammalian cells. Science **143**, 1454–1457 (1964b).

— Sinclair, W. K.: Recovery of X-irradiated mammalian cells. Current topics in radiation research I, 165–220 (1965).

— Sutton-Gilbert, H., Moses, W. B., Alescio, T., Swain, R. W.: Radiation response of mammalian cells grown in culture. V. Temperature dependence of the repair of X-ray damage in surviving cells (aerobic and hypoxic). Radiat. Res. **25**, 359–376 (1965a).

— Swain, R. M., Alescio, T., Sutton, H., Moses, W. H.: Oxygen, nitrogen, recovery and radiation therapy. Cellular Radiation Biology, Baltimore: Williams & Wilkins 1965b.

— Sublethal X-ray damage and its repair in mammalian cells. Radiation Research, ed. by G. Silini. Amsterdam: North Holland 1967.

ELKIND, M. M., WHITMORE, G. F.: The radiobiology of cultured mammalian cells. New York: Gordon & Breach 1967.

— MOSES, W. B., SUTTON-GILBERT, H.: Radiation response of mammalian cells grown in culture. VI. Protein, DNA, and RNA inhibition during the repair of X-ray damage. Radiat. Res. **31**, 156–173 (1967a).

— SUTTON-GILBERT, H., MOSES, W. B., KAMPER, C.: Sub-lethal and lethal radiation damage. Nature **214**, 1088–1092 (1967b).

— SAKAMOTO, K., KAMPER, C.: Age-dependent toxic properties of actinomycin D and X-rays in cultured Chinese hamster cells. Cell Tissue Kinet. **1**, 209–224 (1968).

— SAKAMOTO, K.: Combined effects of X-irradiation and chemotherapeutic drugs (nitrogen mustard and actinomycin D). Front. Radiation Ther. Onc. **4**, 53–75, Basel: Karger 1969.

— KANO, E., SUTTON-GILBERT, H.: Cell killing by actinomycin D in relation to the growth cycle of Chinese hamster cells. J. Cell Biol. **42**, 366–377 (1969).

— Damage and repair processes relative to neutron (and charged particle) irradiation. Current topics in radiation research **VII**, 1–44 (1970).

— KANO, E.: Actinomycin D and radiation fractionation studies in asynchronous and synchronized Chinese hamster cells. Radiat. Res. **44**, 484–497 (1970).

— Summary of general discussion on radiobiological aspects of fast neutrons in radiotherapy. Europ. J. Cancer **7**, 249–257 (1971).

— KANO, E.: Radiation-induced age response changes in Chinese hamster cells. Evidence for a new form of damage and its repair. Int. J. Rad. Biol. **19**, 547–560 (1971).

ELLIS, F.: Modern radiobiology and the radiotherapist. Proc. Roy. Soc. Med. **54**, 1133–1142 (1961).

— The relationship of biological effect to dose-time-fractionation factors in radiotherapy. Current topics in radiation research **IV**, 357–379 (1968).

EMERY, E. W., DENEKAMP, J., BALL, M. M., FIELD, S. B.: Survival of mouse skin epithelial cells following single and divided doses of X-rays. Radiat. Res. **41**, 450–466 (1970).

ERIKSON, R. L., SZYBALSKI, W.: Molecular radiobiology of human cell lines. III. Radiation-sensitizing properties of 5-Iododeoxyuridine. Cancer Res. **23**, 122–130 (1963).

EVANS, R. G., PINKERTON, A., DJORDJEVIC, B., MAMACOS, J., LAUGHLIN, J. S.: Changes in biological effectiveness of a fast neutron beam with depth in tissue-equivalent material. Radiat. Res. **45**, 235–243 (1971).

FAIRCHILD, R. G., DREW, R. M., ATKINS, H. L.: Dose-rate effects for various dose rates of ^{252}Cf radiation on HeLa cells in culture. Radiology **96**, 171–174 (1970a).

— — — The oxygen enhancement ratio for protracted irradiation with ^{252}Cf. Radiology **96**, 661–665 (1970b).

FELL, H. B.: Tissue culture: I – The advantages and limitations as a research method. Brit. J. Radiol. **8**, 27–31 (1935).

FEOLA, J. M., LAWRENCE, J. H., WELCH, G. P.: Oxygen enhancement ratio and RBE of Helium ions on mouse lymphoma cells. Radiat. Res. **40**, 400–413 (1969).

FETNER, H. W., PORTER, E. D.: Multipolar mitosis in the KB (Eagle) human cell line and its increased frequence as a function of 250 kV X-irradiation. Exp. Cell Res. **37**, 429–439 (1965).

FISHER, H. W., YEH, J.: Contact inhibition in colony formation. Science **155**, 581–582 (1967).

FOSTER, C. J., MALONE, J., ORR, J. S., MACFARLANE, D. E.: The recovery of the survival curve shoulder after protracted hypoxia. Brit. J. Radiol. **44**, 540–545 (1971).

FOWLER, J. F., STERN, B. E.: Dose-time relationships in radiotherapy and the validity of cell survival curve models. Brit. J. Radiol. **36**, 163–173 (1963).

FOX, M., GILBERT, C. W.: Continuous irradiation of a murine lymphoma line P 388 F in vitro. Int. J. Rad. Biol. **11**, 339–347 (1966).

— NIAS, A. H. W.: A modification of the sensitivity of mammalian cells surviving treatment with methyl methane sulfonate. Europ. J. Cancer **4**, 325–335 (1968).

— — The influence of recovery from sublethal damage on the response of cells to protracted irradiation at low dose-rate. Current topics in radiation research **VII**, 71–103 (1970).

— GILBERT, C. W., LAJTHA, L. G., NIAS, A. H. W.: The interpretation of "split-dose" experiments in mammalian cells after treatment with alkylating agents. Chem. Biol. Interactions **1**, 241–246 (1970).

FRINDEL, E., CHARRUYER, F., TUBIANA, M., KAPLAN, H. S., ALPEN, E. L.: Radiation effects on DNA synthesis and cell division in the bone-marrow of the mouse. Int. J. Rad. Biol. **11**, 435–443 (1966).

— VALLERON, A. J., VASSORT, F., TUBIANA, M.: Proliferation kinetics of an experimental ascites tumour of the mouse. Cell Tissue Kinet. **2**, 51–65 (1969a).

— BLAYO, M. C., POCIDALO, J. J.: Modifications métaboliques ex vivo des cellules tumorales au cours de la croissance d'une ascite expérimentale de la souris C3H. Europ. J. Cancer **5**, 85–89 (1969b).

FROESE, G.: The respiration of ascites tumour cells at low oxygen concentrations. Biochim. Biophys. Acta **57**, 509–519 (1962).

— The distribution and interdependence of generation times of HeLa cells. Exp. Cell Res. **35**, 415–419 (1964).

— Division delay in HeLa cells and Chinese hamster cells. A time-lapse study. Int. J. Rad. Biol. **10**, 353–367 (1966).

— The factors affecting tumour oxygenation. Front. Radiation Ther. Onc. **1**, 16–26. Basel: Karger 1968.

— CORMACK, D. V.: A correlation between division delay and loss of colony forming ability in Chinese hamster cells irradiated in vitro. Int. J. Rad. Biol. **14**, 589–592 (1968).

GÄRTNER, H.: Vergleichende Untersuchungen über den Primäreffekt nach Einwirkung schneller Elektronen und Röntgenstrahlen auf Gewebekulturen. Strahlentherapie **89**, 26–51 (1953).

Gärtner, H.; Untersuchungen an der Gewebekultur. Strahlenpathologie der Zelle. Hrsg. E. Scherer u. H. S. Stender. Stuttgart, Thieme, 1963.

Gifford, G. E.: Some effects of anaerobiosis on the growth and metabolism of HeLa cells. Exp. Cell Res. **31**, 113–118 (1963).

Gilbert, C. W., Nias, A. H. W.: Distribution of the number of cells in a clone – a Monte Carlo calculation. Nature **211**, 28–30 (1966).

Goldfeder, A.: Further studies on the effect of irradiation on proliferation and metabolic processes of normal and malignant tissues. 4. Effects produced by different dosage rates of X-rays radiation on the proliferation of various tissues grown in vitro. Radiology 35, 210–222 (1940).

Gray, L. H.: The initiation and development of cellular damage by ionizing radiations. Brit. J. Radiol. **26**, 609–618 (1953).

— Conger, A. D., Ebert, M., Hornsey, S., Scott, O. C. A.: The concentration of oxygen dissolved in tissues at the time of irradiation as a factor in radiotherapy. Brit. J. Radiol. **26**, 638–648 (1953).

— Radiobiologic basis of oxygen as a modifying factor in radiation therapy. Am. J. Roentgen. **85**, 803–815 (1961).

— Radiation biology and cancer. Cellular Radiation Biology. Baltimore: Williams & Wilkins 1965.

Griem, M. L., Kannon, W., Malkinson, F. D., Skaggs, L. S.: The effect of variation in dose rate on the survival of Chinese hamster cells grown in tissue culture (Abstr.). Radiat. Res. **39**, 514 (1969).

Haefner, K.: Zum Inaktivierungskriterium für Einzelzellen unter besonderer Berücksichtigung der Teilungsfähigkeit Röntgen- und UV-bestrahlter Saccharomyces-Zellen verschiedenen Ploidiegrades. Int. J. Rad. Biol. **9**, 545–558 (1965).

— Striebeck, U.: Radiation-induced lethal sectoring in Escherichia coli B/r and B/s-1. Mut. Res. **4**, 399–407 (1967).

Hahn, G. M., Boen, J. R., Miller, R. G., Boyle, S. F., Kallman, R. F.: Mathematical models of the recovery of mammalian cells from radiation injury with respect to changes in radiosensitivity. Cellular Radiation Biology, Baltimore: Williams & Wilkins 1965.

— Bagshaw, M. A.: Serum concentration: Effects on cycle and X-ray sensitivity of mammalian cells. Science **151**, 459–461 (1966).

— Kallman, R. F.: State vector description of proliferation of mammalian cells in tissue culture. II. Effects of single and multiple doses of ionizing radiations. Radiat. Res. **30**, 702–713 (1967).

— Failure of Chinese hamster cells to repair sublethal damage when X-irradiated in the plateau phase of growth. Nature **217**, 741–742 (1968).

— Stewart, J.R., Yang, S.-J., Parker,V.: Chinese hamster cell monolayer cultures. I. Changes in cell dynamic and modifications of the cell cycle with the period of growth. Exp. Cell Res. **49**, 285—292 (1968).

— Radiobiology of mammalian cells in the plateau phase of growth. Conference on Time and Dose Relationships in Radiation Biology as Applied to Radiotherapy. Brookhaven National Laboratory BNL-50203, 1969.

Halberstädter, L., Goldhaber, G., Doljanski, L.: Comparative studies on the radiosensitivity of normal and malignant cells in culture. I. The effect of X-rays on cell outgrowth in cultures of normal rat fibroblasts and rat benzpyrene-induced sarcoma. Cancer Res. **2**, 28–31 (1942).

Hall, E. J., Bedford, J. S.: Dose-rate: its effect on the survival of HeLa cells irradiated with Gamma rays. Radiat. Res. **22**, 305–315 (1964).

— — Oliver, R.: Extreme hypoxia: its effect on the survival of mammalian cells irradiated at high and low dose-rates. Brit. J. Radiol. **39**, 302–307 (1966a).

— — Porter, E. H.: The oxygen effect at low dose-rate. Brit. J. Radiol. **39**, 958–959 (1966b).

— Oliver, R., Shepstone, B. J., Bedford, J. S.: On the population kinetics of the root meristem of vicia faba exposed to continuous irradiation. Radiat. Res. **27**, 597–603 (1966c).

— Dose-rate and the oxygen effect. Brit. J. Radiol. **40**, 395–396 (1967a).

— The oxygen effect: pertinent or irrelevent to clinical radiotherapy? Brit. J. Radiol. **40**, 874–875 (1967b).

— Cavanagh, J.: The oxygen effect for acute and protracted radiation exposures measured with seedlings of vicia faba. Brit. J. Radiol. **40**, 128–133 (1967).

— Radiobiological measurements with 14 MeV neutrons. Brit. J. Radiol. **42**, 805–813 (1969a).

— Cell killing at very low dose-rates. Conference on Time and Dose Relationships in Radiation Biology as Applied to Radiotherapy. Brookhaven National Laboratory. BNL-50203, 1969b.

— Diskussionsbemerkung in: Conference on Time and Dose Relationships in Radiation Biology as Applied to Radiotherapy. Brookhaven Nationa Laboratory. BNL-50203, p. 76–79, 1969c.

Hall, D. R., Lewis, L. D., Town, C. D., Fish, P. J., Lindop, P. J.: Radiation response of HeLa cells exposed at very low temperatures. Int. J. Rad. Biol. **16**, 43–50 (1969).

Hall, E. J., Rossi, H. H., Roizin, L. A.: Low-dose-rate irradiation of mammalian cells with radium and californium-252. Radiology **99**, 445–451 (1971).

Han, A., Miletic, B., Petrovic, D., Jovic, D.: Survival properties and repair of radiation damage in L-cells after X-irradiation. Int. J. Rad. Biol. **8**, 201–211 (1964).

Harris, H.: The relationship between the respiration and multiplication of rat connective tissue cells in vitro. Brit J. Exp. Path. **37**, 512–517 (1956).

Harrison, R. G.: Observations on the living developing nerve fiber. Proc. Soc. Exp. Biol. (N. Y.) **4**, 140 (1907).

Hellman, A., Merchant, D. J.: Effects of continuous low-level cobalt-60 Gamma radiation on an in vitro mammalian cell system. 1. Response to varying dose-rates. Radiat. Res. **18**, 437–445 (1963a).

— — Effects of continuous low-level cobalt-60 Gamma radiation on an in vitro mammalian cell system. 2. Recovery and the effect of hypothermia. Radiat. Res. **18**, 580–592 (1963b).

HENDRY, J. H., HOWARD, A.: The response of haemopoietic colony-forming units to single and split doses of Gamma-rays or D–T neutrons. Int. J. Rad. Biol. **19**, 51–64 (1971).

HEWITT, H. B.: Studies of the dissemination and quantitative transplantation of a lymphocytic leukaemia of CBA mice. Brit. J. Cancer **12**, 378–401 (1958).

— WILSON, C. W.: A survival curve for mammalian leukaemia cells irradiated in vivo. (Implications for the treatment of mouse leukaemia by wholebody irradiation). Brit. J. Cancer **13**, 69–75 (1959).

— CHAN, D. P.-S., BLAKE, E. R.: Survival curves for clonogenic cells of a murine keratinizing squamous carcinoma irradiated in vivo or under hypoxic conditions. Int. J. Rad. Biol. **12**, 535–549 (1967).

HOLFORD, R. M.: An investigation of the effect of X-rays on the rate of DNA synthesis in mouse L-cells. Int. J. Rad. Biol. **11**, 367–371 (1966).

HOLTHUSEN, H.: Beiträge zur Biologie der Strahlenwirkung. Untersuchungen an Askarideneiern. Pflügers Arch. ges. Physiol. **187**, 1–24 (1921).

HOOD, S. L., NORRIS, G.: Dosimetry of human cell cultures irradiated at the interface in plastic and in glass dishes. Radiat. Res. **14**, 705–712 (1961).

HOPWOOD, F. L., DONALDSON, M.: A remarkable sequel to an attempt to determine the X-ray lethal dose for tissue cultures growing in vitro. Brit. J. Radiol. **3**, 69–75 (1930).

HOPWOOD, L. E., TOLMACH, L. J.: Deficient DNA synthesis and mitotic death in X-irradiated HeLa cells. Radiat. Res. 70–**46**, 84 (1971).

HORNSEY, S.: The effect of oxygen tension on degeneration in chick avian fibroblasts produced by X-rays. GRAY u. Mitarb. (1953).

— SILINI, G.: Studies on cell-survival of irradiated Ehrlich ascites tumour. II. Dose effect curves for X-rays and neutron irradiations. Int. J. Rad. Biol. **4**, 135–141 (1961).

— The effect of hypoxia on the sensitivity of the epithelial cells of the jejunum. Int. J. Rad. Biol. **18**, 539–546 (1970a).

— The relative biological effectiveness of fast neutrons for intestinal damage. Radiology **97**, 649–452 (1970b).

HOWARD, A., PELC, S. R.: Synthesis of deoxyribonucleic acid in normal and irradiated cells and its relation to chromosome breakage. Heredity **6**, suppl., 261–273 (1953).

— The oxygen requirement for recovery in splitdose experiments with oedogonium. Int. J. Rad. Biol. **14**, 341–350 (1968).

HUG, O.: Die relative biologische Wirksamkeit ionisierender Strahlen. Deutscher Röntgenkongreß 1963, Teil B, 330–337. München: Urban & Schwarzenberg 1963.

— KELLERER, A.: Zur Interpretation der Dosiswirkungsbeziehungen in der Strahlenbiologie. Biophysik **1**, 20–32 (1963).

— Zytologische Aspekte der Strahlentherapie. Radiol. Austr. **15**, 147–159 (1964).

— KELLERER, A. M.: Strahlenbiologische Beiträge zum Problem des Zeitfaktors in der Therapie. Proc. XI. Int. Congr. Radiol., 744–758 (1965).

HUG, O., KELLERER, A. M.: Stochastik der Strahlenwirkung. Berlin: Springer 1966.

— — ZUPPINGER, A.: Der Zeitfaktor. Handbuch der Medizinischen Radiologie II/1, 272–354. Hrsg. A. ZUPPINGER. Berlin: Springer 1966.

HUMPHREY, R. M., DEWEY, W. C., CORK, A.: Effect of oxygen in mammalian cells sensitized to radiation by incorporation of 5-bromodeoxyuridine into the DNA. Nature **198**, 268–269 (1963).

HURWITZ, C., TOLMACH, L. J.: Time-lapse cinemicrographic studies of X-irradiated HeLa S 3 cells. I. Cell progression and cell disintegration. Biophys. J. **9**, 607–633 (1969a).

— — Time-lapse cinemicrographic studies of X-irradiated HeLa S 3 cells. II. Cell fusion. Biophys. J. **9**, 1131–1143 (1969b).

JAMES, A. P., WERNER, M. M.: Radiation-induced lethal sectoring in yeast. Radiat. Res. **29**, 523–536 (1966).

JOHNSON, R. E., HARDY, W. G., SWAIN, R. W.: Radiotherapeutic effects on mammalian tumour cells. I. Modification of leukaemia L 1210 growth kinetics with X-irradiation. Int. J. Rad. Biol. **10**, 243–250 (1966).

KALLMAN, R. F.: Recovery from radiation injury: a proposed mechanism. Nature **197**, 557–560 (1963).

KANNON, W., MALKINSON, F. D., SKAGGS, L. S., GRIEM, M. L.: The effects of high dose-rate electrons on dose response curve of Chinese hamster cells in tissue culture (Abstr.). Radiat. Res. **35**, 564–565 (1968).

KAUFMANN, H.: Skizzen zu einer biochemischen und Systemtheorie der strahleninduzierten Mitosestörungen. Strahlentherapie **141**, 439–445 (1971).

KELLERER, A. M., ROSSI, H. H.: RBE and the primary mechanism of radiation action. Radiat. Res. **47**, 15–34 (1971).

KEMBER, N. F.: An in vivo cell survival system based on the recovery of rat growth cartilage from radiation injury. Nature **207**, 501–503 (1965).

— Cell survival and radiation damage in growth cartilage. Brit. J. Radiol. **40**, 496–505 (1967a).

— Hypoxia and recovery in growth cartilage in vivo. Int. J. Rad. Biol. **13**, 387–390 (1967b).

— Radiobiological investigations with fast neutrons using the cartilage clone system. Brit. J. Radiol. **42**, 595–597 (1969).

KIM, J. H., EVANS, T. C.: Effects of X-irradiation on the mitotic cycle of Ehrlich ascites tumor cells. Radiat. Res. **21**, 129–143 (1964).

— — — Recovery from sub-lethal X-ray damage of mammalian cells during inhibition of synthesis of DNA. Nature **204**, 598–599 (1964).

— EIDINOFF, M. L., KAUGHLIN, J. S.: Recovery from sub-lethal X-ray damage of synchronized HeLa cells during inhibition of protein synthesis. Int. J. Rad. Biol. **11**, 509–511 (1966).

— GELBARD, A. S., PEREZ, A. G.: Action of hydroxyurea on the nucleic acid metabolism and viability of HeLa cells. Cancer Res. **27**, 1301–1305 (1967).

KIMURA, N.: The effects of X-ray irradiation on living carcinoma and sarcoma cells in tissue cultures in vitro. J. Cancer Res. **4**, 95–135 (1919).

Koch, C. J., Kruuv, J.: The effect of extreme hypoxia on recovery after irradiation by synchronized mammalian cells. Radiat. Res. 48, 74–85 (1971).

Krontowski, A. A.: Zur Analyse der Röntgenstrahleneinwirkung auf den Embryo und die embryonalen Gewebe. Strahlentherapie 21, 12–30 (1926).

Kruuv, J., Sinclair, W. K.: X-ray sensitivity of synchronized Chinese hamster cells irradiated during hypoxia. Radiat. Res. 36, 45–54 (1968).

Kuyper, C. M., Liebecq-Hutter, L., Chévremont-Comhaire, S.: Effets de radiations sur l'activité mitotique et les acides desoxyribonucleiques de fibroblasts cultives in vitro. Exp. Cell Res. 28, 459–479 (1962).

Lajtha, L. G., Oliver, R.: Some radiobiological considerations in radiotherapy. Brit. J. Radiol. 34, 252–257 (1961).

Lamerton, L. F.: Cell proliferation under continuous irradiation. Radiat. Res. 27, 119–138 (1966).

Lange, C. S.: On the relative importance of repair and progression in Elkind recovery as measured in synchronous HeLa cells. Int. J. Rad. Biol. 17, 61–79 (1970a).

— On the estimation of survival curve parameters for the cells of organized tissues in vivo from split dose data. Radiat. Res. 44, 390–403 (1970b).

Laser, H.: Strahlenbiologische Untersuchungenan Gewebekulturen. Strahlentherapie 38, 391–437 (1930).

Lasnitzki, I.: The effect of X-rays on cells cultivated in vitro. Brit. J. Radiol. 13, 279–283 (1940).

— Lea, D. E.: The variation with wavelength of the biological effect of radiation. Brit. J. Radiol. 13, 149–162 (1940).

— The response of cells in vitro to variations in X-ray dosage. Brit. J. Radiol. 16, 137–141 (1943a).

— The effect of X-rays on cells cultivated in vitro. Part II: Recovery factor. Brit. J. Radiol. 16, 61–67 (1943b).

— The effect of dose-rate variations on mitosis and degeneration in tissue cultures of avian fibroblasts. Brit. J. Radiol. 19, 250–256 (1946).

Legrys, G. A., Hall, E. J.: The oxygen effect and X-ray sensitivity in synchronously dividing cultures of Chinese hamster cells. Radiat. Res. 37, 161–172 (1969).

Leith, J. T., Schilling, W. A., Welch, G. P.: Survival of mouse-skin epithelial cells after heavy-particle irradiation. Int. J. Rad. Biol. 19, 603–609 (1971).

Levis, A. G.: X-irradiation sensitivity of nitrogen mustard-resistant mammalian cells in vitro. Nature 198, 498–499 (1963).

— Marin, G.: Induction of multipolar spindles by X-radiation in mammalian cells in vitro. Exp. Cell. Res. 31, 448–451 (1963).

Linden, W. A., Prévôt jr., H., Schneider, C., Berg, H., Lügger, A.: Synchronisation des Teilungszyklus von Säugetierzellen in vitro durch fraktionierte Röntgenbestrahlung. Strahlentherapie 140, 706–710 (1970).

Littbrand, B., Révész, L.: Survival of cells in anoxia Brit. J. Radiol. 41, 479–480 (1968).

— — The effect of oxygen on cellular survival and recovery after radiation. Brit. J. Radiol. 42, 914–924 (1969).

Littbrand, B.: Survival characteristics of mammalian cell lines after single or multiple exposures to Roentgen radiation under oxic or anoxic conditions. Acta Radiol. Ther. 9, 257–281 (1970a).

— Multiplication of tumor cells in vitro after oxic or anoxic exposure to Roentgen radiation. Acta Radiol. Ther. 9, 337–352 (1970b).

Little, J. B.: Delayed initiation of DNA synthesis in iradiated human diploid cells. Nature 218, 1064–1065 (1968).

— Repair of sub-lethal and potentially lethal radiation damage in plateau phase cultures of human cells. Nature 224, 804–806 (1969).

— Irradiation of primary human amnion cell cultures: effects on DNA synthesis and progression through the cell cycle. Radiat. Res. 44, 674–699 (1970).

— Repair of potentially lethal radiation damage in mammalian cells: enhancement by conditioned medium from stationary cultures. Int. J. Rad. Biol. 20, 87–92 (1971).

Liversage, W. E.: The oxygen effect at fractionated high dose-rate compared with that at low dose-rate. Brit. J. Radiol, 40, 394–395 (1967).

— A general formula for equating protracted and acute regimes of radiation. Brit. J. Radiol. 42, 432–440 (1969).

Lockart, R. R., Elkind, M. M., Moses, W. B.: Radiation response of mammalian cells grown in culture. II. Survival and recovery characteristics of several subcultures of HeLa S-3 cells after X-irradiation. J. Natl. Cancer Inst. 27, 1393–1404 (1961).

Lozzio, C. B.: Lethal effects of fluordeoxyuridine on cultured mammalian cells at various stages of the cell cycle. J. Cell. Physiol. 74, 57–62 (1969).

Ludovici, P. P., Pock, R. A., Christian, R. T., Miller, N. F.: The effect of X-irradiation on HeLa during different phases of the growth cycle. Radiat. Res. 14, 131–140 (1961).

Lund, E., Rosengren, B.: Survival of HeLa cells after large doses of X-radiation. Int. J. Rad. Biol. 11, 99–102 (1966).

Madoc-Jones, H.: Variations in radiosensitivity of a mammalian cell line with phase of the growth cycle. Nature 203, 983–984 (1964).

— Bruce, W. R.: Sensitivity of L-cells in exponential and stationary phase to 5-fluorouracil. Nature 215, 302–303 (1967).

Mak, S., Till, J. E.: The effects of X-rays on the progress of L-cells through the cell cycle. Radiat. Res. 20, 600–618 (1963).

Malone, J. F., Foster, C. J., Orr, J. S., Solomonides, E.: The effects on the survival of HeLa S-3 cells of independent variations in the sizes of the first and the second X-ray doses in split dose experiments. Int. J. Radiat. Biol. 20, 225–231 (1971).

Marcus, P. I., Ciecura, S. J., Puck, T. T.: Clonal growth in vitro of epithelial cells from normal human tissues. J. Exp. Med. 104, 615–627 (1956).

Marin, G., Levis, A. G.: X-radiation and nitrogen mustard, interaction in mammalian cells grown in vitro. Radiat. Res. 23, 192–202 (1964).

MARIN, G., BENDER, M. A.: Radiation-induced mammalian cell death: time-lapse cinemicrographic observations. Exp. Cell Res. 43, 413–423 (1966).

MASUDA, K.: Survival of synchronized L-cells irradiated with 14 MeV neutrons. Int. J. Rad. Biol. 20, 85–86 (1971).

MAURO, F., ELKIND, M. M., SAKAMOTO, K.: Sulfur mustard and X-ray effects on cultured Chinese hamster cells: a comparison of some survival characteristics. Radiat. Res. 578–579 (1967).

— — Differences in survival variations during the growth cycle of cultured Chinese hamster cells treated with X-rays and sulfur mustard. Cancer Res. 28, 1150–1156 (1968a).

— — Comparison of repair of sublethal damage in cultured Chinese hamster cells exposed to sulfur mustard and X-rays. Cancer Res. 28, 1156–1161 (1968b).

— GROSSO, A., TOLMACH, L. J.: Variations in sulfhydryl, disulfide and protein content during synchronous and asynchronous growth of HeLa cells. Biophys. J. 9, 1377–1397 (1969).

— MADOC-JONES, H.: Age response of cultured mammalian cells to cytotoxic drugs. Cancer Res. 30, 1397–1408 (1970).

MCNALLY, N. J., BEWLEY, D. K.: A biological dosimeter using mammalian cells in tissue culture and its use in obtaining neutron depth dose curves. Brit. J. Radiol. 42, 289–294 (1964).

MICHAEL, B. D., SCOTT, O. C. A., RÉVÉSZ, L.: The removal of oxygen from a liquid medium by flushing with nitrogen. Brit. J. Radiol. 39, 707–708 (1966).

MILETIĆ, B., PETROVIĆ, D., HAN, A., ŠAŠEL, L.: Restoration of viability of X-irradiated L-strain cells by isologous and heterologous highly polymerized deoxyribonuleic acid. Radiat. Res. 23, 94–103 (1964).

MILTENBURGER, H. G.: Über die Proliferation von Säugetierzellen in vitro und deren Reaktion auf Röntgenbestrahlung. 1. Experimentelle Methoden und Messung nicht-letaler Strahlenschäden. Strahlentherapie 138, 429–444 (1969a).

— Über die Proliferation von Säugetierzellen in vitro und deren Reaktion auf Röntgenbestrahlung. II. Phänomene der nicht-letalen Schädigung. Strahlentherapie 138, 595–601 (1969b).

MORKOVIN, D., FELDMAN, A.: End point of one of the actions of radiation on living tissue important in radiation therapy and in acute radiation syndrome. Brit. J. Radiol. 33, 197 (1960).

MOTTRAM, J. C.: A factor of importance in the radiosensitivity of tumours. Brit. J. Radiol. 9, 606–614 (1936).

MUNRO, T. R., GILBERT, C. W.: The relation between tumour lethal doses and the radiosensitivity of tumour cells. Brit. J. Radiol. 34, 246–251 (1961).

— The influence of the oxygen: nitrogen sensitivity ratio on theoretical dose-cure relations. Brit. J. Radiol. 40, 619–626 (1967).

— The absence of "permanent" recovery in certain Chinese hamster fibroblasts. Brit. J. Radiol. 44, 478–480 (1971).

NIAS, A. H. W., LAJTHA, L. G.: Continuous irradiation with tritiated water of mammalian cells in a monolayer. Nature 206, 613–614 (1964).

— GILBERT, C. W., LAJTHA, L. G., LANGE, C. S.: Clone-size analysis in the study of cell growth following single or during continuous irradiation. Int. J. Rad. Biol. 9, 275–290 (1965).

— GREENE, D., FOX, M., THOMAS, R. L.: Effect of 14 MeV monoenergetic neutrons on HeLa and P-388 F cells in vitro. Int. J. Rad. Biol. 13, 449–456 (1967).

— Clone size analysis: a parameter in the study of cell population kinetics. Cell Tissue Kinet. 1, 153–165 (1968).

— FOX, M.: Minimum clone size for estimating normal reproductive capacity of cultured cells. Brit. J. Radiol. 41, 468–474 (1968).

— — Steady state conditions in continuously irradiated mammalian cell cultures (Abstr.). Brit. J. Radiol. 42, 719 (1969).

— EBERT, M.: Effect of single and continuous irradiation of HeLa cells at —196°C. Int. J. Rad. Biol. 16, 31–41 (1969).

— SWALLOW, A. J., KEENE, J. P., HODGSON, B. W.: Effects of pulses of radiation on the survival of mammalian cells. Brit. J. Radiol. 42, 553 (1969).

— — — — Survival of HeLa-cells from 10 nanosecond pulses of electrons. Int. J. Rad. Biol. 17, 595–598 (1970).

— GREENE, D., MAJOR, D.: Constancy of biological parameters in a 14 MeV neutron field. Int. J. Rad. Biol. 20, 145–151 (1971).

— FOX, M.: Synchronization of mammalian cells with respect to the mitotic cycle. 3rd L. H. Gray Memorial Conference, Manchester. Cell Tissue Kinet. 4 (1971) (in Druck).

NORRIS, G., HOOD, S. L.: Some problems in the culturing and radiation sensitivity of normal human cells. Exp. Cell Res. 27, 48–62 (1962).

OHARA, H., TERASIMA, T.: Variations of cellular sulfhydryl content during cell cycle of HeLa cells and its correlations to cyclic change of X-ray sensitivity. Exp. Cell Res. 58, 182–185 (1969).

OLIVER, R.: The influence of anoxia on the recovery of sublethal radiation damage – some possible implications. Brit. J. Radiol. 40, 476–477 (1967).

OPITZ, E.: Die biologischen Grundlagen der Strahlentherapie des Carcinoms. Lehrbuch der Strahlentherapie. Bd. I, 875–911. Hrsg.: H. Meyer. Berlin: Urban & Schwarzenberg 1925.

PACE, D. M., THOMPSON, J. R., VAN CAMP, W. A.: Effects of oxygen on growth in several established cell lines. J. Natl. Cancer Inst. 28, 897–905 (1962).

PAINTER, R. B., ROBERTSON, J. S.: Effect of irradiation and theory of role of mitotic delay on the time course of labeling of HeLa S 3 cells with tritiated thymidine. Radiat. Res. 11, 206–217 (1959).

— Repair of DNA in mammalian cells. Current topics in radiation research VII, 45–70 (1970).

PARKER, R. C.: Methods of tissue culture. New York: Hoeber, 3rd ed. 1960.

PARKHOMENCO, I. M., BURLAKOVA, E. V., BEKENEVA, G. P.: Radiosensitivity of two established mammalian cell lines (M10 and SOC) and its variation during the cell cycle. IVᵉ Congrès international de radiobiologie et de physico-chimie des rayonnements, Evian. Livre des résumés, 647, 1970.

Paskin, A., Bronk, B., Dienes, G. J.: Stochastic models of cell proliferation and cell response to radiation. Recovery and Repair Mechanisms in Radiobiology. Brookhaven Symposia in Biology **20**, 169–178 (1968).

Paul, J.: Cell and tissue culture. Edinburgh: Livingstone. 4th ed. 1970.

Petrović, D., Nias, A. H. W.: Restoration of radiation damage examined by the analysis of HeLa cell clones. Int. J. Rad. Biol. **11**, 609–611 (1966).

— — A comparison of the effects upon HeLa cells of isopropyl methane sulfonate and X-rays during different phases of the cell cycle. Europ. J. Cancer **3**, 321–328 (1967).

— Restoration of radiation-induced damage by nucleic acids. Current topics in radiation research **IV**, 251–292 (1968).

— Ferle-Vidović, A.: Restoration of radiation-induced damage related to the cell cycle. Effects of radiation on cellular proliferation and differentiation. Wien: IAEA 1968.

Phillips, R. A., Tolmach, L. J.: Anomalous X-ray survival kinetics in HeLa cell populations. Int. J. Rad. Biol. **8**, 569–588 (1964).

— — Repair of potentially lethal damage in X-irradiated HeLa cells. Radiat. Res. **29**, 413–432 (1966).

Phillips, T. L.: Qualitative alteration in radiation injury under hypoxic conditions. Radiology **91**, 529–536 (1968).

— Hanks, G. E.: Apparent absence of recovery in endogenous colony-forming cells after irradiation under hypoxic conditions. Radiat. Res. **33**, 517–532 (1968).

— Worsnop, R. B.: Oxygen depletion by ultra-high dose-rate electrons in bacteria and mammalian cells (Abstr.). Radiat. Res. **35**, 545 (1968).

Pomerat, C. M., Logie, L. C., Nakanishi, Y. H.: Irradiation of cells in tissue culture. Radiation biology and cancer. Austin: University of Texas Press 1959.

Porter, E. H.: Extrapolation numbers. Brit. J. Radiol. **36**, 372–377 (1963).

— Dose-rate and survival curves. Brit. J. Radiol. **38**, 607–612 (1965).

Potten, C. S.: Radiation depigmentation of mouse hair: a study of follicular melanocyte populations. Cell Tissue Kinet. **1**, 239–254 (1968).

— Radiation depigmentation of mouse hair: effects of mouse strain. Brit. J. Dermat. **81**, 289–298 (1969).

— Howard, A.: Radiation depigmentation of mouse hair: the influence of local tissue oxygen tension on radiosensitivity. Radiat. Res. **38**, 65–81 (1969).

Powers, W. E., Tolmach, L. J.: Demonstration of an anoxic component in a mouse tumor-cell population by in vivo assay of survival following irradiation. Radiology **83**, 328–335 (1964).

Prévôt, H., Schneider, C., Brunkhorst, H., Lügger, A.: Erhöhung der Strahlensensibilität von Säugetierzellen durch Synchronisation ihres Teilungszyklus mit fraktionierter Röntgenbestrahlung. Strahlentherapie **141**, 446–450 (1971).

Puck, T. T., Marcus, P. I.: A rapid method for viable cell titration and clone production with HeLa cells in tissue culture: the effect of X-irradiated cells to supply conditioning factor. Proc. Natl. Acad. Sci. **41**, 432–437 (1955).

— — Action of X-rays on mammalian cells. J. Exp. Med. **103**, 653–660 (1956).

— — Cieciura, S. J.: Clonal growth of mammalian cells in vitro. J. Exp. Med. **103**, 273–283 (1956).

— Morkovin, D., Marcus, P. I., Cieciura, S. J.: Action of X-rays on mammalian cells. II. Survival curves from normal human tissues. J. Exp. Med. **106**, 485–500 (1957).

— Steffen, J.: Life cycle analysis of mammalian cells. I. A method for localizing metabolic events within the life cycle, and its application to the action of colcemide and sublethal doses of X-irradiation. Biophys. J. **3**, 379–397 (1963).

— Cellular aspects of the mammalian radiation syndrome: nucleated cell depletion in the bone marrow. Proc. Natl. Acad. Sci. **52**, 152–160 (1964a).

— Cellular interpretation of aspects of the acute mammalian radiation syndrome. Symp. Int. Soc. Cell Biol. **3**, 63–77 (1964b).

Pujara, C. M., Whitmore, G. F.: An experimental investigation of the division probability model for cell growth. Cell Tissue Kinet. **9**, 99–118 (1970).

Raju, M. R., Gnanapuran, M., Madhvanath, U., Howard, J., Lyman, J. T.: Relative biologic effectiveness and oxygen enhancement ratio at various depths of a 910 MeV Helium ion beam. Acta Radiol. T her. **10**, 353–357 (1971).

Read, J.: The effect of ionizing radiations on the broad bean root. Part X: the dependence of the X-ray sensitivity on dissolved oxygen. Brit. J. Radiol. **25**, 89–99 (1952).

Reinhold, H. S.: Improved microcirculation in irradiated tumours. Europ. J. Cancer **7**, 273–280 (1971).

Revell, S. H.: Diskussionsbemerkung auf dem 3rd L. H. Gray meeting, Manchester 1971. Current Topics in Radiat. Res. Quarterly **VII**, in Druck (1972).

Révész, L., Littbrand, B.: Variation of the relative sensitivity of closely related neoplastic cell lines irradiated in culture in the presence of absence of oxygen. Nature **203**, 742–744 (1964).

— — Qualitative differences between cellular radiation damage suffered under oxic and anoxic conditions: the dual effect of oxygen. Proc. Int. Conf. Radiat. Biol. & Canc., Kyoto 1966.

— — Fractionated irradiation and the effect of oxygen. Progress in Radiology, ed. by L. Turano. Amsterdam: Excerpta Medica 1967.

— — The dual effect of oxygen. Studia biophys. **15/16**, 197–210 (1969a).

— — Culture age and cellular radiosensitivity. Exp. Cell Res. **55**, 283–284 (1969b).

Roffo, A. H.: Die Wirkung der Röntgenstrahlen auf das „in vitro" gezüchtete Herz. Strahlentherapie **19**, 745–758 (1925).

Rueckert, R. R., Mueller, G. C.: Effect of oxygen tension on HeLa cell growth. Cancer Res. **20**, 944–949 (1960a).

— — — Studies on unbalanced growth in tissue culture. I. Induction and consequences of thymidine deficiency. Cancer Res. **20**, 1584–1591 (1960b).

SAKAMOTO, K., ELKIND, M. M.: X-rays and nitrogen mustard: Indepedent action in Chinese hamster cells. Biophys. J. **9**, 1115–1130 (1969).

SANFORD, K. K., LIKELY, G. D., EARLE, W. T.: The growth in vitro of single isolated tissue cells. J. Natl. Canc. Inst. **9**, 229–252 (1948).

SASAKI, S.: The distribution of the number of post-irradiation cell divisions. Tohoku J. Exp. Med. **97**, 347–361 (1969).

SATO, C. KOJIMA, K.: Irreversible loss of negative surface charge and loss of colony forming ability in Burkitt lymphoma cells after X-irradiation. Exp. Cell Res. **65**, 435—439 (1981).

SCAIFE, J. F., BROHEE, H.: An investignation of factors influencing mitotic G_2 delay in synchronous cultures of human kidney cells after X-irradiation. Canad. J. Biochem. **47**, 237—249 (1969).

— Mitotic G_2 delay induced in synchronized human kidney cells by UV- and X-irradiation and its relation to DNA strand breakage, repair, and transcription. Cell Tissue Kinet. **3**, 229—242 (1970).

SCHNEIDER, D. O., WHITMORE, G. F.: Comparative effects of neutrons and X-rays on mammalian cells. Radiat. Res. **18**, 286–306 (1963).

SCHUBERT, M.: Biologische Röntgenstrahlenwirkung, ihre Erforschung mittels der Gewebeexplantationsmethode. Strahlentherapie **26**, 425–471 (1927).

SCHWARZ, G.: Über Desensibilisierung gegen Röntgen- und Radiumstrahlen. Münch. Med. Wschr. **56**, 1217–1218 (1909).

SCOTT, O. C. A.: Some aspects of the effect of ionizing radiation on tumors in experimental animals. Adv. Biol. Med. Phys. **VI**, 121–173 (1958).

— Some observations on the use of transplanted tumors in radiobiological research. Radiat. Res. **14**, 643–652 (1961).

— DISS, C., STURROCK, J.: The effect of irradiated medium on the growth of L 5178 Y lymphoma cells. Int. J. Rad. Biol. **10**, 617–619 (1966).

SEELIG, K. J., RÉVÉSZ, L.: Effect of lethally damaged tumour cells upon the growth of admixed viable cells in diffusion chambers. Brit. J. Cancer **14**, 126–138 (1960).

SEYDEL, H. G.: Mitotic delay after fractionated irradiation of autotransplants of a spontaneous mouse tumor. Am. J. Roentg. **100**, 938–943 (1967).

SILINI, G., HORNSEY, S.: Studies on cell-survival of irradiated Ehrlich ascites tumour. I. The effect of the host's age and the presence of non-viable cells on tumour takes. Int. J. Rad. Biol. **4**, 127–134 (1961).

— — Studies on cell-survival of irradiated Ehrlich ascites tumour. III. A comparison of the X-ray survival curves obtained with a diploid and a tetraploid strain. Int. J. Rad. Biol. **5**, 147–153 (1962).

SINCLAIR, W. K., MORTON, R. A.: Variations in X-ray response during the division cycle of partially synchronized Chinese hamster cells in culture. Nature **199**, 1158–1160 (1963).

— X-ray-induced heritable damage (small colony formation) in cultured mammalian cells. Radiat. Res. **21**, 584–611 (1964a).

— Survival and recovery after X-irradiation of synchronized Chinese hamster cells in culture. Jap. J. Genet. suppl. **40**, 141–161 (1964b).

SINCLAIR, W. K., MORTON, R. A.: Recovery following X-irradiation of synchronized Chinese hamster cells. Nature **203**, 247–250 (1964).

— Hydroxyurea: differential lethal effects on cultured mammalian cells during the cell cycle. Science **150**, 1729–1731 (1965).

— BISHOP, D. H. L.: Synchronous cultures of strain L mouse cells. Nature **205**, 1272–1273 (1965).

— MORTON, R. A.: X-ray and ultraviolet sensitivity of synchronized Chinese hamster cells at various stages of the cell cycle. Biophys. J. **5**, 1–25 (1965).

— — X-ray sensitivity during the cell generation cycle of cultured Chinese hamster cells. Radiat. Res. **29**, 450–474 (1966).

— X-ray survival and DNA synthesis in Chinese hamster cells. I. The effect of inhibitors added before X irradiation. Proc. Natl. Acad. Sci. **58**, 115–122 (1967a).

— Radiation effects on mammalian cell populations in vitro. Radiation Research, ed. by. G. Silini. Amsterdam: North Holland 1967b.

— Cyclic X-ray responses in mammalian cells in vitro. Radiat. Res. **33**, 620–643 (1968a).

— Radiation survival in synchronous and asynchronous Chinese hamster cells in vitro. Biophysical aspects of radiation quality. 2nd panel report. Wien: IAEA 1968b.

— Protection by cysteamine against lethal X-ray damage during the cell cycle of Chinese hamster cells. Radiat. Res. **39**, 135–154 (1969a).

— Methods and criteria of mammalian cell synchrony. Normal and malignant cell growth, ed. by. R. J. M. Fry et al., Recent Results in Cancer Research, vol. 17. New York: Springer 1969b.

— Dependence of radiosensitivity upon cell age. Conference on Time and Dose Relationships in Radiation Biology as Applied to Radiotherapy. Brookhaven National Laboratory BNL-50203, 1969c.

SIRACKA, E., LITTBRAND, B., RÉVÉSZ, L.: Effect of oxygen on the recovery of lethal and non-lethal radiation damage. Exp. Cell. Res. **58**, 191–194 (1969).

SKARSGARD, L. D., KIHLMAN, B. A., PARKER, L., PUJARA, C. M., RICHARDSON, S.: Survival, chromosome abnormalities, and recovery in heavy-ion- and X-irradiated mammalian cells. Radiat. Res. suppl. **7**, 208–221 (1967).

SPEAR, F. G.: The delayed lethal effect of radiation on tissue cultures in vitro. Proc. Roy. Soc. Lond. B **106**, 44–49 (1930).

— The effect of spaced radiation on tissue cultures in vitro. Proc. Roy. Soc. Lond. B **110**, 224–234 (1932).

— GRIMMETT, L. G.: The biological response to Gamma rays of radium as a function of the intensity of radiation. Brit. J. Radiol. **6**, 387–403 (1933).

— Tissue culture III – its application to radiobiological research. Brit. J. Radiol. **8**, 280–297 (1935).

— GRAY, L. H., READ, J.: Biological effect of fast neutrons. Nature **142**, 1074–1075 (1938).

— Radiations and living cells. London: Chapman & Hall 1953.

STEWART, J. R., HAHN, G. M., PARKER, V., BAGSHAW, M. A.: Chinese hamster cell monolayer cultures. II. X-ray sensitivity and sensitization by 5-bromodeoxycytidine in the exponential and plateau periods of growth. Exp. Cell Res. **49**, 293–299 (1968).

Strangeways, T. S. P.: Observations on the changes seen in living cells during growth and division. Proc. Roy. Soc. Lond. B **94**, 137–141 (1922).

— Oakeley, H. E. G.: The immediate changes observed in tissue cells after exposure to soft X-rays while growing in vitro. Proc. Roy. Soc. Lond. B **95**, 373–381 (1923).

— The technique of tissue culture. Cambridge: Heffer 1924.

— Hopwood, F. L.: The effect of X-rays on mitotic cell division in tissue culture in vitro. Proc. Roy. Soc. Lond. B **100**, 283–293 (1926).

— Fell, H. B.: A study of the direct and indirect action upon the tissues of the embryonic fowl. Proc. Roy. Soc. Lond. B **102**, 9–29 (1927).

Stubblefield, E., Klevecz, R.: Synchronization of Chinese hamster cells by reversal of colcemid inhibition. Exp. Cell Res. **40**, 660–664 (1965).

Stroud, A., Resh, D.: Characteristics of mutant clones of pig-kidney cells several years after X-irradiation. Radiat. Res. **31**, 580–581 (1968).

Suit, H. D.: Radiation Biology: basis for radiotherapy. Textbook of Radiotherapy, ed. by G. H. Fletcher. Philadelphia: Lea & Febinger 1966a.

— Response to X-irradiation of a tumour recurring after a TCD_{95} radiation dose. Nature **211**, 996–997 (1966b).

Sutherland, R. M., Inch, W. R., McCredie, J. A., Kruuv, J.: A multicomponent radiation survival curve using an in vitro tumour model. Int. J. Rad. Biol. **18**, 491–495 (1970).

— McCredie, J. A., Inch, W. R.: Growth of multicell spheroids in tissue culture as a model of nodular carcinomas. J. Natl. Cancer Inst. 46, 113—120 (1971).

Szumiel, I., Ziema-Zak, B., Rosiek, O., Sablinsko, J., Beer, J. Z.: Harmful effects of an irradiated cell culture medium. Int. J. Rad. Biol. **20**, 153–161 (1971).

Terasima, T., Tolmach, L. J.: Changes in X-ray sensitivity of HeLa cells during the division cycle. Nature **190**, 1210–1211 (1961).

— —Variation in several responses of HeLa cells to X-irradiation during the division cycle. Biophys. J. **3**, 11–33 (1963a).

— — X-ray sensitivity and DNA synthesis in synchronous populations of HeLa cells. Science **140**, 490–492 (1963b).

— On the role of DNA in cell killing by radiation. Conference on Time and Dose Relationships in Radiation Biology as Applied to Radiotherapy. Brookhaven National Laboratory BNL-50203, 1969.

Thomlinson, R. H., Gray, L. H.: The histological structure of some human lung cancers and the possible implications for radiotherapy. Brit. J. Cancer **9**, 539–549 (1956).

— The oxygen effect in mammals. Report 675, Brookhaven National Laboratory, 204–215, 1961.

— Oxygen therapy – biological considerations. Modern trends in radiotherapy, ed. by T. J. Deeley and C. A. P. Wood. London: Butterworths 1967.

Thomlinson, R. H., Craddock, E. A.: The gross response of an experimental tumour to single doses of X-rays. Brit. J. Cancer **21**, 108–123 (1967).

Thompson, L. H., Suit, H. D.: Proliferation kinetics of X-irradiated mouse L cells studied with time-lapse photography. I. Experimental methods and data analysis. Int J. Rad. Biol. **18**, 391–397 (1967).

— Humphrey, R. M.: Response of mouse L-P 59 cells to X-irradiation in the G_2 phase. Int. J. Rad. Biol. **15**, 181–184 (1969).

— Suit, H. D.: Proliferation kinetics of X-irradiated mouse L cells studied with time-lapse photography. II. Int. J. Rad. Biol. **15**, 347–362 (1969).

Till, J. E., McCulloch, E. A.: A direct measurement of the radiation sensitivity of normal mouse bone marrow cells. Radiat. Res. **14**, 213–222 (1961).

— — Early repair processes in marrow cells irradiated and proliferating in vivo. Radiat. Res. **18**, 96–105 (1963).

Todd, P.: Heavy-ion irradiation of cultured human cells. Radiat. Res. suppl. **7**, 196–207 (1967).

— Fractionated heavy ion irradiation of cultured human cells. Radiat. Res. **34**, 378–389 (1968a).

— Defective mammalian cells isolated from X-irradiated cultures. Mutat. Res. **5**, 173–183 (1968b).

—, Winchell, H. S., Feola, J. M., Jones, G. E.: Pulsed high-intensity roentgen rays. Acta Radiol. Ther. **7**, 22–26 (1968).

Tolmach, L. J., Marcus, P. I.: Development of X-ray-induced giant HeLa cells. Exp. Cell Res. **20**, 350–360 (1960).

— Growth patterns of X-irradiated HeLa cells. Ann. N.Y. Acad. Sci. **95**, art. 2, 743–757 (1961).

—, Terasima, T., Phillips, R. A.: X-ray sensitivity changes during the division cycle of HeLa S 3 cells and anomalous survival kinetics of developing microcolonies. Cellular Radiation Biology. Baltimore: Williams & Wilkins 1965.

— Diskussionsbemerkung zu Sinclair a.a.O., 1969c.

Town, C. D.: Effect of high dose-rates on survival of mammalian cells. Nature **215**, 847–848 (1967).

Trott, K.-R.: Mortality rate and recovery in pedigrees of irradiated mammalian cells in vitro. Studia biophys. **18**, 127–135 (1969).

—, Hug, O.: Intraclonal recovery of division probability in pedigrees of single X-irradiated mammalian cells. Int. J. Rad. Biol. **17**, 483–486 (1970).

—, Hug, O., Kellerer, A. M.: Proliferation kinetics in pedigrees of irradiated L cells. IVᵉ Congrès international de radiobiologie et de physico-chimie des rayonnements, Evian. Livre des résumés, 867, 1970.

— Jahresbericht der Gesellschaft für Strahlen- und Umweltforschung 1970, München 1971.

— Diskussionsbemerkung auf der 3ʳᵈ L. H. Gray Memorial Conference 1971. Current Topics in Radiat. Res. VII (in Druck, 1972).

Van Putten, L. M., Kallman, R. F.: Oxygenation status of a transplantable tumor during fractionated radiation therapy. J. Natl. Canc. Inst. **40**, 441–451 (1968).

— Lelieveld, P.: Factors determining cell killing by chemotherapeutic agents in vivo — 1. Cyclophosphamide. Europ. J. Cancer 6, 313—321 (1970).

VAN PUTTEN, L. M.: Factors determining cell killing by chemotherapeutic agents in vivo — II. Melphalan, Chlorambucil and nitrogen mustard. Europ. J. Cancer 7, 11—16 (1971).

VOLLMER, H., RAJEWSKY, B.: Mikrokinematographische Studien über die Wirkung von Röntgenstrahlen auf normale und Tumorzellen in Gewebekulturen. Strahlentherapie 60, 524–540 (1937).

VOS, O., SCHENK, H. A. E. M., BOOTSMA, D.: Survival of excess thymidine synchronized cell populations in vitro after X-irradiation in various phases of the cell cycle. Int. J. Rad. Biol. 11, 495–503 (1966).

WALKER, I. G., HELLEINER, C. W.: The sensitivity of cultured mammalian cells in different stages of the division cycle to nitrogen and sulfur mustards. Cancer Res. 23, 734–738 (1963).

—, THATCHER, C. J.: Studies on the lethal effects of sulfur mustard on dividing mammalian cells. Radiat. Res. 34, 110–127 (1968).

WALTERS, R. A., PETERSEN, D. F.: Radiosensitivity of mammalian cells. I. Timing and dose-dependence of radiation-induced division delay. Biophysical J. 8, 1475–1486 (1968).

—, TOBEY, R. A.: Radiosensitivity of mammalian cells. IV. Effect of X-irradiation on the DNA synthetic period in synchronized cells. Biophys. J. 10, 556–562 (1970).

WATANABE, I., OKADA, S.: Deoxyribonucleic acid synthesis during the first post-irradiation life cycle of the lethally irradiated cultured mammalian cells (L 5178 Y). Radiat. Res. 35, 202–212 (1968).

WEED, B. H., RUSS, S.: The effect of roentgen and radium radiations upon the viability of the cells of a mouse carcinoma. J. Pathol. Bacter. 17, 1–11 (1912).

WESTRA, A., BARENDSEN, G. W.: Proliferation characteristics of cultured mammalian cells after irradiation with sparsely and densely ionizing radiations. Int. J. Rad. Biol. 11, 477–485 (1966).

— Non-lethal damage in mammalian cells produced by ionizing radiations, heat, and other agents (Abstr.). Studia biophys. 2, 246 (1967).

WHITFIELD, J. F., RIXON, R. H.: Effects of X-radiation on multiplication and nucleic acid synthesis in cultures of L-strain mouse cells. Exp. Cell Res. 18, 126–137 (1959).

WHITMORE, G. F., GULYAS, S., BOTOND, J.: Radiation sensitivity throughout the cell cycle and its relationship to recovery. Cellular Radiation Biology. Baltimore: Williams & Wilkins 1965.

—, TILL, J. E.: Quantitation of cellular radiation responses. Ann. Rev. Nucl. Sci. 14, 347–374 (1964).

— —, GULYAS, S.: Radiation-induced mitotic delay in L cells. Radiat. Res. 30, 155–171 (1967).

—, BORSA, J., BACCHETTI, S., GRAHAM, F.: Mammalian cell killing by inhibitors of DNA synthesis. Normal and malignant cell growth, ed. by R. J. M. FRY et. al., Recent Results in Cancer Research 17, New York: Springer 1969a.

—, GULYAS, S., KOTALIK, J.: Recovery from radiation damage in mammalian cells. Conference on Time and Dose Relationships in Radiation Biology as Applied to Radiotherapy. Brookhaven National Laboratory, BNL 50203, 1969b.

WILLIAMS, J. F., TILL, J. E.: The radiation sensitivity of normal and polyoma-transformed rat embryo cells. Radiat. Res. 29, 282–294 (1966).

WILLMER, E. N.: Cells and tissues in culture. 3 vol. London: Academic Press 1965.

WILSON, C. W.: Possible implications of recent radiobiological obersvations for tumor-dose-fractionation schedules. Radiology 77, 940–945 (1961).

WITHERS, H. R.: The dose-survival relationship for irradiation of epithelial cells of mouse skin. Brit. J. Radiol. 40, 187–194 (1967a).

— Recovery and repopulation in vivo by mouse skin epithelial cells during fractionated irradiation. Radiat. Res. 32, 227–239 (1967b).

— The effect of oxygen and anaesthesia on radiosensitivity in vivo of epithelial cells of mouse skin. Brit. J. Radiol. 40, 335–343 (1967c).

— ELKIND, M. M.: Dose-survival characteristics of epithelial cells of mouse intestinal mucosa. Radiology 91, 998–1000 (1968).

— Capacity for repair in cells of normal and malignant tissues. Conference on Time and Dose Relationships in Radiation Biology as Applied to Radiotherapy. Brookhaven National Laboratory BNL-50203, 1969.

— ELKIND, M. M.: Radiosensitivity and fractionation response of crypt cells of mouse jejunum. Radiat. Res. 38, 598–613 (1969).

— — Microcolony survival assay for cells of mouse intestinal mucosa exposed to radiation. Int. J. Rad. Biol. 17, 261–267 (1970).

— BRENNAN, J.T., ELKIND, M.M.: The response of stem cells of intestinal mucosa to irradiation with 14 MeV neutrons. Brit. J. Radiol. 43, 796–801 (1970).

— OLIVER, G. D., GLENN, D. W.: Response of mouse jejunal crypt cells to low dose rate irradiation with californium neutrons or radium gamma-rays. Radiat. Res. 48, 484—494 (1971).

WOOD, F. C., PRIME, F.: Die Wirkung des Radiums auf überpflanzte Tiertumoren. Strahlentherapie 12, 1071–1084 (1921).

— — Die tödliche Röntenstrahlendosis für Krebszellen. Strahlentherapie 13, 629–638 (1922).

WU, A. M., SIMINOVITCH, L., TILL, J. E., McCULLOCH, E. A.: Evidence for a relationship between mouse heamopoietic stem cells and cells forming colonies in culture. Proc. Natl. Acad. Sci. 59, 1209–1215 (1968).

XEROS, N.: Deoxyriboside control and synchronization of mitosis. Nature 194, 682–683 (1962).

YAMADA, M., PUCK, T. T.: Action of radiation on mammalian cells. IV. Reversible mitotic lag in HeLa S 3 cells produced by low doses of X-rays. Proc. Natl. Acad. Sci. 47, 1181–1191 (1961).

YOUNG, J. M., FOWLER, J. F.: The effect of X-ray-induced synchrony on two-dose cell survival experiments. Cell Tissue Kinet. 2, 95–110 (1969).

YU, C. K., SINCLAIR, W. K.: Mitotic delay and chromosomal aberrations induced by X-rays in synchronized Chinese hamster cells in vitro. J. Natl. Canc. Inst. 39, 619–629 (1967).

— — Protection by cysteamine against mitotic delay and chromosomal aberrations induced by X-rays in synchronized Chinese hamster cells. Radiat. Res. 43, 357–371 (1970).

C. Strahleninduzierte Chromosomenaberrationen

Von

Manfred Bauchinger

Mit 32 Abbildungen

I. Einführung

Im Jahr 1927 entdeckte H. J. MULLER, daß durch Röntgenstrahlen die spontane Mutationsrate in Drosophila stark erhöht wurde. Fast zum gleichen Zeitpunkt, unabhängig von MULLERs Experimenten, konnte STADLER (1928) in Hordeum vulgare die mutagenen Eigenschaften von Röntgen- und γ-Strahlen des Radiums nachweisen. In den Jahren nach diesen grundlegenden Entdeckungen wurden die Studien zur experimentellen Auslösung von Mutationen in Pflanzen und Tieren rasch vorangetrieben (GOODSPEED u. OLSEN, 1928; ALTENBURG, 1928; MULLER, 1928; STADLER, 1932; MULLER u. ALTENBURG, 1930; OLIVER, 1930, 1932). Dabei ergab sich bald, daß alle ionisierenden Strahlenarten und auch ultraviolettes Licht mutagen wirken können. Beim Studium von Kopplungsgruppen (Gene sind zu Kopplungsgruppen zusammengefaßt; je größer der Abstand zwischen zwei Genen ist, um so größer ist die Chance, daß zwischen ihnen ein Crossing-over, d.h. Rekombination auftritt) in Drosophila fiel MULLER eine weitere Besonderheit der Röntgenstrahlen auf. Er fand, daß nach Bestrahlung die Rekombinationshäufigkeiten von Genen, Gensequenzen und Kopplungsgruppen in einem Ausmaß verändert waren, wie es spontan niemals beobachtet werden konnte. MULLER u. PAINTER (1929) sowie DOBZHANSKY (1929) zeigten, daß diese strukturellen Veränderungen in den Kopplungsgruppen auf entsprechende Veränderungen in den Chromosomen zurückzuführen waren.

Dies war der Beginn umfangreicher Versuche zur experimentellen Auslösung struktureller Chromosomenaberrationen. Die Studien waren zunächst von biophysikalischen Fragestellungen (Übersicht bei LEA, 1946) bestimmt und auf pflanzliche und niedere tierische Objekte beschränkt. Später gewannen auch biochemische Aspekte (WOLFF, 1960a) der Aberrationsinduktion eine immer größere Bedeutung. Durch die Entwicklung und Verfeinerung spezieller Methoden zur Züchtung verschiedenster Gewebe von Säugern, die es erlaubten deren Chromosomen sichtbar zu machen, wurde für die Strahlencytogenetik ein weites Arbeitsfeld eröffnet.

Von besonderem Interesse war natürlich die Erforschung der Wirkung ionisierender Strahlen auf die Chromosomen des Menschen. Dies wurde durch die Entwicklung einer einfachen Technik zur Kultur kleiner Lymphozyten aus dem peripheren Blut durch MOORHEAD u. Mitarb. (1960) ermöglicht. Mit ihrer Hilfe konnten nun auch die im lebenden Organismus induzierten Chromosomenveränderungen in größerem Ausmaß studiert werden.

Eine umfassende Behandlung des Themas „Strahleninduzierte Chromosomenaberrationen" ist im Rahmen dieses Handbuchartikels nicht möglich. Es wurde daher versucht das Thema in 2 Teilen zu bearbeiten. In einem allgemeinen Teil werden grundlegende Fragen der Aberrationsentstehung besprochen. Der spezielle Teil befaßt sich mit der Darstellung experimenteller Befunde über strahleninduzierte Chromosomenaberrationen in menschlichen Lymphozyten, da bis heute die meisten Untersuchungen an diesen Zellen durchgeführt wurden.

II. Allgemeine Interpretation der Entstehungsweise und Struktur strahleninduzierter Chromosomenaberrationen

1. Hypothesen zur Aberrationsentstehung

Die Mechanismen der Aberrationsentstehung sind von komplexer Natur und noch nicht voll aufgeklärt. Heute existieren zwei grundlegende Hypothesen zur Erklärung der Entstehungsweise struktureller Chromosomenaberrationen. Die Bruch-Reunions-Hypothese (breakage-first-Hypothese) wurde ursprünglich von STADLER (1931) vorgeschlagen und durch Arbeiten von SAX (1938, 1939, 1940, 1941) gestützt. Als Alternative zu dieser klassischen Hypothese wurde von REVELL (1954, 1959, 1963, 1966) die sogenannte Austauschhypothese (exchange-Hypothese) formuliert, die durch Arbeiten von EVANS (1962, 1967a), NEWCOMBE (1942), NEARY u. Mitarb. (1964, 1966), NEARY (1965) untermauert wurde.

Es zeigte sich, daß die Ergebnisse verschiedener Bestrahlungsexperimente einmal mit Hilfe des Bruch-Reunions-Modells, ein anderes Mal mit Hilfe des Austauschmodells zu deuten waren. Andererseits waren aber beide Hypothesen unter bestimmten Voraussetzungen unannehmbar (BREWEN, 1963, 1964; EVANS u. SCOTT, 1964; GRANT, 1965; NEARY, 1967; REVELL, 1966; SAVAGE u. Mitarb., 1968; SCOTT u. EVANS, 1964; WOLFF, 1965; HEDDLE u. Mitarb., 1969; BREWEN u. BROCK, 1968). Somit dürfte zum gegenwärtigen Zeitpunkt jede der beiden Hypothesen, wie es in vielen Fällen interpretiert wird, weder ganz korrekt noch ganz falsch sein (HEDDLE u. BODYCOTE, 1970).

Im folgenden werden beide Hpyothesen kurz dargelegt. Ausführlichere Besprechungen siehe in Übersichten bei EVANS (1962), RIEGER u. MICHAELIS (1967), WOLFF (1963, 1960a, 1961b).

a) Bruch-Reunions-Hypothese (Breakage-first-Hypothese)

Nach dieser Hypothese entstehen Aberrationen primär durch direkte oder indirekte Brüche beim Durchgang eines ionisierenden Teilchens (oder spontan) durch die als kontinuierlich angesehene Struktur des Interphasechromosoms oder bei der Passage eines ionisierenden Teilchens in Chromosomennähe. Die Bruchenden können nun entweder a) sich in ihrer ursprünglichen Konfiguration wiedervereinigen (Restitution), b) sich mit anderen Bruchenden zu neuen Konfigurationen vereinigen (Reunion, „illegitimate fusion") oder c) offen bleiben. Sämtliche intra- und interchromosomalen Strukturumbauten (exchange-Aberrationen), zu deren Entstehung mindestens zwei Bruchflächen notwendig sind, werden somit bei diesem „Reunionsprozeß" gebildet. Bei den terminalen Deletionen und azentrischen Fragmenten liegen die ursprünglichen Bruchflächen als stabilisierte Diskontinuitäten der Chromosomenstruktur vor.

b) Austauschhypothese (Exchange-Hypothese)

Die Austauschhypothese ist im wesentlichen eine Hypothese zur Interpretation strahleninduzierter Chromatidaberrationen in der Metaphase. Von FOX (1966, 1967) in Zellen von Locustus-Embryonen sowie BREWEN u. BROCK (1968) in Blutzellen von Wallabia bicolor wurde versucht, sie auch auf die Entstehung von Aberrationen auf chromosomaler Ebene anzuwenden.

Nach der von REVELL an Vicia entwickelten Austauschhypothese sind alle Aberrationen, einschließlich der sogenannten einfachen Chromatidbrüche, als Folge von Austauschprozessen anzusehen. Das Primärereignis ist nicht ein Bruch (Diskontinuität), sondern eine *lokale Instabilisierung* der Chromosomenstruktur, deren Natur aber im Augenblick nicht näher charakterisiert werden kann. Die Primärläsion kann nun entweder direkt repariert werden oder bei einem weiteren Prozeß, der sogenannten *Austauscheinleitung*, mit einer anderen Primärläsion in Wechselwirkung treten. In einer dritten Phase erfolgt der eigentliche *Austausch*, der nach ähnlichen Mechanismen, wie sie beim meiotischen Crossing-over stattfinden, ablaufen könnte. Der Austauschprozeß kann vollständig oder unvollständig sein. Erfolgt ein unvollständiger Austausch zwischen Schwesterchromatiden, so entsteht daraus eine Chromatidendeletion (Chromatidbruch). Eine wichtige Annahme der Austauschhypothese ist, daß der Austausch nur innerhalb einer schleifenförmigen Überlagerung (REVELL-loop) der entspiralisierten Chromatide im Interphasekern erfolgen kann (Abb. 5).

2. Dosis-Wirkungs-Beziehung strahleninduzierter Chromosomenaberrationen

a) Dicht ionisierende Strahlenarten

Bestrahlungsexperimente mit schnellen Neutronen (GILES, 1940, 1943; THODAY, 1942; GILES u. CONGER, 1950; GILES u. Mitarb., 1953; WOLFF u. Mitarb., 1958) und Alpha-Partikeln (KOTVAL u. GRAY, 1947), also dicht ionisierende Strahlenarten, ergaben für sämtliche Aberrationstypen auf chromosomaler und chromatidaler Ebene eine annähernd lineare Dosis-Wirkungs-Beziehung nach der Gleichung:

$$Y = c + kD$$

(Y = Aberrationsausbeute; c = spontane Aberrationsfrequenz; k = Koeffizient der Aberrationsinduktion = Aberrationshäufigkeit pro Zelle pro Dosiseinheit; D = Dosis) LEA u. CATCHESIDE, 1942.

Eine Abhängigkeit von der Dosisleistung der Bestrahlung bestand nicht (Übersichten bei EVANS, 1962; WOLFF, 1960a, b).

b) Locker ionisierende Strahlenarten

Die Ergebnisse aus den Experimenten von SAX (1938, 1939, 1940, 1941) in Tradescantia-Mikrosporen standen mit der Bruch-Reunions-Hypothese im Einklang. Es zeigte sich, daß einfache terminale Deletionen und Isochromatidaberrationen etwa linear mit der Röntgenstrahlendosis zunahmen. Die Ausbeute dieser als „Ein-Treffer" (one-track)-Aberrationen bezeichneten Defekte wurde weder durch eine Veränderung der Dosisleistung noch durch eine Dosisfraktionierung beeinflußt.

Dizentrische Chromosomen und Ringe, also Aberrationen, zu deren Entstehung 2 Bruchereignisse mit einem anschließenden Strukturaustausch notwendig sind, nahmen jedoch — wenn die Expositionszeit im Verhältnis zur sogenannten „Rejoining time" kurz genug war — etwa mit dem Quadrat der Dosis zu.

Mit zunehmender Dauer der Bestrahlung wurde die Ausbeute an Austauschaberrationen jedoch wesentlich geringer. Die dosisleistungsabhängigen Aberrationen wurden deshalb als Folge einer Wechselwirkung zwischen zwei unabhängig voneinander entstandenen Brüchen angesehen und als „Zwei-Treffer" (two-track)-Aberrationen bezeichnet. Aus Dosisleistungs- und Dosisfraktionierungsexperimenten wurde geschlossen, daß nur ein kleiner Teil der ursprünglich induzierten Brüche offen bleibt und als terminale Deletionen stabilisiert wird oder zur Bildung von Austauschaberrationen (Reunion) miteinander in Wechselwirkung tritt. Der überwiegende Teil der primären Brüche bzw. Primärläsionen (nach Schätzungen von LEA [1946] und WOLFF u. Mitarb. [1958] 90—99%) führt Restitutionsprozesse durch, die zur Herstellung der ursprünglichen Konfiguration führen.

Die Austauschhypothese postuliert die Entstehung sämtlicher Aberrationen als Folge von Austausch-Prozessen zwischen den als „labile Regionen" angesehenen Primärereignissen. Diese können voneinander unabhängig oder durch ein einziges ionisierendes Teilchen entstanden sein. REVELL konnte (1963, 1966) in Vicia faba, selbst für terminale Chromatidendeletionen, eine signifikante Abweichung von einer linearen Dosis-Wirkungs-Beziehung ermitteln. Auch in Experimenten anderer Autoren ergab sich bei Verwendung von Strahlenarten mit geringer Ionisationsdichte für Translokationen keine einfache quadratische Dosis-Wirkungs-Beziehung. Die Aberrationsausbeute konnte als Potenzfunktion der Dosis dargestellt werden:

$$Y = c + kD^n .$$

Durch eine log-log-Transformation der Potenzfunktion erhält man eine Gerade, deren Steigung dem Dosisexponenten n entspricht. In Vicia-Wurzelspitzen lag n zwischen 1,5 und 1,8. Allgemein näherte sich der Dosisexponent 2, wenn mit hohen Dosisleistungen bestrahlt wurde.

Somit ist n sehr variabel und eine Dosis-Wirkungs-Beziehung unter ausschließlicher Angabe des Dosisexponenten n meist nicht exakt zu charakterisieren. (Für eine ausführliche Diskussion von Dosis-Wirkungs-Beziehungen sei auf den Artikel von Kellerer u. Hug in diesem Handbuch verwiesen.)

Catcheside u. Mitarb. (1946) berücksichtigten die Überlagerung linearer und quadratischer Komponenten in der Beziehung zwischen Dosis und Aberrationsausbeute und postulierten, daß die beiden Primärläsionen einiger Austausch-Aberrationen zum Teil gleichzeitig durch ein ionisierendes Teilchen induziert werden (lineare Komponente αD), andere aber durch zwei voneinander unabhängige ionisierende Teilchen entstehen (quadratische Komponente βD^2). Dies läßt sich durch ein Polynom zweiten Grades formulieren:

$$Y = c + \alpha D + \beta D^2 .$$

Die Größe der linearen Komponente bestimmt dabei die Abweichung von einer rein quadratischen Beziehung. Bei niederen Dosen überwiegt die lineare Komponente, im höheren Dosisbereich die quadratische. Da nach der klassischen Theorie die Bruchereignisse unmittelbar nach der Bestrahlung auftreten und Brüche nur eine begrenzte Lebenszeit besitzen, nimmt nach diesem Modell die quadratische Komponente mit abnehmender Dosisleistung (entspricht einer Zunahme der Expositionszeit) ebenfalls ab, während die lineare Komponente unverändert bleibt. Für die Entwicklung obiger Gleichung waren folgende Gesichtspunkte ausschlaggebend. Bei locker ionisierenden Strahlenarten ist die Ionisationsdichte entlang der Bahnspur ungleichmäßig, da z.B. das Bahnende dichter ionisiert als die übrigen Bahnabschnitte. (Darüber hinaus kommen überall in der Bahn auch Fluktuationen vor, die sich durch die Statistik der elektronischen Kollisionen ergeben.) Die Ionisationsdichte in diesen Bereichen entspricht somit etwa derjenigen nach Einwirkung von dicht ionisierenden Strahlenarten. Demnach werden z.B. am Bahnende die beiden zu einer Translokation notwendigen Primärläsionen gleichzeitig induziert, d.h. die am Bahnende induzierten Aberrationen folgen einer linearen (αD), die entlang der geringer ionisierenden Bahnabschnitte induzierten Aberrationen jedoch einer quadratischen (βD^2) Kinetik.

Von Neary (1965) stammen Überlegungen, die dem Einfluß von δ-Strahlen (dabei handelt es sich um sekundäre Elektronen, die Bahnspuren erzeugen, in denen die Verteilung der Ionen verschieden von der der Primärpartikel ist) auf die Aberrationsausbeute Rechnung tragen. Es wird auf die Möglichkeit der Bildung von „Zwei-Treffer" (two-track)-Prozessen, verursacht durch die Bahnspur eines primären Teilchens und einer seiner δ-Strahlen oder durch zwei δ-Strahlen des gleichen Primärteilchens, hingewiesen.

Muller (1940, 1954a, b) fand in seinen Drosophila-Experimenten stets einen Dosisexponenten von 1,5, der ihn dazu veranlaßte, die sogenannte „$\frac{3}{2}$-Regel" aufzustellen ($Y = c + kD^{1,5}$). Er versuchte, diese Abweichung mit dem Absterben von Zellen, bedingt durch bestimmte Chromosomenaberrationen, zu erklären. Solche Aberrationstypen sollten bei niederen Dosen weniger häufig entstehen als bei höheren. Da sie aber dann infolge der Zellselektion nicht zu erfassen sind, äußert sich dies in einer Auslöschung der rein quadratischen Dosis-Wirkungs-Beziehung.

3. Zeit- und Raumfaktor der Aberrationsentstehung

Nach beiden Hypothesen der Aberrationsentstehung ist unter bestimmten Bedingungen für die Erzeugung von chromosomalen Strukturumbauten eine Wechselwirkung zwischen *zwei* unabhängig voneinander induzierten und revertierungsfähigen Primärläsionen (Brüche oder labile Zustände) möglich. Sie kann aber nur dann erfolgen, wenn die Primärläsionen innerhalb kurzer Zeit entstehen und räumlich nahe genug beieinander liegen. Die Entstehung von „Zwei-Treffer"- oder „two-track"-Aberrationen wird somit von Zeit- und Raumfaktoren beeinflußt.

In einer Reihe von Experimenten wurde nun versucht, einerseits den Anteil jener Brüche zu ermitteln, die restituierten und andererseits die Zeitdauer zu bestimmen, innerhalb der die Bruchenden ein „Rejoining" unter Bildung von Austausch-Aberrationen durchführen können (SAX, 1941; DE SERRES u. GILES, 1953; WOLFF u. LUIPPOLD, 1955; EVANS, 1967a; CATCHESIDE u. Mitarb., 1946; WOLFF, 1954a; 1956, 1957). Untersucht wurden diese Fragestellungen mit Versuchsanordnungen, in denen die Dosisleistung variiert oder die Dosis fraktioniert in zwei Halbdosen appliziert wurde.

a) Zeitfaktor

Allgemein ist der „Zeitfaktor" als das Verhältnis einer „Langzeitdosis" zu einer „Kurzzeitdosis", die beide den gleichen biologischen Effekt hervorrufen, definiert. Ist ein Effekt unabhängig von der zeitlichen Dosisverteilung, so ist der Zeitfaktor gleich 1; ein Zeitfaktor, der > 1 ist, zeigt an, daß die Kumulation der Einzeleffekte bei Protrahierung oder Fraktionierung der Bestrahlung unvollständig ist.

Nach den vorliegenden experimentellen Daten hat bei Verwendung von *dicht ionisierenden Strahlenarten* (schnelle Neutronen oder Alphateilchen) eine Veränderung der Dosisleistung oder eine Dosisfraktionierung allgemein keinen Einfluß auf die Aberrationsausbeute. Sämtliche Aberrationen folgen hier einer linearen Dosis-Wirkungs-Beziehung. Dies bedeutet, daß die zu einem Austausch notwendigen zwei Primärläsionen gleichzeitig durch die Energiedeposition eines ionisierenden Teilchens induziert werden und zwischen ihnen keine freie Kooperation möglich ist.

Es sei jedoch auf die Befunde von GOOCH u. Mitarb. (1964) verwiesen (siehe Kapitel III 3a), die mit 14,1 MeV-Neutronen an Lymphozyten erarbeitet wurden und darauf hindeuten, daß man auch hier nicht nur mit „one-track"-Aberrationen zu rechnen hat. Wegen der durch 14,1 MeV-Neutronen ausgelösten schnellsten Protonen, die einen sehr niedrigen LET aufweisen, wäre eine gewisse „two-track"-Komponente durchaus zu erwarten.

Bei Verwendung von *locker ionisierenden Strahlen* können, wie schon erwähnt, die beiden Primärläsionen von Austausch-Aberrationen entweder gleichzeitig durch ein einziges ionisierendes Teilchen induziert (linearer Anteil) oder aber durch zwei verschiedene ionisierende Teilchen (quadratischer Anteil) erzeugt werden. In den Experimenten ergab sich nun allgemein, daß bei konstanter Dosis die Ausbeute an „two-track"-Aberrationen mit abnehmender Dosisleistung geringer wurde. Der gleiche Effekt trat auf, wenn bei einer Dosisfraktionierung das Zeitintervall zwischen den beiden Halbdosen eine bestimmte Länge überschritt. Nach der Bruch-Reunions-Hypothese wurde dieses Zeitfaktorphänomen damit erklärt, daß Brüche nur für eine begrenzte Zeit „offen" bleiben und zu einer Wechselwirkung mit anderen Brüchen befähigt sind. Überschreitet z.B. die Zeitspanne zwischen zwei Halbdosen, mit denen jeweils eine bestimmte Anzahl von Brüchen induziert wurde, die „Lebenszeit" der von der ersten Halbdosis erzeugten Brüche, so wird die Bildung von „two-track"-Aberrationen verhindert, da die initialen Brüche schon wieder restituiert sind, ehe sie mit jenen, die von der zweiten Halbdosis induziert wurden, kooperieren können.

Durch die von LEA u. CATCHESIDE (1942), CATCHESIDE u. Mitarb. (1946) entwickelte „G-Funktion" (hier vereinfacht wiedergegeben $G(t) = \frac{2}{t} - \frac{2}{t^2}$; wobei t = Expositionszeit, dividiert durch die „Rejoining-time", bedeutet) kann eine Aussage über den relativen Beitrag der „two-track"-Komponente in der Dosiswirkungskurve gemacht werden. Die Autoren konnten in ihren Experimenten an Tradescantia zeigen, daß die Ausbeute an Translokationen (interchanges) proportional G war, wenn bei konstanter Dosis die Intensität der Strahlung variiert wurde.

Mit Hilfe von Dosisleistungs- und Fraktionierungsexperimenten wurde versucht, die „Lebenszeit" von Brüchen abzuschätzen und so auch einen Einblick in das Restitutions-Reunions-System zu bekommen (Übersicht bei Rieger, 1967). Dabei zeigte sich, daß eine Abhängigkeit sowohl vom Testobjekt als auch von den Versuchsbedingungen besteht. In Tradescantia waren Brüche z.B. ca. 4—30 Minuten kooperationsfähig, in Vica faba mehrere Stunden (Lea u. Catcheside, 1942; Catcheside u. Mitarb., 1946; Kirby-Smith u. Dolphin, 1958; Wolff u. Luippold, 1958, Wolff 1954a), in Lymphozyten zwischen 60 und 90 Minuten (Prempree u. Mitarb., 1969; Prempree u. Merz, 1969), nach Stefanescu u. Mitarb. (1972) wenigstens 20 Stunden, nach Wolff (1972) 4—5 Stunden, in Drosophilaspermien aber mehrere Tage (Muller, 1940).

Wichtige Befunde ergaben dazu auch die Versuche von Wolff (1954a, b, 1960c, 1961c), Wolff u. Luippold (1955, 1956) in Vicia-Samen. Sie zeigten, daß röntgenstrahlen-induzierte Primärläsionen auf Grund ihrer Revertierungsgeschwindigkeit in langlebige und kurzlebige Typen unterteilt werden konnten.

Bei Bestrahlung unter aeroben Bedingungen blieben Brüche ca. 2 Stunden, unter anaeroben Verhältnissen jedoch nur 30 Minuten offen und waren zur Bildung von Austauschaberrationen kooperationsfähig (Sauerstoffeffekt, siehe Kapitel II/5).

Neben diesen relativ langlebigen Bruchtypen konnte Wolff einen zweiten kurzlebigen Bruchtyp mit einer Lebensdauer von nur 1 Minute nachweisen, der jedoch nur bei einer größeren Dosisleistung als 200 R/min und einer Bestrahlungsdauer von weniger als 1 Minute auftrat.

b) Raumfaktor

Verschiedene Beobachtungen über die Häufigkeit von Röntgen- oder γ-Strahlen-induzierten Translokationsschromosomen sowie über ihre intra- und interzelluläre Verteilung ließen vermuten, daß die Aberrationsentstehung nicht nur von der zeitlichen Koexistenz der Primärläsionen abhing, sondern auch von ihrer lagemäßigen Zuordnung. Es zeigte sich, daß in Tradescantia-Mikrosporen intrachromosomale Aberrationen (hier Ring-chromosomen) häufiger auftraten als interchromosomale, z.B. dizentrische Chromosomen (Sax, 1940). Weiterhin ergab sich (Wolff, 1959; Evans, 1961; Atwood, 1963), daß interchromosomale Aberrationen (Translokationen) in Tradescantia, Vicia und Hordeum nach Bestrahlung in der G_1- oder späten G_2-Phase des Zellzyklus nicht zufällig nach Poisson zwischen den Zellen verteilt waren, sondern stets zu viele Zellen mit einer und zu wenig Zellen mit mehreren Translokationen vorhanden waren.

Eine rein zufallsgemäße Kooperation der Primärläsionen bei den „Rejoining-Prozessen" war somit nicht gegeben. Schon 1947 konnte Lea zeigen, daß eine Wechselwirkung nur zwischen räumlich dicht benachbarten Primärläsionen stattfinden kann. Diese Überlegungen waren die Grundlage zur Aufstellung des sogenannten „*site-Konzepts*" (Wolff, 1959, 1963; Atwood, 1963), das im wesentlichen Folgendes beinhaltet:

In einem Zellkern sind nur eine begrenzte Zahl von „sites" (ausdehnungsmäßig begrenzte Volumina) vorhanden, in denen die Chromosomen so nahe zusammenliegen, daß zeitlich kooperationsfähige Primärläsionen, auch aus räumlichen Gründen in der Lage sind, miteinander in Wechselwirkung zu treten, um Austausch-Aberrationen bilden zu können. Mit anderen Worten, es sind nur eine begrenzte Anzahl von Orten im Kern vorhanden, in denen sich die Chromosomen innerhalb einer sogenannten „Rejoining-distance" zueinander befinden.

Nach einer Schätzung von Lea (1946) sollte die Länge der „Rejoining-distance" h = 1 μ betragen. Spätere Überlegungen ergaben für den „site"-Durchmesser 0,1—0,3 μ (Wolff u. Mitarb., 1958) bzw. 0,2 μ (Neary u. Mitarb., 1967). Chmelevsky u. Mitarb.

(1971) errechneten für menschliche Lymphocyten nach ^{60}Co-γ-Bestrahlung 0,5 μ, READ (1966) in Tradescantia Mikrosporen sowie BAUCHINGER und SCHMID (1973) in Lymphocyten, kommen jedoch wieder zu Wechselwirkungsdistanzen in der Größenordnung von wenigstens 1 μ.

Fragen zur Objektspezifität der „sites" sowie der Abhängigkeit ihrer Anzahl von verschiedenen Faktoren, wie z. B. der Geometrie des Zellkerns, dem Replikationszustand der Chromosomen und dem Aberrationstyp — der wiederum im Zusammenhang mit dem Zellzyklus steht — wurden von verschiedenen Arbeitsgruppen analysiert (GARCIA-BENITENZ u. WOLFF, 1962; EVANS u. SAVAGE, 1963; READ, 1965, 1966; SAVAGE, 1965, 1970; SAVAGE u. PAPWORTH, 1966).

Im Gegensatz zu WOLFF vertritt READ (1965) die Ansicht, daß jeder Bruch innerhalb eines Chromosoms, ein sog. „Exchange-site" etabliert. Unter diesen Umständen sollte die Zahl der „sites", in denen ein Strukturaustausch erfolgen kann, sehr groß sein. HEDDLE (1965) fand, daß die Rekombination freier Chromosomenenden innerhalb eines „sites" zufällig erfolgt. NORMAN u. SASAKI (1966) glauben, in ihren Experimenten mit menschlichen Lymphocyten die READsche Vorstellung bestätigt zu finden. Sie konnten zeigen, daß die Wahrscheinlichkeit, mit der ein Chromosom in ein dizentrisches Chromosom miteinbezogen wird, direkt proportional zu seiner Länge in der Interphase ist. Außerdem war die Zahl der dizentrischen und Ringchromosomen pro Zelle in erster Linie durch die Anzahl der Centromere begrenzt und nicht durch die Anzahl möglicher „sites". Von SAVAGE (1965) wird für die Annahme des „site"-Konzepts die Existenz von sog. „site-determining factors" gefordert.

4. Relative biologische Wirksamkeit verschiedener Strahlenarten (RBW)

Im Abschnitt 2 wurde erläutert, daß für die Erzeugung von Chromosomenveränderungen durch dicht ionisierende und locker ionisierende Strahlen unterschiedliche Dosiswirkungsbeziehungen bestehen. Zur Charakterisierung dieser unterschiedlichen biologischen Wirksamkeit verschiedener Strahlenqualitäten wurde der Begriff der relativen biologischen Wirksamkeit (RBW) eingeführt.

LEA u. CATCHESIDE (1942) fanden an Tradescantia-Pollenschläuchen bei vergleichenden Untersuchungen über die Aberrationsauslösung durch verschiedene Strahlenarten oder einer Strahlenart mit unterschiedlichen Energien, daß bei einer gegebenen Dosis schnelle Neutronen wirksamer waren als Röntgenstrahlen. GILES u. TOBIAS (1954) konnten ebenfalls bei Tradescantia zeigen, daß die durch verschiedene Strahlenarten verursachten unterschiedlichen Aberrationshäufigkeiten auf eine verschieden starke Energieposition entlang der Bahnspur eines ionisierenden Teilchens zurückgeführt werden können. Die RBW verschiedener Strahlenarten wird somit von ihrem „linearen Energietransfer" (LET = mittlere lineare Energieverlustrate eines ionisierenden Teilchens pro μ-Bahnlänge) bestimmt. GILES u. TOBIAS fanden, daß verschiedene Strahlenarten, aber mit gleichem LET-Bereich — sie benutzten 30 MeV-Alphateilchen, 190 MeV-Deuteronen und 100 KeV-Röntgenstrahlen — etwa gleichviel Chromosomenaberrationen auslösten. Strahlenarten mit verschiedenem LET erzeugten auch unterschiedliche Aberrationsfrequenzen.

Der LET eines ionisierenden Teilchens ist um so größer, je dichter die Ionisationen entlang seiner Bahn erfolgen. In der Regel gilt, daß bei gleichartigen Versuchsbedingungen Strahlen mit höherem LET jeweils eine höhere RBW aufweisen (LEA, 1955; READ, 1959; BORA, 1958, 1961; KIRBY-SMITH u. DANIELS, 1953).

CONGER u. Mitarb. (1958) konnten jedoch zeigen, daß RBW-Kurven nach Erreichen eines Maximums wieder absinken können. So fanden sie beim Vergleich verschiedener Strahlenarten (250 KeV-Röntgenstrahlen, 3 MeV- und 14 MeV- Neutronen) mit ^{60}Co-Gamma-Strahlen in Tradescantia, — getestet wurden Chromosomen- und Chromatid-Aberrationen — daß maximale RBW-Werte etwa bei einem LET von 60 KeV pro μ auftraten, die Kurve dann abfiel und im Bereich von 120—220 keV/μ verflachte. Der Kurvenverlauf wurde durch das Wirksamwerden eines Sättigungseffektes erklärt, der dadurch zustande kommt, daß z.B. nach Eintritt eines Bruchs oder einer Primärläsion zusätzliche Ionisationen in einem kritischen Bereich keinen zusätzlichen Effekt mehr nach sich ziehen können. Neary u. Mitarb. (1963) konnten schließlich in ihren Versuchen zeigen, daß die RBW von schnellen Neutronen, im Vergleich zu Gamma-Strahlen, viel höhere Werte erreichen kann, als sie bis dahin angegeben wurden. Sie fanden bei einem Vergleich von ^{60}Co-Gamma-Strahlen mit schnellen Neutronen der Energie 0,7 und 3 MeV, RBW-Werte, die sich einem Grenzwert der Größenordnung 100 nähern mußten.

Die Experimente zur Klärung der Beziehung zwischen LET und RBW für Chromosomenveränderungen sind außerordentlich zahlreich und können an dieser Stelle weder voll aufgezählt noch interpretiert werden. Es sei deshalb auf Übersichten bei Bora (1961, tabellarische Zusammenstellung), Rieger u. Michaelis (1967) sowie Evans (1962) verwiesen. Nur ein Experiment von Savage (1968) sei hier aufgeführt, das den unterschiedlichen Einfluß des LET auf den Typ der beobachtbaren Chromosomenaberrationen veranschaulicht. Im Gegensatz zu einer Strahlung mit niedrigem LET erzeugten α-Partikel in Tradescantia Pollen in zunehmendem Maße unvollständige Isochromatid-interchanges.

Es muß noch erwähnt werden, daß sowohl LET- als auch RBW-Werte durch verschiedene physikalische und biologische Faktoren beeinflußt werden. So hängt die RBW einer bestimmten Strahlenart von dem untersuchten Aberrationstyp ab und es ist keineswegs gleichgültig, ob z.B. Chromatiddeletionen, Translokationen oder Gaps analysiert werden. Als weitere Punkte seien die Dosis sowie die Dosisleistung genannt. Neary u. Mitarb. (1963) fanden bei einem Vergleich von ^{60}Co-Gamma-Strahlen und schnellen Neutronen (0,7 und 3 MeV) ihre hohen RBW-Werte bei kleinen Dosen oder langen Bestrahlungszeiten. Entscheidend ist auch die physiologische Reaktionslage der Zellen und dabei vor allem die Sauerstoffspannung in den Zellen zur Zeit der Bestrahlung. Die Wirksamkeit dicht ionisierender Strahlen wird z.B. durch Sauerstoff kaum beeinflußt, während Strahlenarten mit geringem LET unter aeroben Bedingungen etwa um einen Faktor 3 wirksamer sind als unter anaeroben Bedingungen (Conger, 1956; Evans u. Neary, 1959; Hornsey u. Mitarb. 1960). Schließlich seien noch die Befunde von Rosenzweig u. Rossi (1959), Rossi u. Rosenzweig (1956) zitiert, nach denen das Spektrum der tatsächlichen Energiekonzentration in mikroskopischen Bereichen nicht stets dem LET-Spektrum gleichgesetzt werden kann und von der Größe des bestrahlten Volumens abhängt. Gray (1956) und Rossi (1959) haben darauf hingewiesen, daß auch den δ-Strahlen besondere Bedeutung für die Variabilität der RBW-Werte zukommt.

Das Konzept RBW und LET steht auch in engem Zusammenhang mit der Interpretation fundamentaler Prozesse der Aberrationsentstehung. So glaubten Catcheside u. Lea (1943) aufgrund ihrer Experimente annehmen zu können, daß zur Erzeugung eines Bruchs eine Energie von etwa 600 eV (17 Ionisationsereignisse) notwendig sei. Die Zunahme der RBW mit steigendem LET wäre somit durch eine kumulative Wirkung vieler Energiedepositionen zu erklären. Demgegenüber haben Neary (1965), Neary u. Savage (1966), Neary u. Mitarb. (1964, 1967) in ihren Arbeiten eine Theorie der RBW entwickelt, nach der die Primärläsion in einer lokalen Region des Interphasechromosoms (z.B. die DNS-Doppelhelix mit ihrem angelagerten Protein) in der Regel durch eine einzige Ionisation verursacht wird. Als prinzipielle Ursache für eine ausgesprochene LET-Abhängigkeit der Chromosomenaberrationen ist die Tatsache anzusehen, daß nun Paare solcher makromolekularer Bereiche (targets) geschädigt werden müssen, die dann miteinander in Wechselwirkung treten. Werden diese beiden Primärläsionen durch voneinander unabhängige Bahnspuren (tracks) induziert, so ist die Aberrationshäufigkeit unter der Voraussetzung, daß Dosis und LET nicht zu hoch sind, etwa proportional zum Quadrat der Dosis und unabhängig vom LET. Werden beide Primärläsionen durch die gleiche Bahnspur erzeugt, ist die Häufigkeit etwa proportional der Dosis und auch dem LET. Entscheidend für die Möglichkeit einer Wechselwirkung zwischen beiden Primärläsionen ist, daß sie sich innerhalb eines kritischen Bereichs von etwa 0,2 μ befinden (siehe dazu auch Abschn. 3b).

5. Veränderungen der Aberrationsausbeute durch den Sauerstoff (Sauerstoffeffekt)

Die Aberrationsausbeute wird durch verschiedene physikalische und chemische Modifikatoren beeinflußt. Der wohl wichtigste Faktor ist die zum Zeitpunkt der Bestrahlung in den Zellen vorherrschende Sauerstoffspannung. Da eine sehr große Zahl von Arbeiten über den Sauerstoff als Modifikator der Aberrationsentstehung vorliegt, kann hier nur auf die prinzipiellen Befunde eingegangen werden. Ausführlichere Darstellungen finden sich bei GILES (1954), READ (1959), ALPER (1960), HOLLAENDER (1960), EVANS (1962), SOBELS (1963), RIEGER u. MICHAELIS (1967).

THODAY u. READ (1947, 1949) konnten in Vicia faba-Wurzelspitzen als Erste einen Sauerstoffeffekt beobachten. Es zeigte sich, daß nach Bestrahlung mit Röntgenstrahlen und in Gegenwart von Luft die Zahl der abnormen Anaphasen etwa dreimal so groß war als nach einer Bestrahlung unter Sauerstoffmangel. Bei Verwendung von dicht ionisierenden Alphateilchen (hoher LET) wird die Aberrationshäufigkeit jedoch kaum oder gar nicht beeinflußt. Neutronen nehmen eine Mittelstellung zwischen Röntgenstrahlen und Alphateilchen ein (GILES u. Mitarb., 1952).

Bei Experimenten mit Strahlenarten sehr geringer Ionisationsdichte zeigte sich, daß trotz vollständiger Anoxie die Aberrationsinduktion nicht vollständig verhindert werden kann. Es wäre denkbar, daß hier die auch bei locker ionisierenden Strahlen stets vorhandenen Komponenten hoher Energiekonzentrationen entlang einer Bahnspur — darauf wurde bereits in einem vorausgegangenem Abschnitt hingewiesen — eine Rolle spielen.

Aus den Experimenten von GILES u. RILEY (1949, 1950), GILES u. BEATTY (1950), RILEY u. Mitarb. (1952), NEARY (1957), GRAY (1957) war ersichtlich, daß ein Sauerstoff-Effekt nur bei unmittelbarer Gegenwart von O_2 während der Bestrahlung auftrat. Eine Verringerung der O_2-Spannung während der Bestrahlung ergab eine geringere Aberrationsausbeute. GILES u. BEATTY (1950) fanden auch, daß bei einer gegebenen Strahlendosis die Aberrationsrate mit zunehmender O_2-Konzentration in der Gasphase signifikant anstieg. Bei Partialdrucken von $> 21\%$ war jedoch keine weitere wesentliche Erhöhung zu erzielen. Um also bei Bestrahlung unter anoxischen Bedingungen (N_2) eine etwa gleichgroße Aberrationsausbeute wie bei Bestrahlung in Luft (21 % O_2) zu bekommen, ist es notwendig, bei Anoxie eine zweieinhalb- bis dreifach höhere Dosis zu applizieren.

Es sei noch darauf hingewiesen, daß der Sauerstoff-Effekt bei einer Bestrahlung in feuchten Testsystemen durch die Gegenwart von Stickoxyd (NO) nachgeahmt werden kann (KIHLMAN, 1958, 1959; GRAY u. Mitarb., 1958). In trockenen Systemen zeigt NO jedoch Strahlenschutzeigenschaften (SPARRMANN u. Mitarb., 1959; POWERS u. Mitarb., 1959, 1960).

Auf Grund zahlreicher Experimente, vor allem von GILES u. Mitarb. (siehe dazu GILES, 1954) wurde die sensibilisierende Wirkung des Sauerstoffs bei der Aberrationsinduktion durch eine Zunahme der Zahl primärer Brüche gedeutet. Darüber hinaus wird auch die Restitutionsrate der induzierten Brüche durch O_2 beeinflußt (WOLFF u. ATWOOD, 1954). Unter anaeroben Bedingungen induzierte Brüche haben eine kürzere „Rejoining-time" (WOLFF u. LUIPPOLD, 1955, 1958).

Im Abschnitt 3 wurde bereits darauf hingewiesen, daß Brüche, die unter anaeroben Bedingungen induziert werden, eine wesentlich kürzere Lebensdauer (Zeitraum, in dem die Brüche reaktionsfähig sind) haben als jene, die unter aeroben Verhältnissen induziert werden. Daraus haben WOLFF u. LUIPPOLD (1956) versucht, die Existenz eines selbst strahlensensiblen Reunions-Restitutions-Systems abzuleiten, das unabhängig von der Bruchinduktion unter Sauerstoff und hohen Dosen stärker geschädigt wird als unter anaeroben Bedingungen und niedrigen Dosen.

Nach SWANSON (1954) kommt der Sauerstoff-Effekt dadurch zustande, daß potentielle Brüche unter anaeroben Verhältnissen repariert werden. ALPER (1956) glaubt, daß durch Sauerstoff potentielle Brüche bevorzugt in echte Brüche transformiert werden.

6. Aberrationstypen

a) Strukturelle Chromosomenaberrationen

Strahleninduzierte strukturelle Chromosomendefekte können in drei Gruppen eingeordnet werden:

a) Chromosomenaberrationen,
b) Chromatidaberrationen,
c) Subchromatidaberrationen.

Bei diesen strukturellen Veränderungen lassen sich im allgemeinen zwei Grundtypen unterscheiden: 1. die einfache Deletion (Bruchstückverlust), 2. der Strukturumbau, der innerhalb ein und desselben Chromosoms bzw. der Chromatide (intrachange) oder zwischen verschiedenen Chromosomen bzw. Chromatiden (interchange) erfolgen kann.

Welcher dieser drei Aberrationstypen nun beobachtet werden kann, hängt davon ab, in welcher Phase des Zellzyklus bestrahlt wurde. Nach Howard u. Pelc (1951) wird das Interphasestadium in drei Phasen eingeteilt. Die Präsynthese- oder G_1-Phase, die DNS-Synthese- oder S-Phase sowie die Postsynthese- oder G_2-Phase. Die Chromosomen liegen

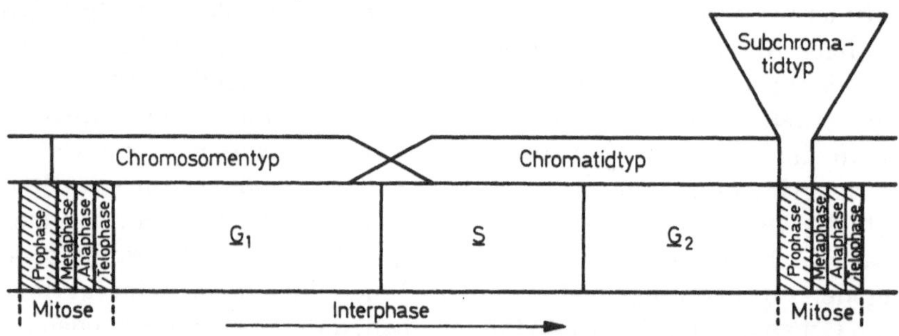

Abb. 1. Beziehung zwischen dem Typ der strahleninduzierten Aberrationen und den verschiedenen Stadien des Zellzyklus. (Nach Evans, 1962)

in diesen Phasen in einem unterschiedlichen Replikationszustand vor. Dies bedeutet u. a., daß sie eine verschiedenartige Lateraldifferenzierung aufweisen (Wolff, 1969b). Werden Zellen in G_1 bestrahlt, so reagiert das unreduplizierte Chromosom als sei es funktionell „einsträngig", und es entstehen Aberrationen vom Chromosomentyp. Werden Zellen in der S- oder G_2-Phase bestrahlt, d. h. werden beide durch die Reduplikation entstandenen Chromatiden erfaßt, so entstehen Aberrationen vom Chromatidtyp (Abb. 1).

Experimente an Pflanzen (Wolff, 1961a; Wolff u. Luippold, 1964; Evans u. Savage, 1963), tierischen Zellkulturen (Hsu u. Mitarb., 1962; Monesi u. Mitarb., 1967) und menschlichen Lymphozyten (Wolff, 1969a) haben gezeigt, daß der Übergangspunkt, von dem an die Chromosomen auf eine Bestrahlung an Stelle von Chromosomenaberrationen mit Chromatidaberrationen reagieren, in der späten G_1-Phase liegt. Wolff leitet daraus für menschliche somatische Chromosomen eine vielsträngige Struktur ab, die in der späten G_1-Phase gelockert wird, um dann funktionelle Chromatiden zu bilden. Die Aufspaltung erfolgt also noch vor der DNS-Synthese.

Subchromatidaberrationen werden nicht im Interphasekern induziert, sondern während der Mitose. Im Gegensatz zur Interphase sind hier die Chromosomen mikroskopisch sichtbar. Werden Zellen in der frühen Prophase bestrahlt, so werden Halbchromatidaberrationen erzeugt, die sich als Seitenarmbrücken in der Anaphase manifestieren (Crouse, 1954; Wilson u. Mitarb., 1959). Somit vermag auch die Prophasechromatide auf die Bestrahlung als Doppelstruktur zu reagieren.

Es sei noch darauf hingewiesen, daß bei Applikation identischer Strahlendosen die verschiedenen Stadien der Interphase in bezug auf die Aberrationsentstehung eine unterschiedliche Strahlensensibilität aufweisen können. So wurde von Evans u. Savage (1963) in Pflanzen für die G_1-Phase eine relativ geringe Empfindlichkeit beobachtet, sie stieg dann im Verlauf der S- zur G_2-Phase an und verringerte sich wiederum vor der Metaphase.

Brewen (1965) fand dagegen, daß in menschlichen Lymphozyten die G_1-Phase mehr als dreimal empfindlicher war als die G_2- und siebzehnmal so empfindlich als die S-Phase (erfaßt wurden nur asymmetrische Austauschaberrationen). Die Unterschiede wurden auf räumliche Beziehungen zwischen den Chromosomen innerhalb des untransformierten (nach Lajtha (1963) befinden sich dort die Zellen in einer G_0-Phase) Zellkerns der peripheren kleinen Lymphozyten zurückgeführt. Heddle u. Mitarb. (1967) glauben, daß auf Grund ihrer Befunde aus 2-Tage-Kulturen G_1 sogar 5—6mal empfindlicher als G_2 und mehr als 25 mal empfindlicher als S sein müßte. Sheppard u. Ferrari (1970) konnten Brewens Befunde für „interchange"-Aberrationen bestätigen. Wurde jedoch als Maß für die Empfindlichkeit die prozentuale Häufigkeit der gestörten Zellen angenommen, war das G_2-Stadium viermal empfindlicher als G_0. Die Strahlenempfindlichkeit der S-Phase lag dazwischen.

Gewissermaßen eine Feinstruktur der Empfindlichkeit innerhalb einer bestimmten Phase konnte ebenfalls bereits nachgewiesen werden. So von Ma u. Wolff (1965) in Tradescantia-Mikrosporen (Wolff, 1968) und von Scott u. Evans (1967) in Vicia-faba-Wurzelspitzenzellen jeweils für G_2.

α) *Chromosomenaberrationen*

Sie werden in der G_1-Phase des Zellzyklus induziert und können in der folgenden Metaphase in verschiedenen Typen auftreten. Ihre Vielfalt hängt nach den Vorstellungen der Bruch-Reunions-Hypothese davon ab, wie viele der induzierten Brüche offen bleiben (Deletionen) oder miteinander in Wechselwirkung treten (Austausch-Aberrationen). Austausch-Prozesse können sowohl intra- als auch interchromosomal erfolgen. Dabei können sämtliche vier Bruchenden (vollständiger Austausch) oder nur zwei (unvollständiger Austausch) beteiligt sein. Ein intrachromosomaler Austausch kann innerhalb eines Chromosomenarmes (intra-arm-intrachange) oder zwischen beiden Schenkeln (inter-arm-intrachange) erfolgen. Evans (1962) unterteilt den zuletzt genannten Typ noch in zwei Gruppen, wobei er einen sogenannten U-Typ (die Fusion der Bruchenden erfolgt proximal zu proximal) und einen X-Typ (distal zu proximal) unterscheidet. Ein Austausch nach dem U-Typ führt z. B. zu zentrischen Ringen und Fragmenten und wird als asymmetrisch bezeichnet (Abb. 2). Austauschprodukte nach dem X-Typ können zu einer Deletion führen oder eine Inversion ergeben. Letztere bleibt cytologisch meist unentdeckt. Sie werden als symmetrische Konfigurationen bezeichnet. Interchromosomale, asymmetrische Translokationsprodukte sind z. B. dizentrische Chromosomen mit ihren dazugehörigen azentrischen Fragmenten. Bei symmetrischen reziproken Translokationen entstehen atypische monozentrische Chromosomen. Komplexere Austauschfiguren lassen sich auf die beschriebenen Grundtypen zurückführen.

β) *Chromatidaberrationen*

Sie werden im allgemeinen in der S- und G_2-Phase des Zellzyklus, nach Aufspaltung des Chromosoms in zwei Chromatiden induziert. Verschiedene Chemikalien, wie z. B. alkylierende Substanzen, führen jedoch auch bei Einwirkung in der präreplikativen Phase (G_1) zu Chromatidaberrationen. Lindahl-Kiessling u. Mitarb. (1970) erhielten durch eine Pulsbehandlung (90 Min.) von Lymphozytenkulturen mit ³H-Uridin kurz vor oder nach PHA-Applikation (Zellen sind in G_0 oder früher G_1) ebenfalls bevorzugt Chromatiddefekte. Zu ähnlichen Ergebnissen kam Wolff (1970) nach Röntgenbestrahlung von Lymphozyten, die 15—30 Minuten mit Glycerin vorbehandelt waren.

Die Klassifikation der Chromatidaberrationen wird nach gleichartigen Kriterien, wie sie für die Aberrationen vom Chromosomentyp gelten, vorgenommen. Zu einer besseren

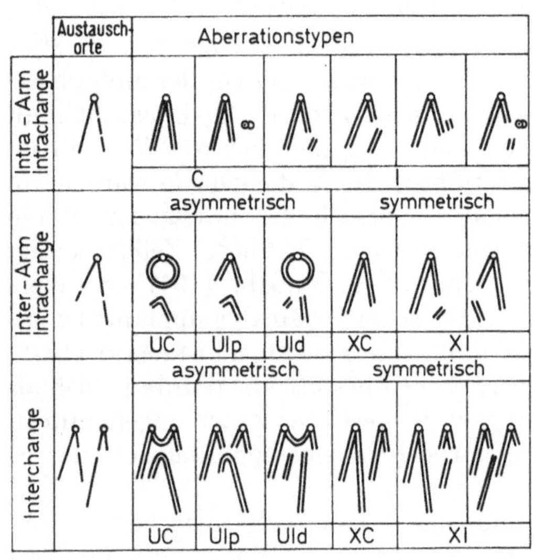

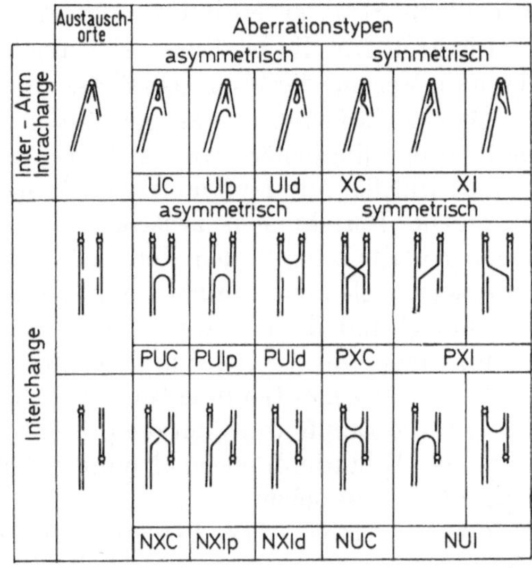

Abb. 2   Abb. 3

Abb. 2. Durch einen Strukturumbau entstandene Aberrationen vom Chromosomentyp. Bei der Klassifikation wird zwischen einem vollständigen (complete, C) bzw. einem unvollständigen (incomplete I) Austausch unterschieden, der U- oder X-förmig erfolgen kann. p bzw. d bezeichnet die proximale bzw. distale Lage der offen gebliebenen Bruchstellen. (Nach Evans, 1962)

Abb. 3. Durch einen Strukturumbau entstandene Aberrationen vom Chromatidtyp. Mit P bzw. N wird das Auftreten von polarisierten bzw. nichtpolarisierten Centromeren bezeichnet. Weitere Erklärung der Symbole siehe Abb. 2. (Nach Evans, 1962)

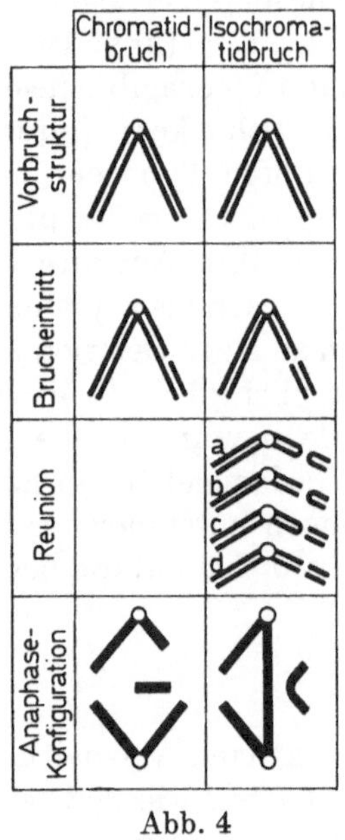

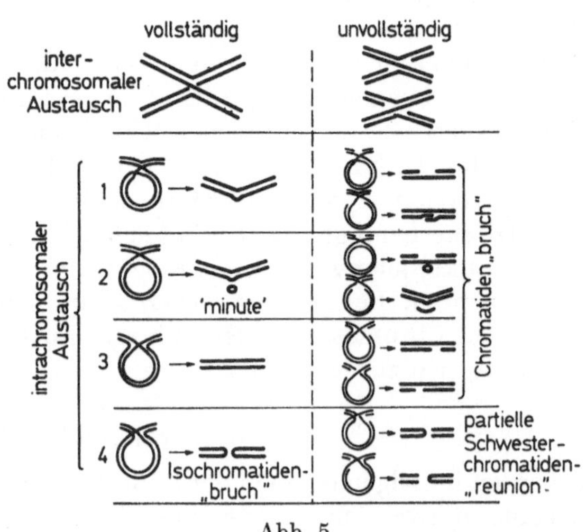

Abb. 4   Abb. 5

Abb. 4. Schematische Darstellung der Entstehungsweise eines Chromatid- bzw. Isochromatidbruchs. a–d zeigt die verschiedenen Formen von Schwesterchromatiden-Reunionen, wie sie in den proximalen (p) und distalen (d) Chromosomenabschnitten erfolgen können. Sie werden folgendermaßen bezeichnet: a = sister-union; b = non-union proximal, NUp; c = NUd; d = NUpd. (Nach Lea, 1947)

Abb. 5. Entstehung von Chromatidaberrationen nach der Austausch-Hypothese. Die dünneren Linien zeigen eine vollständige Chromatidenpaarung innerhalb eines sogenannten „Revell-loops" zur Zeit des Austausches während der Interphase. Die dickeren Linien kennzeichnen die entsprechenden Metaphasekonfigurationen; die Schleifen sind während der Chromosomenkontraktion verschwunden. (Nach Revell, 1959)

Charakterisierung der chromatidalen Interarm-Austauschfiguren (Inter-arm-interchanges) wurde von EVANS (1961) zusätzlich noch die Lagebeziehung der Centromeren (polarisiert bzw. nichtpolarisiert) beider Translokationschromosomen berücksichtigt. Im Gegensatz zu Chromosomenaberrationen zeigen Chromatidaberrationen eine weitaus größere Variabilität der Formen, sind aber trotzdem cytologisch gut identifizierbar. Ein Grund dafür ist die während der Metaphase persistierende enge parallele Lage der Schwesterchromatiden, die es erlaubt, selbst vollständige symmetrische Chromatidtranslokationen zu erkennen. Schemen, in denen die verschiedenen Typen von Chromatidaberrationen auf der Grundlage des Bruch-Reunions-Modells eingeordnet sind, zeigen Abb. 3 und 4. Nach der Austauschhypothese sind Chromatidbrüche jedoch als unvollständige „intra-arm intrachanges" anzusehen. Abb. 5 zeigt ein Schema dieser Aberrationstypen, wie es von REVELL (1959) auf der Grundlage dieses Modells aufgestellt wurde.

γ) *Subchromatidaberrationen*

Sie werden in der Prophase induziert und können in der Anaphase als Seitenarmbrücken beobachtet werden. Da sie bisher in menschlichen Zellen nach Bestrahlung nicht gefunden wurden, soll hier nicht näher auf sie eingegangen werden.

b) Achromatische Lücken (gaps)

Neben den besprochenen drei Grundtypen struktureller Chromosomenaberrationen können nach Bestrahlung oft noch sog. „gaps" oder achromatische Lücken beobachtet werden. Dabei handelt es sich um feulgennegative Regionen in den Chromatiden, die in verschiedenen Längen und Durchmessern auftreten können und als einfache oder Isolocus-gaps klassifiziert werden (Abb. 6f, g). Im Gegensatz zu Chromatidbrüchen führen sie in der Anaphase nicht zu azentrischen Fragmenten und stellen somit keine echten Diskontinuitäten der Chromosomenstruktur dar (REVELL, 1959, 1963; EVANS, 1963a, b, 1967a; SCOTT u. EVANS, 1967). Dies wird auch durch neuere elektronenoptische Befunde bestätigt

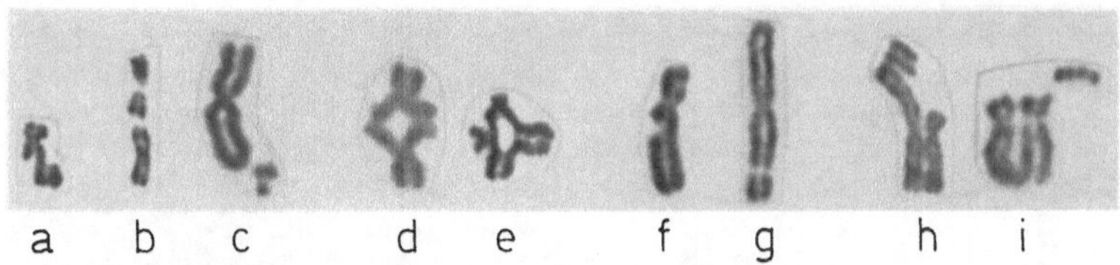

Abb. 6. Verschiedene Chromosomendefekte in menschlichen Lymphozyten. a–e Aberrationen vom Chromatidtyp. a) einfacher Chromatidbruch, b) Isochromatidbruch NUpd, c) Isochromatidbruch NUd, d + e Chromatidaustausch, d) symmetrisch, e) asymmetrisch, f + g Achromatische Lücken (gaps), f) zwei einfache gaps verschiedener Größe im kurzen und langen Arm des Chromosoms, g) iso-gap, h + i Diplochromosomen als Folge einer Endoreduplikation mit h) Fragmentation eines Chromosoms, i) mit Fragmentation beider Chromosomen

(BRØGGER, 1971; SCHEID u. TRAUT (1971a, b), in denen mehrere Chromatinfibrillen innerhalb der „Lücken" festgestellt wurden.

REVELL (1959) konnte zeigen, daß die Zahl der echten Diskontinuitäten, wie sie in früheren Experimenten von THODAY (1951) und LEA u. CATCHESIDE (1942) angegeben wurde, zu hoch war, weil gaps als Chromatiddeletionen gezählt worden waren. Gaps werden vor allem in der G_2-Phase, selten auch in der G_1-Phase des Zellzyklus induziert und zeigen eine etwa lineare Dosis-Wirkungs-Beziehung. Für ihre Entstehung existiert eine Reihe von Erklärungen. Die wichtigsten stammen von EVANS, der sie 1963 (a, b) als Folge von lokalen Entspiralisierungen der Chromosomenstruktur oder DNS-Verlusten, 1967 (a) als in der Metaphase manifestierte Primärläsionen, die in keinen Austauschprozeß miteinbezogen und nicht repariert wurden, interpretierte.

c) Numerische Aberrationen

Neben den strukturellen Chromosomendefekten können auch Abweichungen von der modalen Chromosomenzahl (beim Menschen 46) beobachtet werden. Zellen mit solchen numerischen Aberrationen lassen sich in aneuploide und polyploide Formen einteilen.

α) *Aneuploidie*

Abweichungen von der modalen Zahl nach unten werden als hypodiploid, nach oben als hyperdiploid charakterisiert. In einer Reihe von Arbeiten (Zusammenfassung im UNSCEAR-Bericht, 1969) wurde sowohl nach Bestrahlung in vivo als auch in vitro, in menschlichen peripheren Lymphozyten über eine Zunahme von hypodiploiden Zellen berichtet. Diese Beobachtungen sind vielfach auf Kritik gestoßen. Dabei wurde angeführt, daß die Aneuploidie erst durch die Kulturbedingungen induziert würde oder als Präparationsartefakt anzusehen sei. Sicherlich kann das Auftreten aneuploider Zellen nicht prinzipiell auf diese Art und Weise erklärt werden. Man darf annehmen, daß bei einer Bestrahlung sowohl Centromer als auch Centriolen und Spindelapparat in Mitleidenschaft gezogen werden, was zu Fehlverteilungen der Chromosomen und damit zu aneuploiden Tochterzellen führen kann. Trotzdem sind die Bewertungsgrundlagen für aneuploide Zellen mit einem relativ großen Unsicherheitsfaktor behaftet. Als quantitativer Indikator für eine Strahlenexposition sind sie kaum geeignet.

β) *Polyploidie*

In polyploiden Zellen ist die diploide Chromosomenzahl um einen oder mehrere Chromosomensätze erhöht. Die Entwicklung solcher Zellen ist auf einen gestörten Mitoseablauf zurückzuführen. Dieser kann durch einen Defekt im Spindelapparat verursacht werden oder dadurch zustande kommen, daß asymmetrische Chromosomenaberrationen eine re-

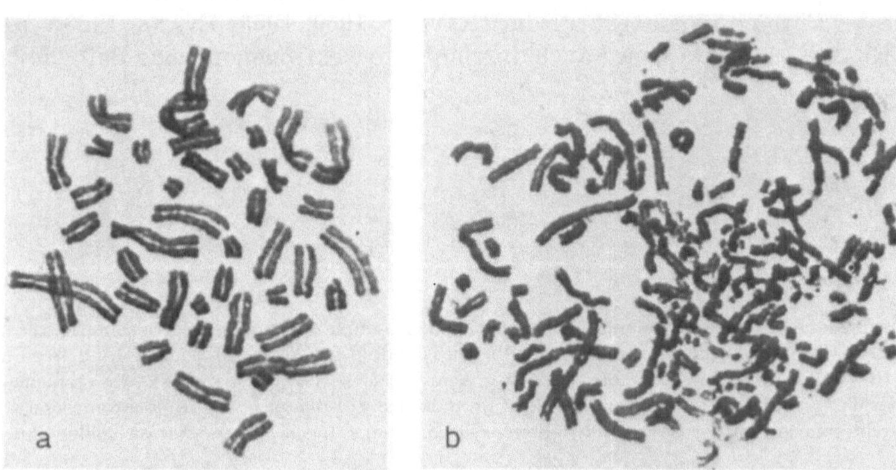

Abb. 7. Polyploide Metaphasen menschlicher Lymphozyten. a) Zelle mit 42 Diplochromosomen nach Endoreduplikation, b) Tetraploide Zelle mit multiplen Chromosomendefekten; Strukturumbauten, Fragmentation, Entspiralisierungsvorgänge

guläre Kern- und Zellteilung be- oder verhindern. Als Folgeerscheinungen kommt es zur Fusion der Tochterkerne, zur Restitutionskernbildung, zur Bildung vielkerniger Zellen oder zu Endoreduplikationen (Abb. 7). Cytologisch beobachtbar wird die Polyploidisierung meist erst im Verlauf der folgenden Mitose. Die Zahl der polyploiden Zellen hängt somit auch von der Zellkinetik des untersuchten Gewebes und von den Kulturbedingungen ab. In Lymphozytenkulturen steigt z.B. der Tetraploidindex bei einer Verlängerung der Kulturzeit von 48 auf 72 Stunden an (siehe Kapitel III/2). Obschon das Auftreten polyploider Zellen gewisse Hinweise auf eine vorausgehende Strahlenexposition gibt, kann es jedoch nicht als ein exaktes Maß derselben verwendet werden. Berichte über Polyploidie in menschlichen peripheren Lymphozyten nach Bestrahlung in vitro und in vivo sind im UNSCEAR-Report (1969) zusammengestellt.

7. Klassifikation der Aberrationen

Chromosomenaberrationen lassen sich zweckmäßig in die beiden Hauptgruppen der strukturellen und der numerischen Aberrationen unterteilen.

Da sich jedoch zur Aufstellung von quantitativen Dosiswirkungsbeziehungen in der Regel nur strukturelle Veränderungen eignen, soll hier nur diese Gruppe besprochen werden. Strukturelle Chromosomenaberrationen kommen in einer Vielfalt von Formen vor (Abb. 8—10), die in verschiedenen Ordnungsschemen klassifiziert wurden. Die Beurteilung und Klassifikation der Aberrationen kann nach verschiedenen Gesichtspunkten erfolgen:

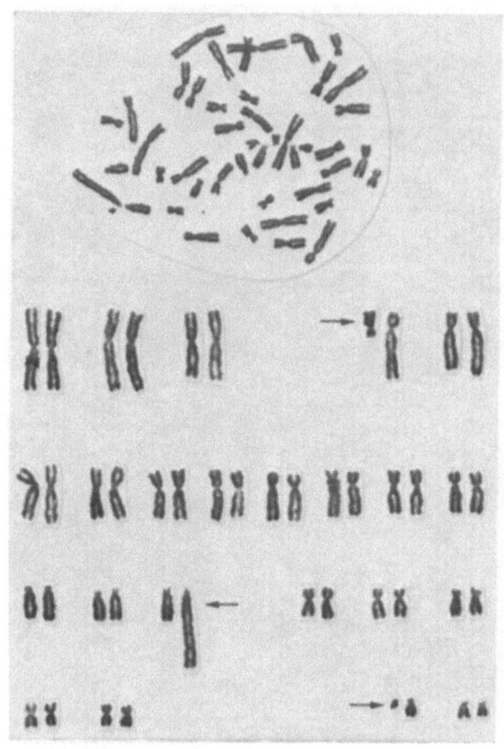

Abb. 8. Chromosomenmuster eines menschlichen Lymphozyten mit atypischem Chromosom (Translokation t [Bq −; Dq +] nach Chicago Conference 1966) und Defizienz (Gq −)

1. Nach dem Entstehungsmechanismus der Aberrationen.
Ein diesbezüglich ursprünglich von DARLINGTON u. UPCOTT (1941) in ihren Arbeiten über Chromosomenaberrationen in Pflanzenzellen vorgeschlagenes Schema wurde jedoch durch beschreibende Klassifikationen verdrängt.

2. Nach Zellen, die bestimmte Aberrationstypen enthalten und deren funktionellem Verhalten bei der Mitose (BUCKTON u. Mitarb., 1962; BUCKTON u. PIKE, 1964b; BUCKTON u. Mitarb., 1967a). Es werden drei Zelltypen unterschieden:

A-Zellen: Normale Zellen ohne strukturelle Chromosomendefekte. Zusätzlich werden noch modale und nicht-modale Formen erfaßt.

B-Zellen: Zellen, die nur Aberrationen vom Chromatidtyp enthalten.

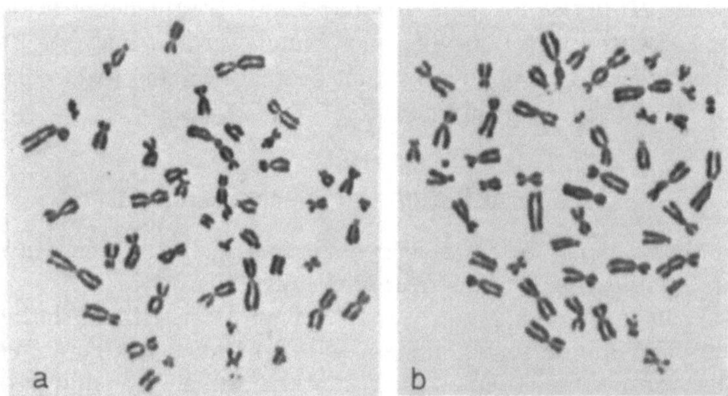

Abb. 9. Metaphasen menschlicher Lymphozyten mit multiplen chromosomalen Strukturdefekten. a) 1 dizentrisches, 1 trizentrisches, 1 atypisches Chromosom, azentrische Fragmente, 1 Chromatidbruch, b) 2 dizentrische Chromosomen, azentrische Fragmente

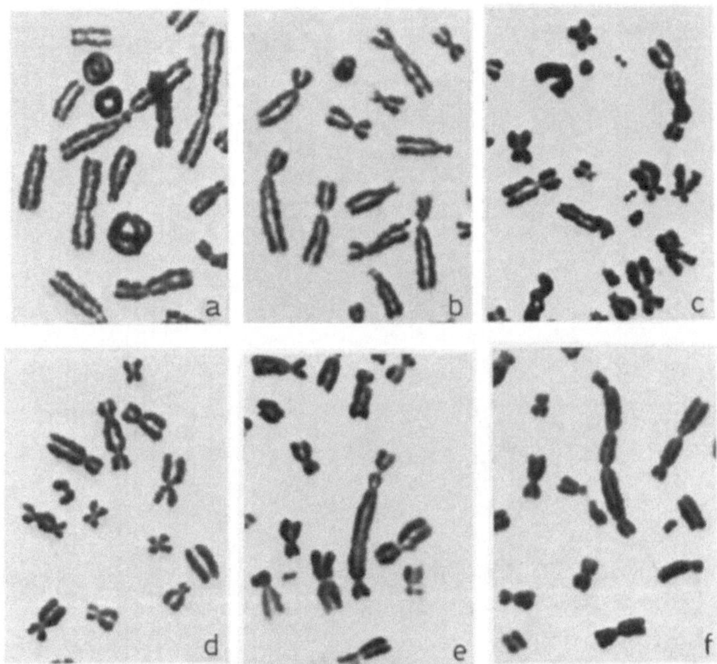

Abb. 10. Ausschnitte aus Metaphaseplatten menschlicher Lymphozyten mit Aberrationen vom Chromosomentyp. a) Zentrischer Ring, 2 azentrische Ringe, azentrisches Fragment, b) azentrischer Doppelring, c) dizentrisches Chromosom, interstitielle Deletionen (double minutes), d) dizentrisches Chromosom, azentrisches Fragment, e) trizentrisches Chromosom, azentrisches Fragment, f) tetrazentrisches Chromosom, dizentrisches Chromosom, azentrische Fragmente

C-Zellen: Zellen, die Aberrationen vom Chromosomentyp enthalten. Sie werden nach ihren Überlebensaussichten bei weiteren Teilungen in zwei Kategorien, die sogenannten C_u- und C_s-Zellen unterteilt.

C_u-Zellen enthalten sogenannte „*unstabile*" Chromosomenaberrationen, wie Ringe, dizentrische Chromosomen oder azentrische Fragmente. Je nach dem, ob sich eine C_u-Zelle in ihrer ersten oder zweiten Teilung nach Bestrahlung befindet, werden X_1- oder X_2-Zellen unterschieden. X_2-Zellen werden z.B. dadurch erkannt, daß sie dizentrische oder Ringchromosomen ohne azentrische Fragmente enthalten oder daß identische Aberrationstypen auftreten.

C_s-Zellen enthalten sogenannte „*stabile*" Chromosomenaberrationen, die durch einen vollständigen symmetrischen Stückaustausch entstanden sind.

3. Nach der morphologischen Struktur der Aberrationen.

Eine Form der Klassifikation, die primär weder Annahmen über den präzisen Entstehungsmechanismus der Aberrationen noch über deren Verhalten bei weiteren Zellteilungen macht. Die Aberrationen werden in verschiedenen Ordnungsschemen erfaßt. Bei einem von BAUCHINGER u. HUG (1966), SCHMID u. BAUCHINGER (1969) vorgeschlagenen Schema werden vier Zellklassen unterschieden:

N-Zellen sind Zellen mit *normalem* Chromosomenmuster. Sie können modal oder nichtmodal ($\pm$ 2 Centromere) sein.

S-Zellen sind Zellen mit *strukturellen* Chromosomendefekten. Sie können Chromosomen- bzw. Chromatidaberrationen enthalten, die sich in zwei Grundtypen aufgliedern lassen:

Aberrationen vom $S_1\text{-}Typ$:

Sie können auf *Bruchstückverluste, ohne sichtbare Strukturumbauten* zurückgeführt werden (Chromatidbrüche Abb. 6a—c, Defizienzen Abb. 8, azentrische Fragmente Abb. 6h, i, 10a, b, interstitielle „minute"-Deletionen Abb. 10c).

Aberrationen vom $S_2\text{-}Typ$:

Sie können auf chromosomale *Strukturumbauten* zurückgeführt werden (Chromatidaustauschfiguren Abb. 6d, e, multizentrische Chromosomen Abb. 10 c—f, 9, Ringchromosomen Abb. 10a, atypische nicht klassifizierbare Chromosomen Abb. 8, 9a).

U-Zellen sind Zellen mit *unspezifischen Chromosomendefekten*, die nicht mit einer echten Diskontinuität der Chromosomenstruktur verbunden sind (gaps, Fusionen, pyknotische Chromosomen Abb. 6f, g).

D-Zellen sind Zellen mit *diffusen Chromosomenaberrationen* (Pulverisierung, „break-constrictions", Entspiralisierungen).

III. Experimentelle Befunde über strahleninduzierte Chromosomenaberrationen in menschlichen peripheren Lymphozyten

Eine Literaturübersicht zu diesem Thema ist auch im UNSCEAR-Bericht (1969) enthalten.

1. Die Lymphozytenkultur

OSGOOD u. KRIPPAEHNEs (1955) „gradient tissue culture"-Technik zur Züchtung menschlicher Leukozyten wurde von NOWELL (1960), HUNGERFORD u. Mitarb. (1959), MOORHEAD u. Mitarb. (1960) so weit entwickelt, daß man damit menschliche Chromosomen relativ einfach sichtbar machen konnte. Heute ist die Kurzzeitkultur von peripheren Lymphozyten bereits zu einer Routinemethode geworden. Es ist daher auch verständlich, daß die meisten Erfahrungen über strahleninduzierte Chromosomenaberrationen an diesem Testobjekt gewonnen wurden. Die Technik der Lymphozytenkultur und Chromosomenpräparation sei kurz erläutert.

Aus 10—20 ccm heparinisiertem Armvenenblut wird durch Sedimentation der Erythrozyten das lymphozytenhaltige Plasma gewonnen. Zusammen mit einem speziellen Nährmedium und Phytohämagglutinin (PHA; einem mitogenen Extrakt aus Phaseolus vulgaris) wird es zwei bis drei Tage bei 37° C im Brutschrank gehalten. Durch das Phytohämagglutinin werden die kleinen Lymphozyten (CARSTAIRS, 1962; MACKINNEY u. Mitarb., 1962; MARSHALL u. ROBERTS, 1963; TANAKA u. Mitarb., 1963; ELVES u. WILKINSON, 1963), die in der G_1-Phase (möglicherweise in einer G_0-Phase) des Zellzyklus vorliegen, in blastenartige Zellen transformiert und treten in die Mitose ein. Einige Stunden vor Beendigung der Kultur wird zur Anreicherung der Metaphasen dem Medium kurzzeitig Colcemid oder Colchicin zugesetzt. Durch die Behandlung mit einer hypotonischen Salzlösung kommt es nach einer Schwellung der Zellen zu einer Auflockerung des Kernchromatins. In diesem Zustand werden die Zellen fixiert und auf einen Objektträger gebracht. Durch einen Trocknungsprozeß werden sie auf der Glasoberfläche flach ausgebreitet. Abschließend erfolgt die Färbung und das Eindecken der Präparate.

Neben dieser als Makromethode bezeichneten Lymphozytenkultur wurden auch Mikromethoden unter Verwendung von nur wenigen Tropfen Vollblut entwickelt, z.B. Arakaki u. Sparkes (1963), Evans (1965).

Kritische Diskussionen über prinzipielle Fragen der Lymphozytenkulturtechnik finden sich bei Mellmann (1965), Moorhead (1967), Sharpe u. Mitarb. (1969).

2. Die Abhängigkeit der Aberrationshäufigkeit von der Kulturdauer

Buckton u. Pike (1964a, b) hatten als erste beobachtet, daß in Lymphozytenkulturen von Strahlenpatienten die Zahl der Zellen mit dizentrischen Chromosomen, Ringen und azentrischen Fragmenten (sogenannte C_u-Zellen) bei Verlängerung der Kulturdauer von 48 auf 72 Stunden abnahm. Zudem fehlten in vielen Zellen mit asymmetrischen Austauschaberrationen die korrespondierenden azentrischen Fragmente. Zu ähnlichen Ergebnissen kamen Ishihara u. Kumatori (1965) bei Thorotrastpatienten und bei in vitro-Studien. Darüber hinaus fanden beide Arbeitsgruppen in 72 Stunden-Kulturen mehr polyploide Zellen als in 48 Stunden-Kulturen. Tetraploide Zellen enthielten dabei oft Chromosomenaberrationen paarweise oder in octoploiden Zellen sogar vierfach (Ishihara u. Kumatori, 1966). Auf Grund detaillierter Untersuchungen von Sasaki u. Norman (1967), Heddle u. Mitarb. (1967), Bender u. Brewen (1969) sowie Antoshina u. Mitarb. (1969) ergab sich dann übereinstimmend, daß nach dreitägiger Kulturzeit sehr viele Zellen bereits in ihrer zweiten (X_2) oder einer späteren Teilung in vitro beobachtet wurden. Die Ausbeute an C_u-Zellen war nach 48 Stunden etwa doppelt so hoch als nach 72 Stunden (Buckton u. Mitarb., 1962; Buckton u. Pike, 1964a, b, 1967a; Norman u. Mitarb., 1966; Sasaki u. Norman, 1967; Heddle u. Mitarb., 1967; Schmid u. Bauchinger, 1969).

Die Abnahme der C_u-Zellen wird darauf zurückgeführt, daß es diesen nicht möglich ist, mehrere Zellteilungen, die bei längerer Kulturzeit erfolgen können, zu überleben. So kann z.B. durch dizentrische oder Ring-Chromosomen ein normaler Zell- und Kernteilungsablauf be- oder verhindert werden. Es kommt zur Ausbildung von Anaphasebrücken, welche die mechanische Trennung der beiden Tochterkerne stark beeinflussen. Gelingt keine Trennung, entstehen tetraploide Restitutionskerne, die in der Regel nur begrenzt lebensfähig sind. Wenn Zellen in der Metaphase liegenbleiben, können sie nach dem Durchlaufen eines weiteren Zellzyklus durch Endoreduplikation polyploidisiert werden (Abb. 7a). Azentrische Fragmente werden bei der Zellteilung entweder eliminiert oder zufällig in die Tochterzellen miteingeschlossen. Dadurch entstehen unbalancierte Genverhältnisse, die die Lebensfähigkeit dieser Zellen beeinträchtigen können.

Keine wesentliche Behinderung der Mitose sollte durch atypische monozentrische Chromosomen erfolgen, die bei symmetrischen Translokationsvorgängen meist ohne zusätzlichen Bruchstückverlust entstehen (Abb. 8). Es ist jedoch zu bedenken, daß es durch Austauschvorgänge zwischen nicht homologen Chromosomen immerhin zu Umlagerungen des genetischen Materials kommt, deren Folgen sich unter Umständen erst in späteren Zellgenerationen negativ auf diese Zellen auswirken können.

Verschiedene Aberrationstypen können bei der Mitose auch unterschiedlich schnell eliminiert werden. Nach Sasaki u. Norman (1967) beträgt z.B. die Wahrscheinlichkeit für ein dizentrisches Chromosom, durch die erste Teilung in vitro zu kommen, etwa 0,5, dafür daß zwei Teilungen überstanden werden, jedoch nurmehr 0,25. Für abnorme monozentrische Chromosomen liegt der erste Wert bei 0,9. Die Wahrscheinlichkeit, daß eine C_u-Zelle gegenüber einer C_s-Zelle überlebt, entspricht etwa 0,35.

Im Gegensatz zu den bisher erwähnten Autoren fanden ISHIHARA u. KUMATORI (1967), HONDA u. Mitarb. (1969) sowie BENDER u. BREWEN (1969) keine signifikanten Unterschiede für die Aberrationshäufigkeit in Zwei- bzw. Drei-Tage-Kulturen.

Schließlich sei noch darauf hingewiesen, daß durch eine Verlängerung der Kulturzeit nicht nur die Aberrationshäufigkeit beeinflußt werden kann, sondern auch die Gefahr einer falschen Beurteilung der Aberrationstypen wächst. So kann z. B. ein einfacher Chromatidbruch aus der ersten Teilung nach Bestrahlung, nach der Replikation in der folgenden

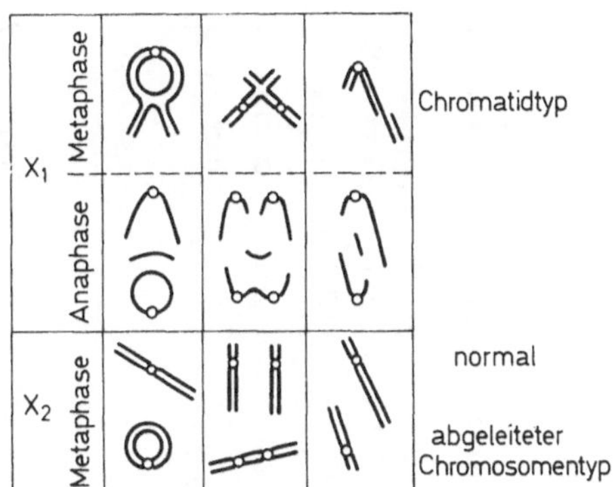

Abb. 11. Schematische Darstellung der Entstehungsweise sogenannter abgeleiteter (derived) Aberrationen vom Chromosomentyp. Aberrationen vom Chromatidtyp können nach Durchlaufen der X_1-Anaphase und Replikation in der folgenden Interphase, in X_2-Metaphasen einer der Tochterzellen als abgeleitete Aberrationen vom Chromosomentyp (Ringchromosom, dizentrisches Chromosom, atypisches Chromosom) beobachtet werden. Im vorliegenden Fall wurde jeweils angenommen, daß das azentrische Fragment verloren ging

Interphase, bei Beobachtung in der X_2-Metaphase, als atypisches monozentrisches Chromosom auftreten. Ein asymmetrischer Chromatidaustausch kann unter der Voraussetzung, daß die X_1-Anaphase ungestört ablaufen kann, nach der Replikation, in der X_2-Metaphase als dizentrisches Chromosom erscheinen. Aberrationen vom Chromatidtyp können somit in späteren Teilungen als sogenannte abgeleitete („derived") Aberrationen vom Chromosomentyp erscheinen und zur Auswertung gelangen (Abb. 11).

Zur Aufstellung von quantitativen Dosiswirkungsbeziehungen ist es daher zweckmäßig, die Kulturbedingungen so einzurichten, daß die Zellen möglichst in ihrer ersten (X_1) Teilung nach der Bestrahlung beobachtet werden können.

3. Strahleninduzierte Chromosomenaberrationen in vitro

a) Untersuchungen der Dosiswirkungsbeziehung

α) *Röntgen- und Gammastrahlen*

Vergleicht man die Dosiswirkungsbeziehungen, wie sie nach akuter Bestrahlung von menschlichen peripheren Lymphozyten in vitro mit Strahlenarten von geringem LET ermittelt wurden, mit jenen, wie sie von SAX, LEA und CATCHESIDE (Kap. II) an Pflanzen gefunden wurden, so zeigen sich teilweise einige unerwartete Unterschiede.

Nach Arbeiten von EVANS (1967a, b, c, 1968) weicht die Dosiswirkungsbeziehung für Austauschaberrationen in Lymphozyten nach akuter Röntgenbestrahlung (250 kV) stark von einer einfachen D^2-Beziehung ab. In der Potenzfunktion $Y = kD^n$ ergab sich für dizentrische Chromosomen und Ringe der niedrige Dosisexponent $n = 1,17 \pm 0,04$ ($n \neq 1$; $n \neq 2$). Die Ergebnisse konnten auch dem linear-quadratischen Modell $Y = c + \alpha D + \beta D^2$ angepaßt werden. Der Koeffizient β der „two-track"-Komponente war signifikant von 0 verschieden.

Tabelle 1. *Koeffizienten des quadratischen Modells $Y = c + \alpha D + \beta D^2$ für dizentrische Chromosomen bzw. dizentrische Chromosomen und Ringe. * Die Anpassung an das quadratische Modell wurde von* Evans (1967) *durchgeführt. — Keine Angaben vorhanden.*

Aberration	Kulturzeit	$Y = c + \alpha D + \beta D^2$		Dosisleistung rad/Min.	Strahlenart	Literatur
		$\alpha \times 10^{-3}$	$\beta \times 10^{-6}$			
Dizentrische Chromosomen	50–54	(2,51 ± 0,15)	(2,22 ± 0,58)	17,5–230,5	250 kV Röntgen	Evans (1967)
,,	50; 60	(0,66 ± 0,30)	(2,17 ± 1,62)	23,4	230 kV Röntgen	Watson u. Gillies (1970)
,,	50; 55	(2,50 ± 0,74)	(1,35 ± 2,24)	98–200	250 kV Röntgen	Scott u. Mitarb. (1970)
,,	51	(1,34 ± 0,93)	(5,72 ± 2,10)	110	180 kV Röntgen ⎫	Bajerska u. Liniecki (1969a)
,,	51	(2,53 ± 0,29)	(0,97 ± 0,61)	15,8	180 kV Röntgen ⎬	
,,	48	(0,69 ± 0,07)	(4,92 ± 0,18)	50	220 kV Röntgen	Schmid u. Mitarb. (1971)
,,	50–55	(1,78 ± 0,20)	(2,30 ± 0,53)	19–292 (akut)	1,2 MeV ^{60}Co γ ⎫	Scott u. Mitarb. (1970)
,,	50–55	(0,52 ± 0,13)	(1,72 ± 0,27)	0,04–0,55 (chronisch)	1,2 MeV ^{60}Co γ ⎬	
Dizentrische Chromosomen + Ringe	50–54	(3,42 ± 0,17)	(3,51 ± 0,68)	17,5–230,5	250 kV Röntgen	Evans (1967)
,,	72	(0,36 ± 0,19)	(3,07 ± 1,26)	60	250 kV Röntgen	Bender u. Gooch (1962)*
,,	52	(0,91 ± 0,20)	(6,0 ± 0,7)	12,5–100 (akut)	250 kV Röntgen ⎫	Brewen u. Luippold (1971)
,,	52	(0,68 ± 0,10)	(0,68 ± 0,23)	– (chronisch)	^{137}Cs γ ⎬	
,,	48	(0,73 ± 0,05)	(5,42 ± 0,20)	50	220 kV Röntgen	Schmid u. Mitarb. (1972)

Ähnlich niedrige Dosisexponenten für dizentrische Chromosomen fanden Bajerska u. Liniecki (1969a) nach akuter Bestrahlung mit 180 kV-Röntgenstrahlen (n = 1,15 ± 0,11) sowie Scott u. Mitarb. (1970) nach 250 kV-Röntgenstrahlen (n = 1,16 ± 0,23). Darüber hinaus ergab die statistische Analyse in beiden Fällen gesicherte Hinweise für eine lineare Dosiswirkungsbeziehung, da sich die Dosisexponenten nicht signifikant von 1 unterschieden und bei Scott die Ergebnisse am besten dem linearen Modell Y = kD angepaßt werden konnten.

Scotts Experimente mit akuter Gammastrahlung konnten am besten durch das linear-quadratische Modell beschrieben werden, in dem sowohl die lineare als auch die quadratische Komponente signifikant > 0 war. In der Potenzfunktion war der Dosisexponent n = 1,24 ± 0,06. Für den Vergleich der beiden Strahlenarten ergab sich ein RBW-Wert von 0,82 ± 0,03 für ^{60}Co-Gammastrahlen.

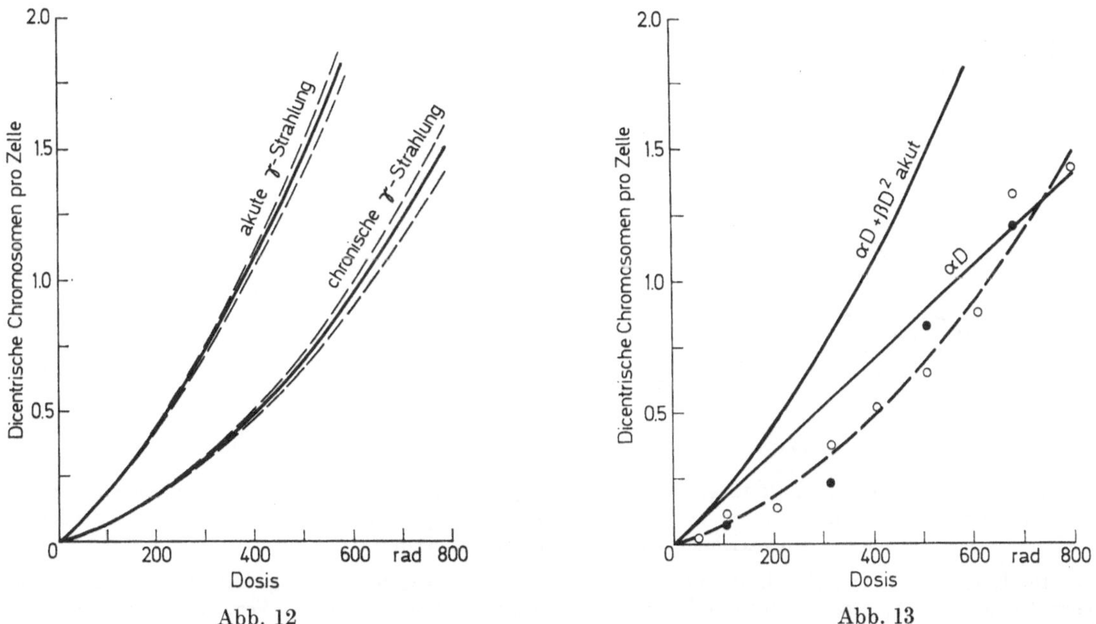

Abb. 12. In vitro-Bestrahlung. Bestangepaßtes Polynom 2. Grades (mit Standardfehler) für akute und chronische (24 h) ^{60}Co-Gammabestrahlung. (Nach Scott u. Mitarb., 1970)

Abb. 13. In vitro-Bestrahlung. Bestangepaßtes Polynom 2. Grades für eine akute ^{60}Co-Gammabestrahlung und dessen lineare Komponente (αD). Die gestrichelte Linie (······) zeigt das entsprechende Polynom für eine chronische (24 h) Gammabestrahlung von + PHA-(○) und —PHA-(●)-Zellen. (Nach Scott u. Mitarb., 1970)

Ein überraschendes Ergebnis erbrachten Scotts Versuche mit chronischer Gammastrahlung. Bei einer 24stündigen Exposition war der Dosisexponent mit n = 1,52 ± 0,01 höher als bei akuter Bestrahlung. Die Dosiswirkungsbeziehung konnte am besten dem linear quadratischen Modell angepaßt werden, in dem α und β hoch signifikant > 0 waren. Abb. 12 zeigt die linear-quadratischen Dosiswirkungskurven für die akute und chronische Exposition. Es ist ersichtlich, daß nach chronischer Bestrahlung die Aberrationshäufigkeit gegenüber der akuten Exposition bei einer Dosis von 500 rad etwa auf die Hälfte, bei 50 rad etwa auf ein Drittel verringert ist. Abb. 13 zeigt, daß abgesehen von den beiden höchsten Dosen, die Ausbeute an dizentrischen Chromosomen nach der chronischen Bestrahlung, noch unter dem Niveau der linearen (αD) Komponente der „akuten"-Kurve liegt. Dies widerspricht den bisher an Pflanzen gewonnenen Ergebnissen. Danach wäre durch eine verringerte Dosisleistung (durch Zunahme der Expositionszeit) im linear-quadratischen Modell eine Verringerung der „two-track"-(βD²)-Komponente zu erwarten gewesen, während die „one-track"-Komponente im wesentlichen nicht beeinflußt wird (siehe Kapitel II 2).

Bajerska u. Liniecki (1969a), Brewen u. Luippold (1971) fanden dies auch für das in vitro-Lymphozyten-System bestätigt. Bei Bajerska u. Liniecki war die Dosiswirkungsbeziehung für dizentrische Chromosomen bei 180 kV Röntgenstrahlen, die mit einer Dosisleistung von 15,8 rad/min appliziert wurden, linear (n = 1,15). Bei 110 rad pro Minute wich die Regressionsfunktion knapp von der Linearität ab (n = 1,23 ± 0,13). Im Polynom 2. Grades hatte die Verringerung der Dosisleistung eine Verminderung der quadratischen Komponente um eine Größenordnung zur Folge (Tabelle 1). Der gleiche Effekt wurde für Ringe, azentrische Fragmente und interstitielle Deletionen beobachtet. Die von Brewen und Luippold berechneten Dosiswirkungsbeziehungen für zentrische Ringe + dizentrische Chromosomen nach akuter Röntgenstrahlung (250 kV) und chronischer ^{137}Cs-γ-Strahlung (24 Stunden) waren am besten durch eine linear-quadratische Funktion zu beschreiben (Tabelle 1). Aus Abb. 14 ist ersichtlich, daß nur die „two-track"-Komponente signifikant durch die Dosisleistung beeinflußt wird. Unter Verwendung der linearen

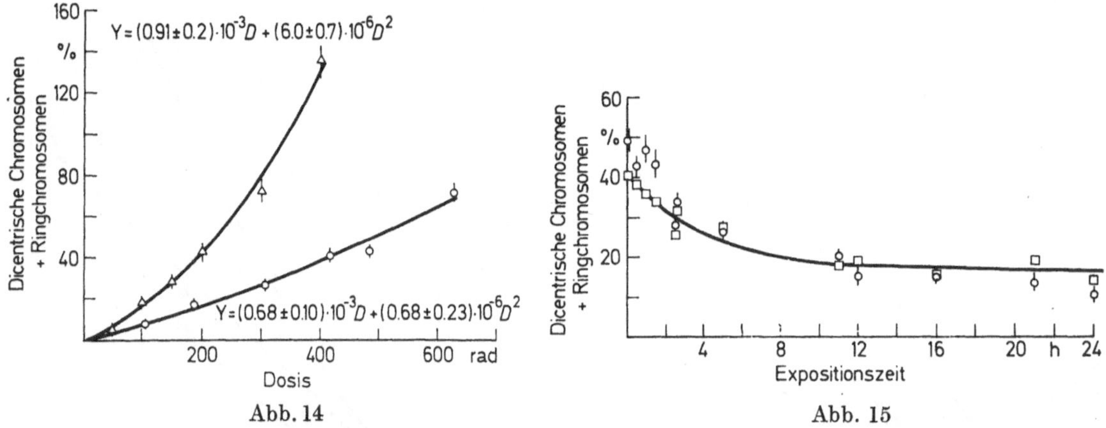

Abb. 14   Abb. 15

Abb. 14. In vitro-Bestrahlung. Bestangepaßte Polynome 2. Grades für eine akute Röntgenbestrahlung ($\triangle$) und chronische (24 h) ^{137}Cs-Gammastrahlung ($\bigcirc$). Bei den empirischen Werten sind die Standardfehler eingezeichnet. (Nach Brewen u. Luippold, 1971)

Abb. 15. Empirische Werte für die Häufigkeit dizentrischer Chromosomen + Ringe nach einer etwa einheitlichen Dosis von 200 R aber unterschiedlichen Expositionszeiten. Die empirischen Werte ($\bigcirc$) werden mit den theoretischen Werten ($\square$) bei der gemessenen Dosis und der theoretischen Kurve (———) für eine Bestrahlung mit einer konstanten Dosis von 200 R verglichen. (Nach Brewen u. Luippold, 1971)

Koeffizienten ergab sich ein RBW-Wert von 0,75 für Gammastrahlen im Vergleich zu 250 kV-Röntgenstrahlen. In Abb. 15 ist die Häufigkeit der dizentrischen Chromosomen + Ringe als Funktion der Bestrahlungsdauer bei einer konstanten Dosis dargestellt. Brewen und Luippold konnten nachweisen, daß in ihren Versuchen mit zunehmender Expositionszeit diese Aberrationstypen in weitgehender Übereinstimmung mit der von Lea u. Catcheside (1942), Catcheside u. Mitarb. (1946) aufgestellten „G-Funktion" (unter Annahme einer „rejoining-time" von 90 Minuten; siehe Kapitel II/3) abnahmen. Die Abweichung der beobachteten Werte von der theoretischen Kurve, die bei den kurzen Expositionszeiten auftrat (Abb. 15), wurde darauf zurückgeführt, daß bei Zimmertemperatur bestrahlt wurde (siehe dazu Kap. IV 1). Bender konnte in allen seinen Experimenten (Bender u. Gooch [1962a], Gooch u. Mitarb. [1964], Bender u. Barcinski [1969], Bender u. Brewen [1969]) die Befunde für Ringe und dizentrische Chromosomen stets dem Modell $Y = kD^2$ am besten anpassen. Als Beispiel sei ein Experiment von Bender u. Barcinski (1969) mit 250 kV Röntgenstrahlen angeführt, in dem die Proportionalitätskonstante k = $(12,74 ± 0,15) \cdot 10^{-6}$ dizentrische Chromosomen und Ringe pro Zelle pro rad² betrug. Deletionen nahmen dagegen linear mit der Dosis zu, im Modell $Y = c + kD$ ergab sich für k = $(2,48 ± 0,12) \cdot 10^{-3}$ Deletionen pro Zelle pro rad. In der Potenzfunktion war der

Tabelle 2. *Dosisexponenten und Koeffizienten der Potenzfunktion* $Y = kD^n$ *sowie Koeffizienten des Modells* $Y = kD^2$ *für dizentrische Chromosomen bzw. dizentrische Chromosomen + Ringe. – Keine Angaben vorhanden.*

Aberration	Kulturzeit	$Y = kD^n$		Dosisleistung rad/Min.	Strahlenart	Literatur
		k	n			
Dizentrische Chromosomen	66	–	1,2	3.5	^{60}Co γ	Mouriquand u. Mitarb. (1971)
„	50–55	$(6,65 \pm 2,40) \cdot 10^{-4}$	$1,24 \pm 0,06$	19–292 (akut)	^{60}Co γ	Scott u. Mitarb. (1970)
„	50–55	$(5,70 \pm 3,64) \cdot 10^{-5}$	$1,52 \pm 0,10$	0,04–0,55 (chronisch) 24 h	^{60}Co γ	
„	54	$8,4 \cdot 10^{-5}$	$1,59 \pm 0,10$	45,0	^{60}Co γ	Sevankayev u. Bochkov (1968)
„	?	$3,95 \cdot 10^{-5}$	$1,66 \pm 0,04$	?	^{60}Co γ	Chmelevsky u. Mitarb. (1971)
Diz. Chromos. + Ringe	50	$(25,5 \pm 0,41) \cdot 10^{-6}$	$1,78 \pm 0,03$	81.6–86,0	^{60}Co γ	Sasaki u. Mitarb. (1970)
„	48	$1,77 \cdot 10^{-5}$	$1,89 \pm 0,28$	—	^{60}Co γ	Visfeldt (1966)
Diz. Chromos.	50–55	$(1,17 \pm 1,54) \cdot 10^{-3}$	$1,16 \pm 0,23$	98–200 (akut)	250 kV Röntgen	Scott u. Mitarb. (1970)
„	50–54	$(1,35 \pm 0,28) \cdot 10^{-3}$	$1,17 \pm 0,04$	17,5–230,5	250 kV Röntgen	Evans (1967)
„	51	$8,18 \cdot 10^{-4}$	$1,23 \pm 0,13$	110,0	180 kV Röntgen	Bajerska u. Liniecki (1969 a)
„	51	$1,23 \cdot 10^{-3}$	$1,15 \pm 0,11$	15,8	180 kV Röntgen	
„	48	–	$1,58 \pm 0,03$	30,0	250 kV Röntgen	Shepard u. Ferrari (1970)
„	48	$1,63 \cdot 10^{-5}$	$1,88 \pm 0,10$	50,0	220 kV Röntgen	Schmid u. Mitarb. (1972)
Diz. Chromos. + Ringe	48	$2,91 \cdot 10^{-5}$	$1.78 \pm 0,07$	50,0	220 kV Röntgen	
„	48	$0.30 \cdot 10^{-5}$	1,82	100,0	250 kV Röntgen	Dolphin (1969)
„	50	$8,5 \cdot 10^{-6}$	1,94	—	1,5-1,9 MeV Röntgen	Sasaki (1969)
„	50	$81,4 \cdot 10^{-6}$	1,66	—	200 kV Röntgen	
„	50	–	2,04	10–200,0	1,9 MeV Röntgen	Norman (1966, 1967)
„	72	–	1,90	10–200,0	1,9 MeV Röntgen	
„	45–54	$(0,86–1,51) \cdot 10^{-5}$	$1,95 \binom{1,76}{2,13}$	12,0	2,0 MeV Röntgen	Buckton u. Mitarb. (1969, 1971)
„	45–54	–	$2,01 \binom{1,82}{2,20}$	12,0	2,0 MeV Röntgen	
„	56	–	$2,15 \pm 0,07$	50,0	250 kV Röntgen	Bender u. Barcinski (1969)

$$Y = kD^2$$

Aberration	Kulturzeit	k	n	Dosisleistung rad/Min.	Strahlenart	Literatur
Diz. Chromos.	72–90	$0,9 \cdot 10^{-6}$	2	—	200 kV Röntgen	Kelly u. Brown (1965)
„	72–96	$(2,7 \pm 1,4) \cdot 10^{-5}$	2	100—200	100 kV–1,9 MeV Röntgen	Norman u. Mitarb. (1964)
„	72	$8,2 \cdot 10^{-6}$	2	100	160 kV Röntgen	Mouriquand u. Mitarb. (1966)
„	48	$(4,73 \pm 0,21) \cdot 10^{-6}$	2	30	250 kV Röntgen	Shepard u. Ferrari (1970)
Diz. Chromos. + Ringe	72	$0,75 \cdot 10^{-5}$	2	52	240 kV Röntgen	Edgren (1970)
„	72	$(0,52 \pm 0,07) \cdot 10^{-5}$	2	60	250 kV Röntgen	Bender u. Gooch (1962)
„	72	$(0,60 \pm 0,05) \cdot 10^{-5}$	2	10	250 kV Röntgen	Gooch u. Mitarb. (1964)
„	42–66	$(7,58 \pm 0,4) \cdot 10^{-6}$	2	50	1,9 MeV Röntgen	Bender u. Brewen (1969)
„	56	$(12,74 \pm 0,15) \cdot 10^{-6}$	2	50	250 kV Röntgen	Bender u. Barcinski (1969)
„	50	$(5,7 \pm 0,5) \cdot 10^{-6}$	2	10–200	1,9 MeV Röntgen	Norman u. Sasaki (1966, 1967)
„	50	$(3,1 \pm 0,5) \cdot 10^{-6}$	2	10–200	1,9 MeV Röntgen	

Dosisexponent für Deletionen n = 1,10 ± 0,08, für Ringe und dizentrische Chromosomen n = 2,15 ± 0,07.

Benders Ergebnisse stehen in guter Übereinstimmung mit den Befunden von Ohnuki u. Mitarb. (1961), Bell u. Baker (1962), Kelly u. Brown (1965), Norman u. Sasaki (1966), Norman (1967). Die Dosiswirkungsbeziehung für dizentrische Chromosomen bzw. dizentrische Chromosomen und Ringe konnte in eigenen Versuchen mit 220 kV Röntgenstrahlen (Schmid u. Mitarb., 1972) stets am besten durch das linear-quadratische Modell beschrieben werden, wobei α und β signifikant von 0 verschieden waren. Eine Anpassung an das Modell $Y = kD^2$ war nicht möglich (Tabelle 1).

Die Abb. 16, 31, 32 zeigen nochmals anschaulich, daß zwischen den Ergebnissen aus verschiedenen Laboratorien teilweise beträchtliche Diskrepanzen bestehen, sowohl was die Gesamtaberrationsrate als auch den Verlauf der Dosiswirkungskurve betrifft. In den

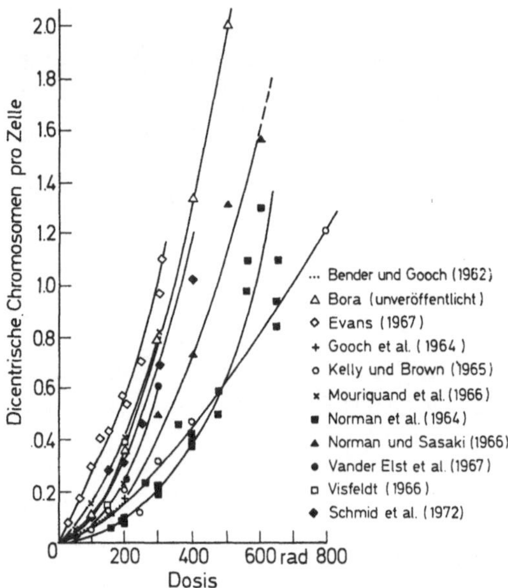

Abb. 16. In vitro-Bestrahlung. Dosis-Wirkungs-Beziehung für dizentrische Chromosomen (+ Ringe) aus verschiedenen Laboratorien. (Nach Abbatt, 1971; ergänzt)

Tabellen 1, 2 sind Koeffizienten der Aberrationsentstehung und Dosisexponenten für die getesteten Modelle der Dosiswirkungsbeziehung zusammengestellt.

Evans (1967b) versuchte vor allem die voneinander abweichenden Befunde zwischen seinen und Benders Experimenten durch die unterschiedliche Kulturdauer (52—54 Stunden bzw. 72 Stunden) zu erklären (siehe dazu auch Kap. III 2). Er glaubt, daß insbesondere bei hohen Dosen, in 72stündigen Kulturen wegen der strahleninduzierten Mitoseverzögerung, mehr X_1-Zellen mit einer hohen Aberrationsrate vorhanden sind als dies bei niederen Dosen der Fall ist. Die Dosiswirkungsbeziehung $Y = kD^2$ für dizentrische Chromosomen und Ringe würde somit nur infolge der längeren Kulturzeit zustande kommen. Norman u. Sasaki (1966) und Norman (1967) konnten jedoch selbst bei kürzeren Kulturzeiten als sie Evans anwandte, ebenso Bender u. Barcinski (1969) bei einer Wiederholung von Evans' Versuchen unter gleichen experimentellen Bedingungen, ihre Befunde stets diesem Modell am besten anpassen. Bender u. Brewen (1969) glauben aufgrund ihrer Experimente annehmen zu können, daß in Lymphozytenkulturen wenigstens zwei Lymphozytenpopulationen mit einer unterschiedlichen Strahlenempfindlichkeit vorhanden sein müssen, die zudem mit verschiedenen Geschwindigkeiten den Transformationsprozeß bis zur Mitose durchlaufen. Somit wäre gewissermaßen ein Zellklon für die Ergebnisse nach 48stündiger, der andere für jene nach 72stündiger Kulturzeit verantwortlich.

Weitere Gründe für die Variabilität der verschiedenen in vitro-Befunde werden in Kapitel IV 1 besprochen.

β) Schnelle Neutronen

Bisher liegen nur wenige Untersuchungen der Dosiswirkungsbeziehung nach Bestrahlung von peripheren Lymphozyten mit schnellen Neutronen (hoher LET) vor. GOOCH u. Mitarb. (1964) fanden nach Bestrahlung mit 14,1 MeV DT-Neutronen, bei einer Dosisleistung von 6 rad/min, in 72-Stunden-Kulturen für „Chromosomenbrüche" (terminale und interstitielle? Deletionen) eine geringe Abweichung von einer linearen Beziehung. Die Dosis-Wirkungs-Beziehung für dizentrische Chromosomen und Ringe wich zwar nicht signifikant von dem linearen Modell ab, konnte jedoch weit besser dem rein quadratischen Modell angepaßt werden (k = 12,1 · 10^{-6} dizentrische Chromosomen + Ringe pro Zelle pro rad²). SCOTT u. Mitarb. (1969) errechneten mit BENDERS Daten (Abb. 18) für die Potenzfunktion einen Exponenten von n = 1,42 ± 0,20. Die RBW für die Erzeugung dieser beiden Aberrationstypen beträgt gegenüber 250 kV-Röntgenstrahlen nur 1,4.

Diese Befunde stehen im Gegensatz zu jenen, wie sie an Pflanzen erarbeitet wurden und in denen sich für sämtliche Aberrationstypen eine lineare Zunahme mit steigender Dosis

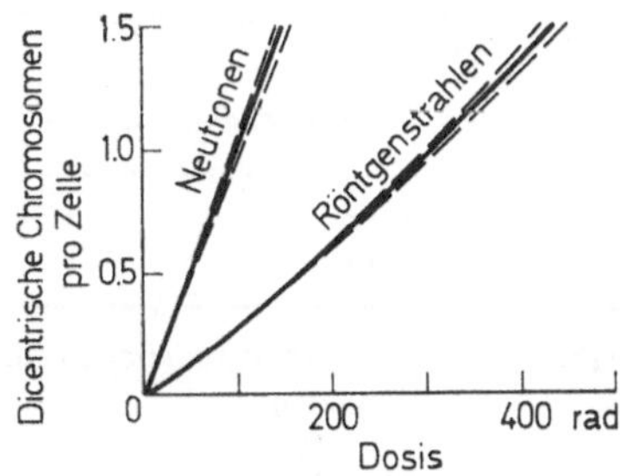

Abb. 17. In vitro-Bestrahlung. Dosiswirkungskurve mit Standardfehler für Röntgen- und Neutronenbestrahlung. Die Beziehung für Röntgenstrahlen wurde aus kombinierten Ergebnissen von SCOTT u. Mitarb. (1969) und EVANS (1967), die Beziehung für Neutronen aus Befunden von SCOTT u. Mitarb. (1969) jeweils mit PHA-stimulierten Zellen berechnet. (Nach SCOTT u. Mitarb., 1969)

ergab (Kapitel II 2). Im Vergleich zu GOOCH fand SASAKI (1971) mit 14,1 MeV TD-Neutronen, jedoch nach nur 50 stündiger Kulturzeit, einen Dosisexponenten von 1,24 (Abb. 30). Vorläufige Ergebnisse von GOOCH mit 2,5 MeV DD-Neutronen ergaben eine lineare Dosis-Wirkungs-Beziehung für sämtliche Aberrationstypen und eine RBW im Vergleich zu 250 kV-Röntgenstrahlen von 4—5 für Deletionen. Mit 2,03 MeV Neutronen erhielt SASAKI einen Dosisexponenten n = 1,09.

SCOTT u. Mitarb. (1967, 1969) benutzten zu ihren Versuchen schnelle Spalt-Neutronen, für die sie eine mittlere Energie von ca. 0,7 MeV angeben. Die Lymphozyten wurden vor oder nach der Stimulation mit Phytohämagglutinin (PHA) bestrahlt und in Mikrokulturen bei einer Kulturzeit zwischen 48—56 Stunden gehalten. Es zeigt sich, daß die Aberrationshäufigkeit in Zellen, die nach der PHA-Stimulierung bestrahlt worden waren, selbst bei einer um den Faktor 1000 veränderten Neutronendosisleistung (0,057—50 rad/min, bei Dosen bis 150 rad) nicht verändert wurde. In zwei von fünf Experimenten ergab sich bei Zellen, die im nichtstimulierten Zustand bestrahlt worden waren, ein geringfügiger Dosisleistungseffekt. Dieser wird jedoch nur als Folge einer unterschiedlichen PHA-Stimulation von weniger stark strahlengeschädigten Zellen angesehen. Für sämtliche Aberrationstypen konnte bei steigender Neutronendosis eine lineare Dosiswirkungsbeziehung ermittelt werden. Im Vergleich zu 250 kV-Röntgenstrahlen ergab sich für dizentrische Chromosomen ein RBW-Wert von ca. 3,5 (Abb. 17, 18).

DOLPHIN u. PURROT (1970) fanden, daß bei Bestrahlung mit Spaltungsneutronen die Ausbeute an dizentrischen Chromosomen etwa linear mit der Dosis zunahm. Im Gegensatz zu Scott u. Mitarb. (1969) war in bezug auf 250 kV-Röntgenstrahlen der RBW-Wert nicht konstant. Vielmehr ergaben sich hier bei geringerer Aberrationsausbeute (dizentrische Chromosomen/Zelle) höhere RBW-Werte als bei einer größeren Aberrationsrate (Tabelle 3).

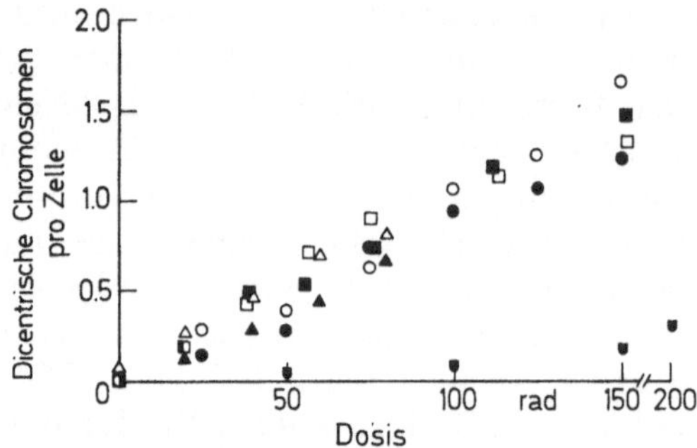

Abb. 18. In vitro-Bestrahlung. Dosiswirkungsbeziehung nach Bestrahlung stimulierter Zellen mit Neutronen bei einer Dosisleistung von 50 rad/min (○), 6,75 rad/h (□) und 3,41 rad/h (△) und für nichtstimulierte Zellen bei einer Dosisleistung von 50 rad/min (●), 6,75 rad/h (■) und 3,41 rad/h (▲). Mit dem Symbol ▼ ist die Dosis-Wirkungs-Beziehung nach einer Bestrahlung von nichtstimulierten Zellen mit 14,1 MeV-Neutronen bei 6 rad/min aus den Befunden von Gooch u. Mitarb. (1964) dargestellt. (Aus Scott u. Mitarb., 1969)

Tabelle 3. *RBW für Spaltungsneutronen hoher Dosisleistung bei verschiedenen Aberrationsraten*

Diz. Chr. pro Zelle	Dosis (rad)		RBW
	Röntgenstrahlen	Spaltungsneutronen	
0,1	120	14	8,5
1,0	375	120	3,1

Chmelevsky u. Mitarb. (1971) sowie Biola u. Mitarb. (1971) konnten nach einer gemischten γ- und Neutronenbestrahlung für dizentrische Chromosomen ebenfalls eine lineare Dosiswirkungsbeziehung der Form $Y = 0,726 \cdot 10^{-2}\,D$ bzw. $Y = 1,027 \cdot 10^{-2}D$ errechnen.

γ) Protonen

Experimente an Lymphozyten wurden bisher nur mit 50 MeV Protonen (Dosisleistung 0,62 rad/min) von Todorov u. Mitarb. (1972) durchgeführt. Sie konnten ihre Daten einer Potenzfunktion $Y = (12,6 \pm 1,6) \cdot 10^{-5}\,D^{1,36 \pm 0,27}$ anpassen. Im Vergleich zu 180 kV Röntgenstrahlen [$Y = (7,9 \pm 0,35) \cdot 10^{-5}\,D^{1,47 \pm 0,012}$] ergab sich in einem Dosisbereich von 100—500 rad für Protonen eine RBW von $0,88 \pm 0,01$.

4. Strahleninduzierte Chromosomenaberrationen in vivo

Es hatte sich rasch gezeigt, daß die von Moorhead u. Mitarb. (1960) angegebene Methode zur Züchtung von peripheren Lymphozyten und zur Präparation der menschlichen Chromosomen hervorragend geeignet war. In der Strahlencytogenetik des Menschen wurden daher auch bis heute nahezu alle Befunde an peripheren Lymphozyten erarbeitet. Für die Chromosomenpräparation aus Haut- oder Knochenmarkszellen existieren ebenfalls ausgezeichnete Techniken. Da aber in diesen Geweben Zellpopulationen in verschiedenen Entwicklungsstadien auftreten, werden bei einer Bestrahlung gleichzeitig sämtliche Stadien des Zellzyklus erfaßt. Dies hat zur Folge, daß sich sowohl Zahl und Art der Chromosomendefekte nach einer Strahlenexposition rasch ändern.

Chromosomenaberrationen bei bestrahlten Personen wurden nach den verschiedenartigsten Expositionsbedingungen gefunden. Sie sollen im Folgenden behandelt werden.

a) Medizinische Strahlenanwendung

Zusammenfassung und kritische Diskussion der Literatur bis einschließlich 1966 bei
BAUCHINGER (1967).

α) Strahlendiagnostische Maßnahmen

Obwohl bei der Strahlendiagnostik nur Teile des Körpers mit Dosen von Bruchteilen
eines rad bis zu mehreren rad bestrahlt werden, wurde schon über Chromosomendefekte
nach diagnostischer Bestrahlung berichtet. So fanden STEWART u. SANDERSON (1961)
nach mehreren Röntgenaufnahmen an den Extremitäten bei einem Klinefelter-Patienten,
in zwei Zellen von 31 untersuchten, „möglicherweise" zwei dizentrische Chromosomen.
CONEN (1963) beschrieb zwei dizentrische Chromosomen in 121 Zellen und vermutlich
Chromatidaberrationen bei einem mißgebildeten Kind, das eine Woche nach einer Serie
von diagnostischen Bestrahlungen untersucht worden war. Chromosomendefekte wurden
auch von BLOOM u. TJIO (1964) nach Röntgenkontrastdarstellung des Magen-Darm-Kanals
bei 5 Personen und 30 Minuten nach einer Herzkatheterisierung unter Röntgenbeobach-
tung bei einem von acht Fällen festgestellt. MARSCH u. Mitarb. (1965) haben auf ähnliche
Effekte bei neun Patienten sowie MASSIMO u. Mitarb. (1965) bei zehn Kindern nach „wenigen bis zahlreichen" diagnostischen Röntgenaufnahmen hingewiesen. Da die Zahl der
beobachteten Chromosomenaberrationen in sämtlichen Fällen nur sehr gering war, konnten
quantitative Dosiswirkungsbeziehungen bisher noch nicht aufgezeigt werden. Es sei aber
an dieser Stelle auf die Arbeit von SCHMICKEL (1967) hingewiesen, in der gezeigt wird,
daß nach in vitro-Bestrahlung von Lymphozyten (100 kV-Röntgenstrahlen) mit Dosen,
die im strahlendiagnostischen Bereich lagen, eine signifikant höhere Aberrationsrate auftrat als in Kontrollen.

β) Strahlentherapie mit externaler Bestrahlung bzw. Radiumeinlagen

α_1) Teilkörperbestrahlung

Die meisten Untersuchungen über cytogenetische Veränderungen bei Strahlenpatienten
wurden nach Strahlenexpositionen bei therapeutischen Maßnahmen, insbesondere bei der
Bestrahlung von Geschwülsten gemacht. Der erste Befund stammt von TOUGH u.
Mitarb. (1960). Sie fanden bei zwei Patienten, die wegen ankylosierender Spondylitis bestrahlt worden waren, schwere Strukturveränderungen an den Chromosomen, wie azentrische Fragmente, dizentrische Chromosomen und Ringchromosomen. Die Zahl der gestörten Zellen war gegenüber der bei Kontrollen signifikant erhöht.

Nach diesen ersten Ergebnissen wurden in rascher Folge weitere Studien über karyo-
logische Befunde bei Patienten nach Röntgen- bzw. ^{60}Co-γ-Therapie veröffentlicht
(MOORE u. Mitarb., 1964; DOIDA u. Mitarb., 1965; MARSCH u. Mitarb., 1965; MILLARD,
1965; BRANCADORO u. SICILIANO, 1965; WARREN u. MEISNER, 1965; DUBROVA, 1967;
AMAROSE u. Mitarb., 1967; AMAROSE u. BAXTER, 1965; TSARANOVA, 1970). Erfolgt die
Chromosomenanalyse kurze Zeit nach Abschluß der Strahlenbehandlung, so konnten im
Mittel in 25—35 % der ausgewerteten Zellen strukturelle Chromosomendefekte beobachtet
werden.

Von verschiedenen Arbeitsgruppen wurde besonders das zeitliche Verhalten strahleninduzierter Chromosomenaberrationen intensiver untersucht. Ganz allgemein konnte
dabei beobachtet werden, daß mit zunehmendem Zeitabstand von der Strahlenexposition
die Zahl der Zellen mit Chromosomenaberrationen stark abnimmt. Die Edinburgher
Gruppe (BUCKTON u. Mitarb., 1962, 1967a, c, e; COURT-BROWN, 1965, 1968) untersuchte
Patienten, die wegen Spondylarthritis ankylopoetica partiell bestrahlt worden waren.
Es wurde ein Zeitraum bis zu 10 Jahren nach der Bestrahlung erfaßt. Sie fanden, daß innerhalb der ersten zwei Jahre die Zahl der sog. C_u-Zellen (dizentrische Chromosomen, Ringe,
azentrische Fragmente) stark und danach nur noch geringfügig abnahm, nach 10 Jahren
jedoch noch viermal höher als in den Kontrollen war. Die Häufigkeit von sog.

C_s-Zellen (reziproke Translokationen) war jedoch nach 10 Jahren nicht signifikant geringer als unmittelbar nach Bestrahlung (Abb. 19). Obgleich C_u-Zellen als unstabil definiert sind, können solche Zellformen noch Jahre nach der Strahlenexposition und zudem in ihrer ersten Teilung (X_1) nach der Induktion der Aberrationen beobachtet werden. Durch eine Analyse der Abnahmegeschwindigkeit der X_1C_u-Zellen in Blutproben, die zu späteren Zeitpunkten als vier Jahre nach Bestrahlung gewonnen wurden, haben die Autoren versucht, die mittlere Lebenszeit der kleinen Lymphozyten abzuschätzen. Dabei ergab sich ein Wert von 1574 Tagen mit einem Vertrauensbereich von 891—6743 Tagen. Norman u. Mitarb. (1965, 1966) kamen durch eine Untersuchung der Häufigkeit von Zellen mit azentrischen Fragmenten bei Frauen, die wegen Cervixcarcinomen bestrahlt worden waren, auf eine mittlere Lebenszeit der Lymphozyten von 530 ± 64 Tagen.

Aus einer Reihe von zytogenetischen Befunden ergibt sich, daß X_1C_u-Zellen, noch Monate bis Jahrzehnte nach der Strahlenexposition, in PHA-stimulierten Kulturen beobachtet werden können. Fitzgerald (1964, 1967) glaubt, daß diese Zellen einer langlebigen Lymphozytenpopulation angehören müssen und eine immu-

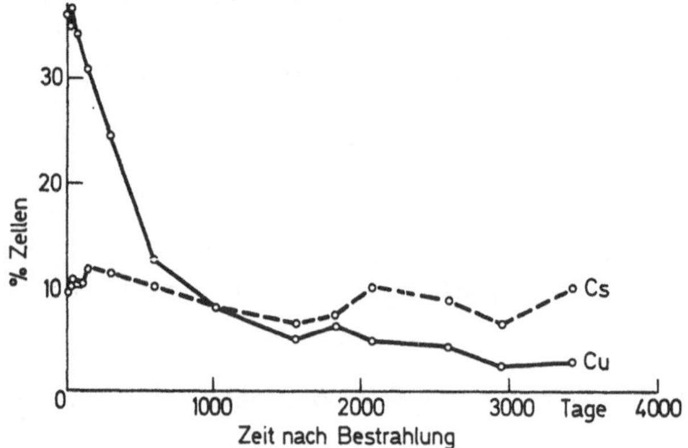

Abb. 19. Strahlentherapie. Zeitliche Veränderung von C_s- und C_u-Zellen in peripheren Lymphozyten nach Röntgen-Therapie ankylosierender Spondylitis. (Nach Buckton u. Mitarb., 1967)

nologische Funktion besitzen. Dabei würden solche Zellen nach der Bestrahlung in einer Art Ruhezustand im Körper verweilen, ohne sich zu teilen. Die ersten Mitosen laufen erst in der Kultur nach PHA-Stimulation ab. Gestützt werden die Überlegungen dieser sogenannten „long-lived cell"-Hypothese von der Immunologie her. Antigene können ein immunologisches Gedächtnis induzieren; dabei entstehen spezifische Lymphozyten, die sogenannten „memory-cells". Diese immunkompetenten Zellen können nun jahrelang ohne Teilung im Körper leben, bewahren aber dabei eine latente Fähigkeit zur Proliferation bis zum Augenblick des erneuten Auftretens des spezifischen Antigenreizes, der dann eine Teilung auslöst. Nowell (1965, 1967) vermutet, daß die Aberrationshäufigkeit zu verschiedenen Zeitpunkten nach der Bestrahlung von den Antigentypen und der Häufigkeit der Antigenstimulierung abhängt, der eine bestrahlte Person in diesen Zeiträumen ausgesetzt ist.

Goh, Goh u. Sumner (1968a, b) glauben nicht, daß alle Aberrationen, die in peripheren Lymphozyten lange Jahre nach der Bestrahlung beobachtet werden, unmittelbar bei dem Bestrahlungsvorgang entstanden sind. Sie fanden, daß in ihren Experimenten Plasma von bestrahlten Personen in Kulturen normaler Blutlymphozyten Chromosomendefekte auslösen kann, selbst wenn die Plasmaspender schon vor sieben Jahren bestrahlt worden waren. Zu ähnlichen Ergebnissen kamen Hollowell u. Littlefield (1968) bei einem analogen Kulturansatz. Goh entwickelte aus diesen Befunden eine alternative Erklärung zur sogenannten „long-lived cell"-Hypothese. Danach sollen die Aberrationen durch einen „Plasmafaktor" unbekannter Art ausgelöst werden, der durch die Bestrahlung erzeugt oder aktiviert wird und für lange Zeit wirksam bleibt, um die Chromosomen zu schädigen. Bei einer experimentellen Nachprüfung durch Scott (1969) zeigte sich, daß tatsächlich ein solcher „Plasmafaktor" sowohl in in vitro als auch in vivo bestrahltem Blut induziert werden kann. Aber sowohl die in diesem Versuch erzeugten, als auch die von den zuerst genannten Autoren beschriebenen Aberrationen können nur als Defekte vom Chromatidtyp oder als sogenannte abgeleitete oder „derived" Aberrationen vom Chromosomentyp interpretiert werden (Abschn. 2). Ein einwandfreier Nachweis, daß durch einen „Plasmafaktor" „echte" Aberrationen vom Chromosomentyp erzeugt werden können, konnte bisher nicht geführt werden.

Schließlich sei noch darauf hingewiesen, daß die Reproduktion und Weitergabe auch von solchen als unstabil bezeichneten Aberrationen prinzipiell möglich ist. Beispiele für eine solche Persistenz von Aberrationen sind die Chromosomenverhältnisse, die in manchen Tumoren vorherrschen oder selbstreduplizierende Ringchromosomen, wie sie gelegentlich in Fällen von kongenitalen Anomalien beschrieben wurden. Ähnliche Befunde für dizentrische Chromosomen stammen von DARLINGTON bzw. DAVIDSON (1963) in Vicia faba und von SIDOROV u. SOKOLOV (1963) für azentrische Fragmente in Crepis capillaris.

In den Lymphozyten dürfte jedoch eine ständige Neubildung unstabiler Aberrationen wegen der bereits erwähnten Störungen des Mitoseablaufes nur selten vorkommen. Wenn nach Bestrahlung Zellklone beobachtet werden (ISHIHARA u. KUMATORI, 1965; COURT-BROWN u. Mitarb., 1967; HONDA u. Mitarb., 1969), sind sie in der Regel durch atypische monozentrische Chromosomen charakterisiert, d.h. in den betreffenden Zellen dürften wohl relativ balancierte Genverhältnisse vorherrschen.

Von BAUCHINGER u. HUG (1966), BAUCHINGER (1968), SCHMID u. BAUCHINGER (1969) wurde die zeitliche Veränderung von Chromosomenaberrationen nach einer kombinierten Radium-Röntgen-Therapie verschiedener gynäkologischer Tumoren über einen Zeitraum von 25 Jahren hinweg verfolgt. Die Zahl der Zellen mit strukturellen Chromosomendefekten (S-Zellen) war im ersten Jahr nach Bestrahlung noch nicht signifikant vermindert (ähnliche Befunde erhielt KUCEROVA (1970) bei Patienten nach fraktionierter Röntgenbestrahlung von Mamma Carcinomen), nahm aber dann zwischen 1 und 3,5 Jahren sehr rasch (annähernd exponentiell) bis auf 25 % des Ausgangswertes ab. Ein weiteres Ab-

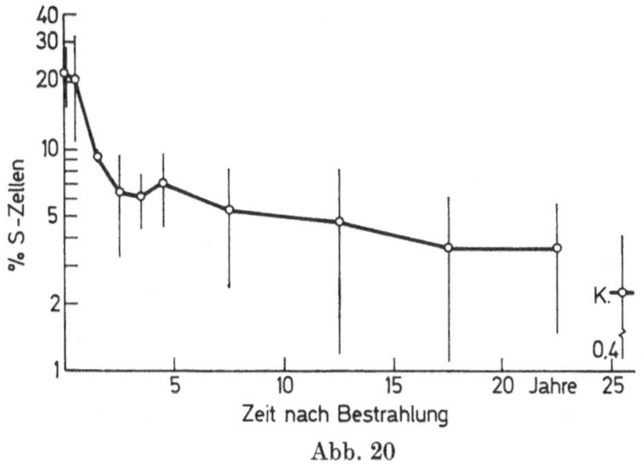
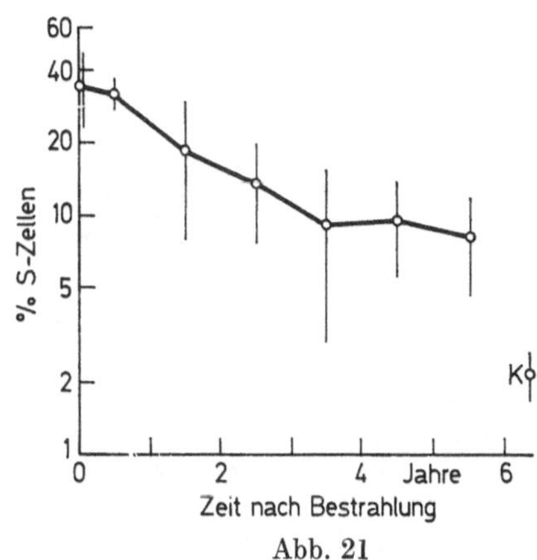

Abb. 20   Abb. 21

Abb. 20. Radium-Röntgentherapie. Zeitliche Veränderung strahleninduzierter Chromosomenaberrationen. Prozentuale Häufigkeit von Zellen mit strukturellen Chromosomenaberrationen (S-Zellen), Kulturzeit 68 Stunden. K = Kontrollwerte. Die vertikalen Linien entsprechen den Standardabweichungen. (Nach BAUCHINGER, 1968)

Abb. 21. Radium-Röntgen-Therapie. Zeitliche Veränderung strahleninduzierter Chromosomenaberrationen. Prozentuale Häufigkeit von S-Zellen in den ersten 6 Jahren nach einer kombinierten Radium-Röntgen-Therapie (Kulturzeit 48 Stunden). K = Kontrollwert. Die vertikalen Linien entsprechen den Standardabweichungen. (Nach SCHMID u. BAUCHINGER, 1969)

sinken erfolgte nun wesentlich langsamer; erst nach 15 Jahren war die Zahl der S-Zellen wiederum um die Hälfte vermindert, ohne jedoch die Kontrollwerte zu erreichen (Abb. 20, 21).

Es zeigte sich ferner, daß verschiedene Typen von S-Zellen unterschiedlich schnell eliminiert wurden. Aus den Kurven der Abb. 22 ist ersichtlich, daß die Zahl der Zellen mit dizentrischen Chromosomen bzw. azentrischen Fragmenten in den ersten vier Jahren am schnellsten abnimmt. Dabei werden Zellen mit dizentrischen Chromosomen aber bereits im ersten Jahr um 50 % vermindert. Bei Zellen mit azentrischen Fragmenten wird dieser Wert erst im dritten Jahr erreicht. Eine solche Elimination konnte bei allen Aberrationstypen beobachtet werden. Selbst Zellen mit atypischen monozentrischen Chromosomen bzw. Defizienzen (sog. C_s-Zellen), die bei BUCKTON u. Mitarb. (1962, 1967a, b) stets in einer konstanten Häufigkeit vorkamen, zeigten eine signifikante Abnahme mit zunehmendem Zeitabstand von der Bestrahlung (Abb. 22, 23). Hinsichtlich des zeitlichen Verhaltens von sog. C_s- und C_u-Zellen dürfte somit kein prinzipieller, sondern nur ein gradueller Unterschied bestehen; letztere werden wesentlich schneller eliminiert. Weiter ergab sich, daß Zellen mit multiplen Chromosomenaberrationen rascher eliminiert wurden als solche, die weniger Aberrationen enthielten (Abb. 24). Auch die Zahl der „Zwei-Bruch‟-Aberrationen (hierher gehören sämtliche Strukturbauten) nahm mit zunehmendem Zeitabstand von der Bestrahlung rascher ab, als die der „Ein-Bruch‟-Aberrationen. Die Eliminationsprozesse werden im Zusammenhang mit gestörten Kern- und Zellteilungsabläufen diskutiert.

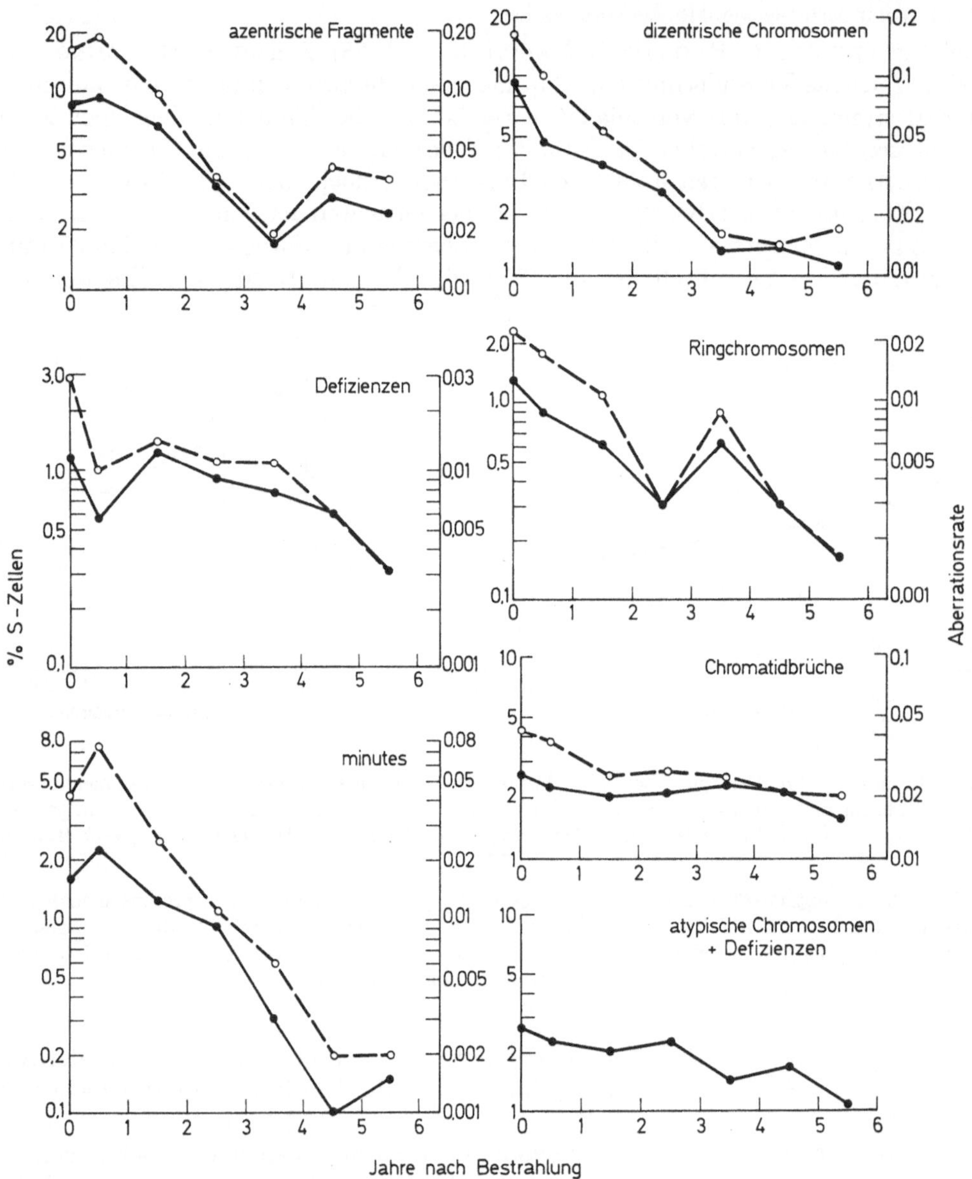

Abb. 22. Radium-Röntgen-Therapie. Häufigkeit von Zellen mit *nur einem* spezifischen Aberrationstyp in Abhängigkeit von der Zeit nach Bestrahlung in Prozent aller ausgewerteten Zellen (●——●) und Gesamthäufigkeit der verschiedenen Aberrationstypen als Rate pro ausgewertete Zelle (○------○). (Nach Schmid u. Bauchinger, 1969)

Wegen der allgemein bei einer medizinischen Teilkörperbestrahlung vorherrschenden inhomogenen räumlichen und zeitlichen Dosisverteilung ist die Aufstellung von quantitativen Dosiswirkungsbeziehungen beträchtlich erschwert oder meist ganz unmöglich gemacht. Buckton u. Mitarb. (1967 c) konnten nach Bestrahlung von Spondylitis-Patienten, bei relativ übersichtlichen Dosisverhältnissen (100—700 rad; 250 kV-Röntgenstrahlen

HVL = 2,7 mm Cu) eine Beziehung zur Oberflächendosis ableiten. Blutproben wurden stets 24 Stunden nach der Strahlenexposition, in einigen Fällen auch unmittelbar danach abgenommen. In den nach 24 Stunden entnommenen Blutproben fanden sich mehr Aberrationen als in jenen unmittelbar nach Bestrahlung. Trotz einer beträchtlichen Streuung der Einzelwerte nahmen, zumindest im Dosisbereich bis 300 rad, in der Beziehung

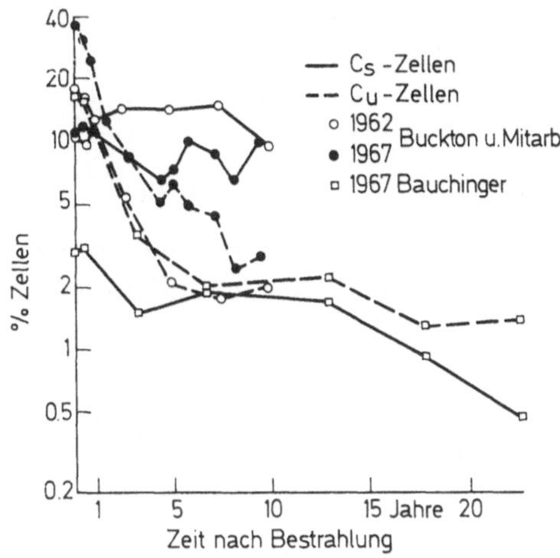

Abb. 23. Strahlentherapie. Vergleich der zeitlichen Veränderung von C_s- und C_u-Zellen nach therapeutischer Teilkörperbestrahlung bei BUCKTON u. Mitarb. (1962, 1967) sowie BAUCHINGER (1967). (Nach BAUCHINGER, 1968)

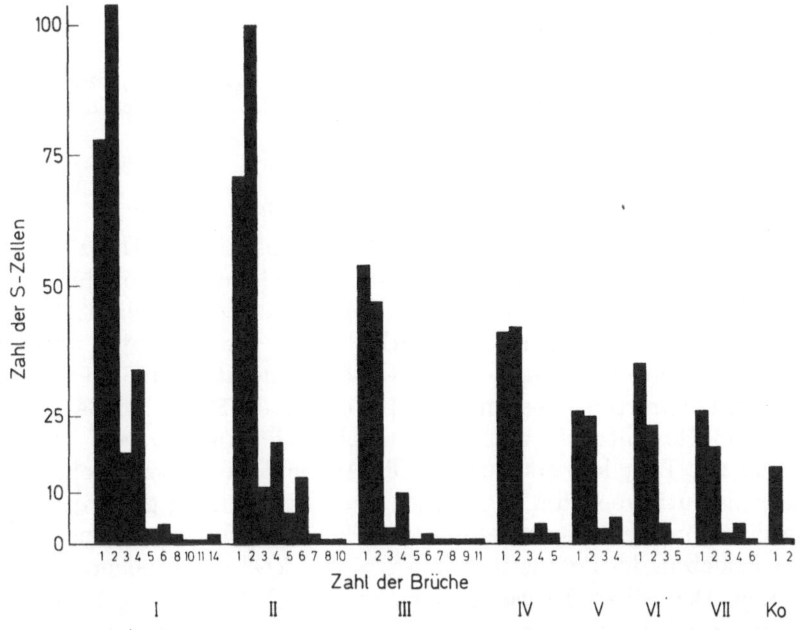

Abb. 24. Radium-Röntgen-Therapie. Häufigkeit von Zellen mit n Brüchen zu verschiedenen Zeitpunkten nach der Bestrahlung. Die Ziffern I–VII bezeichnen verschiedene Personengruppen, die 0–6 Jahre nach der Bestrahlung untersucht wurden. Ko = Kontrollgruppe. (Nach SCHMID u. BAUCHINGER, 1969)

$Y = c + kD^n$ dizentrische Chromosomen, Ringe und azentrische Fragmente mit dem Exponenten $n = 1,97$ (Konfidenzbereich 1,5—2,4) der Dosis zu. Unter Einbeziehung der Befunde nach einer Dosis von 700 rad, konnte jedoch die Dosiswirkungsbeziehung nicht mehr diesem Modell angepaßt werden, da der Dosisexponent n beträchtlich vermindert war. Nach einer fraktionierten Bestrahlung von Spondylitis-Patienten (10 Fraktionen mit jeweils 150 rad in 12—14 Tagen) ergab sich für dizentrische Chromosomen + Ringe sowie für azentrische Fragmente über den gesamten Dosisbereich hinweg eine lineare Beziehung und kein Hinweis auf einen Sättigungseffekt im Bereich der hohen akkumulierten Dosen (Abb. 25).

Von Stenman u. Mitarb. (1970) wurde die Dosis-Wirkungs-Beziehung in Lymphozyten von 26 Frauen, die wegen Mamma-Carcinom einer Röntgentherapie (250 kV) ausgesetzt waren, untersucht. Unter Verwendung der akkumulierten Oberflächendosis erhielten sie für azentrische Fragmente einen Dosisexponenten $n = 0,61 \pm 0,12$, für dizentrische Chromosomen und Ringe $n = 0,88 \pm 0,13$, aus denen sie jeweils eine lineare Dosis-Wirkungs-Beziehung ableiteten:

$$Y = 0,22 + 1,68\,(\pm\,0,17) \cdot 10^{-5}\,D \quad \text{bzw.} \quad 0,0086 + 1,53\,(\pm\,0,15) \cdot 10^{-5}\,D\;.$$

Es zeigte sich weiter, daß zwar die Zahl der Aberrationen pro Zelle mit zunehmender Dosis anstieg, daß aber ab einer Dosis von 6000 rad die Zahl der geschädigten Zellen 22 % nicht mehr überstieg.

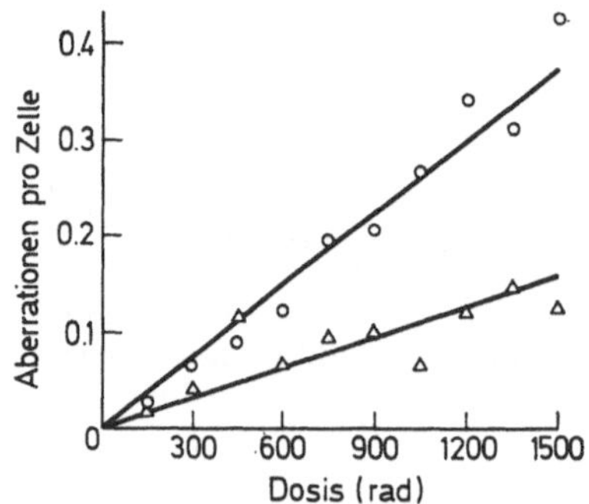

Abb. 25. Strahlentherapie. Dosis-Wirkungs-Beziehung für azentrische Fragmente △, dizentrische Chromosomen und Ringe ○, im Verlauf einer Strahlentherapie (Teilkörperbestrahlung) von Spondylitis-Patienten. (Nach Buckton u. Mitarb., 1967)

β_1) *Ganzkörperbestrahlung*

Abgeschlossene Chromosomenanalysen nach therapeutischer Ganzkörperbestrahlung liegen bisher nur von insgesamt 22 Patienten mit ausgedehnten Bronchialcarcinomen vor. Die Befunde sind in vier Arbeiten der Edinburgher Gruppe publiziert (Buckton u. Mitarb., 1967c, 1969, 1971; Langlands u. Mitarb., 1968). Die Patienten wurden mit Röntgenstrahlen, die mit Hilfe eines 2 MeV-Van de Graaff-Generators erzeugt wurden, bei einem durchschnittlichen Fokus-Haut-Abstand von 160 cm, in ca. 30 min in Bauch- und Rückenlage bestrahlt. Die Gesamtdosis variierte zwischen 17 und 50 rad. Die Befunde von 16 Patienten sind aus Tabelle 4 ersichtlich. Die Ausbeute an dizentrischen Chromosomen und Ringen war in Blutproben, die 24 Stunden nach Bestrahlung gewonnen wurden, höher als in jenen unmittelbar nach Bestrahlung. Aus den zusammengefaßten Daten von 1968 und 1969 ergaben sich in der Potenzfunktion $Y = c + kD^n$ entsprechend Dosisexponenten von 0,86 bzw. 1,59. Der höhere Dosisexponent aus der Untersuchung 24 Stunden nach Bestrahlung ist im wesentlichen auf eine signifikant erhöhte Aberrationsrate bei zwei Patienten zurückzuführen, die mit 50 rad bestrahlt worden waren (ähnlich den Befunden nach Teilkörperbestrahlung).

In einem weiteren Experiment (Buckton u. Mitarb., 1969) wurden sechs Personen einer Ganzkörperbestrahlung mit Dosen zwischen 36 und 50 rad ausgesetzt und die Aberrationsrate (dizentrische Chromosomen und Ringe) in Blutproben, die unmittelbar nach Bestrahlung gewonnen wurden, festgestellt. Eine Blutprobe, die vor der Strahlenexposition gewonnen wurde, erhielt jeweils die gleiche Strahlendosis in vitro und wurde auf die gleichen Chromosomendefekte hin untersucht. Ein direkter Vergleich der Häufigkeiten von dizentrischen Chromosomen und Ringen, die nach Bestrahlungen von peripherem Blut in vivo

Tabelle 4. *Häufigkeit von dizentrischen Chromosomen + Ringen in peripheren Blutkulturen unmittelbar oder 24 Stunden nach Ganzkörperbestrahlung von Patienten mit 2 MeV-Röntgenstrahlen.*
a) *1 Zelle mit einem dizentrischen und einem trizentrischen Chromosom wurde bewertet als ob 3 dizentrische Chromosomen vorhanden wären.*
b) *7 Ringe und dizentrische Chromosomen in 75 ausgewerteten Zellen.*
(Nach LANGLANDS u. Mitarb., 1968)

Fall Nr.	Dosis (rad)	Kontrolle (100 Zellen)	Unmittelbar nach Bestrahlung (200 Zellen)	24 Stunden nach Bestrahlung
1	25	1	5	3
2	25	0	2	8
3	25	0	9	5
4	25	0	6	7
5	25	0	8	4
6	25	0	5	3
7	50	0	4	15
8	50	0	14	14
9	50	3[a]	10	15
10	50	1	9	9
11	50	0	11	15
12	50	1	9	7[b]
13	17	0	2	1
14	28	0	1	4
15	36	0	5	7
16	40	0	8	7

Tabelle 5. *Vergleich der Häufigkeit von dizentrischen Chromosomen und Ringen nach 2 MeV-Röntgen-Ganzkörper und in vitro-Bestrahlung.* (Nach BUCKTON u. Mitarb., 1969)

Fall Nr.	Alter (Jahre)	Dosis (rad)	Kontrollen		in vitro		Unmittelbar nach Bestrahlung in vivo	
			Ausgew. Zellen	diz. Chr. + Ringe	Ausgew. Zellen	diz. Chr. + Ringe	Ausgew. Zellen	diz. Chr. + Ringe
I	63	30	200	0	200	5	200	6
II	69	36	100	0	200	7	200	4
III	56	40	100	2	100	3	100	4
IV	64	44	100	3	200	6	200	6
V	67	45		mißlungen	200	5	300	15
VI	75	50	100	0	100	8	100	2

oder in vitro erzeugt wurden, ergab keine statistisch signifikanten Unterschiede (Tabelle 5).

Dies bestätigte sich auch bei eigenen Untersuchungen (BAUCHINGER, 1971) von bisher sechs Krebspatienten nach therapeutischer Ganzkörperbestrahlung und identischer Bestrahlung von Blutproben in vitro mit ^{60}Co γ-Strahlen (Dosis 10 und 20 R). Im Gegensatz zur Edinburgher Gruppe fanden sich aber mehr Aberrationen bei Untersuchungen unmittelbar nach Bestrahlung als 24 Stunden nach Bestrahlung.

Aus beiden Studien läßt sich ableiten, daß ein Vergleich von in vitro- und in vivo-Befunden im Hinblick auf eine biologische Dosimetrie somit prinzipiell sinnvoll ist. Da aber in Dosisbereichen unterhalb von 50 rad die Zahl der Chromosomenaberrationen sehr gering ist (die automatisierte Auswertung einer größeren Anzahl von Zellen durch Computer kann gegenwärtig noch nicht mit der gewünschten Zuverlässigkeit durchgeführt werden), ist eine Extrapolation auf niedere Dosisbereiche auf der Grundlage der verfügbaren in vitro-Befunde (allgemein 50—500 rad) nur begrenzt möglich.

γ_1) *Extrakorporale Bestrahlung*

Von Winkelstein u. Mitarb. (1967) wurden Chromosomenanalysen bei drei Patienten durchgeführt, deren Blut vor einer Nierentransplantation extrakorporal bestrahlt worden war. Das Blut wurde durch einen Quinton-Scribner-Shunt geleitet und dabei einem β-Strahler (^{90}Sr — ^{90}Y) exponiert. Bei einer Durchflußgeschwindigkeit von 100 ml/min betrug die Transitdosis 25 rad. Nach 4—8 Stunden Expositionszeit wurden Lymphozyten-kulturen angelegt. Zusätzlich erfolgten in vitro-Untersuchungen, in denen Blut nach einer einzigen Passage durch das Bestrahlungssystem kultiviert wurde. In beiden Fällen wurde die Häufigkeit von Zellen mit dizentrischen Chromosomen bestimmt. Die durch chemische Dosimetrie bestimmte Dosis wurde mit jener Dosis verglichen, die sich mit Hilfe der in Norman u. Sasakis (1966) in vitro-Experimenten, für das Modell $Y = kD^2$ ermittelten Proportionalitätskonstante k [$(5{,}7 \pm 0{,}5)\,10^{-6}$ dizentrische Chromosomen + Ringe/Zelle/

Tabelle 6. *Extrakorporale Bestrahlung. Physikalische Dosis und Dosisabschätzung auf Grund der Häufigkeit dizentrischer Chromosomen in peripheren Lymphozyten.*

a) *Physikalische Dosis, berechnet auf Grund der Durchflußgeschwindigkeit und des Blutvolumens bei der Passage durch das Bestrahlungssystem.*

b) *Physikalische Dosis, abgeschätzt auf Grund des Blutvolumens, der Durchflußgeschwindigkeit und der Bestrahlungsdauer.*

c) *Dosisabschätzung auf Grund der Häufigkeit von dizentrischen Chromosomen in 200–300 Metaphasen von Blutlymphozyten unmittelbar nach Bestrahlung.*

(Nach Winkelstein u. Mitarb., 1967)

	Berechnete physikalische Gesamtdosis	Dosisabschätzung auf Grund der Häufigkeit diz. Chromos. (80% Vertrauensbereich)
A. *In vitro*-Untersuchung: Blutprobe nach einer	450[a]	440–490
Passage durch das Bestrahlungssystem (^{90}Sr–	565[a]	510–565
^{90}Y). Durchflußgeschwindigkeit 3,0–15,7 ml/min	295[a]	245–310
	148[a]	115–175
B. *In vivo*-Untersuchung: Blutprobe unmittelbar nach	120[b]	145[c]
einer 4–8 stündigen extrakorporalen Bestrahlung	120[b]	180[c]
(mehrere Passagen)	240[b]	230[c]

rad^2)] berechnen ließ. Obgleich keine detaillierten Angaben über die Aberrationsausbeute vorliegen, ergaben sich für beide Dosisabschätzungen relativ gut übereinstimmende Werte (Tabelle 6).

Sharpe u. Mitarb. (1967) fanden dagegen bei einem extrakorporal bestrahlten Patienten mit Reticulumzellsarkom, daß sich die physikalischen und biologischen Dosisabschätzungen um einen Faktor 2,7 unterschieden. Für diese Differenz wurden Austauschprozesse zwischen peripherem Blut und extravaskulären Orten verantwortlich gemacht. Bei einem Patienten mit Hodgkinscher Krankheit konnten dieselben Autoren (1968) auf Grund der Häufigkeit von Zellen mit dizentrischen Chromosomen feststellen, daß bei einer extra-korporalen Bestrahlung nur etwa 20 % der Lymphozyten bestrahlt werden, während der Rest in den extravaskulären Depots des Körpers verbleibt.

γ) *Medizinische Radioisotopenanwendung*

Von besonderem Interesse ist die Auswirkung chronischer internaler Bestrahlung über mehrere Jahre hinweg, wie sie durch inkorporierte langlebige Radionuklide hervorgerufen wird. Dies ist der Fall bei Patienten, denen vor Jahrzehnten Thorotrast (Handelsname einer stabilisierten kolloidalen Suspension von ^{232}Thoriumdioxyd) als Röntgenkontrastmittel appliziert wurde. Es wird bevorzugt im retikulo-endothelialen System gespeichert und kaum aus dem Körper ausgeschieden. Auf diese Weise stellt es eine ständige innere Strahlenquelle für α-Teilchen mit hohem LET dar. In sämtlichen vorliegenden Untersuchungen ergab sich, daß in Blutlymphozyten (72 h-Kulturen) von Thorotrast-Patienten signifikant mehr Chromosomenaberrationen auftraten als bei Kontrollpersonen (KUMATORI u. ISHIARA, 1963; ISHIARA u. KUMATORI, 1966; FISCHER u. Mitarb., 1966, 1967). BUCKTON u. Mitarb. (1967d) fanden bei 48stündiger Kulturzeit, daß viele Zellen mehr als eine Aberration enthielten. Dizentrische Chromosomen kamen in einer Häufigkeit von 3,8/100 Zellen vor. Die internale Strahlenbelastung wurde durch Ganzkörperzählung gemessen. Eine eindeutige Dosiswirkungsbeziehung konnte bisher nicht ermittelt werden.

Über analoge Chromosomenaberrationen, wie sie nach externaler Bestrahlung auftreten, wird auch nach therapeutischer Anwendung von Radiojod berichtet (BOYD u. Mitarb. [1961], OISHI u. POMERAT [1964], MACINTYRE u. DOBYNS [1962], NOFAL u. BEIERWALTES [1964], AMAROSE u. BAXTER [1965], YUGE [1968]). Die durch Inkorporation von ^{131}J hervorgerufene Knochenmarkdosis liegt in der Größenordnung von 1 rad/appliziertes mCi. Sie kann aber je nach Schilddrüsenaktivität ganz erheblich schwanken (EMRICH u. KEIDERLING, 1963; HUG, 1964; SCHULTE-BRINKMANN, 1966). Chromosomenaberrationen fanden auch MACDIARMID (1965), KAY u. Mitarb. (1966), ILBERY u. Mitarb. (1971) nach Behandlung von Polycythaemia vera mit ^{32}P (10 mCi ^{32}P können dabei eine Ganzkörperbelastung von 50—100 rad erzeugen). VISFELDT u. Mitarb. (1970, 1971), VISFELDT (1971) beobachteten nach ^{32}P-Therapie in Knochenmarkszellen eine Klonbildung mit abnormalen Chromosomenmustern.

b) Berufliche Strahlenexposition

Chromosomenuntersuchungen bei Personen, die während ihrer beruflichen Tätigkeit chronisch strahlenexponiert waren, ergaben in vielen Fällen eine Zunahme von Zellen mit Chromosomendefekten. Als besonderer Hinweis auf eine Strahlenexposition konnte jeweils das Auftreten von Zellen mit dizentrischen Chromosomen oder Ringen gewertet werden, da speziell diese Typen in unbestrahlten Kontrollpersonen äußerst selten auftreten (ca. 1/2000 Zellen in 48 Stunden —, 1/8000 in 72 Stunden Kulturen). Die Befunde sind schwer miteinander zu vergleichen, da die akkumulierten Strahlendosen über verschieden lange Zeiträume hinweg aufgenommen wurden, und unterschiedliche Expositionsbedingungen mit verschiedenen Strahlenarten vorlagen. Von besonderer Bedeutung für die Strahlenschutzüberwachung ist die Tatsache, daß in einigen Fällen eine erhöhte Zahl von Chromosomendefekten beobachtet wurde, obwohl die aufgenommene Strahlendosis noch unterhalb der erlaubten Schwelle lag.

Chromosomenaberrationen in peripheren Lymphozyten wurden bei Strahlenarbeitern in Reaktoren und Strahlenkliniken nach externaler Bestrahlung mit Röntgen- bzw. γ-Strahlen festgestellt (SASAKI u. Mitarb., 1963; NORMAN u. Mitarb., 1964a, b; COURT-BROWN u. Mitarb., 1965; SUGAHARA u. Mitarb., 1965; DOIDA u. Mitarb., 1965; GORIZONTOWA, 1966; BUCKTON u. Mitarb., 1967b; FORNI u. Mitarb., 1969; SEVANJKAYEV u. Mitarb., 1969; POPESCU u. STEFANESCU, 1971); ebenso nach zusätzlicher internaler Bestrahlung infolge einer Inkorporation verschiedener radioaktiver Nuklide (EL-ALFI, 1967; WALD u. Mitarb., 1967; BROWN u. MCNEILL, 1969; BAUCHINGER u. Mitarb., 1970).

Bei ersten Untersuchungen von Personen, die im Thermalstollen und in der Inhalationshalle des Mineralbads Badgastein tätig sind und dabei ständig ^{222}Rn, ^{220}Rn und deren Tochterprodukte einatmen, konnten POHL-RÜLING u. Mitarb. (1970) azentrische Fragmente und dizentrische Chromosomen (3/3720 Zellen) beobachten. MOURIQUAND u. Mitarb. (1965), VISFELDT (1967), EBENEZER u. SADASIVAN (1968), KILIBARDA u. Mitarb. (1968) fanden Chromosomenveränderungen bei Röntgenärzten, -Technikern und -Schwestern. Die zuletzt genannten Autoren konnten eine Korrelation zwischen Aberrationshäufigkeit und Expositionszeit feststellen. BAUCHINGER u. HUG (1968), BAUCHINGER u.

Mitarb. (1970) untersuchten 34 Schwestern einer Strahlenklinik, die bei der Handhabung von Radiumeinlagen zur Krebstherapie der γ-Strahlung ausgesetzt waren. Sowohl über den gesamten Dosisbereich von 0,1—92 rem (Filmplakettenwerte) als auch in einem Bereich bis zu 20 rem konnte eine lineare Dosiswirkungsbeziehung (für Bruchrate und Zahl der Zellen mit Chromosomendefekten) ermittelt werden (Abb. 26).

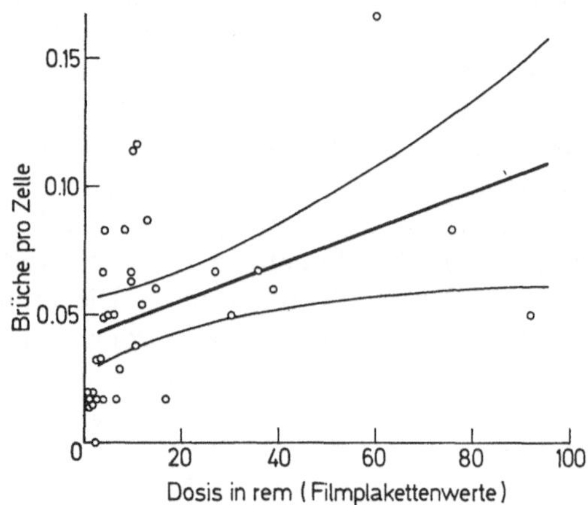

Abb. 26. Berufliche Strahlenexposition. Dosis-Wirkungs-Beziehung für eine Gruppe von 34 Radium-Schwestern. Die gebogenen Linien stellen den 95% Vertrauens-Bereich für die Regressionslinie dar (Y = 0,042 + 0,0007 D). (Nach Bauchinger u. Mitarb., 1970)

Eine besondere Gruppe von beruflich strahlenbelasteten Personen bilden die Leuchtzifferblattmaler der Uhrenindustrie. Bei diesem Personenkreis können hohe Körperaktivitäten von inkorporiertem ^{226}Ra und ^{90}Sr festgestellt werden. Von Tuscany u. Müller (1967), Boyd u. Mitarb. (1966, 1967), Brown u. Mitarb. (1968) wurden in peripheren Lymphozyten, von Tuscany u. Müller auch in Zellen des Knochenmarks dieser Arbeiter eine erhöhte Aberrationsfrequenz nachgewiesen. Boyd u. Mitarb. fanden außerdem, daß die Zahl der Aberrationen mit steigender Körperaktivität · von ^{226}Ra (0,04 mCi— 0,56 mCi) zunahm.

c) Strahlenunfälle

Über Chromosomenaberrationen in peripheren Blutzellen von Personen, die an Strahlenunfällen beteiligt waren, wurde von folgenden Autoren berichtet: von Bender u. Gooch (1962b, 1963, 1966), Gooch u. Mitarb. (1964), Goh (1968a) bei insgesamt 11 Personen, von Lejeune u. Mitarb. (1967), Biola u. Lego (1966) bei jeweils einem Fall sowie von Pendic u. Djordjevic (1968) bei drei Fällen nach einer gemischten Strahlenexposition mit γ-Strahlen und Neutronen. Nach Strahlenunfällen mit γ-Strahlen untersuchten Buckton u. Mitarb. (1967b), Sugahara u. Mitarb. (1967), Dolphin u. Mitarb. (1970) jeweils zwei Personen, Lejeune u. Mitarb. (1967), Caratzali u. Mitarb. (1967) jeweils drei Personen sowie Lisco u. Lisco (1969) zwei Personen mit zusätzlicher γ-Strahlenexposition. Es liegen auch Befunde über Inkorporation von radioaktiven Nukliden vor. So berichtet Sugahara u. Mitarb. (1967) über drei Arbeiter, die Uranylfluorid und Wald u. Mitarb. (1967) über 7 Arbeiter, die ^{125}J eingeatmet hatten. Gabay u. Mitarb. (1968) untersuchten eine Person, bei der es neben einer Exposition mit ^{210}Po zu einer Inkorporation von ^{226}Ra kam.

Allgemein war bei den betroffenen Personen gegenüber unbestrahlten Kontrollen die Zahl der Zellen mit Chromosomenaberrationen erhöht. Mit Ausnahme des zuletztgenannten Falles war wiederum das Auftreten von dizentrischen Chromosomen und Ringen auffällig. In einigen Fällen wurde auf Grund der Häufigkeit dieser Aberrationstypen eine biologische Dosisabschätzung versucht, die relativ gut mit der physikalisch gemessenen Dosis korrelierte.

d) Kernwaffenexplosionen

Chromosomenuntersuchungen bei Überlebenden der Atombombenexplosionen in Hiroshima und Nagasaki wurden von DOIDA u. Mitarb. (1965), ISHIHARA u. KUMATORI (1965, 1967), BLOOM u. Mitarb. (1966, 1967a, b, 1968), AWA u. BLOOM (1968), HONDA u. Mitarb. (1969), SASAKI u. MIYATA (1968) durchgeführt.

Während DOIDA in den 7 untersuchten Fällen nur eine erhöhte Aneuploidie-Rate feststellen konnte, fanden ISHIHARA u. KUMATORI in 3 von 6 Fällen dizentrische Chromosomen sowie in einem Fall ein Ringchromosom bei einer Gesamtstörungsrate von 3,5—6,5%. BLOOM (1967b) führte vergleichende Untersuchungen bei zwei verschiedenen Altersgruppen durch. In einer Gruppe wurden 94 Personen erfaßt, die bis zum Zeitpunkt der Explosion jünger als 30 Jahre, in der zweiten Gruppe 77 Personen, die älter als 30 Jahre waren. Die relative Häufigkeit von dizentrischen Chromosomen, Ringen und azentrischen Fragmenten war in den beiden Gruppen sehr ähnlich. In der Gruppe der älteren Überlebenden fanden sich jedoch mehr symmetrische Translokationen und Inversionen. Bei neun Personen von 188 konnte eine Klonbildung von Zellen mit jeweils der gleichen Aberration nachgewiesen werden. Hierzu ist bemerkenswert, daß eine solche Klonbildung bei 48stündiger Kulturzeit häufiger entdeckt wurde als bei 66—77stündiger Inkubation (HONDA u. Mitarb., 1969). Nach physikalischen Schätzungen waren die betroffenen Personen einer Dosis von 204—991 rad einer gemischten γ- und Neutronen-Strahlung ausgesetzt. Vorläufige Versuche, eine Korrelation zwischen der Aberrationshäufigkeit und der Dosis herzustellen, scheinen auf eine lineare Dosiswirkungsbeziehung hinzudeuten.

Chromosomenuntersuchungen von 128 Personen, vor deren Geburt mindestens ein Elternteil bei der Atombombenexplosion einer Strahlendosis von wenigstens 100 rad ausgesetzt war, ergaben keine signifikant erhöhte Aberrationsrate im Vergleich zu Kontrollpersonen, die bereits vor der Explosion geboren waren (BLOOM u. Mitarb., 1968). Bei 38 Überlebenden, die bei einer Strahlenexposition ihrer Mütter (geschätzter Bereich 104—477 rad) in utero betroffen worden waren, zeigte sich im Vergleich zu den Kontrollen jedoch eine geringe (0,52 %), aber signifikante Zunahme von Lymphozyten, die komplexe chromosomale Umbauten enthielten (0,04 %) (BLOOM u. Mitarb., 1967a, 1968).

Die bisher umfangreichste Untersuchungsreihe stammt von SASAKI u. MIYATA (1968). Ca. 22 Jahre nach der Atombombenexplosion wurden 51 Überlebende erfaßt. 11 unbestrahlte Personen dienten als Kontrollen. Insgesamt wurden 83506 Zellen analysiert. Bei den bestrahlten Personen betrug die Rate der dizentrischen Chromosomen und Ringe 0,0024/Zelle (201 in 73996 Zellen), bei den Kontrollen 0,0002 (2 in 9510 Zellen). Auch die Zahl der Zellen mit stabilen symmetrischen Austauschaberrationen war erhöht. Es zeigte sich, daß Personen, die dem Hypozentrum am nächsten waren, auch die höchsten Störungsraten aufwiesen (Abb. 27, 28). Ebenso ergaben sich bei den direkt exponierten Personen höhere Werte als bei solchen, die durch Holz oder Beton relativ abgeschirmt waren.

Zu einer Abschätzung der absorbierten Dosis wurde die Häufigkeit der C_s-Zellen (Abb. 27) und die Zahl der dizentrischen Chromosomen + Ringe in X_1C_u-Zellen (Abb. 28) benützt. Diese Werte wurden zu entsprechenden Befunden nach in vitro-Studien mit 1,5 und 2 MeV-Röntgenstrahlen in Beziehung gebracht. Abb. 29 zeigt die daraus resultierende Abschätzung der durchschnittlichen absorbierten Ganzkörperdosis in verschiedenen Abständen vom Hypozentrum. Die gestrichelte Linie T66D gibt die von AUXIER u. Mitarb. (1966) nach physikalischen Methoden abgeschätzte Dosis in Luft an. Die unerwartet hohen Werte, die bei einigen Personen in einer Entfernung von mehr als 2,4 km vom Hypozentrum gefunden wurden, werden darauf zurückgeführt, daß die betreffenden zusätzlich noch einer anderen als der primären Strahlung ausgesetzt waren. Auf Grund der biologischen Dosimetrie wurden, im Vergleich zur physikalischen Dosimetrie, in Bereichen nahe des Hypozentrums höhere Werte, in entfernteren niedrigere Werte ermittelt. Die Autoren glauben, daß sich daraus für Personen, die sich zum Zeitpunkt der Explosion nahe am Hypozentrum aufhielten, eine selektive Sterblichkeit ableiten läßt. Demzufolge wären die am stärksten Strahlenexponierten im Verlauf von 22 Jahren verstorben, während nur die gut abgeschirmten und somit auch einer geringeren Strahlenbelastung ausgesetzten Personen überlebten.

Eine erhöhte Zahl von Zellen mit Chromosomenaberrationen wurde auch bei Personen beobachtet, die dem radioaktiven Niederschlag von thermonuklearen Testexplosionen ausgesetzt waren.

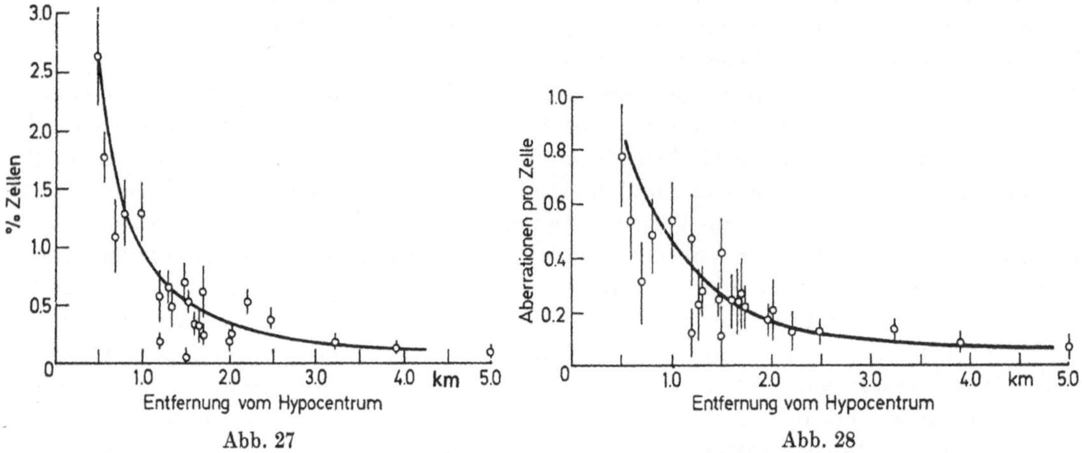

Abb. 27. Kernwaffenexplosionen. Häufigkeit von C_8-Zellen unter sämtlichen (ausgenommen C_u-Zellen) Zellen in verschiedenen Abständen vom Hypozentrum. (Nach Sasaki u. Miyata, 1968)

Abb. 28. Kernwaffenexplosionen. Zahl der dizentrischen Chromosomen + Ringe pro X_1C_u-Zelle in verschiedenen Abständen vom Hypozentrum. (Nach Sasaki u. Miyata, 1968)

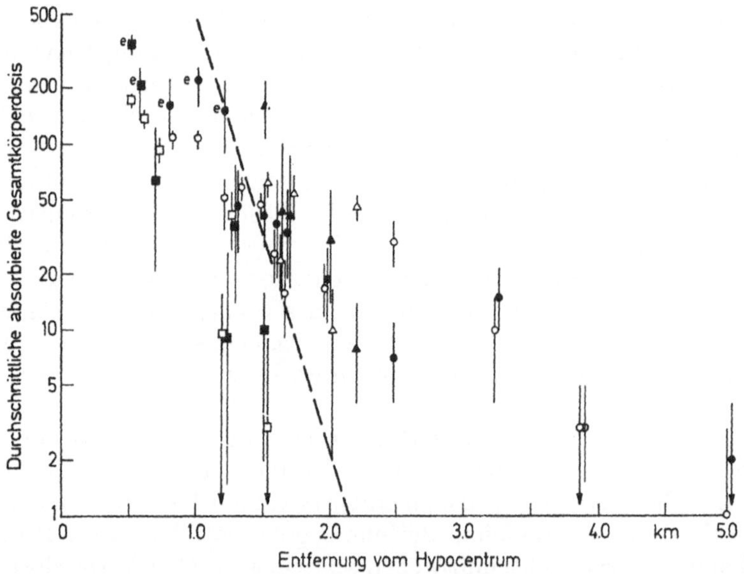

Abb. 29. Kernwaffenexplosionen. Durchschnittliche absorbierte Gesamtkörperdosis, abgeschätzt nach der Häufigkeit von Chromosomenaberrationen. Die vertikalen Linien durch jeden Punkt entsprechen den 50% Konfidenzbereichen. Die gestrichelte Linie T66D gibt die nach physikalischen Methoden abgeschätzte Dosis in Luft an. e kennzeichnet Überlebende mit einer Epilation. Durch Dreiecke, Kreise und Quadrate sind die direkt Exponierten bzw. durch Holz- oder Betonhäuser abgeschirmten Überlebenden bezeichnet. Dosisabschätzungen nach den C_8-Zellen-Befunden (Abb. 27) sind mit offenen Symbolen, Dosisabschätzungen nach Befunden in X_1C_u-Zellen (Abb. 28) sind mit geschlossenen Symbolen dargestellt. (Nach Sasaki u. Miyata, 1968)

Von ISHIHARA u. KUMATORI (1966, 1967) liegen zwei Arbeiten über Befunde bei 20 Fischern vor, die 1954 auf Bikini einer externalen Bestrahlung von 220—600 rad ausgesetzt waren und zusätzlich radioaktives Material in unbekannter Menge inkorporiert hatten. Bei Verlaufsstudien konnten im Knochenmark von drei Personen Zellklone mit abnormalen Chromosomen entdeckt werden. Die Aufstellung einer Dosiswirkungsbeziehung war nicht möglich.

LISCO u. CONARD (1967) untersuchten Bewohner der Marshall-Inseln, die dem radioaktiven „fall-out" der in rund 160 km Entfernung auf Bikini gezündeten Bombe ausgesetzt waren. Bei 30 Personen wurde eine Ganzkörperbelastung mit γ-Strahlen von ca. 175 rad, bei 13 eine solche mit ca. 70 rad geschätzt. Zusätzlich lag eine Inkorporation von radioaktivem Jod und Strontium vor. Acht nichtexponierte Personen dienten als Kontrolle. Ein überraschender Befund der Chromosomenanalyse war, daß bei den Kontrollpersonen mehr azentrische Fragmente gefunden wurden als bei den bestrahlten Leuten. Chromatidaberrationen waren jedoch in der exponierten Personengruppe vermehrt, darüber hinaus konnten auch asymmetrische und symmetrische Translokationen beobachtet werden.

e) Erhöhte natürliche Strahlenbelastung

Bestimmte geographische Regionen der Erde (Guarapary, Brasilien; Kerala, Indien) sind durch das Vorkommen von Monazitsand charakterisiert. Bei diesen Ablagerungen handelt es sich um Phosphate seltener Erden, die Thorium und Uran enthalten. Die Bevölkerung in diesen Gebieten ist somit ständig einer erhöhten natürlichen Strahlenbelastung ausgesetzt:

1. durch externale β- und γ-Strahlung, verursacht durch das natürliche Uran und Thorium im Monazit;

2. durch β- und γ-Strahlung des Radons und Thorons sowie deren Zerfallsprodukte in der Luft;

3. durch eine internale Exposition dieser in den Körper aufgenommenen und abgelagerten radioaktiven Stoffe.

Messungen mit Lithium- und Calciumfluorid-Dosimetern, die ständig um den Hals getragen wurden, erbrachten bei 500 Personen in Guarapary (an der Atlantikküste, 340 Meilen nordöstlich von Rio de Janeiro) eine durchschnittliche Strahlenbelastung von 740 mR/Jahr (BARCINSKI u. Mitarb., 1971). Im Küstenstreifen von Kerala betrug die mittlere pro-Kopf-Belastung bei 16 600 Personen 397 mR/Jahr, bei Spitzenwerten bis > 2 R/Jahr (57 Personen), (GOPAL-AYENGAR u. Mitarb., 1971).

Während für die Monazit-Region in Indien bisher nur demographische und dosimetrische Studien vorliegen, wurden in Brasilien bereits bei 131 Personen, im Alter von 20—60 Jahren Chromosomenuntersuchungen in peripheren Lymphozyten durchgeführt. Als Kontrollen dienten 104 Personen derselben sozial-ökonomischen und rassischen Bevölkerungsstruktur, die jedoch in Regionen mit normaler natürlicher Strahlenbelastung leben. Befunde aus 72 h-Kulturen (ausgewertete Zellen 9 092) erbrachten für Personen aus Guarapary signifikant mehr Deletionen (0,73 %) und dizentrische Chromosomen + Ringe (0,19 %) als in den Kontrollen (0,20 bzw. 0,02).

IV. Die Verwendung strahleninduzierter Chromosomenaberrationen in menschlichen Lymphozyten zur biologischen Dosimetrie

Für den Strahlenschutz ist es außerordentlich wichtig, über ein wirksames Überwachungssystem zu verfügen, um etwa bei beruflich strahlenexponierten Personen die aufgenommene Strahlendosis möglichst exakt abschätzen zu können. Zu diesem Zweck werden meist physikalische Dosimeter, wie etwa Filmplaketten, verwendet. Es wurde aber auch schon versucht, eine biologische Dosimetrie durchzuführen, indem man z. B. quantitative und qualitative Veränderungen des Blutbildes analysierte. Einer biologischen Dosisabschätzung kommt vor allem auch nach Strahlenunfällen eine große Bedeutung zu, wenn Personen betroffen wurden, die keine physikalischen Dosimeter trugen. Bender u. Gooch (1962a) schlugen vor, die Häufigkeit von Chromosomenaberrationen in peripheren Lymphozyten für eine biologische Dosimetrie zu verwenden. In den vorausgehenden Kapiteln wurde gezeigt, daß dieser Vorschlag schnell Anklang gefunden hatte und Dosisabschätzungen nach den verschiedensten Expositionsbedingungen auf der Grundlage des Chromosomenschadens versucht wurden. In diesem Kapitel sollen Probleme besprochen werden, die sich bei dieser Form der biologischen Dosimetrie ergeben (siehe dazu auch Sharpe, 1969; Evans, 1970; Dolphin u. Purrot, 1970; UNSCEAR-Report 1969; Abbatt, 1971; Silberstein u. Mitarb., 1971).

1. Dosiswirkungsbeziehung bei in vitro-Versuchen

Die Voraussetzung für eine sinnvolle Dosisabschätzung einer in vivo-Bestrahlung ist die Kenntnis der Dosiswirkungsbeziehung bei definierten und übersichtlichen Bestrahlungsbedingungen in vitro. Aus den in verschiedenen Laboratorien durchgeführten Bestrahlungsversuchen in vitro (Kapitel III 3) ist ersichtlich, daß prinzipiell klare Beziehungen zwischen der induzierten Aberrationshäufigkeit und der absorbierten Dosis bestehen. Ein Vergleich dieser Befunde zeigt jedoch, daß bei gleichen Dosen weder das Ausmaß der Störungen noch der Verlauf der Dosiswirkungskurven einheitlich ist (Abb. 16, 31, 32; Tabellen 1, 2). Darüber hinaus lassen sich die experimentellen Befunde verschiedenen mathematischen Modellen der Dosiswirkungsbeziehung anpassen, und es ist gegenwärtig noch nicht endgültig zu entscheiden, mit welchem dieser Modelle die Verhältnisse in dem komplexen System der kleinen Lymphozyten am besten beschrieben werden können (siehe dazu auch Kapitel II 2 und Handbucharartikel Kellerer u. Hug). Bis zu einem gewissen Grad werden die unterschiedlichen Resultate verschiedener Autoren daher auch von der jeweiligen mathematisch-statistischen Behandlung der Versuchsdaten beeinflußt sein.

Es wurde bereits angedeutet, daß solche Diskrepanzen von den verschiedensten Faktoren hervorgerufen werden können. So wurden in einigen Laboratorien zur Aufstellung von Dosiswirkungskurven verschiedene Strahlenqualitäten benutzt. Aus Sasakis Befunden (Abb. 30) ist jedoch klar ersichtlich, daß dies bei konstanten Kulturbedingungen zu völlig unterschiedlichen Dosiswirkungsbeziehungen führt. 1,9 MeV-Röntgenstrahlen waren z. B. weniger wirksam als ^{60}Co-Gamma-Strahlen, diese aber wiederum selbst weniger wirksam als 200 kV-Röntgenstrahlen. Die höchste Aberrationsausbeute an dizentrischen Chromosomen + Ringen wurde mit schnellen Neutronen von 14,1 MeV T(d, n) und 2,03 MeV ^{10}Be(d,n)^{9}B erzielt. In der Potenzfunktion ergaben sich in gleicher Reihenfolge wie oben für die einzelnen Strahlenqualitäten die Dosisexponenten n = 2,04; 1,78; 1,66, 1,24 und 1,09. Diskrepanzen lassen sich auch aus unterschiedlichen Kulturbedingungen ableiten. So war die Aberrationsausbeute bei einer Kulturzeit von 72 Stunden (Abb. 31) geringer als bei einer Kulturzeit von 52—54 Stunden (Abb. 32). Bisher wurde dieses Phänomen ausschließlich mit der Elimination bestimmter Aberrationstypen bei Zellteilungen, die erst in der Kultur ablaufen, erklärt. Nach neueren Befunden muß jedoch auch das Vorhandensein verschiedener Lymphozytenpopulationen mit unterschiedlicher Strahlenempfindlichkeit sowie unterschiedlicher Empfindlichkeit gegenüber dem den Transformationsprozeß auslösenden Phytohämagglutinin in Betracht gezogen werden (Bender u. Brewen, 1969; Sharpe, 1969). Siehe dazu auch Kapitel III 2.

Es zeigt sich auch, daß der Dosisexponent entscheidend von den Bestrahlungsbedingungen abhängt. Werden nämlich die Zellen bereits im Vollblut vor dem Kulturansatz bestrahlt (Abb. 32a, b), so ergeben sich höhere Dosisexponenten als bei Bestrahlung von stimulierten Zellen im Kulturmedium (Abb. 32c, d). Die Unterschiede entstehen durch eine höhere Aberrationsausbeute im niederen Dosisbereich bei Bestrahlung stimulierter Kulturen. Bei Dosen > 250 rad ist die Aberrationsausbeute bei diesen Bestrahlungsbedingungen etwa gleich groß. BAJERSKA u. LINIECKI (1969b), BENDER u. BREWEN (1969) haben darauf hingewiesen, daß sowohl die Temperatur während der Bestrahlung als auch die Inkubationstemperatur als kritischer Faktor hinsichtlich der Beeinflussung der Aberrationsfrequenz anzusehen ist. Sie fanden, daß bei niederen Inkubationstemperaturen einerseits der Mitoseindex geringer war und andererseits bei Erniedrigung der Bestrahlungstemperatur von 37°C auf 20°C eine Verminderung der Zahl der dizentrischen Chromosomen und azentrischen Fragmente etwa um den Faktor 2 auftrat. BORA u. SOPER (1971) vertreten die Ansicht, daß die Strahlenempfindlichkeit menschlicher Chromosomen unabhängig von

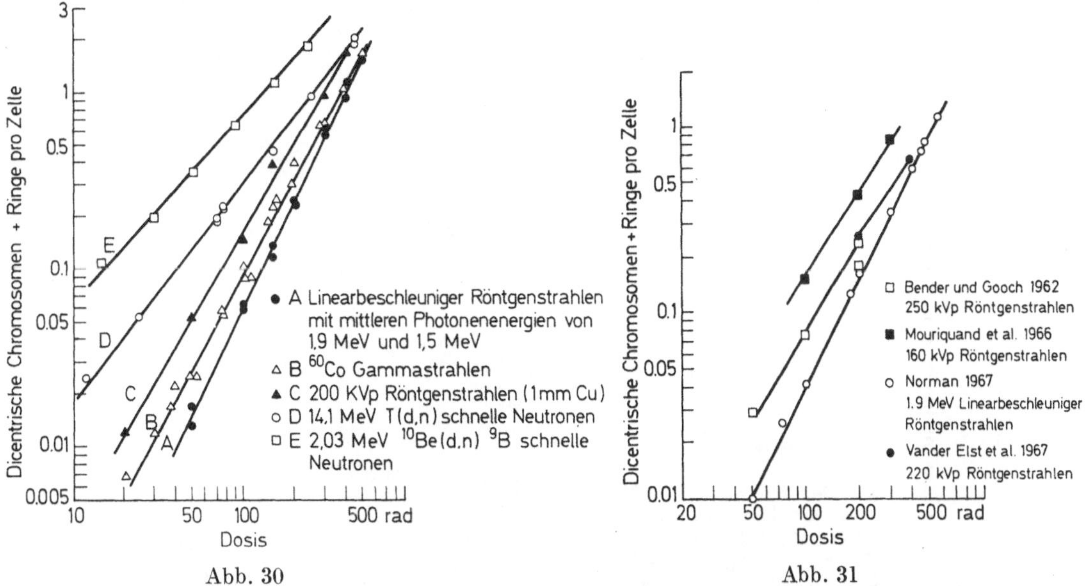

Abb. 30. In vitro-Bestrahlung. Dosis-Wirkungs-Beziehung für dizentrische Chromosomen + Ringe für Strahlenarten mit unterschiedlichem LET. Die Zellen wurden vor dem Kulturansatz bestrahlt. Kulturzeit 50 Stunden. (Nach SASAKI, 1971)

Abb. 31. In vitro-Bestrahlung. Dosis-Wirkungs-Beziehung für dizentrische Chromosomen + Ringe. Die Zellen wurden mit Röntgenstrahlen verschiedener Energie vor dem Kulturansatz bestrahlt und 72 Stunden kultiviert. (Nach UNSCEAR-Report, 1968)

der Temperaturvariation (5—37 °C in ihren Versuchen) ist. Vielmehr soll es bei niederen Temperaturen zu einer Begünstigung der Restitutionsprozesse kommen.

Ergänzend seien an dieser Stelle auch die Experimente von WATSON u. GILLIES (1970) angeführt, in denen zum ersten Mal der Sauerstoffeffekt bei bestrahlten Lymphozytenkulturen untersucht wurde. Während die Dosiswirkungskurve für Lymphozyten, die in Gegenwart von Sauerstoff bestrahlt worden waren, einem linear-quadratischen Modell angepaßt werden konnte, ergab sich für die Bestrahlung unter anaeroben Bedingungen eine lineare Dosiswirkungsbeziehung. Im Gegensatz zu den Befunden an anderen Zellsystemen zeigte jedoch der Sauerstoff hier keine ausgesprochen dosismodifizierende Wirkung.

Man sollte annehmen, daß auch unterschiedliche Kulturtechniken, wie sie die Mikro- bzw. Makromethode der Lymphozytenkultur darstellen, zu den beschriebenen Diskrepanzen beitragen. Von BUCKTON u. Mitarb. (1971) wurde auch in Makrokulturen eine höhere Aberrationsrate als in Mikrokulturen gefunden, es zeigte sich aber, daß dadurch die Form der Dosiswirkungskurve nicht signifikant beeinflußt wurde. Dieser Befund sowie die Arbeiten von SHARPE u. Mitarb. (1969), BENDER u. BARCINSKI (1969) zeigen somit, daß die Diskrepanzen zwischen den verschiedenen in vitro-Befunden primär nicht durch unterschiedliche Kulturmethoden hervorgerufen werden. Einem anderen Faktor, der individuellen Strahlenempfindlichkeit, muß dabei sicher eine größere Bedeutung beigemessen werden, obwohl gegenwärtig auch hierzu noch widersprüchliche Befunde vorliegen. Keine signifikanten Unterschiede in der Strahlenempfindlichkeit von Lymphozyten verschiedener Blut-

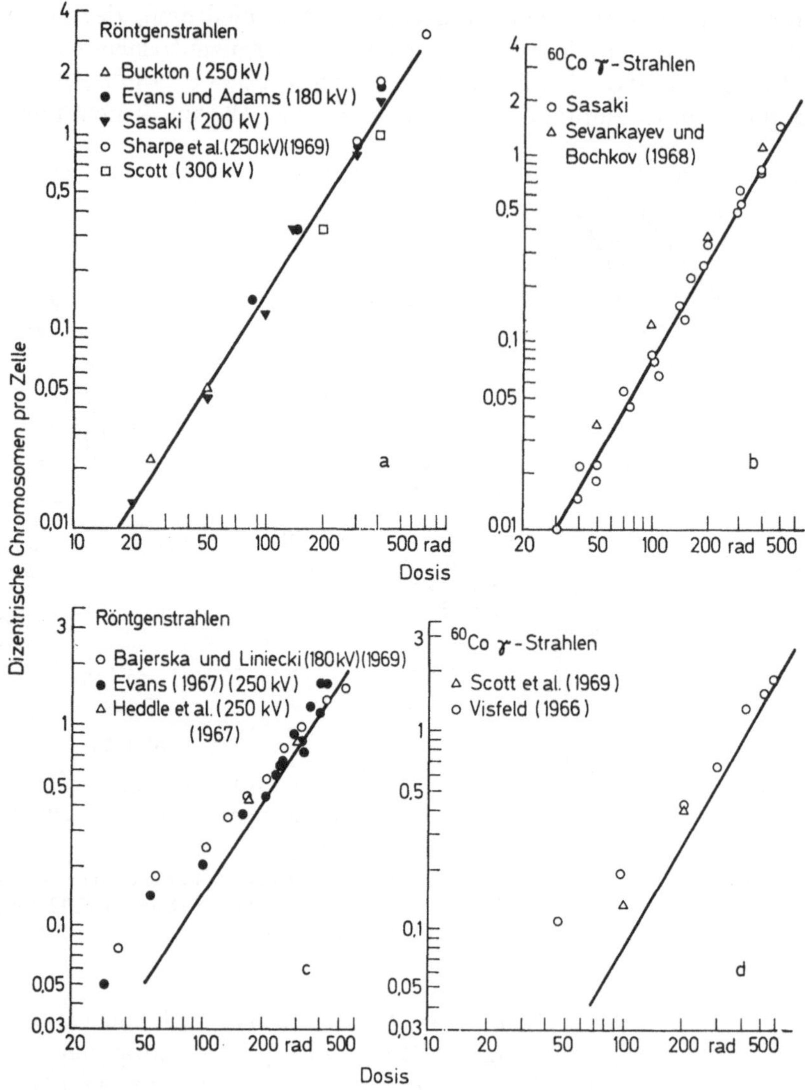

Abb. 32. In vitro-Bestrahlung. Vergleich der Häufigkeiten von dizentrischen Chromosomen in Lymphozyten, die im Vollblut vor der Kultur (a, b) bzw. nach dem Kulturansatz im Kulturmedium (c, d) bestrahlt wurden. Die Regressionslinien, die den Ergebnissen der Figuren a und b angepaßt sind, wurden zum Vergleich auch in die beiden Figuren c und d eingezeichnet. Beachte hier die höhere Aberrationsausbeute im niederen Dosisbereich sowohl nach Röntgen- als auch nach ^{60}Co γ-Bestrahlung, die dann auftritt, wenn die Zellen im Kulturmedium bestrahlt wurden. (Nach UNSCEAR-Report, 1969)

spender nach Bestrahlung mit der gleichen Dosis fanden Bender u. Gooch (1962a, 1966), Dekaban u. Mitarb. (1966), Gooch u. Mitarb. (1964), Bajerska u. Liniecki (1969a), Sharpe u. Mitarb. (1969) sowie Scott u. Mitarb. (1969). Bender u. Brewen (1969) konnten ausgeprägte Unterschiede zwischen verschiedenen Spendern hinsichtlich der Zeit, die notwendig war, um die erste Mitose zu erreichen, feststellen. Auch bei Sheppard u. Ferrari (1970) waren individuelle Unterschiede vorhanden.

Von verschiedenen Autoren wurde der sogenannte „Alterseffekt" untersucht. Dies geschah durch in vitro-Bestrahlung peripherer Lymphozyten von Blutspendern verschiedenen Alters mit einer konstanten Dosis. Evans u. Adams (1970) stellten für alle Aberrationen sowohl eine starke intraindividuelle als auch interindividuelle Variabilität fest. Die Aberrationshäufigkeit, ausgedrückt als Zahl der dizentrischen Chromosomen pro Zelle, nahm in den frühen Lebensjahren bis zu einem Minimum bei 36 ± 9 Jahren ab und stieg dann wieder an. Bochkov u. Pilosov (1968) fanden eine höhere Strahlenempfindlichkeit bei Kindern und älteren Leuten als bei Personen mittleren Alters (20—40 Jahre). Von Sasaki u. Mitarb. (1970) wurde eine erhöhte Aberrationsrate nur bei Neugeborenen ($<$ 12 Monate) beobachtet. Liniecki u. Mitarb. (1971) fanden für dizentrische Chromosomen eine negative lineare Korrelation mit dem Alter der Blutspender. Wurde als Bezugswert die Aberrationsrate bei Neugeborenen verwendet, so ergab sich eine altersbedingte Verminderung um 0,4 % pro Altersjahr. Kein Alterseffekt konnte für azentrische Chromosomen, Ringe und minutes festgestellt werden. Eine individuelle Varianz konnte nach Korrektur für das Lebensalter nur für azentrische Fragmente gefunden werden. Übereinstimmend wurden in sämtlichen Befunden keine Geschlechtsunterschiede in der Strahlenempfindlichkeit beobachtet.

Von verschiedenen Untersuchern konnte schließlich gezeigt werden, daß auch der Genotyp einer Zelle deren Strahlenempfindlichkeit beeinflussen kann. So fanden Chudina u. Mitarb. (1966), Dekaban u. Mitarb. (1966), Kucérova (1967) sowie Evans u. Adams (1970) nach in vitro-Bestrahlung in Lymphozyten von Patienten mit Down's Syndrom (G-Trisomie) eine höhere Aberrationsrate als in Lymphozyten von Normalpersonen. Sasaki u. Mitarb. (1970) untersuchten in einer detaillierten Studie verschiedene Typen angeborener Chromosomenanomalien, um nähere Aufschlüsse über die genotypischen Unterschiede der Strahlenempfindlichkeit zu bekommen. Dabei stellten sie fest, daß Lymphozyten, die für Teile einzelner Chromosomen oder für komplette Chromosomen trisom waren, eine größere Strahlenempfindlichkeit besaßen als Zellen mit einem normalen Karyotyp. Monosomien, reziproke Translokationen und Inversionen wirkten sich dagegen nicht aus.

2. Der Einfluß physikalischer und biologischer Faktoren auf die Aberrationsausbeute in vivo

Buckton u. Mitarb. (1969), Bauchinger (1971) fanden, daß die Aberrationsrate (dizentrische Chromosomen + Ringe) in peripheren Lymphozyten nach therapeutischer Ganzkörperbestrahlung von Carcinompatienten nicht signifikant von jener verschieden war, wie sie in Blutproben auftrat, welche unter gleichen Expositionsbedingungen mit gleicher Dosis in vitro bestrahlt worden waren (siehe Kapitel III 4a).

Dies kann als ein Hinweis dafür angesehen werden, daß es prinzipiell sinnvoll ist, nach einer in vivo-Bestrahlung eine Dosisabschätzung mit Hilfe von Dosiswirkungskurven, die bei in vitro-Versuchen erstellt wurden, zu versuchen. Es muß jedoch betont werden (Bauchinger u. Mitarb., 1970), daß nach einer Strahlenexposition in vivo eine einfache Beziehung zwischen der Aberrationsausbeute und der Dosis nicht ohne weiteres zu erwarten ist. Die Entstehung von Chromosomenaberrationen hängt wesentlich von der räumlichen Dosisverteilung innerhalb des Körpers ab. Dabei kommt wohl der lokalen Dosis im Blut und den Geweben, in denen die Lymphozyten erzeugt und gespeichert werden, besondere Bedeutung zu. Es ist aber heute noch nicht bekannt, ob die integrale Dosis in diesen Geweben als kritisch angesehen werden muß, oder ob sich die Dosis in den verschiedenen Depots unterschiedlich auf die Erzeugung von Chromosomenaberrationen auswirkt. Ferner ist zu bedenken, daß eine vollkommen homogene Dosisverteilung praktisch niemals vorliegt. Selbst unter den Expositionsbedingungen bei einer therapeutischen Ganzkörperbestrahlung wird durch die unterschiedliche Absorption in Weichteilen und Knochen eine Variabilität der lokalen Dosis verursacht.

Es ist verständlich, daß die Situation noch weit unübersichtlicher wird, wenn eine Teilkörperbestrahlung vorliegt, die meist noch mit einer inhomogenen Dosisverteilung erfolgte. Sicherlich wird durch Austauschprozesse, die zwischen den lymphatischen Geweben und dem peripheren Blut ablaufen, die Aberrationsausbeute entscheidend beeinflußt. Einer unterschiedlichen Strahlenempfindlichkeit verschiedener Entwicklungsstadien oder ganzer Subpopulationen von Lymphozyten kommt entscheidende Bedeutung zu. Selbstverständlich kann analog zu den in vitro-Verhältnissen mit einer unterschiedlichen Effektivität verschiedener Strahlenarten und -energien gerechnet werden. Auch eine interne Bestrahlung nach Inkorporation langlebiger radioaktiver Nuklide dürfte sich hier mit Sicherheit noch zusätzlich auswirken. Schließlich muß noch in Betracht gezogen werden, daß die Aberrationsausbeute auch von der zeitlichen Verteilung der Dosis und vom Zeitpunkt der Chromosomenanalyse nach der Bestrahlung abhängt. Dies kann aus den Studien der zeitlichen Veränderung strahleninduzierter Chromosomenaberrationen abgeleitet werden. Sie haben gezeigt, daß mit zunehmendem Zeitabstand von der Bestrahlung die Zahl der Zellen mit Chromosomendefekten auf Grund von Erholungs- und Selektionsprozessen abnimmt.

Zusammenfassend läßt sich sagen, daß die Aberrationsausbeute nach einer Bestrahlung in vivo von komplexen physikalischen und biologischen Faktoren bestimmt wird, die auf den ersten Blick ihre Verwendung als biologisches Dosimeter als wenig geeignet erscheinen lassen. Es ist jedoch mit Sicherheit anzunehmen, daß die „Chromosomendosimetrie" in ihrer heutigen Form noch präzisiert werden kann, wenn die folgenden Punkte intensiv bearbeitet werden:

1. Erstellung von Dosiswirkungskurven nach in vitro-Bestrahlung (besonders auch in niederen Dosisbereichen) unter standardisierten Expositions- und Kulturbedingungen.

2. Systematische Untersuchungen der Korrelation zwischen Aberrationsausbeute und Dosis sowie der zeitlichen und räumlichen Dosisverteilung unter möglichst übersichtlichen und homogenen Bestrahlungsbedingungen in vivo.

3. Standardisierung der Auswertungskriterien hinsichtlich der Aberrationstypen sowie der Zahl auszuwertender Zellen unter Einbeziehung von automatisierten Chromosomenanalysen.

4. Untersuchung der unterschiedlichen Strahlenempfindlichkeit verschiedener Personen.

5. Analyse der Zellkinetik des Lymphozytensystems.

Wenn die Forschungen in dieser Richtung konsequent vorangetrieben werden, wird die „Chromosomendosimetrie" sicher zu einer sinnvollen Ergänzung der physikalischen Strahlenschutzüberwachung.

Literatur

Abbatt, J. D.: Cytogenetic indicators of radiation (and other) damage-calibration-present and future practical applications. Biochemical indicators or radiation injury in man. Proc. Symp. Vienna 149–180, 1971.

Alper, T.: The modification of damage caused by primary ionization of biological targets. Radiat. Res. 5, 573–586 (1956).

— Cellular radiobiology. Ann. Rev. Nuclear Sci. 10, 489–530 (1960).

Altenburg, E.: The limit of radiation frequency effective in producing mutations. Amer. Nat. 62, 540–554 (1928).

Amarose, A. P., Baxter, D. H.: Chromosomal changes following surgery and radiotherapy in patients with pelvic cancer. Obstet. Gynecol. 25, 828–843 (1965).

— Plotz, E. J., Stein, A. A.: Residual Chromosomal Aberrations in Female Cancer Patients after Irradiation Therapy. Exp. and Molec. Pathol. 7, 58–91 (1967).

Antoshina, M. M., Kozlov, V. M., Bochkov, N. P.: Effect of γ-rays on human chromosomes. IV. Dynamics of chromosome aberrations in a leukocyte culture in a course of several mitotis. Genetika (Leningrad) 5/7, 114–120 (1969).

ARAKAKI, D. T., SPARKES, R. S.: Microtechnique for culturing leukocytes from whole blood. Cytogenetics 2, 57–60 (1963).

ATWOOD, K. C.: Number of nuclear sites for aberration formation and the distribution of aberrations. WOLFF, S. (Ed.) "Radiation-induced chromosome aberrations". New York: Columbia Univ. Press 73–86, 1963.

AUXIER, J. A., CHEKA, J. S., HAYWOOD, F. F., JONES, T. D., THORNGATE, J. H.: Free-field radiation dose distribution from the Hiroshima and Nagasaki bombings. Health Physics 12, 425–429 (1966).

AWA, A., BLOOM, A. D., YOSHIDA, M. C.: Cytogenetic study of the offspring of atomic bomb survivors. Nature 218, 367–368 (1968).

BAUCHINGER, M.: Chromosomenaberrationen durch medizinische Strahlenanwendung. Münchner Med. Wschr. 109, 1008–1014 (1967).

— Chromosomenaberrationen und ihre zeitliche Veränderung nach Radium-Röntgentherapie gynäkologischer Tumoren. Strahlentherapie 135, 553–564 (1968).

— HUG, O.: Chromosomenaberrationen nach Radium-Röntgentherapie gynäkologischer Tumoren. Strahlentherapie 131, 109–121 (1966).

— — Chromosomenaberrationen bei beruflicher Strahlenbelastung in der Radiumtherapie. Fortschritte auf dem Gebiet der Röntgenstr. 109, 97–103 (1968).

— Chromosomenaberrationen in menschlichen peripheren Lymphozyten nach Einwirkung von ionisierenden Strahlen und Endoxan. Bericht B 309 der Gesellschaft für Strahlen und Umweltforschung München 1—80, 1971.

— SCHMID, E., HUG, O.: The relevance of chromosome aberration yields for biological dosimetry after low level occupational irradiation. Int. Atomic Energy Agency. Symposium on new developments in physical and biological radiation detectors. Vienna SM-143/13, 23.—27. 11. 1970.

— SCHMID, E.: Chromosomenaberrationen menschlicher Lymphocyten nach Röntgenbestrahlung in vitro. II. Analyse der Primärprozesse. Mutat. Res. in Vorbereitung (1973).

BAJERSKA, A., The influence of X-ray dose and time of its delivery in vitro upon the yield of chromosomal aberrations in the peripheral blood lymphocytes. Int. J. Rad. Biol. 16, 467–481 (1969a).

— LINIECKI, J.: The influence of temperature at irradiation in vitro on the yield of chromosomal aberrations in peripheral blood lymphocytes. Int. J. Rad. Biol. 16, 483–493 (1969b).

BARCINSKI, M. A., ALMEIDA, J. C. C., ABREU, M. C., KAYATH, H. C.: Chromosome studies on inhabitants of high-background radiation areas in Brazil. Persönliche Mitteilung. 1971.

BELL, A. G., BAKER, D. G.: Irradiation-induced chromosome aberrations in normal human leukocytes in culture. Canad. J. Genet. Cytol. 4, 340–351 (1962).

BENDER, M. A., BARCINSKI, M. A.: Kinetics of two-break aberration production by X-rays in human leukocytes. Cytogenetics 8, 241–246 (1969).

BENDER, M. A., BREWEN, J. G.: Factors influencing chromosome aberration yields in the human peripheral leukocyte system. Mutat. Res. 8, 383–399 (1969).

— GOOCH, P. C.: Persistent chromosome aberrations in irradiated human subjects. Radiat. Res. 16, 44–53 (1962b).

— — Persistent chromosome aberrations in irradiated human subjects. II. Three and one half year investigation. Radiat. Res. 18, 389–396 (1963).

— — Types and rates of X-ray induced chromosome aberrations in human blood irradiated in vitro. Proc. nat. Acad. Sci. Wash. 48, 522–532 (1962a).

— — Somatic chromosome aberrations induced by human whole-body irradiation: The "Recuplex" Criticality Accident. Radiat. Res. 29, 568–582 (1966).

BIOLA, M. T., LE GO, R.: Utilisation des analyses chromosomiques en tant que dosimetrie biologique. 1st International Congress of the International Radiation Protection Association, Rome, 5–10 September 1966.

— — DUCATEZ, G.: Formation de chromosomes dicentriques dans les lymphocytes humains soumis in vitro a un flux de rayonnement mixte (gamma, neutrons). Advances in physical and biological radiation detectors. Vienna SM-142/48, 633–645, 23.–27. 1970 (1971).

BLOOM, A. D., TJIO, J. H.: In vivo effects of diagnostic X-irradiation on human chromosomes. New England J. Med. 270, 1341–1344 (1964).

— NERIISHI, S., KAMADA, N., ISEKI, T., KEEHN, R. J.: Cytogenetic investigation of survivors of the atomic bombings of Hiroshima and Nagasaki. Lancet 2, 672–674 (1966).

— AWA, A. A., NERIISHI, S., HONDA, T., ARCHER, P. G.: Chromosome aberrations in leukocytes of older survivors of the atomic bombings of Hiroshima and Nagasaki. Lancet 11, 802–805 (1967a).

— NERIISHI, S., ARCHER, P. G.: Cytogenetics of the in utero exposed of Hiroshima and Nagasaki. Lancet 2, 10–12 (1968).

— — KAMADA, N., ISEKI, T.: Leucocyte chromosome studies in adult and in utero exposed survivors of Hiroshima and Nagasaki, 136–143. Human Radiation Cytogenetics, EVANS, H. J., COURT-BROWN, W. M., McLEAN, A. S., eds. Amsterdam: North Holland Publishing Co., 1967b.

BOCHKOV, N. P., PILOSOW, R. A.: The effect of gamma-rays on human chromosomes. II. The dependence of chromosome aberration frequency upon sex and age. Genetika 4, 144 (1968).

BORA, K. C.: Relative biological efficiencies of 220 Kvp X-rays and 14,1 MeV neutrons in the induction of aberrations in chromosomes of Tradescantia at low temperature. Proc. Second Int. Conf. on peaceful Uses of Atomic energy 22, 342–350 (1958).

— Relative biological efficiencies of ionizing radiations on the induction of cytogenetic effects in plants "Effects of ionizing radiations on seeds". Int. Atomic Agency, Vienna, 345–357, 1961.

— unveröffentlicht. Siehe aber dazu ABATT 1971.

— SOPER, R.: Influence of temperature on the induction and repair of radiation induced aberrations in the human chromosome. Can. J. Genet. Cytol. 13, 364–368 (1971).

Boyd, J. T., Court-Brown, W. M., Vennart, J., Woodcock, G. E.: Chromosome studies on women formerly employed as luminous dial painters. Brit. Med. J. 1, 377–382 (1966).

— — Woodcock, G. E., Veomett, R. C.: Relationship between external radiation exposure and chromosome aberration among luminous dial painters, pp. 208–214 in Human Radiation Cytogenetics. Evans, H. J., Court-Brown, W. M., McLean, A. S. (eds.), Amsterdam: North Holland Publishing Co., 1967.

— Buchmann, W., Lennox, B.: Damage to chromosomes by therapeutic doses of radioiodine, Lancet 1, 977–978 (1961).

Brancadoro, P., Siciliano, A.: Sulle anomalie indotte delle radiazioni ionizzanti nei chromosomi umani. Munt. radiol. (Firenze) 31, 1217–33 (1965).

Brewen, J. G.: Dependence of frequency of X-ray-induced chromosome aberrations on dose rate in the Chinese Hamster. Proc. Nat. Acad. Sci. (U.S.) 50, 322–329 (1963).

— Kinetics of X-ray-induced chromatid aberrations in Vicia faba and studies relating aberration frequencies to the cell cycle. Mutat. Res. 1, 400–408 (1964).

— Cell-cycle and radiosensitivity of the chromosomes of human leucocytes. Int. J. Rad. Biol. 9, 391–397 (1965).

— Luippold, H. E.: Radiation-induced human chromosome aberrations: In vitro dose rate studies. Mutat. Res. 12, 305–314 (1971).

— Brock, R. D.: The exchange hypothesis and chromosome-type aberrations. Mutat. Res. 6, 245–255 (1968).

Brøgger, A.: Apparently spontaneous chromosome damage in human leukocytes and the nature of chromatid gaps. Humangenetik 13, 1–14 (1971).

Brown, J. K., McNeill, J. R.: Aberrations in leukocyte chromosomes of personnel occupationally exposed to low levels of radiations. Radiat. Res. 40, 534–543 (1969).

— Porter, J.H., Gabay, J. J.: Chronic effects from radium-226 body burden on human chromosomes cultured in vitro. N.Y. St. J. Med. 68, 2641–47 (1968).

Buckton, K. E., Jacobs, P. A., Court-Brown, W. M., Doll, R.: A study of the chromosome damage persisting after X-ray therapy for ankylosing spondylitis. Lancet 2, 676–682 (1962).

— Pike, M. C.: Chromosome investigations on lymphocytes from irradiated patients: Effect of time in culture. Nature 202, 714–715 (1964a).

— Pike, M. C.: Time in culture. An important variable in studying in vivo radiation-induced chromosome damage in man. Int. J. Rad. Biol. 8, 439–452 (1964b).

— Court-Brown, W. M., Smith, P. G.: Lymphocyte survival in men treated with X-rays for ankylosing Spondylitis. Nature 214, 470–473 (1967a).

— Dolphin, G.W., McLean, A. S.: "Studies of chromosome aberrations in cultures of peripheral blood from men employed at UKAEA establishments". Human Radiation Cytogenetics (Evans, H. J., Court-Brown, W. M., McLean, A. S., Eds.). Amsterdam: North Holland Publishing Co., 174–182, 1967b.

Buckton, K. E., Langlands, A. O., Smith, P. G., McLelland, J.: Chromosome aberrations following partial- and whole body X-irradiation in man. Dose response relationships, pp. 122–135 in Human Radiation Cytogenetics. Evans, H. J., Court-Brown, W. M., McLean, A. S., eds., Amsterdam: North Holland Publishing Co., 1967c.

— — Woodcock, G. E.: Cytogenetic changes following Thorotrast administration. Int. J. Rad. Biol. 12/6, 565–577 (1967d).

— Smith, P. G., Court-Brown, W.M.: The estimation of lymphocyte lifespan from studies on males treated with X-rays for ankylosing spondylitis, 106–114. Human Radiation Cytogenetics, Evans, H. J., Court-Brown, W. M., McLean, A. S., eds., Amsterdam: North Holland Publishing Co., 1967e.

— — Smith, P. G., Looby, P. C., Woodcock, G. E.: Chromosome aberrations iduced in human peripheral blood by 2 MeV-X-irradiation to the whole-body and in vitro. Radiation induced cancer. Proc. Symp. Athens Int. Atomic Energy Agency 135–146, 1969.

— Langlands, A. O., Smith, P. G., Woodcock, G. E., Looby, P. C., McLelland, J.: Further studies on chromosome aberration production after whole body irradiation in man. Int. J. Rad. Biol. 19, 369–378 (1971).

Caratzali, A., Stefanescu, D. T., Popescu, H.: Chromosome abnormalities after irradiation with small doses of γ-rays, Presse med. 75, 1637–1638 (1967).

Carstairs, K., The small lymphocyte, its possible pluripotential quality. Lancet 1, 829 (1962).

Catcheside, D. G., Lea, D. E., Thoday, J. M.: Types of chromosome structural change induced by the irradiation of Tradescantia microspores. J. Genet. 47, 113–136 (1946).

— — Effect of ionization distribution on chromosome breakage by X-rays. J. Genet. 45, 186–196 (1943).

Chicago Conference: Standardization in Human Cytogenetics. Birth Defects: Original Article Series II, 2 (1966). The National Foundation, New York.

Chudina, A. P., Lalyutina, T. C., Pogosyane, E. E.: Sravneniye radiochustvitelnosti kromosom v kultivirumyemikh leukocitakh perifericheskoy v norme i sindrome Downa. Genetica 4, 51–63 (1966).

Chmelevsky, D., Chemtob, M., Parmentier, N. C.: Microdosimetrie et formation de chromosomes dicentriques dans les lymphocytes humains irradies in vitro. Third Symposion on Microdosimetry, Stresa october 18–22, 1971.

Conger, A. D.: Radiations effects on ascites tumor chromosomes. Ann. N.Y. Acad. Sci. 63, 929 (1956).

— Randolph, M. C., Sheppard, W. C., Luippold, H. E.: Quantitative relation of RBE in Tradescantia and average LET of gamma-rays, X-rays and 1,3-, 2,5- and 14,1-MeV fast neutrons. Radiat. Res. 9, 525–547 (1958).

Conen, P. E., Bell, A. G., Aspin, N.: Chromosomal aberration in an infant following the use of diagnostic X-rays. Pediatrics 31, 72–79 (1963).

Court-Brown, W. M.: Studies on chromosome damage following in vivo human radiation exposure. Proc. roy. Soc. Edinb. **70**, 125–131 (1968).

— Buckton, K. E., McLean, A. S.: Quantitative studies of chromosome aberrations in man following acute and chronic exposure to X-rays and γ-rays. Lancet **1**, 1239–1241 (1965).

— — Langlands, A. O.: The identification of lymphocyte clones with chromosome structural aberrations in irradiated men and women. Int. J. Rad. Biol. **13**, 155–169 (1967).

Crouse, H. V.: X-ray breakage of lily chromosomes at first meiotic metaphase. Science **119**, 485–487 (1954).

Darlington, C. D.: Zitiert von Chu, E. H. Y.: Radiation induced chromosome aberrations ed. S. Wolff, New York: Columbia Univ. Press 217, 1963.

— Upcott, M. B.: Spontaneous chromosome change. J. Genet. **41**, 275–296 (1941).

Davidson, D.: Zitiert von Chu, E. H. Y.: Radiation induced chromosome aberrations, ed. Wolff, S. New York: Columbia Univ. Press 217, 1963.

Dekaban, A. S., Thron, R., Steusing, J. K.: Chromosomal aberrations in irradiated blood and blood cultures of normal subjects and of selected patients with chromosomal abnormalities. Radiat. Res. **27**, 50–63 (1966).

Dobzhansky, T.: Genetical and cytological proof of translocations involving the third and fourth chromosome of Drosophila melanogaster. Biol. Zbl. **49**, 408–419 (1929).

Doida, J., Sugahara, T., Horikawa, M.: Studies on some radiation-induced chromosome aberrations in man. Radiat. Res. **26**, 69–83 (1965).

Dolphin, G. W., Bolton, D., Humphreys, D. H. O., Speight, D. L., Stradling, G. N.: Biological and Physical Dosimetry after a Radiation Accident, Nature **227**, 165 (1970).

— Purrott, R. J.: Thes use of radiation induced chromosome aberrations in human lymphocytes as a dosimeter. Int. Atomic Energy Agency. Symposium on new developments in physical and biological radiation detectors. Vienna SM-143/8, 23.—27. 11. 1970.

Dubrova, S. E.: Исследование кариотипа клеток крови и костного мозга у двух больных миеломной болезнью в связи с рентгенотерапией. Генетика **6**, 54–61 (1967).

Ebenezer, L. N., Sadasivan, G.: Chromosome damage in X-ray technicians. Indian. H. Med. Res. **56**, 1023–1027 (1968).

Edgren, J.: Effect of Cysteine on chromosome aberrations induced by radiation of human lymphocytes in vitro. Acta Radiologica Supplement **198** (1970).

El-Alfi, O. S., Rugab, A. S., Eassa, E. H. M.: Detection of radiation damage in exposed personnel by chromosome study. Brit. J. Radiol. **40**, 760–764 (1967).

Van der Elst, E., Gimenez, J. C., Beninson, D.: Utilizacion del indice de aberraciones chromosomicas como dosimetro biologico. Report of Comision Nacional de Energia, Buenos Aires, 1967.

Elves, M. W., Wilkinson, J. F.: The effects of PHA on normal and leukaemic leukocytes when cultured in vitro. Exp. Cell Res. **30**, 200–203 (1963).

Emrich, D., Keiderling, W.: Strahlenexposition und Strahlenschutz bei Anwendung offener radioaktiver Isotope in der Medizin. Dtsch. med. Wschr. **88**, 515–520 (1963).

Evans, H. J.: Chromatid aberrations induced by gamma irradiation. I. The structure and frequency of chromatid interchanges in diploid and tetraploid cells of Vicia faba. Genetics **46**, 257–275 (1961).

— Chromosome aberrations induced by ionizing radiation, in Bourne, G. H., Danielli, J. F. (Eds.). International Review of Cytology 13, 221–231 (1962). New York and London: Academic Press.

— Chromosome aberrations and the target theory. Wolff, S. (Ed.) "Radiation Induced Chromosome Aberrations"; New York: Columbia Univ. Press, 8–40, 1963a.

— Possible reasons for variation in chromosome radiosensitivity during mitotic and meiotic cycles. Sobels, F. (Ed.) "Repair from Genetic Radiation Damage". Oxford: Pergamon Press, 31–49, 1963b.

— A simple microtechnique for obtaining human chromosome preparations with some comments on DNA replication in sex chromosomes of the goat, cow, and pig. Exp. Cell Res. **38**, 511–156 (1965).

— Repair and recovery from chromosome damage induced by fractionated X-ray exposures, pp. 482–501. Radiation research 1966, Amsterdam: North Holland Publ. Co., 1967a.

— Dose-response relations from in vitro studies, pp. 20–36. Evans, H. J., Court-Brown, W. M., McLean, A. S., eds.: Human radiation cytogenetics. Amsterdam: North Holland Publ. Co., 1967b.

— Actions of radiations on Chromosomes, pp. 321–339. The scientific bases of medicine. Annual reviews 1967. London: Athlone Press, 1967c.

— The response of human chromosomes to ionizing radiations in vitro. Proc. Roy. Soc. B **70**, 132–151 (1968).

— The use of Chromosome aberration frequencies for biological dosimetry in man. Int. Atomic Energy Agency. Symposium on new developments in physical and biological radiation detectors, Vienna SM-143/77, 23—27. 11. 1970.

— Adams, A.: Influence of cell stage on X-ray induced chromosomal aberrations in human peripheral blood leucocytes. "Radiation Research" Proc. 5th Int. Congr. Radiat. Res. Evian 1970.

— Neary, G. J.: The influence of oxygen on the sensitivity of Tradescantia pollen tube chromosomes to X-rays. Radiat. Res. **11**, 636–641 (1959).

— Savage, J. R. K.: The relation between DNA synthesis and chromosome structure as resolved by X-ray damage. J. Cell. Biol. **18**, 525–540 (1963).

— Scott, D.: Influence of DNA synthesis on the production of chromatid aberrations by X-rays and maleic hydrazide in Vicia faba. Genetics **49**, 17–38 (1964).

Fischer, P., Golob, E., Kunze-Muehl, E., Haimben A., Dudley, R. A., Muellner, T., Parr, R. M., Vetter, H.: Chromosome aberrations in peripheral blood cells in man following chronic irradiation from internal deposits of Thorotrast. Radiat. Res. **29**, 505–515 (1966).

Fischer, P., Golob, E., Kunze-Muehl, E., Muellner, T.: Chromosome aberrations in persons with thorium dioxide burdens, pp. 194–202 in Human Radiation Cytogenetics. Evans, H. J., Court-Brown, W. M., McLean, A. S., eds. Amsterdam: North Holland Publishing Co., 1967.

Fitzgerald, P. H.: The immunological role and life-span of small lymphocytes. J. theoret. Biol. **6**, 13–17 (1964).

— The life-span and role of the small lymphocyte. pp. 94–98 in Human Radiation Cytogenetics. Evans, J. H., Court-Brown, W. M., McLean, A. S., eds. Amsterdam: North Holland Publishing Co., 1967.

Forni, A., Ghezzi, J., Cappelini, J.: Cytogenetic studies in subjects with chronic occupational exposure to low doses of ionizing radiations. Med. Lavoro (Milano) **60**, 169–174 (1969).

Fox, D. P.: The effects of X-rays on the chromosomes of Locust embryos. II. Chromatid interchanges and the organisation of the interphase nucleus. Chromosoma **20**, 173–194 (1966).

— The effects of X-rays on the chromosomes of Locust embryos. III. The chromatid aberration types. Chromosoma **20**, 386–412 (1967).

Gabay, J., Sax, N., Brown, C.: The establishment and effects of a 226 Ra body burden. 13. Meeting on Bioassay and Analytical Chemistry, Berkeley, Calif. UCRL-18140, 197–212, 1968.

Garcia-Benitez, C., Wolff, S.: On the increase of sites for chromosome exchange formation after chromosome duplication. Science **135**, 438–439 (1962).

Giles, N. H.: The effect of fast neutrons on the chromosomes of Tradescantia. Proc. nat. Acad. Sci. Wash. **26**, 567–575 (1940).

— Comparative studies of the cytogenetical effects of neutrons and X-rays. Genetics **28**, 398–418 (1943).

— Beatty, A. V.: The effect of X-irradiation in oxygen under pressure on chromosome aberration frequency in Tradescantia microspores. Genetics **35**, 666–667 (1950).

— Conger, A. D.: Chromosomal interchanges induced in Tradescantia microspores by fast neutrons from uranium fission. J. cell. comp. Physiol. **35**, Suppl. 1, 83–88 (1950).

— Beatty, A. V., Riley, H. P.: The effect of oxygen on the production by fast neutrons of chromosomal aberrations in Tradescantia microspores. Genetics **37**, 641–649 (1952).

— De Serres, F. J., Beatty, A. V.: The effect of radiation dose fractionation on the chromosome aberration frequencies in Tradescantia microspores. II. Studies with fast neutrons, Genetics **38**, 416–420 (1953).

— Riley, H. R.: The effect of oxygen on the frequency of X-ray induced chromosomal rearrangements in Tradescantia microspores. Proc. Natl. Acad. Sci. U.S. **35**, 640–646 (1949).

— — Studies on the mechanism of the oxygen effect on the radiosensitivity of Tradescantia chromosomes. Proc. Natl. Acad. Sci. U.S. **36**, 337–344 (1950).

Giles, N. H., Tobias, C. A.: The effect of linear energy transfer on radiation-induced chromsome aberrations in Tradescantia microspores. Science **120**, 993–994 (1954).

— Radiation-induced chromosome aberrations in Tradescantia. Hollaender (Ed.), "Radiation Biology". New York: McGraw-Hill, **1**, 713–761 (1954).

Goh, K. O.: Total-body irradiation and human chromosomes: Cytogenetic studies of the peripheral blood and bone marrow leukocytes seven years after total-body irradiation. Radiat. Res. **35**, 155–170 (1968a).

— Summer, H.: Breaks in normal human chromosomes: Are they induced by a transferable substance in the plasma of persons exposed to total-body irradiation. Radiat. Res. **35**, 171–181 (1968b).

Gooch, P. C., Bender, M. A., Randolph, M. L.: Chromosome aberrations induced in human somatic cells by neutrons, pp. 325–432. Biological effects of neutron and proton irradiation, Vol. I. International Atomic Energy Agency, Vienna 1964.

Goodspeed, T. H., Olsen, A. R.: The production of variations in Nicotiana by X-ray treatment. Proc. Natl. Acad. Sci. U.S. **14**, 66–69 (1928).

Gopal-Ayengar, A. R., Sundaram, K., Mistry, K. B., Sunta, C. M., Nambi, K. S. V., Kathuria, S. P., Basu, A. S., David, M.: Evaluation of the long-term effects of high background radiation on selected population groups of the Kerala coast, Fourth United Nations Conference on the peaceful uses of atomic energy. Geneva, Switzerland, A/Conf. 49/P/535, 6–16 September 1971.

Gorisontova, M. N.: Некоторые показатели митотической активности костного мозга при воздействии на организм ионизирующей радиации. Мед. радиол. **11**, 55–56 (1966).

Grant, C. J.: Chromosome aberrations and the mitotic cycle in Trillium root tips after X-irradiation. Mutat. Res. **2**, 246–262 (1965).

Gray, L. H.: Primary Sites of Energy Deposition associated with radio-biological lesions. Cell Metabolism. London 1956.

— The influence of oxygen on the radiosensitivity of cells and tissues. Haissinsky, M. (Ed.). "Organic Peroxides in Radiobiology" 104, 1957.

— Green, F. O., Hawes, C. A.: Effect of nitric oxide on the radio-sensitivity of tumour cells. Nature, Lond. **182**, 952–953 (1958).

Heddle, J. A.: Randomness in the formation of radiation-induced chromosome aberrations. Genetics **52**, 1329–1334 (1965).

— Evans, H. J., Scott, D.: Sampling time and the complexity of the human leucocyte system, pp. 6–19 in Human Radiation Cytogenetics. Evans, H. J., Court-Brown, W. M., McLean, A. S. (eds.). Amsterdam: North Holland Publishing Co., 1967.

— Whissell, D., Bodycote, D. J.: Changes in chromosome structure induced by radiations: a test of the two chief hypotheses. Nature **22**, 1159–1160 (1969).

— Bodycote, D. J.: On the formation of chromosomal aberrations. Mutat. Res. **9**, 117–126 (1970).

Hollaender, A.: Radiation Protection and Recovery. Oxford: Pergamon Press 1960.

Hollowell, J. G., Littlefield, G. L.: Chromosome damage induced by plasma of X-rayed patients: An indirect effect of X-ray. Proc. Soc. exp. Biol. (N.Y.) 129, 240–244 (1968).

Honda, T., Kamada, N., Bloom, A. D.: Chromosome aberrations and culture time. Cytogenetics 8, 117–124 (1969).

Hornsey, S., Howard-Flanders, P., Moore, D.: The effects of oxygen on the sensitivity of mammalian tumour cells to neutrons and X-rays. Int. J. Rad. Biol. 2, 37–44 (1960).

Howard, A., Pelc, S. R.: Nuclear incorporation of 32 P as demonstrated by autoradiographs. J. Exp. Cell. Res. 2, 178–187 (1951).

Hsu, T. C., Dewey, W. C., Humphrey, R.: Radiosensitivity of cells of Chinese Hamster in vitro in relations to the cell cycle. Exp. Cell. Res. 27, 441–452 (1962).

Hug, O.: Strahlenbelastung der Schilddrüse und mögliche nachteilige Folgen der Radiojodanwendung. Gemeinsame Tagung der dtsch. Ges. Inn. Med. und der dtsch. Röntgen-Ges. Wiesbaden 9. 4. 1964.

Hungerford, D. A., Nowell, P. C., Beck, S.: The chromosome constitution of a human phenotypic intersex. Am. J. Human Genet. 11, 215–236 (1959).

Ilbery, P. L. T., Chee, C. A., Rickinson, M. A.: The assessment of radiation damage in lymphocytes following radiophosphorus treatment in vivo. Vortrag 3. Human Cytogenetics Conference. Australian Atomic Energy Commission, Sydney 1971.

Ishihara, T., Kumatori, T.: Chromosome aberrations in human leukocytes irradiated in vivo and in vitro. Acta Haem. Jap. 28, 291–307 (1965).

— — Polyploid cells in human leukocytes following in vivo and in vitro irradiation. Cytologia 31, 59–68 (1966).

— — Chromosome studies on Japanese exposed to radiation resulting from nuclear bomb explosion, pp. 144–166. Human Radiation Cytogenetics. Evans, H. J., Court-Brown, W. M., McLean, A. S., eds. North Holland Publishing Co., Amsterdam 1967.

Kelly, S., Brown, C. D.: Chromosome aberrations as a biological dosimeter. Amer. J. publ. Health 55, 1419–1429 (1965).

Kay, H. E. M., Lawler, S. D., Millard, R. E.: The Chromosome in Polycythemia vera, Brit. J. Haemat. 12, 507—513 (1966).

Kihlman, B. A.: The effect of oxygen, nitric oxyde, and respiratory inhibitors on the production of chromosome aberrations by X-rays. Exp. Cell. Res. 14, 639–642 (1958).

— Effect of nitric oxide on the production of chromosomal aberrations by X-rays. Exp. Cell. Res. 17, 588–590 (1959).

Kilibarda, M., Markovic, B., Panov, D.: Studies of chromosome aberrations in persons exposed to ionizing radiation (X-ray ^{226}Ra and ^{222}Rn). Stud. Biophys. (Berl.) 6, 179–186 (1968).

Kirby-Smith, J. S., Dolphin, G. W.: Chromosome breakage at high radiation dose-rates. Nature, Lond. 182, 270–271 (1958).

Kirby-Smith, J. S., Daniels, D. S.: The relative effects of X-rays, gamma rays and beta rays on chromosomal breakage in Tradescantia. Genetics 38, 375–388 (1953).

Kotval, J. P., Gray, L. H.: Structural changes produced in microspores of Tradescantia by α-radiation. J. Genet. 48, 135–154 (1947).

Kucerova, M.: Comparison of radiation effects in vitro upon chromosomes of human subjects. Acta Radiol. 6, 441–448 (1967).

— Chromosome aberrations after X-ray therapy. J. Genet. Hum. 18/1, 21–29 (1970).

Kumatori, T., Ishihara, T.: Chromosome abnormalities of leucocytes observed in Thorotrast injected cases. Ann. Rep. Natl. Inst. Radiol. Sci. 3, 62 (1963).

Lajtha, L. G.: On the concept of the cell cycle. J. Cellular Comp. Physiol. Suppl. 1, 143–145 (1963).

Langlands, A. O., Smith, P. G., Buckton, K. E., Woodcock, G. E.: Chromosome Damage Induced by Radiation. Nature 218, 1133–1135 (1968).

Lea, D. E.: The induction of chromsome structural changes by radiation: detailed quantitative interpretation. Brit. J. Radiol., Suppl. 1, 75–83 (1947).

— Actions of radiations on living cells. Univ. Press, Cambridge 1946.

— Catcheside, D. G.: The mechanism of the induction by radiation of chromosome aberrations in Tradescantia. J. Genet. 44, 216–245 (1942).

Lejeune, J., Berger, R., Levy, C. I.: Analyse caryotypique de quatre cas d'irradiation accidentelle. Ann. de Genet. 10, 118–123 (1967).

Lindahl-Kiessling, K. B., Santesson, Böök, J. A.: Chromosome and chromatid-type aberrations induced by 60 Co irradiation and tritiated uridine in human leukocyte cultures. Chromosoma 31, 280–284 (1970).

Liniecki, J., Bajerska, A., Andryszek, C.: Chromosomal aberrations in human lymphocytes irradiated in vitro from donors (males and females) of varying age. Int. J. Rad. Biol. 19, 349–360 (1971).

Lisco, H., Lisco, E.: Personal communication 1969.

— Conard, R. A.: Chromosome studies on Marshall islanders exposed to fallout radiation. Science 157, 445–447 (1967).

Ma, T. H., Wolff, S.: Far red induced mitotic delay and the apparent increase of X-ray induced chromatid aberrations in Tradescantia microspores. Radiation Botany 5, 293–298 (1965).

MacDiarmid, W. D.: Chromosomal changes following treatment of Polycythaemia with radioactive Phosphorus. Quart. J. Med. 34, 133–143 (1965).

MacKinney, A. A., Stohlman, F., Brecher, G.: The kinetics of cell proliferation in cultures of human peripheral blood. Blood 19, 349–358 (1962).

MacIntyre, M. N., Dobyns, B. M.: Anomalies in chromosomes of the circulating leukocytes in man following large dose of radioactive iodine. J. Clin. Endocr. 22, 1171–1181 (1962).

Marsch, W., Niederalt, G., Gropp, A.: Chromosomenanomalien nach Strahlenbelastung. Dtsch. med. Wschr. 90, 2205–2208 (1965).

Marshall, W. H., Roberts, K. B.: The growth and mitosis of human small lymphocytes after incubation with a phytohaemagglutinin. Quart. J. Exptl. Physiol. **48**, 146–155 (1963).

Massimo, L., Vianello, M. G., Dagna-Bricarelli, F.: Alterazioni cromosomiche dei Leucociti indotte nel bambino da irradiazioni diagnostiche. Acta geneticae medicae et gemellologiae **14**, 282–294 (1965).

Mellmann, W. J.: Human peripheral blood leukocyte cultures, pp. 21–49 in Human Chromosome Methodology. J. J. Yunis, ed. New York: Academic Press 1965.

Millard, R. E.: Abnormalities of human chromosomes following therapeutic irradiation. Cytogenetics **4**, 277–294 (1965).

Monesi, V., Crippa, M., Zito-Bignami, R.: The stage of chromosome duplication as revealed by X-ray breakage and H3-thymidine labeling. Chromosoma **21**, 369–386 (1967).

Moore, J. G., Van Campenhout, J. L., Brandkamp, W. W.: Effects of ionizing irradiation and chemotherapeutic agents on human chromosomes. Amer. J. Obstet. Gynecol. **88**, 985–1000 (1964).

Moorhead, P. S.: Comments on the human leukocyte culture, pp. 1–5 in Human Radiation Cytogenetics. Evans, H. J., Court-Brown, W. M., McLean, A. S. (eds.). Amsterdam: North Holland Publishing Co. 1967.

— Nowell, P. C., Mellman, W. J., Battips, D. M., Hungerford, D. A.: Chromosome preparations of leukocytes cultured from human peripheral blood. Exp. Cell. Res. **20**, 613–616 (1960).

Mouriquand, C., Patet, J., Darnault, J., Gilly, C., Jalbert, P., Wolff, Ch.: Chromosomes et radiations: Étude de 12 sujets professionellement exposés et porteurs de radiodermites. Extrait du Bulletin d'Informations Scientifiques et Techniques du Commissariat a l'Energie Atomiques, No. **94**, 1–23 (1965).

— Gilly, C., Wolf, C., Patet, J.: Étude in vitro de l'effet du rayonnement γ sur les chromosomes humains. Int. J. Rad. Biol. **19**, 263–279 (1971).

— Patet, J., Gilly, C., Jalbert, P., Wolff, Ch.: Chromosomes et radiations: Étude in vitro de l'action des rayons X sur les lymphocytes humains. Raport CEA-R 3007, Commissariat a l'Energie atomique, France 1966.

Muller, H. J.: Artificial transmutation of the gene. Science **66**, 84–87 (1927).

— The measurement of gene mutation rate in Drosophila, its high variability and its dependence upon temperature. Genetics **13**, 279–357 (1928).

— An analysis of the process of structural change in chromosomes of Drosophila. J. Genet. **40**, 1–66 (1940).

— The nature of the genetic effects produced by radiation, Hollaender, A. (Ed.), "Radiation Biology". New York: McGraw-Hill **1**, 351–473 (1954a).

— The manner of production of mutations by radiation. Hollaender, A. (Ed.), "Radiation Biology"; New York: McGraw-Hill **1**, 475–626 (1954b).

— Painter, T. S.: The cytological expression of changes in gene alignment produced by X-rays in Drosophila. Am. Nat. **63**, 193–200 (1929).

Muller, H. J., Altenburg, E.: The frequency of translocations produced by X-rays in Drosophila. Genetics **15**, 283–311 (1930).

Neary, G. J.: Dependence on oxygen and temperature of the sensitivity of broad bean roots to gamma radiation. Nature, Lond. **180**, 248 (1957).

— Chromosome aberrations, cell killing, and the molecular basis of relative biological effectiveness of ionizing radiations. Radiation Research 1966, Amsterdam: North Holland 445–454 (1967).

— Chromosome aberrations and the theory of RBE 1. General considerations. Int. J. Rad. Biol. **9**, 477–502 (1965).

— Savage, J. R. K., Evans, H. J., Whittle, J.: Ultimate maximum values of RBE of fast neutrons and gamma rays for chromosome aberrations. Int. J. Rad. Biol. **6**, 127–136 (1963).

— Savage, J. R. K., Evans, H. J.: Chromatid aberrations in Tradescantia pollen tubes induced by monochromatic X-rays of quantum energy 3 and 1.5 keV. Int. J. Rad. Biol. **8**, 1–19 (1964).

— — Chromosome aberrations and the theory of RBE. II. Evidence from track-segment experiments with protons and alpha particles. Int. J. Rad. Biol. **11**, 209–223 (1966).

— Preston, R. J., Savage, J. R. K.: Chromosome aberrations and the theory of RBE. III. Evidence from experiments with soft X-rays, and a consideration of the effects of hard X-rays. Int. J. Rad. Biol. **12**, 317–345 (1967).

Newcombe, H. B.: The action of X-rays on the cell. II. The external variable. J. Genet. **43**, 237–248 (1942).

Nofal, M. M., Beierwaltes, W. H.: Persistent chromosomal aberrations following radio-iodine therapy. J. Nuclear Med. **5**, 480–485 (1964).

Norman, A.: Multihit aberrations, pp. 53–57. Evans, H. J., Court-Brown, W. M., McLean, A. S., eds.: Human radiation cytogenetics. Amsterdam: North Holland Publ. Co. 1967.

— Ottoman, R. E., Sasaki, M., Veomett, R. C.: The frequency of dicentrics in human leukocytes irradiated in vivo and in vitro. Radiology **83**, 108–110 (1964a).

— Sasaki, M., Ottoman, R. E., Veomett, R. C.: Chromosome aberrations in radiation workers. Radiat. Res. **23**, 282–289 (1964b).

— — — Fingerhut, A. G.: Lymphocyte Lifetime in Women. Science **147**, 745–747 (1965).

— — Chromosome exchange aberrations in human lymphocytes. Int. J. Rad. Biol. **11**, 321–328 (1966).

— — Ottoman, R. E., Fingerhut, A. G.: Elimination of chromosome aberrations from human lymphocytes. Blood **27**, 706–714 (1966).

Nowell, P. C.: Phytohemagglutinin: An initiator of mitosis in cultures of normal human leukocytes. Cancer Res. **20**, 462–466 (1960).

— Unstabile chromosome changes in tuberculin-stimulated leukocyte cultures from irradiated patients. Evidence from immunologically committed, long-lived lymphocytes in human blood. Blood **26**, 798–804 (1965).

— Chromosome aberrations and immunological memory pp. 99–105. Human Radiation Cytogenetics. Evans, H. J., Court-Brown, W. M., McLean,

A. S. (eds.). Amsterdam: North Holland Publishing Co. 1967.

OHNUKI, Y., AWA, A., POMERAT, C. M.: Chromosomal studies on irradiated leukocytes in vitro. Ann. N. Y. Acad. Sci. **95**, 882–900 (1961).

OISHI, H., POMERAT, C. M.: Chromosomal studies on human leukocytes following treatment with Radioactive Iodine in vivo and in vitro. Symp. Inst. Soc. for Cell Biol. **3**, 137–154 (1964).

OLIVER, C. P.: The effect of varying the duration of X-ray treatment upon the frequency of mutations. Science **71**, 44–46 (1930).

— An analysis of the effect of varying the duration of X-ray treatment upon the frequency of mutations. Zschr. indukt. Abstamm.- u. Vererb.-Lehre **61**, 447–488 (1932).

OSGOOD, E. E., KRIPPAEHNE, M. L.: The gradient tissue culture method. Exptl. Cell Res. **9**, 116–127 (1955).

PENDIC, B., DJORDJEVIC, O.: Chromosome aberrations in human subjects five years after whole body irradiation. Jugosl. physiol. et pharmacol. Acta **4**, 231–237 (1968).

POHL-RÜLING, J., POHL, E., FISCHER, P., SAHU, N. K.: Dose estimation for workers exposed to radon 222 inhalation and an investigation of chromosome aberrations in their peripheral blood lymphocytes. Health Physics **19**, 157 (1970).

POPESCU, H. J., STEFANESCU, D. T.: Cytogenetic investigation of industrial workers occupationally exposed to γ-rays. Radiat. Res. **47**, 562–570 (1971).

POWERS, E. L., KALETA, B. F., WEBB, R. S.: Nitric oxide protection against radiation damage. Radiat. Res. **11**, 461 (Abstr.) (1959).

— WEBB, R. S., KALETA, B. F.: Oxygen and nitric oxide as modifiers of radiation injury in spores of Bacillus megaterium. Proc. nat. Acad. Sci. Wash. **46**, 984–992 (1960).

PREMPREE, T., MERZ, T.: Radiosensitivity and repair time: The repair time of chromosome breaks produced during different stages of the cell cycle. Mutat. Res. **7**, 441–451 (1969).

— MICHELSEN, A., MERZ, T.: The repair time of chromosome breaks induced by pulsed X-rays of ultra-high dose rate. Int. J. Rad. Biol. **15**, 571–574 (1969).

READ, J.: Radiation Biology of Vicia faba in Relation to the General Problem. Oxford: Blackwell 1959.

— The induction of chromosome exchange aberrations by ionizing radiations: The "site concept". Int. J. Rad. Biol. **9**, 53–65 (1965).

— Dependence of the numbers of 2-break chromosome aberrations on the size of the dose of ionizing radiation. Radiat. Bot. **6**, 489–498 (1966).

REVELL, S. H.: A new hypothesis for chromatid exchanges. BACQ, Z. M., ALEXANDER, P. (Ed.). Proceedings of the Radiobiological Symposium, Liège. London: Butterworths, pp. 243–253, 1954.

— The accurate estimation of chromatid breakage, and its relevance to a new interpretation of chromatid aberrations induced by ionizing radiations. Proc. Roy. Soc. B. **150**, 563–589 (1959).

— Chromatid aberrations – the generalized theory. WOLFF, S. (Ed.). "Radiation induced chromosome aberrations". New York: Columbia Univ. Press 41–72 (1963).

REVELL, S. H.: Evidence for a dose-squared term in the doseresponse curve for real chromatid discontinuities induced by X-rays, and some theoretical consequences thereof. Mut. Res. **3**, 34–53 (1966).

RIEGER, R., MICHAELIS, A.: Die Chromosomenmutationen. Jena: VEB Gustav Fischer Verlag 1967.

RILEY, H. P., GILES, N. H., BEATTY, A. V.: The effect of oxygen on the induction of chromatid aberrations in Tradescantia microspores by X-irradiation. Am. J. Botany **39**, 592 (1952).

ROSENZWEIG, W., ROSSI, H. H.: Determination of the quality of the absorbed dose delivered by monoenergetic neutrons. Radiat. Res. **10**, 532–544 (1959).

ROSSI, H. H.: Specification of radiation quality. Radiat. Res. **10**, 522 (1959).

— ROSENZWEIG, W.: Limitations of Concept of linear Energy Transfer (LET). Radiology **66**, 105 (1956).

SASAKI, M. S.: Radiation induced chromosome aberrations in lymphocytes. Possible biological dosimeter in man. In Biol. Aspects of radiation protection (SUGAHARA, T., HUG, O. Eds.), Proc. Int. Symp. Kyoto 1969. Igaku Shoin Ltd. Tokyo, 1971.

— MIYATA, H.: Biological dosimetry in atomic bomb survivors. Nature **220**, 1189–1193 (1968).

— NORMAN, A.: Selection against chromosome aberrations in human lymphocytes. Nature **214**, 502–503 (1967).

— OTTOMAN, R. E., NORMAN, A.: Radiation-induced chromosome aberrations in man. Radiology **81**, 652–656 (1963).

— TONOMURA, A., MATSUBARA, S.: Chromosome constitution and its bearing on the chromosomal radiosensitivity in man. Mutat. Res. **10**, 617–633 (1970).

SAVAGE, J. R. K.: Chromosome-exchange sites in Tradescantia paludosa microspores. Int. J. Rad. Biol. **9**, 81–96 (1965).

— Chromatid aberrations induced by 14.1 Mev neutrons in Vicia faba root meristem cells. IAEA Tech. Rep. Ser. **92**, 9 (1968).

— Sites of radiation induced chromosome exchanges. Current topics in Rad. Res. **7** EBERT M., HOWARD A. (Ed.) North Holland Publ. Comp. Amsterdam, London 129–194, 1970.

— PAPWORTH, D. G.: The site distribution parameter for radiation induced chromosome exchanges. J. theoret. Biol. **11**, 1–9 (1966).

— PRESTON, R. J., NEARY, G. J.: Chromatid aberrations in Tradescantia bracteata and a further test of Revell's hypothesis. Mutat. Res. **5**, 47–56 (1968).

SAX, K.: Chromosome aberrations induced by X-rays. Genetics **23**, 494–516 (1938).

— The time factor in X-ray production of chromosome aberrations. Proc. Nat. Acad. Sci. (U.S.) **25**, 225–233 (1939).

— An analysis of X-ray induced chromosomal aberrations in Tradescantia. Genetics **25**, 41–68 (1940).

— Types and frequencies of chromosomal aberrations induced by X-rays. Cold Spring Harbor Symp. Quant. Biol. **9**, 93–101 (1941).

Scheid, W., Traut, H.: Ultraviolet-microscopical studies on achromatic lesions (gaps) induced by X-rays in the chromosomes in Vicia faba. Mutat. Res. 10, 159–161 (1971a).

— — Visualisation by scanning electron microscopy of achromatic lesions (gaps) induced by X-rays in chromosomes of Vicia faba. Mutat. Res 11, 253–255 (1971b).

Schmickel, R.: Chromosome aberrations in leukocytes exposed in vitro to diagnostic levels of X-rays. Am. J. Human Genetics 19, 1–11 (1967).

Schmid, E., Bauchinger, M.: Über das zeitliche Verhalten strahleninduzierter Chromosomenaberrationen beim Menschen. Mutat. Res. 8, 599–611 (1969).

— —Hug,O.: Chromosomenaberrationen menschlicher Lymphocyten nach Röntgenbestrahlung in vitro. I. Qualitative und quantitative Aspekte der Dosis-Wirkungs-Beziehung. Mutat. Res. 16, 307–317 (1972).

Schulte-Brinkmann, W.: Dosisprobleme bei Strahlenschäden des Menschen. Die Medizinische Welt 17, 1567–1575 (1966).

Scott, D., Evans, H. J.: On the non-requirement for deoxyribonucleic acid synthesis in the production of chromosome aberrations by 8-ethoxycaffeine. Mutat. Res. 1, 146–156 (1964).

— — X-ray-induced chromosomal aberrations in Vicia faba: Changes in response during the cell cycle. Mutat. Res. 4, 579–599 (1967).

— The effect of irradiated plasma on normal human chromosomes and its relevance to the long-lived lymphocyte hypothesis. Cell Tissue Kinet. 2, 295–305 (1969).

— Batchelor, A. L., Sharpe, H., Evans, H. J.: RBE for fast neutrons and dose rate studies using fast neutron irradiation. Human Radiation Cytogenetics. Evans, J., Court-Brown, W. M., McLean, A. S., eds. Amsterdam: North Holland Publishing Co., 37–52, 1967.

— Sharpe, H. B., Batchelor, A. L., Evans, H. J., Papworth, D. G.: Radiation-induced chromosome damage in human peripheral blood lymphocytes in vitro. I. RBE and dose-rate studies with fast neutrons. Mutat. Res. 8, 367–381 (1969).

— — — — — Radiation-induced chromosome damage in human peripheral blood lymphocytes in vitro. II. RBE and dose-rate studies with 60 Co γ-X-rays. Mutat. Res. 9, 225–237 (1970).

De Serres, F., Giles, N. H.: The effect of radiation dose fractionation on chromosome aberration frequencies in Tradescantia microspores. I. Studies with X-rays. Genetics 38, 407–415 (1953).

Sevankayev, A. V., Bochkov, N. P.: The effect of gamma rays on human chromosomes. I. The dependence of chromosome aberration frequency upon the dose with irradiation in vitro. Genetika 4, 130–137 (1968).

— Bykhovsky, A. V., Bochkov, N. P.: Investigation of chromosomal aberrations in persons subjected to repeated irradiation associated with their profession. Genetika 5, 126 (1969).

Sharpe, H. B. A., Dolphin, G. W., Dawson, K. B., Field, E. O.: Chromosomal aberration in lymphocytes from an extracorporeally irradiated patient. Lancet II, 1338–1339 (1967).

Sharpe, H. B. A., Dolphin, G. W., Dawson, K. B., Field, E. O.: Methods for computing lymphocyte kinetics in man by analysis of chromosomal aberrations sustained during extracorporeal irradiation of the blood. Cell Tissue Kinet. 1, 263–271 (1968).

— Pitfalls in the use of chromosome aberration analysis for biological radiation dosimetry. Brit. J. Radiol. 42, 943–944 (1969).

— Scott, D., Dolphin, G. W.: Chromosome aberrations induced in human lymphocytes by X-irradiation in vitro: The effect of culture techniques and blood donors on aberration yield. Mutat. Res. 7, 453–461 (1969).

Sheppard, J. S., Ferrari, I.: Stage sensitivity and dose response in human leukocytes. Radiat. Res. 44, 855–866 (1970).

Sidorov, B. N., Sokolov, N. N.: The radiation analysis of chromosome discreteness in the process of autoreproduction. Translation Series: Radiobiology 3, 3 (1963). AEC-tr. 5436, 122–128.

Silberstein, B., I-Wen, Chen, Saenger, E. L.: Cytologic-biochemical radiation dosimeter in man. Biochemical indicators of radiation injury in man. Proc. Symp. Vienna 181–214 (1971).

Sobels, F. H.: Repair and differential radiosensitivity in developing germ cells of Drosophila males. Sobels, F. H. (Ed.), "Repair from Genetic Radiation Damage". Oxford: Pergamon Press 179–197, 1963.

Sparrman, B., Ehrenberg, L., Ehrenberg, A.: Scavenging of free radicals and radiation by nitric oxide in plant seeds. Acta Chem. Scand. 13, 199–200 (1959).

Stadler, L. J.: Mutations in barley induced by X-rays and radium. Science 68, 186–187 (1928).

— The experimental modification of heredity in crop plants. I. Induced chromosomal irregularities. Sci. Agr. 11, 557–572 (1931).

Stadler, L. J.: On the genetic nature of induced mutations in plants. Proceedings 6. Int. Congr. Genetics 1, 274–294 (1932).

Stefanescu, D. T., Teodorescu, M., Popescu, H.J., Brucher, J.: Lack of recovery from radiation induced chromosome damage in G_0 human lymphocytes. Exp. Cell Res. 71, 156–160 (1972).

Stenman, S., Nordling, S., Holsti, L. R., Saksela, E.: Chromosome aberrations induced by X-ray therapy and myxovirus infection in human peripheral leukocytes. Mutat. Res. 10, 607–616 (1970).

Stewart, J. S., Sanderson, A.: Chromosomal aberration after diagnostic X-irradiation. Lancet 1, 978–979 (1961).

Sugahara, T., Doida, Y., Ueno, Y., Hashimoto, T.: Biological dose estimation by means of radiation induced chromosome aberrations in human blood. Nippon Acta Radiologica 25, 42–49 (1965).

— — Sakurai, M.: Chromosome aberrations in accidentally irradiated human subjects. Nippon Acta Radiologica 27, 129–133 (1967).

Swanson, C. P.: The effect of oxygen tension on the production of chromosome breakage by ionizing radiations: An Interpretation. Bacq, Z. M., Alexander, P. (Ed.), "Radiobiology Symp.". London: Butterworth 254–261, 1954.

TANAKA, Y., EPSTEIN, L. B., BRECHER, G., STOHLMAN, F.: Transformation of lymphocytes in cultures of human peripheral blood. Blood **22**, 614–629 (1963).

THODAY, J. M.: The effects of ionizing radiations on the chromosomes of Tradescantia bracteata. A comparison between neutrons and X-rays. J. Genet. **43**, 189–210 (1942).

— The effect of ionizing radiations on the broad bean root. IX. Chromosome breakage and the lethality of ionizing radiations to the root meristem. Brit. J. Radiol. **24**, 572–576, 622–628 (1951).

— READ, J.: Effect of oxygen on the frequency of chromosome aberrations produced by X-rays. Nature **160**, 608 (1947).

— — Effect of oxygen on the frequency of chromosome aberrations produced by alpha-rays. Nature **163**, 133–134 (1949).

TODOROV, S. L., GRIGOR'EV, YU. G., RIZHOV, N. J., IVANOV, B. A., MALYUTINA, T. S., MILEVA, M. S.: Dose response relationship for chromosome aberrations induced by X-rays or 50 MeV protons in human peripheral lymphocytes. Mutat. Res. **15**, 215–220 (1972).

TOUGH, I. S., BUCKTON, K. E., BAIKIE, A. G., COURT-BROWN, W. M.: X-ray induced chromosome damage in man. Lancet **2**, 849–851 (1960).

TSARANOVA, L. L.: A study of chromosomal aberrations in peripheral blood leukocytes after therapeutic irradiation. Medicinskaj Radiologij **4**, 23–30 (1970).

TUSCANY, R., MULLER, J.: Chromosomal study of bone marrow and peripheral blood in persons carrying body burdens of 226 Ra and 90 Sr, pp. 203–207 in Human Radiation Cytogenetics. EVANS, H. J., COURT-BROWN. W. M., MCLEAN, A. S. (eds.). Amsterdam: North Holland Publishing Co. 1967

UNSCEAR-REPORT: Report of the United Nations Scientific Committee on the effects of atomic radiation. General Assembly. 24th Session. Radiation-induced Chromosome aberrations in human cells. Supplement No. 13 (A/7613) United Nations. New York 98–155, 1969.

VISFELDT, J.: Radiation-induced chromosome aberrations in human cells. Doctoral Thesis, published as Risö report No. 117. Danish Atomic Energy Commission, 1966.

— Chromosome aberrations in occupationally exposed personnel in a radiotherapy department. Human Radiation Cytogenetics, EVANS, H. J., COURT-BROWN, W. M., MCLEAN, A. S. (Eds.). Amsterdam: North Holland Publishing Co. 167–173, 1967.

— FRANZEN, S., TRIBUKAIT: Cytogenetic studies in myeloproliferative syndrome and some atypical myeloid disorders. Acta Path. et Microbiol. Scand. **78**, 80–84 (1970).

— — — Primary Polycythaemia. Correlations between the histologic appearences and the chromosome pattern of the bone marrow cells during the disease. Acta Radiologica **10**, 86–114 (1971).

— Primary Polycythaemia. 2. Types of chromosome aberrations in 21 clones found in bone marrow samples from 50 patients. Acta Path. et Microbiol. Scand. Sect. A **79**, 513–523 (1971).

WALD, N., KOIZUMI, A., PAN, S.: A pilot study of the relationship between chromosome aberrations and occupational external and internal radiation exposure. Human Radiation Cytogenetics (EVANS, H. J., COURT-BROWN, W. M., MCLEAN, A. S. (Eds.). Amsterdam: North Holland Publishing Co. 183–193, 1967.

WARREN, S., MEISNER, L. M. A.: Chromosomal Changes in Leukocytes of Patients Receiving Irradiation Therapy. Am. J. Med. Assoc. **193**, 351–358 (1965).

WATSON, G. E., GILLIES, N. E.: The oxygen enhancement ratio for X-ray-induced chromosomal aberrations in cultured human lymphocytes. Int. J. Rad. Biol. **17**, 279–283 (1970).

WILSON, G. B., SPARROW, A. H., POND, V.: Subchromatid rearragements in Trillium erectum. I. Origin and nature of configurations induced by ionizing radiation. Amer. J. Bot. **46**, 309–316 (1959).

WINKELSTEIN, A., CRADDOCK, C. G., MARTIN, D. C., LIBBY, R. L., NORMAN, A., SASAKI, M. S.: 90 Sr 90 Y extracorporeal irradiation in goats and man. Radiat. Res. **31**, 215–229 (1967).

WOLFF, S.: Delay of chromosome rejoining in Vicia faba induced by irradiation. Nature, Lond. **173**, 501 (1954a).

— Some aspects of the chemical protection against radiation damage to Vicia faba chromosomes. Genetics **39**, 356–364 (1954b).

— Progress in radiobiology (ed. MITCHELL, J. S., HOLMES, B. E., SMITH, C. L.) p. 217. Edingburgh: Oliver and Boyd 1956.

— Advances in Radiobiology (Ed.), DE HEVESEY, G. C., FORSSBERG, A. G., ABBATT, J. D., p. 463 Edinburgh: Oliver and Boyd 1957.

— Interpretation of induced chromosome breakage and rejoining. Radiat. Res. Suppl. **1**, 453–462 (1959).

— Chromosome aberrations. HOLLAENDER, A. (Ed.), "Radiation Protection and Recovery", Oxford: Pergamon Press 157–174, 1960a.

— Problems of energy transfer in radiation-induced chromosome damage. Radiat. Res. Suppl. **2**, 122–132 (1960b).

— Radiation studies on the nature of chromosome breakage. Am. Nat. **94**, 85–93 (1960c).

— The doubleness of the chromosome before DNA synthesis as revealed by combined X-ray and tritiated thymidine treatments. Radiat. Res. **14**, 517–518 (1961a).

— Radiation Genetics. ERRERA, M., FORSSBERG, A. (Ed.), "Mechanisms in Radiobiology". New York: Academic Press **1**, 419–476 (1961b).

— Some postirradiation phenomena that affect the induction of chromosome aberrations. J. cell. comp. Physiol. **58** (Suppl. 1), 151–162 (1961c).

— Radiation induced chromosome aberrations. New York and London: Columbia Univ. Press (1963).

— Radiation effects as measured by chromosome damage. Cellular Radiation Biology. Baltimore: William and Wilkins 167–183, 1965.

— Chromosome aberrations and the cell cycle. Radiat. Res. **33**, 609–619 (1968).

— The Splitting of human chromosomes into chromatids in the absence of either DNA- or Protein synthesis. Mutat. Res. **8**, 207–214 (1969a).

Wolff, S.: Strandedness of chromosomes. Intern. Rev. Cytol. **25**, 279–296 (1969b).
— On the "tertiary" structure of chromosomes. Mutation Res. **10**, 405–414 (1970).
— The repair of X-ray-induced chromosome aberrations in stimulated and unstimulated human lymphocytes. Mutat. Res. **15**, 435–444 (1972).
— Atwood, K. C.: Independent X-ray effects on chromosome breakage und reunion. Proc. nat. Acad. Sci., Wash. **40**, 187–192 (1954).
— Luippold, H. E.: Metabolism and chromosome-break rejoining. Science **122**, 231–232 (1955).
— — The production of two chemically different types of chromosomal breaks by ionizing radiations. Proc. nat. Acad. Sci. (Wash.) **42**, 510–514 (1956).
Wolff, S., Luippold, H. E.: Modification of chromosomal aberration yield by postirradiation treatment. Genetics **43**, 493–501 (1958).
— — Chromosome splitting as revealed by combined X-ray and labeling experiments. Exp. Cell Res. **34**, 548–556 (1964).
— Atwood, K. C., Randolph, M. C., Luippold, H. E.: Factors limiting the number of radiation induced chromosome exchanges. I. Distance: Evidence from noninteraction of X-ray-and neutron-induced breaks, J. Biophys. Biochem. Cytol. **4**, 365–372 (1958).
Yuge, J.: Chromosome aberrations induced by internally administered 131 J in man. Ann. Progr. Report **6**, 64–65 (1968).

D. Strahlenwirkung auf extrakaryotische Zellbestandteile

Von

Etta Ullrich-Greve

Mit 20 Abbildungen

I. Relative Empfindlichkeit des extranukleären Zellanteils

1. Direkter Vergleich der Strahlenempfindlichkeit von Plasma und Kern

a) Physiologische Untersuchungen

Wir müssen zunächst die Frage stellen, ob das Cytoplasma überhaupt von Strahlen geschädigt wird, da im allgemeinen die Kernschäden so stark im Vordergrund stehen, daß dem Cytoplasma kaum Aufmerksamkeit geschenkt wird.

Tatsächlich ergaben die ersten Untersuchungen den Eindruck, das Plasma sei völlig strahlenunempfindlich. Zu diesem Schluß kam zunächst G. HERTWIG (1916; zitiert bei PACKARD, 1918) durch einen Versuch mit Froscheiern, die er vor der Befruchtung bestrahlte. Nach schwachen Dosen war die Larvenentwicklung gestört. Nach hohen Dosen verlief sie dagegen normal, nur waren die Larven kleiner und weniger aktiv. Offenbar waren also nach schwachen Dosen strahlengeschädigte weibliche Kerne vorhanden, die die Entwicklung störten, während nach starken Dosen der weibliche Kern ganz ausgeschaltet war, so daß sich androgene Larven mit dem unbestrahlten männlichen Kern ungestört entwickeln konnten. Das besagte aber, daß das bestrahlte Eiplasma nicht geschädigt war. ASTAUROV (1947) kam mit der gleichen Versuchsführung an Seidenspinnerlarven zu demselben Schluß.

Mittlerweile ist es aber WHITING (1949 u. 1955) gelungen, mit einer ähnlichen Versuchsanstellung an Eiern der Schlupfwespe *Habrobracon* auch Plasmaschäden nachzuweisen. Sie bekam zunächst die gleichen Effekte wie HERTWIG und ASTAUROV. Steigerte sie die Strahlendosis aber weiter, so war schließlich auch die Entwicklung der androgenen Männchen gestört, obgleich der männliche Kern nicht bestrahlt war. Dabei kann es sich nur um strahleninduzierte Plasmaschädigungen handeln. Allerdings war die Strahlendosis 20 mal größer als die zur Abtötung des weiblichen Kerns verwendete. Die von HERTWIG und ASTAUROV applizierten Dosen waren demnach vermutlich lediglich zu gering, um einen Effekt am Plasma zu erzielen.

VINTEMBERGER (1928a, b) arbeitete wie HERTWIG an Froscheiern, aber mit einer anderen Versuchsanordnung. Er bestrahlte die Eier im 2-Blastomeren-Stadium zu Beginn der Furchung. Zu diesem Zeitpunkt sind 2 kleine Kerne in einer großen Plasmamenge vorhanden. Da die Lage der Kerne aus der Furchungsebene abzuleiten ist, war es möglich, mit Blei entweder die Kerne abzuschirmen und nur das Plasma zu bestrahlen, oder aber das Plasma abzuschirmen und die Kerne mit nur einer kleinen Menge Plasma zu bestrahlen. Wurde das gesamte Ei oder nur der kernhaltige Teil mit 115 R bestrahlt, starb es am Ende der Furchung. Wurde dagegen nur das Plasma bestrahlt, riefen 350 R noch keine Störung der Entwicklung hervor. Die Dosis war nach WHITINGs Erfahrungen auch zweifellos zu gering. Zum gleichen Ergebnis wie VINTEMBERGER kam HENSHAW (1938) bei partieller Bestrahlung von Seeigel-Eiern, deren Mitose bei Mitbestrahlung des Kerns durch 5700 R verzögert wurde, während bei alleiniger Bestrahlung des Plasmas die gleiche Dosis noch keinen Effekt hatte. Ebenso lokalisierte schließlich Bojansky (1942) bei selektiver Kernbestrahlung in Farnsporen mindestens 95 % der Schädigung im Kern.

Auch diesen Ergebnissen stehen aber eine Reihe entsprechender Untersuchungen an gleichen oder ähnlichen Objekten gegenüber, bei denen sich bei partieller Bestrahlung eine Plasmaschädigung zeigte. So betonte schon Zirkle (1932), daß er bei der Keimung von Farnsporen deutliche Schädigungen beobachtete, auch wenn der Kern nicht getroffen wurde. Miwa u. Mitarb. (1939) bestrahlten wieder Seeigeleier. Sie verwendeten wie Zirkle α-Strahlen, deren Reichweite sie so variierten, daß der Kern in einigen Versuchen nicht mitbestrahlt wurde. Sie fanden bei alleiniger Plasmabestrahlung ebenfalls, daß die Furchung verzögert wurde, falls die Dosis ausreichend hoch gewählt wurde. Petrova (1942a u. b) fand bei der Alge *Zygnema*, daß das 700fache der Dosis, die zum Kerntod führt, bei ausschließlicher Plasmabestrahlung mit α-Strahlen deutliche Letalschäden setzt. — Ulrich (1959), der *Drosophila*-Zygoten mit Röntgenstrahlen behandelte, exponierte jeweils die vordere kernhaltige und die hintere kernfreie Hälfte durch Abschirmung getrennt. Wurde nur das Plasma bestrahlt, war zwar die embryonale und die postembryonale Entwicklung weniger gehemmt, als wenn auch der Kern bestrahlt wurde. Ein Effekt auf das Plasma war aber deutlich erkennbar. Das Verhältnis von Kern- : Plasmaempfindlichkeit betrug an diesem Objekt etwa 1 : 300. Außerdem fand Ulrich auch Unterschiede im zeitlichen Eintritt der strahleninduzierten Letalität. Er lag nach alleiniger Plasmabestrahlung deutlich später.

Die Widersprüche in den Ergebnissen sind also offenbar nur scheinbar und beruhen darauf, daß in den zuerst genannten Arbeiten die verwendeten Dosen zu gering waren, um einen Effekt am Plasma zu erzielen. Es wäre zwar auch denkbar, daß die Unterschiede im Material liegen. Da aber in einigen Fällen die untersuchten Organismen die gleichen waren, fällt diese Möglichkeit weitgehend aus. Es ist noch zu erwägen, ob die Strahlenart eine Rolle spielt, da bei den Versuchen, die einen Effekt auf das Plasma ausübten, meist lokal mit den dichtionisierenden α-Strahlen behandelt wurde. Die einzige Ausnahme von dieser Regel bilden die Versuche H. Ulrichs.

Weitere Hinweise auf die Strahleneffekte auf das Plasma geben die Arbeiten, die wir im Abschnitt über die Wirkung des bestrahlten Plasmas auf den Kern besprechen werden. Versuche, die 2 verschiedene Arbeitsgruppen mit der Alge *Acetabularia* durchführten, geben sogar den Anschein, als ob das Plasma bedeutend strahlenempfindlicher sei als der Kern, was hier zweifellos am untersuchten Material liegt. Es liegen insofern Spezialverhältnisse vor, als es sich um eine Riesenzelle handelt, deren Plasma z. T. räumlich mehrere Zentimeter vom Kern entfernt ist. Wird dieses kernfreie Plasma allein bestrahlt, so degeneriert es bei Dosen, die im Bereich des Kernes noch keine Schädigungen hervorrufen (Bacq u. Mitarb., 1957). Nach denselben Autoren führen Dosen bis 240 R, auf den kernhaltigen Teil gegeben, sogar zu einer Degeneration des kernfernen Plasmas, während der bestrahlte kernhaltige Teil die Regenerationsfähigkeit behält. Six (1956), der ebenfalls eine Degeneration des kernfreien Plasmas, und zwar proportional zur applizierten Dosis, beobachtete, vermutet, daß die Enzyme des Plasmas zerstört werden. Diese Theorie wird durch den Befund gestützt, daß kernfreie Plasmastücke ohne Bestrahlung nach langer Abtrennung vom kernhaltigen Teil die gleichen Degenerationserscheinungen zeigen. Plasmadegenerationserscheinungen nach Kernbestrahlung, die Bacq u. Mitarb. beschreiben, müßten dann auf einer zumindest vorübergehend gehemmten Enzymlieferung aus der Kernregion beruhen. Jedenfalls scheint der Kern in diesem Objekt aber ungewöhnlich strahlenresistent zu sein.

b) Cytologische Untersuchungen

Bislang befaßten wir uns mit Schädigungen, die sich in physiologischen Vorgängen bemerkbar machten. Von verschiedenen Autoren wurde aber auch das cytologische Bild nach getrennter Kern- und Plasmabestrahlung beobachtet. Zirkle u. Bloom (1953),

Bloom u. Mitarb. (1955) und Bloom (1959) konnten durch lokalisierte Bestrahlung mit „microbeams" einzelne Chromosomen oder begrenzte Plasmapartien bestrahlen. Sie konnten bereits mit sehr geringen Dosen Veränderungen an den bestrahlten Chromosomen feststellen, während die 100fache Strahlenmenge am Cytoplasma keine sichtbare Veränderung hervorrief. — Munro (1959) beobachtete allerdings bei zwar sehr starker, aber auch streng lokalisierter Bestrahlung, daß die betroffenen Plasmapartien granulär wurden.

2. Wechselwirkung zwischen bestrahlten und unbestrahlten Zellteilen

a) Plasma-Plasma-Wirkung

Es ist ersichtlich, daß bei streng lokaler Plasmabestrahlung weniger Plasmaschäden auftreten als bei Ganzzellbestrahlung, und zwar sowohl physiologisch als auch cytologisch. Dafür gibt es 2 Erklärungen: Entweder wirkt sich bei Mitbestrahlung des Kerns dessen Schädigung sekundär auch auf das Plasma aus (diese Reaktionen gehören aber nicht in den Rahmen dieses Kapitels) oder es wirkt auf der anderen Seite bei streng lokaler Plasmabestrahlung das reichlich vorhandene, unbestrahlte Plasma kompensierend.

Einen solchen kompensierenden Effekt konnte Daniels (1951, 1952, 1954) an Amoeben nachweisen. Er stellte fest, daß bei Mischung von bestrahltem und unbestrahltem Plasma die Zellen sich wie unbestrahlte verhielten, während bestrahltes Plasma allein deutlich geschädigt war. Hier liegt also eine Art heilende Wirkung vor. Daniels u. Roth (1961) konnten durch fraktioniertes Zentrifugieren des unbestrahlten Plasmas diesen heilenden Effekt sogar lokalisieren, und zwar in der Fraktion, die Mitochondrien und Pinozytosebläschen enthält. Sie vermuten, daß die heilende Wirkung den Mitochondrien zukommt. Zur gleichen Vermutung gelangte Goldfeder (1961), die eine höhere Strahlenempfindlichkeit spindelförmiger gegenüber epithelförmigen Tumorzellen der Maus fand und sie mit der geringeren Mitochondrienzahl der spindelförmigen Zellen erklärte.

b) Plasma-Kern-Wirkung

Aus einer größeren Zahl von Versuchen läßt sich auch auf eine indirekte Schädigung des Kerns durch das bestrahlte Plasma schließen. Zwar konnte Munro (1959) an Kükenfibroblasten nach streng lokaler Plasmabestrahlung keine Veränderung am Kern feststellen, ebensowenig wie Zirkle u. Bloom (1953) und Bloom u. Mitarb. (1955). In diesen Fällen war aber reichlich unbestrahltes Plasma vorhanden, das also wieder eine heilende Wirkung ausüben konnte. Duryee (1949—1950), der Kern und Plasma von Amphibien-Eizellen getrennt bestrahlte, wobei das gesamte Plasma getroffen wurde, beobachtete dann auch nach Injektion des unbestrahlten Kerns in bestrahltes Plasma pyknotische Veränderungen des Kerns.

Zu entsprechenden Ergebnissen führten Versuche von Patterson (1931), von Bonnier u. Lüning (1951, 1952) und Bonnier (1952) an *Drosophila melanogaster*. Sie fanden eine verstärkte Eliminierung des unbestrahlten männlichen x-Chromosoms in bestrahltem Eiplasma. Außerdem fanden Bonnier u. Lüning (1952) an *Drosophila* und Nakao (1953) an Seidenspinnerlarven eine erhöhte Mutationsrate im männlichen x-Chromosom, wenn nur das Ei bestrahlt war. — Whiting (1950a u. b) untersuchte allerdings an *Habrobracon* wiederholt die Möglichkeit, daß vom bestrahlten Plasma Mutationen im androgenen Männchen erzeugt würden, immer mit einem vollkommen negativen Ergebnis. Möglicherweise ist das aber damit zu erklären, daß bei *Habrobracon* die Zeitspanne zwischen Bestrahlung des Eis und Eintritt des Spermiums zu lang war. Versuche von Ord u. Danielli (1956) zeigten nämlich, daß der schädigende Einfluß des bestrahlten Plasmas auf den Kern nur vorübergehend zu bestehen braucht. Wenn sie in eine kernfreie Zelle von *Amoeba proteus* während der ersten 18 Stunden nach Bestrahlung einen unbestrahlten Kern injizierten, kam es zu keiner Klonbildung[1]. Wurde der Kern erst nach 18—48 Stunden injiziert, waren 80 % der Zellen wieder zur Klonbildung[1] fähig. Das Plasma scheint demnach nur während der ersten Stunden nach Bestrahlung schädigend auf den Kern zu wirken. Allerdings scheint der Zeitraum von 1 Stunde zwischen Bestrahlung und Befruchtung des *Habrobracon*-Eies bei Whiting reichlich kurz für das völlige Abklingen des Effektes.

Insgesamt läßt sich einwandfrei feststellen, daß das Plasma bedeutend strahlenresistenter ist als der Kern, daß es aber eindeutig zu schädigen ist. Für die höhere Resistenz ist eine Reihe von Erklärungen anzuführen. So sind die einzelnen Plasmakomponenten im Gegensatz zu den Chromosomen des Kerns meist in großer Zahl vorhanden und die Schädigung eines Teils von ihnen braucht keine feststellbare Wirkung auf die Gesamtzelle zu haben. Außerdem ist vielleicht keine der Plasmakomponenten so streng durchkonstruiert und damit so leicht aus dem Normalzustand zu bringen wie die Chromosomen des Kerns. — Schließlich führen Schjeide u. Mitarb. (1956) noch die Möglichkeit an, daß die Enzyme der Atmungskette, die im Plasma reichlich vorhanden sind, strahleninduzierte oxydierende Radikale sofort wieder abbauen, ehe sie einen Schaden verursacht haben, während dem Kern diese Enzyme fehlen, so daß die Radikale dort zur Wirkung kommen könnten. Dem widerspricht allerdings der Befund Nickels (1961), der bei *Paramaecium* die ersten Schädigungen ausgerechnet an den Mitochondrien, die ja die Enzyme der Atmungskette tragen, gesehen haben will. Darauf sollen die Plasma- und zuletzt die Kernschäden erst folgen. Dieser letzte Punkt widerspricht allerdings allen anderen Angaben. Eine wichtige Rolle der Mitochondrien bei der Strahlenschädigung der Zelle vermuten allerdings auch Scherer u. Völker (1960), indem sie angeben, daß die später zu beschreibenden Strukturänderungen der Mitochondrien, Änderungen im Enzymsystem nach sich ziehen, die dann sekundär den gesamten Energiehaushalt der Zelle stören würden. Mit diesen Befunden scheint auch die bereits beschriebene heilende Wirkung der unbestrahlten Mitochondrienfraktion auf das Cytoplasma übereinzustimmen (s. S. 183).

II. Das Grundplasma

Das Grundplasma, das die Zellorganelle umgibt, erscheint lichtoptisch strukturlos und im elektronenoptischen Bereich jedenfalls ohne distinkte Strukturen. Änderungen durch ionisierende Strahlen können sich daher entweder außerhalb des sichtbaren Bereiches als Änderungen der physikalisch-chemischen Eigenschaften bemerkbar machen oder im optischen Bereich in Form neu auftretender Ablagerungen, Entmischungen oder Ähnlichem.

1. Viskositätsänderung

a) Allgemein

Im physikalisch-chemischen Bereich äußert sich der Strahlenschaden in veränderter Plasma-Viskosität. Im typischen Fall wird die Viskosität gesteigert. Nach sehr schwachen Bestrahlungen kann sie aber auch abnehmen. So ergab auch die erste Viskositätsmessung nach Bestrahlung mit Röntgenstrahlen (Lopriore, 1897) eine Minderung. Dieser Befund wurde in der Folge an verschiedensten Objekten bestätigt (Williams, 1925; Zuelzer u. Philipps, 1925; Feichtinger, 1933). Northen u. McVicar (1940) fanden bei der Alge *Spirogyra* sogar bis 5000 R eine verminderte Viskosität. Offenbar kann die Viskosität eventuell sogar bis zur Verflüssigung herabgesetzt sein (Feichtinger, 1933). Durch starke Bestrahlung wird der entgegengesetzte Effekt bewirkt, und im Extremfall erstarrt das Plasma. Diese Beobachtung machte Feichtinger ebenfalls, und zwar wieder an *Spirogyra* in einem Vergleich zu dem Versuch mit schwacher Bestrahlung. Weber (1923) hatte einen solchen Effekt am gleichen Objekt bereits beschrieben. Er konnte allerdings weder

---

1 Klon = Population, die aus einer Einzelzelle hervorgegangen ist.

an *Phaseolus*-Stärkescheiden noch an *Vicia faba*-Wurzelhauben eine Viskositätsänderung feststellen. Offenbar waren diese Objekte aber ungeeignet, entweder wegen höherer Strahlenresistenz oder — wahrscheinlicher — weil die angewendete Meßmethode hier ungünstig war. (WEBER benutzte die Zentrifugierungsmethode, wobei sich Stärkekörner oder sonstige Einschlüsse in der Zelle verlagern. Möglicherweise ist aber die Stärke in diesen Objekten zu dicht gepackt.)

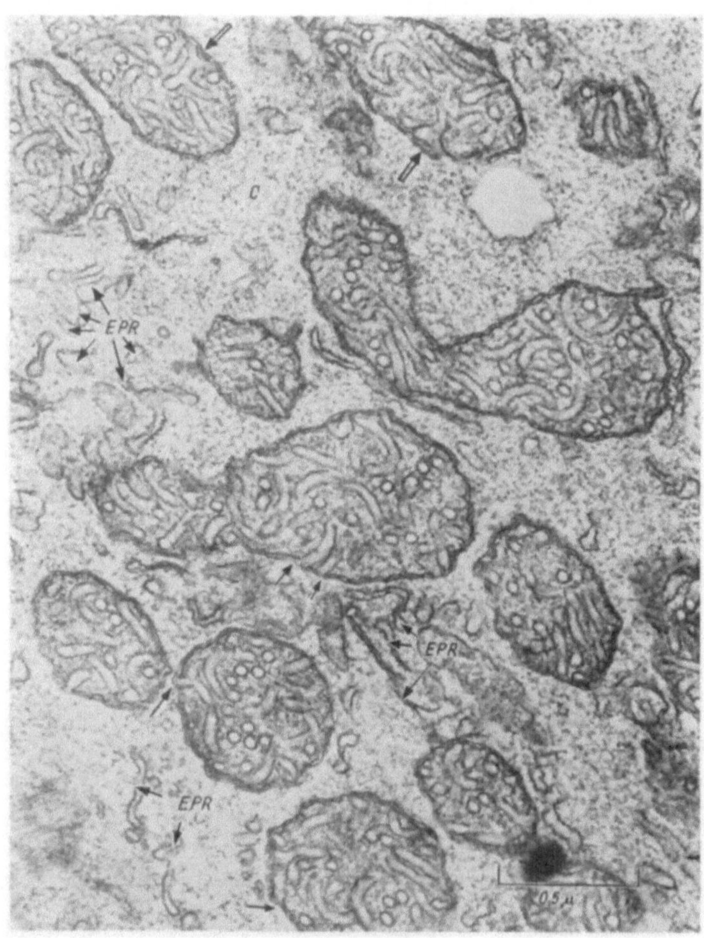

Abb. 1. Normalstruktur der Mitochondrien im unbestrahlten Cytoplasma von *Paramaecium* (Kontrollpräparat). Die Mitochondrien zeigen das bei Protisten allgemein verbreitete, tubuläre Bauprinzip. Die Membranen der *Tubuli mitochondriales* inserieren am inneren Blatt der doppelten Mitochondrien-Hüllmembran (Pfeilmarkierungen). Die Querschnitte der *Tubuli* ergeben, daß es sich dabei um kreisrunde Schläuche handelt. Verzweigungen der Schläuche können gelegentlich gefunden werden (Doppelpfeilmarkierung). Das Grundcytoplasma (C) läßt den nach Vestopal-Einbettung beschriebenen Aufbau (SCHNEIDER, 1959a) aus „granulär-fädigen" Elementen erkennen. Es wird durchzogen von schlauchförmigen, polymorphen Elementen des „Endoplasmatischen Retikulums" (EPR). *Paramaecium aurelia*, Präparationstechnik s. Text. Fixationsgemisch pH 7,07. Elektronenoptisch (E.O.) 13200:1; Endvergrößerung (E.V.) 36800:1. Aus WOHLFAHRT-BOTTERMANN u. SCHNEIDER, Strahlenther. **116**, 25 (1961)

In verschiedenen Arbeiten wird als Frühwirkung starker Bestrahlung eine vorübergehende Viskositätsabnahme beschrieben, der eine Zunahme folgt (WILLIAMS, 1923; ROCHLIN-GLEICHGEWICHT, 1930; NADSON u. ROCHLIN, 1934; SEIFRIZ, 1936).

In manchen Fällen wird auch ein wiederholter Wechsel von Viskositätszu- und -abnahme beobachtet (HERČIK, 1938; NORTHEN u. McVICAR, 1940). Sowohl HERČIK als auch NORTHEN und McVICAR beobachteten aber im Endeffekt immer eine erhöhte Viskosität.

Den bisher erwähnten Untersuchungen lagen lichtoptische Beobachtungen zugrunde. Nach Altmann (1955) sind Viskositätsänderungen des Plasmas aber auch im Elektronenmikroskop festzustellen, und zwar erscheint hochvisköses Plasma dichter als niedervisköses. Entsprechende Änderungen der Strukturdichte wurden vor allem von Schneider (1960, 1961a, b) an *Paramaecium* nach hohen Dosen sowohl als Früh- als auch als Spätschaden beschrieben (Abb. 1 u. 2). Wichtermann u. Figge beschrieben eine größere

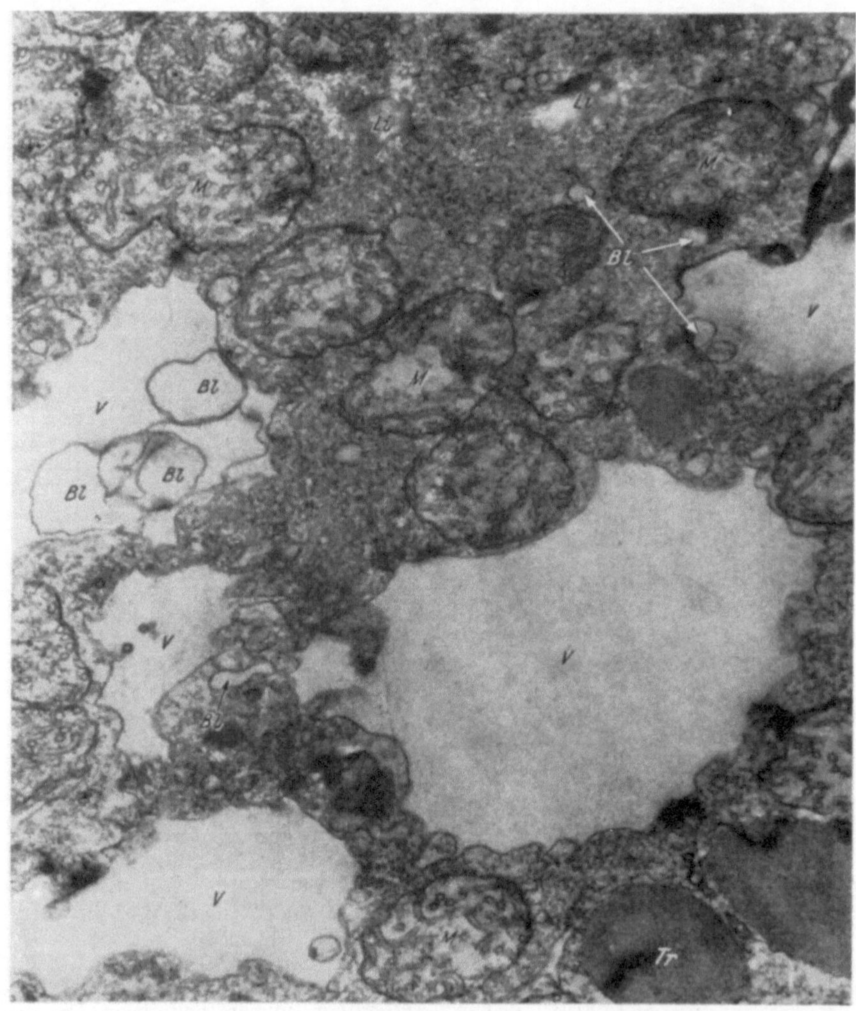

Abb. 2. Cytoplasma nach Einwirkung einer letalen Röntgendosis von 250000 R (= 62½ min Bestrahlungsdauer) im Stadium der Strahlenlähmung. Das Cytoplasma zeigt eine auffallende Strukturdichte (Koagulationsnekrose), unterbrochen von auffallend großen Vakuolen V (Entmischung), die anscheinend teils aus Fusion mehrerer kleiner Bläschen (Bl. links oben) entstanden sind. Die Mitochondrien (M) sind angeschwollen. Li Lipoidtropfen, Tr Trichozysten, Bl Röntgenbläschen. Fixationsgemisch pH 7,08. E.O. 6800:1; E.V. 22800:1. Aus: Schneider, Protoplasma **53**, 530 (1961a)

Strukturdichte des Plasmas am gleichen Objekt bereits 1954 und ebenso Nickel 1961. Braun u. Müller (1961) fanden die gleiche Wirkung auch an Leberzellen der Maus.

Schneider (1961a, b) beschreibt außerdem Plasmaareale, die von Doppelmembranen umschlossen werden und in denen zunächst eine besonders starke Plasmaverdichtung festzustellen ist (s. S. 192 zu Abb. 7).

Nach Parchwitz (1963) können elektronenoptisch wahrnehmbare Strukturverdichtungen des Cytoplasmas von Tumorzellen der Ratte als Folge verstärkter Ausschleusung

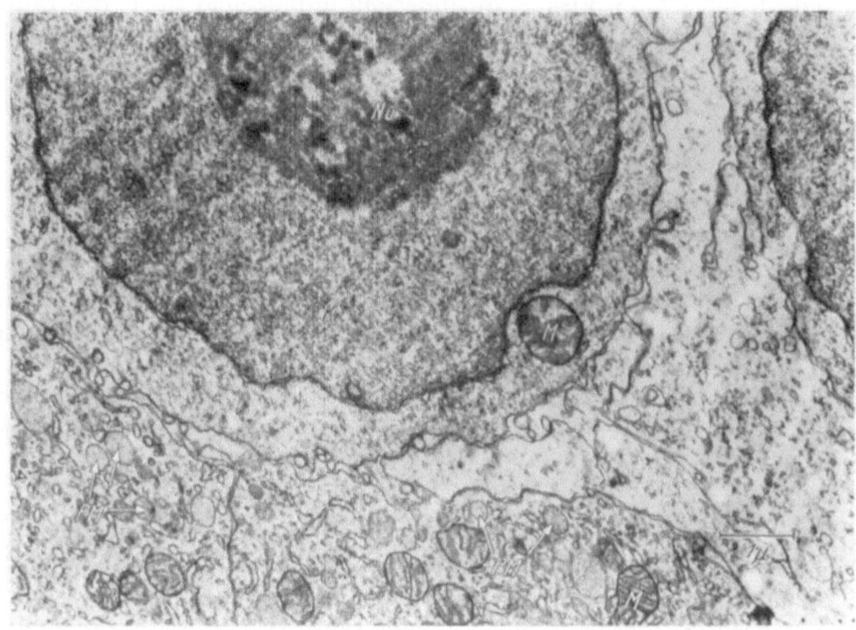

Abb. 3. Walker-Carcinomzelle, unbestrahlt; annähernd runder Kern (K) mit zentralständigem Nukleolus (Nu);
im Cytoplasma Mitochondrien (M) mit meist gut ausgebildeten Cristae mitochondriales und Promitochondrien
(PM); relativ geringe Entwicklung des Ergastoplasmas. E.O. 6100:1; E.V. 10000:1. Aus: PARCHWITZ, in:
SCHERER u. STENDER, Strahlenpathologie der Zelle. (G. Thieme, Stuttgart 1963)

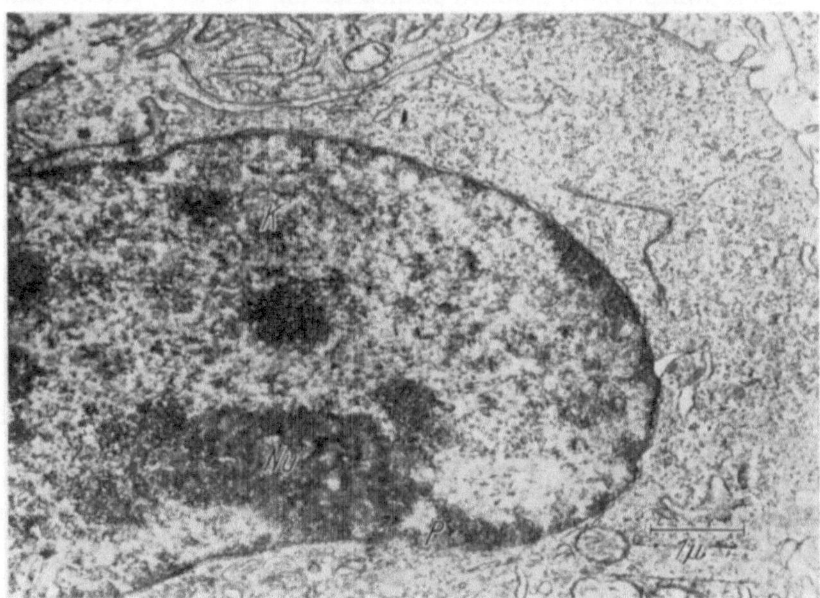

Abb. 4. Walker-Carcinomzelle, 6 Stunden nach Bestrahlung (5000 R HD); Extrusion nukleären Materials durch
einen Porus (P) in der Kernmembran; starke Vermehrung der Ribosomen im Cytoplasma. E.O. 6100:1; E.V.
13000:1. Aus: PARCHWITZ, in: SCHERER u. STENDER, Strahlenpathologie der Zelle. (G. Thieme, Stuttgart 1963)

von Ribosomen aus dem Kern während der ersten Stunden nach Bestrahlung (Abb. 3 u. 4)
auftreten. Später gab der Kern überhaupt keine Ribosomen mehr an das Plasma ab, so
daß es an RNS verarmte (6 Tage nach Bestrahlung). Diese Strukturverdichtungen dürften
kaum etwas mit Viskositätszunahme zu tun haben und bieten also möglicherweise Anlaß
zu Verwechslungen.

Ganz allgemein scheint die Viskositätsänderung unmittelbar nach Bestrahlung innerhalb weniger Minuten einzusetzen und dann über Stunden anzuhalten, sofern sie überhaupt reversibel ist.

Es gibt verschiedene Möglichkeiten, die beschriebenen Viskositätsänderungen zu erklären. Durch Ionisation können die Molekularstrukturen verändert werden. Da es sich beim Cytoplasma um Strukturviskosität handelt, wäre allein dadurch eine Viskositätsänderung möglich. Hinzu kommt, daß die Hydratur mit den Ladungs- und Strukturänderungen der Eiweißmoleküle variiert und damit der Anteil freien Wassers. Tatsächlich sind die Faktoren, welche die Viskosität bedingen, zu zahlreich, als daß man die Reaktionen im einzelnen klären könnte. Daß das gleiche Agens, — hier die ionisierenden Strahlen — in geringen Dosen zur Verminderung, in hohen Dosen zur Erhöhung der Viskosität führt, läßt sich zweifellos auch aus diesem Umstand herleiten.

Auf eine weitere Möglichkeit, den Viskositätswechsel zu erklären, weist Heilbrunn (1958) hin. Er nimmt an, daß Calcium, das normalerweise nicht in die Zelle eindringen kann, sondern in der Plasmamembran festgehalten wird, durch die Bestrahlung aus seiner Bindung gelöst und in das Plasma abgegeben wird. Geringe Mengen Ca^{++} im Plasma würden zu einer Viskositätsverminderung führen, große Mengen zur Vakuolenbildung und damit zur Viskositätssteigerung. Auch so wäre die entgegengesetzte Wirkung von schwacher und starker Bestrahlung erklärbar, zumal Vakuolenbildung auch als Folge von Bestrahlung beobachtet wird (S. 189). Heilbrunn sieht seine Hypothese außerdem durch den Befund Rochlin-Gleichgewichts (1930) bestätigt, die nach Bestrahlung der Pflanzen *Elodea* und *Pteridophyllum* in den oxalsäurehaltigen Vakuolen Ca-Oxalatkristalle fand. Heilbrunn macht allerdings selbst die Einschränkung, daß diese Deutung nur zutreffen kann, falls das Ca^{++} ursprünglich an strahlenempfindliche Moleküle gebunden ist.

Virgin u. Ehrenberg (1953) nehmen schließlich an, daß die Viskositätsänderung auf einer stimulierenden Wirkung der ionisierenden Strahlen beruht. Sie führten der Wasserpflanze *Elodea* radioaktive Isotope zu, woraus sich eine andauernde Bestrahlung mit sehr geringen Dosen ergab. Mit ^{35}S und ^{22}Na normalisierte sich die Viskosität nach einmaligem Wechsel von niedrig zu hoch innerhalb von 2 Stunden wieder, obgleich die Bestrahlung weiter anhielt. Bei stärkerer Bestrahlung durch ^{32}P folgte ein 2. Viskositätswechsel. Nach 12 Stunden waren die Verhältnisse aber auch hier wieder normal. Virgin u. Ehrenberg schließen aus diesem Gewöhnungseffekt, daß diese Reaktion hormonell gesteuert sein könnte.

b) Viskositätsänderung während der Zellteilung

Noch eine besondere Form der strahleninduzierten Viskositätssteigerung wurde an den Eiern verschiedener Meerestiere beobachtet. Unbefruchtete Eier von *Arbacia*, *Chaetopteris* und *Nereis* ändern ihre Viskosität nach Bestrahlung zunächst nicht. Wenn die bestrahlten Eier aber befruchtet werden, wird die Viskosität, die normalerweise während der nun folgenden Mitose zunimmt, stärker und anhaltender gesteigert als bei der Kontrolle (Wilson, 1950; Wilbur u. Recknagel, 1943; Forbes u. Thacher, 1925). Rieser (1955), der mit unbefruchteten Eiern arbeitete, fand bei *Arbacia* und *Chaetopteris* ebenfalls keine Viskositätsänderung, dagegen aber wohl bei unbefruchteten *Asterias*-Eiern. In diesen Eiern läuft die Reifeteilung erst nach der Ablage ab. Sie steigert demnach die Viskosität in der gleichen Weise wie die späteren Mitosen.

Auch in diesem Fall ist der Strahleneffekt noch nicht endgültig zu erklären. Wilson (1950) vermutet, daß durch die Strahlen eine Substanz zerstört wird, die die Gelation in normalen Zellen auflöst. Rieser u. Kaye (1953), die an bestrahlten Muskelzellen der Muschel *Spisula* ähnliche mitose-abhängige Viskositätsänderungen fanden, nehmen an, daß solch ein gelationsauflösender Stoff infolge Bestrahlung aus der Zelle ausgeschieden wird. Diese Erklärungen gewinnen durch einen weiteren Befund Wilsons noch an Wahrscheinlichkeit, der feststellte, daß auch die Befruchtung unbestrahlter Eier mit bestrahlten Spermien zu einer anormal gesteigerten Viskosität führt. Die gelationslösenden Stoffe sollen aber normalerweise von den Chromosomen abgegeben werden.

2. Plasmakoagulation

Bei starker Bestrahlung und daraus folgender starker Ionisation der Proteinmoleküle kann letzten Endes das Eiweiß denaturiert werden, wie RAJEWSKY (1929) in vitro zeigte. In der Zelle muß diese Denaturierung zu Plasmaausflockungen führen. Dementsprechend wurden Plasmakoagulationen, auch körniger Zerfall oder Granulation genannt, beschrieben. An Pflanzenzellen wurde diese Erscheinung schon sehr früh beobachtet, so von FEICHTINGER (1932) an *Crepis*-Wurzeln, von BIEBL (1935) und HERČIK (1938) an *Allium*-Epidermen, von SEIFRIZ (1936) an Myxomyzeten. SCHERER u. WICHMANN (1954) stellten dann auch an Milzzellen der Maus nach Applikation verschiedener Dosen von 100—800 R Koagulation fest, die um so früher einsetzte, je stärker bestrahlt wurde. Bei irreversibler Schädigung von *Paramaecium caudatum* fanden auch WICHTERMANN u. FIGGE (1954) Plasmakoagulation. FEICHTINGER beobachtete, daß bei Verwendung von β-Strahlen die Koagulation erst nach höheren Dosen einsetzte als bei α-Strahlen, zweifellos eine Folge der größeren Ionisationsdichte von α-Strahlen.

Auch die Größe der Granula variiert in Abhängigkeit von der Dosis. BIEBL (1935) fand nach relativ schwacher Bestrahlung einen grobkörnigeren Zerfall als nach starken Dosen. Entsprechend beobachtete SEIFRIZ (1936) in der Nähe des radioaktiven Präparates, also dort, wo die Bestrahlung am stärksten war, eine feinere Granulierung als in größerer Entfernung.

Einige Autoren beschreiben auch lokale Koagulation, obgleich die ganze Zelle bestrahlt wurde. So tritt nach HERČIK die Granulation zuerst in Kernnähe auf. Nach STRUGGER u. Mitarb. (1953) kann sie ebenfalls streng lokal sein und braucht sich nicht über die ganze Zelle auszubreiten. Eine Korrelation zur Lage des Kernes fanden sie aber nicht. FEICHTINGER (1933) gibt andererseits an, daß nach lokaler α-Bestrahlung, die nur etwa $^1/_5$ der Zelle trifft, der Strahleneffekt sich mit einiger Verzögerung über die ganze Zelle ausbreitet. Im allgemeinen scheint das Plasma nur nach starken Dosen zu koagulieren. Diese Schädigung ist dann offenbar meist irreversibel. Nach NADSON (1925) kommt aber offenbar auch eine Erholung von Zellen mit koaguliertem Plasma vor.

3. Vakuolisation

Etwa gleichzeitig mit der Koagulation, manchmal aber auch bei nur gesteigerter Viskosität, erscheinen vermehrte und vergrößerte Vakuolen im Plasma (WILLIAMS, 1923 u. 1925; NADSON, 1925; LEVINE, 1926; FEICHTINGER, 1932; POMERAT, 1958).

SCHNEIDER (1960, 1961a) fand im elektronenmikroskopischen Bild bereits unmittelbar nach Bestrahlung kleine Röntgenbläschen. Dabei war es gleichgültig, ob er mit verträglichen Dosen etwa 20 Minuten oder mit der extrem hohen Dosis von 10^6 R/min 1 Minute lang bestrahlte. Die Bläschen waren unmittelbar nach Bestrahlung zumindest schon zu erkennen. Nach 4 Minuten mit 4 Millionen R waren sie mit Membranen fertig ausgebildet. Aus der Lagerung der Bläschen zueinander schließt SCHNEIDER, daß sie später zu Vakuolen zusammenlaufen, die lichtoptisch sichtbar sind. Die Vakuolen können dann mehrere Tage erhalten bleiben, ehe sie vom Plasma wieder resorbiert werden, was auch nur geschieht, sofern kein Letalschaden induziert wurde (Abb. 5). Während lichtoptisch die Vakuolen erst zu beobachten sind, wenn zumindest die Viskosität des Plasmas gesteigert ist, fand SCHNEIDER eine Strukturverdichtung des Plasmas nur nach sehr hohen Dosen, die Bläschen aber schon nach den niedersten der verwendeten Dosen.

Außerdem konnten GLAUSER (1956) an Rattenleberzellen und später WOHLFAHRT-BOTTERMANN (1959) an Paramaecien mit Hilfe des Elektronenmikroskops winzige Bläschen von $0,5\,\mu$ Durchmesser beobachten, die häufig in Reihen entlang einer Doppelmembran angeordnet waren (Abb. 6).

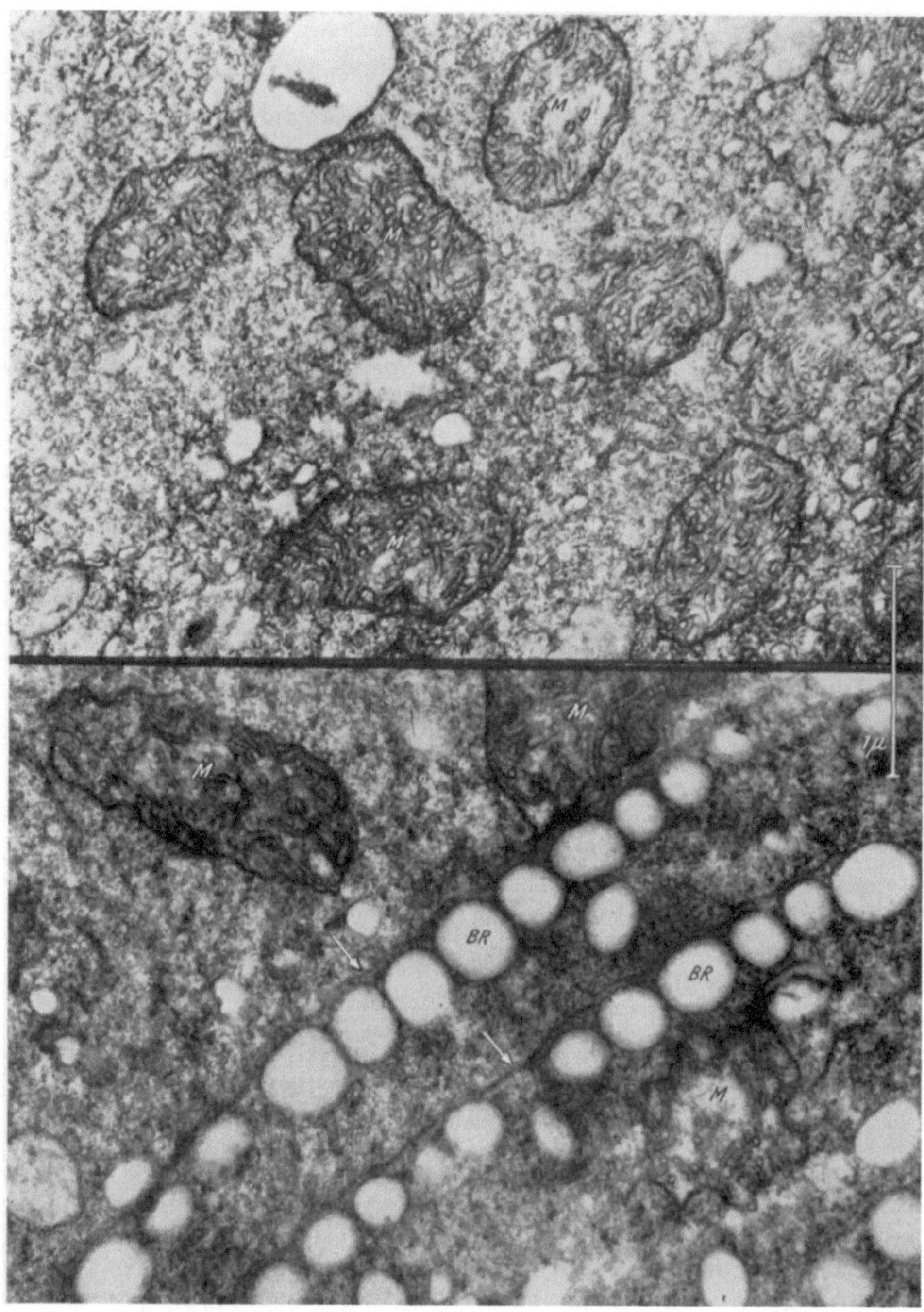

Abb. 5. Oben: Kontrollpräparat. Normale Mitochondrien (M) und Cytoplasma einer unbehandelten Zelle. Unten: Mitochondrien und Cytoplasma nach Einwirkung einer letalen Röntgendosis. Alle Strukturen mit verringertem Elektronenkontrast. Mitochondrien (M) strukturell unverändert. Im Cytoplasma zwei längs angeschnittene Bläschenreihen (BR). Fixation unmittelbar nach Beginn der Lähmungsphase. Elektronenoptisch 11 400 : 1. Endvergrößerung 23 200 : 1. Aus Wohlfahrt-Bottermann, Protoplasma **50**, 82 (1959)

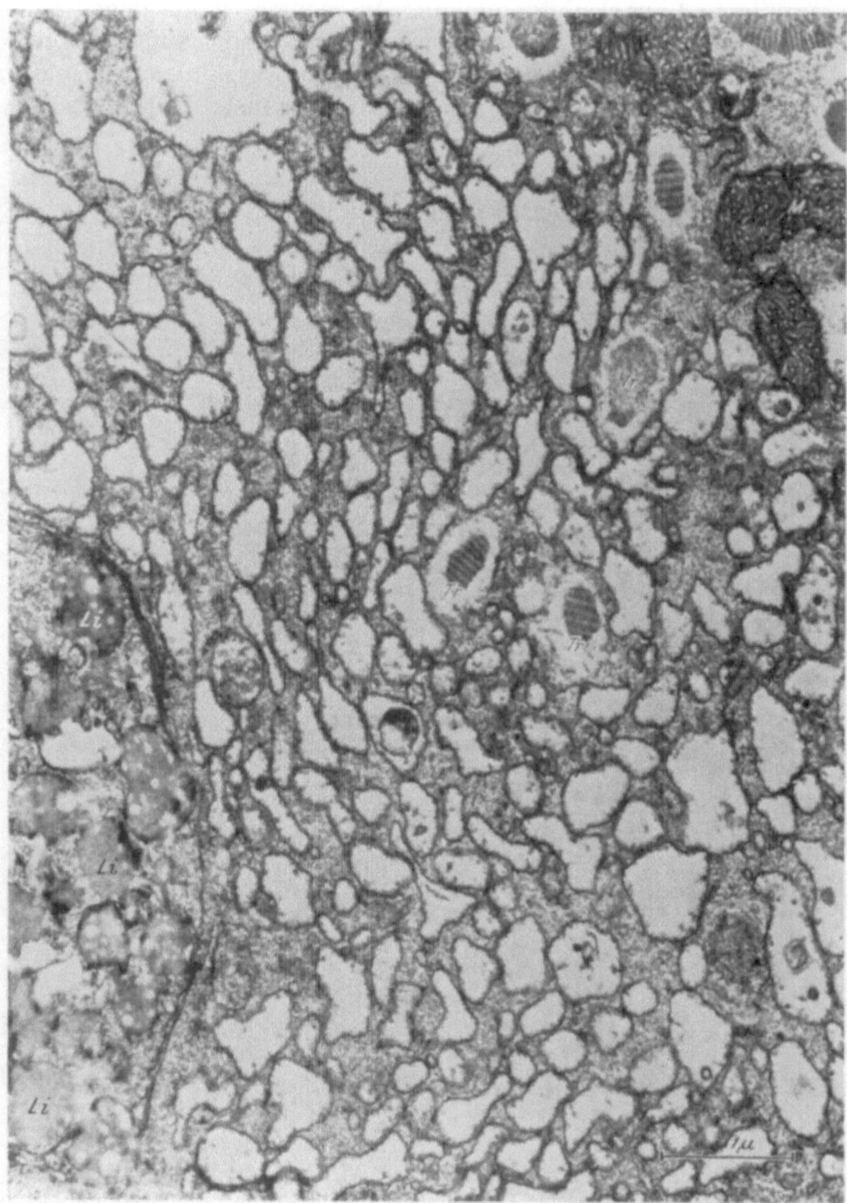

Abb. 6. Cytoplasma 10 Stunden nach Einwirkung einer verträglichen Röntgendosis (150000 R) fixiert. Die Ansammlung von Röntgenbläschen, Vakuolen und Degenerationsvakuolen liegen jetzt in der Mitte der Paramaecienzellen. Sie stehen mit ihren Membranen oftmals in engem Kontakt, was auf ein späteres Verschmelzen zu großen Vakuolen hindeutet.
Tr: Triochcysten, Li: Lipoidtropfen. Fixationsgemisch pH 6,98. E.O. 6900:1; E.V. 22000:1. Aus: SCHNEIDER, Protoplasma **53**. 554 (1961 b)

In dem bereits erwähnten Sonderfall WOHLFAHRT-BOTTERMANNs u. SCHNEIDERs (Abb. 1) und SCHNEIDERs (1961 b), daß Plasmaareale von Doppelmembranen umgeben werden, folgt auf die beschriebene anfängliche Strukturverdichtung des eingeschlossenen Plasmas eine Auflösung, und zwar ausnahmslos (Abb. 7). So bleiben schließlich Flüssigkeitsvakuolen zurück. SCHNEIDER vermutet, daß auch diese Vakuolen resorbiert werden. Er hält diesen Weg jedenfalls für wahrscheinlicher als die andere Möglichkeit, daß sie durch den Cytopharynx entleert werden, da er diesen Vorgang nie beobachten konnte.

Für die verstärkte Vakuolenbildung kommen mehrere Erklärungen in Frage. Wir wiesen schon im Zusammenhang mit der Viskositätsänderung auf 2 Möglichkeiten hin, das waren die veränderte Wasserbindungsfähigkeit der Eiweißmoleküle und die Abgabe von Ca-Ionen ins Zellinnere, wo sie Wasser um sich sammeln. Eine weitere Möglichkeit

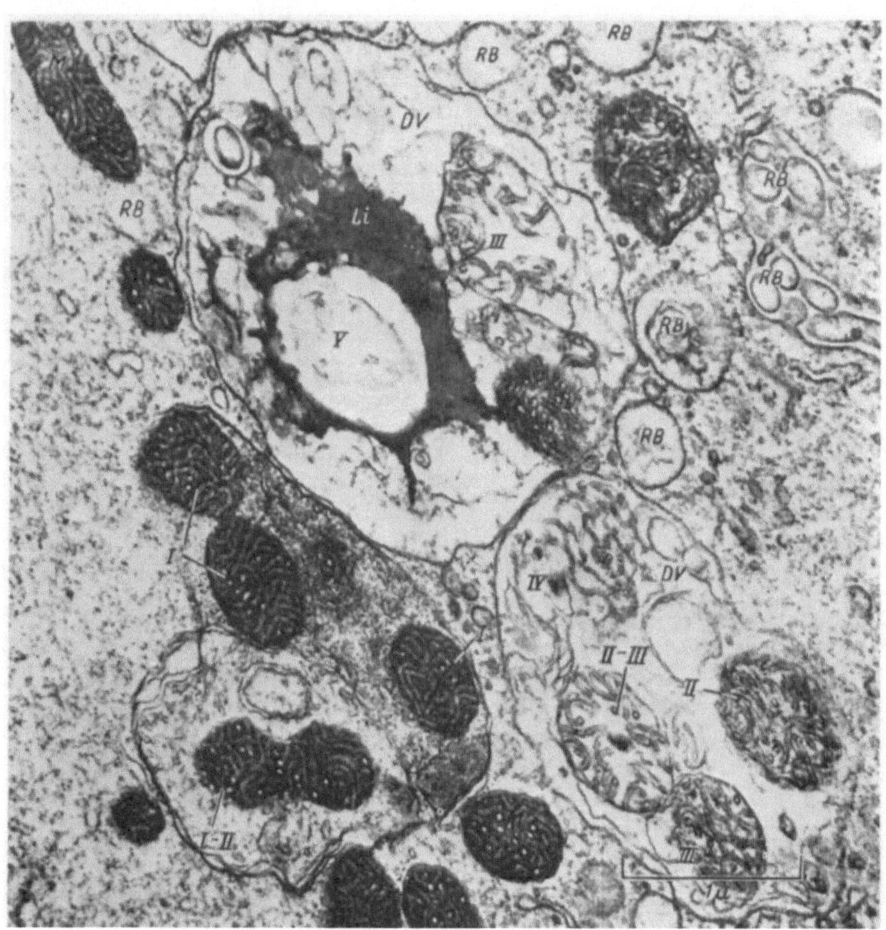

Abb. 7. Mitochondrien, 2 Stunden nach Einwirkung einer verträglichen Röntgendosis (150 000 R). Neben einigen „frei" im Cytoplasma liegenden „normalen" Mitochondrien (M) finden sich vermehrt die charakteristischen Anfangsstadien (I) einer Degeneration in Form von Mitochondrien, die in verdichtetes, von Membranen umgebenes Cytoplasma eingeschlossen sind. Bei der darauf einsetzenden Degeneration wird anscheinend zuerst das Grundcytoplasma abgebaut, denn in den nun entstandenen „Degenerationsvakuolen" (DV) lassen sich elektronenoptisch keine Cytoplasmaelemente mehr nachweisen. Dadurch können die verschiedenen Zerfallsstadien der Mitochondrien besonders gut erfaßt werden. Bei dieser Art der Mitochondrien-Degeneration wird zunächst das äußere Blatt der doppelten Hüllmembran aufgelöst (II), dann folgt das innere Blatt (III), wodurch nur noch die „losen" Tubuli *mitochondriales* übrigbleiben (IV), die aber letztlich auch noch völlig abgebaut werden (V). Häufig findet man in den Degenerations-Vakuolen Lipoid-Anhäufungen (Li), die auf eine Entmischung der Mitochondrien-Bausteine schließen lassen. RB Röntgenbläschen im Grundcytoplasma. *P. aurelia*; Fixationsgemisch pH 6,98. E.O. 6900:1; E.V. 24000:1. Aus: Wohlfahrt-Bottermann und Schneider, Strahlenther. **116**, 25 (1961)

liegt in der veränderten Permeabilität der Plasmamembran, die zu einer erhöhten Wasseraufnahme führt. Wir werden darauf noch im nächsten Kapitel zu sprechen kommen. Schließlich ist es denkbar, daß der Stoffwechsel der Zelle derart gestört ist, daß Wasser im Überschuß gebildet wird.

4. Fettablagerung

Neben den wäßrigen Vakuolen treten nach Bestrahlung häufig auch vermehrte und vergrößerte Fettropfen auf, offenbar meist gleichzeitig mit den Vakuolen. NADSON (1925) beobachtete 10 min nach Bestrahlung Vakuolen und Fettropfen. Die Fettropfen nahmen

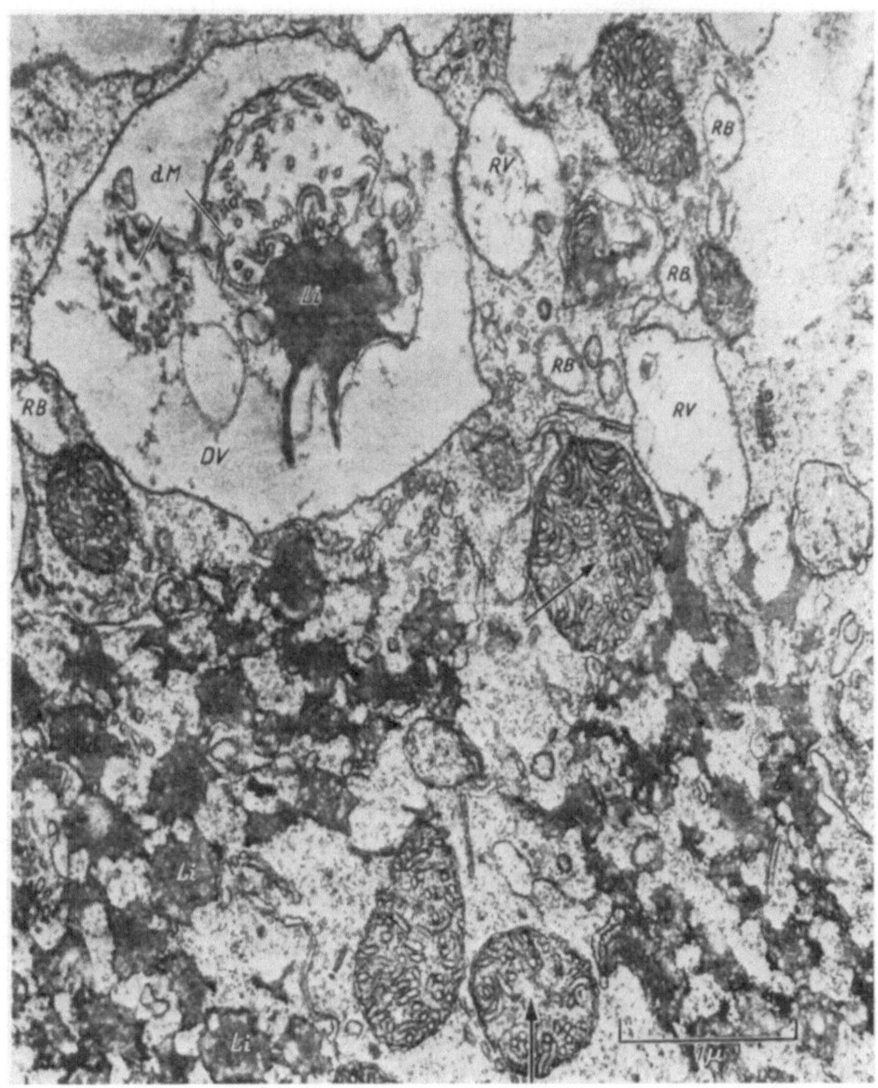

Abb. 8. Mitochondrien 4 Stunden nach Einwirkung einer verträglichen Röntgendosis (150000 R). Auch in diesem Stadium finden sich zahlreiche Degenerationsvakuolen (DV) mit degenerierenden Mitochondrien (dM). In dem großen Mitochondrium in der linken oberen Bildecke liegt wiederum ein Lipoidtropfen (Li). Auch im Grundcytoplasma zeigen sich Ansammlungen von Lipoidtropfen (Li), die auf einen gestörten Fettstoffwechsel (Zellverfettung) schließen lassen. Neben „morphologisch normalen" Mitochondrien kommen auch noch Mitochondrien mit zentraler Aufhellung (Pfeilmarkierungen) vor, die auf eine leichte Schwellung hindeutet. RV Röntgenvakuolen, RB Röngenbläschen. *P. aurelia*; Fixationsgemisch pH 6,98. E.O. 6900:1; E.V. 24000:1. Aus: WOHLFAHRT-BOTTERMANN u. SCHNEIDER, Strahlenther. **116**, 25 (1961)

24 Stunden nach Bestrahlung noch weiter zu. NADSON u. ROCHLIN (1934) fanden diese Erscheinungen an *Allium*-Epidermiszellen 2—3 Stunden nach Bestrahlung und WOHLFAHRT-BOTTERMANN u. SCHNEIDER (1961) bei *Paramaecium* 4 Stunden nach Bestrahlung, wenn mit verträglichen Dosen bestrahlt worden war. Nach WOHLFAHRT-BOTTERMANN u. SCHNEI-

der können die Lipoidtropfen in sich wieder vakuolisiert sein (Abb. 8). Fetttropfen nehmen häufig über Tage zu. Hampton u. Quastler (1958) fanden noch 3 Tage nach Bestrahlung in Darmepithelzellen der Maus zahlreiche Fetttropfen. Glauser konnte dagegen an Rattenlebern keine Fettabsonderung feststellen.

Die Ursache der Fettabscheidung kann wieder eine Entmischung infolge der Eiweiß-koagulation sein. Das häufig gleichzeitige Auftreten beider könnte als eine Bestätigung dieser These gelten. Die Fettabsonderung kann aber auch auf einer Stoffwechselstörung beruhen, also wiederum eine Möglichkeit, die auch für die Vakuolenbildung in Frage kam und das gleichzeitige Auftreten rechtfertigen würde.

Speziell bei der Fetttropfenbildung spricht für die Annahme eines gestörten Metabolismus noch die Tatsache, daß nach Bestrahlung Fetttropfen auch in den Mitochondrien beobachtet wurden (S. 208), in denen die Fette normalerweise oxydiert werden.

Zusammenfassend sei noch einmal darauf hingewiesen, wie unterschiedlich die Plasmareaktionen sein können. Sie können sich bereits in den verschiedenen Organen des gleichen Tieres unterscheiden, wie besonders gut aus Tab. 1 hervorgeht.

III. Membranstrukturen

1. Die äußere Plasmamembran

Die cytologische Struktur der Plasmamembran ist erst durch die Elektronenmikroskopie geklärt worden. Sie stellt sich als Doppelmembran von etwa 150—180 Å Dicke dar. Wie weit diesem Bild die Verhältnisse in vivo entsprechen, ist ebenso fraglich wie bei allen anderen cytologischen Bildern fixierter Präparate. Die Tatsache, daß sich ähnliche Doppelmembranstrukturen auch im Plasma in Form des endoplasmatischen Retikulums und vor allem in so regelmäßig gebauten Strukturen wie den Mitochondrien wiederfinden, spricht allerdings für eine in vivo-Präformation.

a) Cytologische Beobachtungen

Cytologische Beobachtungen an äußeren Zellmembranen nach Bestrahlung liegen noch kaum vor. Nur Glauser (1956) gibt an, daß der Abstand der Lamellen sich stellenweise vakuolär erweitert. Elektronenoptische Aufsichtsbilder speziell von bestrahlten Erythrozyten-Membranen sind nicht sehr befriedigend, da die Membranen schon unter normalen Bedingungen verschiedene Bilder ergeben (Hoffmann, 1956). Zacek u. Rosenberg (1956) wollen allerdings nach Bestrahlung Löcher in den Membranen der ungeschwollenen Erythrozyten beobachtet haben, während Lessler (1959) Faltungen beschreibt, die aber eine Sekundärreaktion auf das veränderte Volumen der Erythrozyten nach Bestrahlung sein dürften. Daß die Zelloberfläche sich ändert, geht außerdem aus veränderten Eigenschaften, wie erhöhter Brüchigkeit und Klebrigwerden, hervor (Rieser, 1955; Ord u. Danielli, 1956). In einer weiteren Arbeit von Lessler u. Herrera (1962) bemerken die Autoren kurz, daß in Dünnschnitten von Froscherythrozyten die äußere Membran geklumpt aussieht. (Erythrozyten-Dünnschnitte sind sonst noch nicht gelungen.)

b) Permeabilitätsänderungen

Um über den Strahlenschaden an Zellmembranen mehr zu erfahren, sind wir auf indirekte Indizien angewiesen, wie sie sich aus Änderungen der physiologischen Wirksamkeit der Membran, also ihrer Permeabilität, ableiten lassen.

Allerdings wird die Aussagekraft dieses Testes dadurch beeinträchtigt, daß es bislang noch nicht möglich war, die passive und aktive, energieabhängige Permeation von Stoffen durch die Zellmembran klar zu unterscheiden. Außerdem herrscht auch über die Wege der aktiven Stoffaufnahme noch Unklarheit.

Tabelle 1. *Effekt von 100 R Röntgen-Ganzkörperbestrahlung auf verschiedene Organe der Maus.* Aus SCHERER u. VOGELL (1958)

	1 Stunde	24 Stunden	3 Tage	7 Tage
Leber *Kern:*	Geringe Chromatinvergröberung. Kernmembran verdichtet. Randständige Nukleolarsubstanz.	Starke Quellung, Kernmembran aufgelockert und teilweise unterbrochen.	Große, oft randständige Nukleolen, Knäuel- und Radspeichenstruktur der Nukleolen. Membran gewellt, teilweise sehr dicht oder aufgerissen.	Struktur fast normalisiert, ebenso Kernmembran. Nukleolen noch teilweise grob klumpig.
Mitochondrien:	Struktur erhalten, Klumpenbildung, Anlagerung an den Kern.	Plump. Struktur teilweise zerstört. Klumpenbildung.	Vakuolenbildung, Doppelkonturierung, Septen zerstört.	Eher kleiner als vorher, verdichtet. Struktur meist wiederhergestellt.
Plasma:	Grundplasma grobwabiger.	Zunehmende Vakuolisierung, dichtes endoplasmatisches Netzwerk um die M. herum.	Weitere Vergröberung, ausgeprägte Doppellamellen sichtbar.	Immer noch deutl. Netzwerk kleinvakuolig verändert.
Niere *Kern:*	Aufgelockert, Kernmembran etwas gewellt und verdichtet.	Nukleolen meist vermindert oder verteilte Nukleolarsubstanz. Kernmembran wie bei 1 Stunde, nur an wenigen Stellen etwas aufgefasert.	Kernwand verdichtet, Membran wellig, aufgerissen. Kerne ödematös.	Weitgehende Normalisierung im Nukleolenbild. Kernmembran glatt.
Mitochondrien:	Tendenz zur Verklumpung, Quellungsneigung, Septen oft deutlicher, zuweilen kleinste Vakuolen.	Vergrößert. verklumpt, doppelkonturiert. Mitochondrienstruktur unregelmäßig, aber noch erhalten. Auch kleinste Vakuolen.	Kleine Vakuolen, Doppelkonturierung. Septenstruktur unregelmäßig. grob. teils verwaschen.	M. haben noch etwas verwaschene Struktur, aber sonst normale Form und Größe. Selten noch Vakuolen. Einzelne M. in Auflösung begriffen.
Plasma:	Bürstensaum unversehrt, Doppellamellen nicht verändert.	Zellgrenzflächen unversehrt. Plasmaretikulum tritt stärker hervor.	Insgesamt zerrissen, vakuolig. Bürstensaum unscharf, aufgefasert.	Grenzflächen wiederhergestellt, auffallend kräftig dargestellte Doppellamellen.
Milz *Kern:*	Grobe Zerstörung vieler Kerne, randständige Nukleolen.	Kernmembran bei erhaltenen Kernen recht dicht und deutlich.	Dichte Kernwand, wandständige große Nukleolen, aber insgesamt starke Zerstörung, Retikulumzellen besser erhalten.	Kernregeneration, glattere Kernwand, Normalisierung des Nukleolarapparates.
Mitochondrien:	In der Nähe stark zerstörter Kerne keine sichtbaren M. Sonst plumpe M., vereinzelt noch Struktur.	Sehr wenig zahlreich, gestaltlos, „ballonartig“, vereinzelte Vakuolisierung.	Nur gelegentlich Innenstruktur, sonst unscharfe, aufgetriebene, ballonförmige Körperchen. Bei Retikulumzellen besser erhaltene M.	Teilweise schon fast normale, teils aber noch reichlich grobvakuolig veränderte geblähte M.
Plasma:	Zerreißt bei der Fixation im Gegensatz zu den parenchymatösen Organen, Mitochondrien frei in Zellkernnähe zu beobachten.			

13*

Das bestuntersuchte Objekt in bezug auf strahleninduzierte Permeabilitätsänderung sind die Säugetier-Erythrozyten. Es war schon seit den frühesten Zeiten der Röntgenologie bekannt, daß Bestrahlungen zur Hämolyse führen können. Holthusen (1923) beobachtete dann erstmals, daß der Eintritt der Strahlenhämolyse von der Zusammensetzung des Mediums, in dem die Erythrozyten suspendiert sind, abhängt. Dieser Befund wurde von Lehmann u. Wels (1926) dahingehend präzisiert, daß nach Bestrahlung in isotonischer Kochsalzlösung zwar Hämolyse stattfindet, aber nicht nach Bestrahlung in isotonischer Glucose-Lösung. Von Ting u. Zirkle (1940a, b) wurde dieser Befund bestätigt und dahingehend ergänzt, daß speziell die Kationen-Abgabe aus den Zellen, vor allem diejenige von K^+, gesteigert ist. Da man damals noch einen rein passiven Stoffaustausch voraussetzte, rechneten sie mit einer entsprechenden beschleunigten K^+-Aufnahme. Von diesem Standpunkt aus waren alle vorausgehenden Befunde mit einer erhöhten Permeabilität für passiv ausgetauschte Ionen vereinbar. Sheppard u. Beyl (1951) wendeten dann erstmals radioaktives ^{42}K für die Untersuchungen der Strahlenhämolyse an. Dabei fanden sie, entsprechend Ting u. Zirkle, die K^+-Abgabe gesteigert. Im Gegensatz zu den bis dahin geltenden Annahmen war aber die ^{42}K-Aufnahme nach Bestrahlung unverändert. Sheppard u. Beyl schlossen daraus auf einen gestörten K^+-Akkumulationsmechanismus. Damit wurde erstmals die Möglichkeit ins Auge gefaßt, daß ein energieabhängiger Prozeß gestört sei. Sheppard u. Steward konnten die Energieabhängigkeit des Austausches dadurch nachweisen, daß sie die Erythrozyten niederen Temperaturen aussetzten, bei denen die energieliefernden Vorgänge verlangsamt wurden. Unter diesen Bedingungen fanden sie wieder eine beschleunigte K^+-Abgabe, allerdings offenbar auch eine beschleunigte Na^+-Abgabe. Daß bei Kältebehandlung von Erythrozyten die K^+-Abgabe verstärkt ist, hatte auch Maizel (1951) schon festgestellt. Er hatte außerdem beobachtet, daß Zuckermangel, also der Mangel einer Energiequelle, den gleichen Effekt hat. Allerdings nimmt er nicht an, daß die Energie zur K^+-Akkumulation benutzt wird, sondern seine Versuche zeigen, ebenso wie die von Hodgkin (1947), daß die Energie vor allem zur Na^+-Ausscheidung aus der Zelle verwendet wird, woraus zwangsläufig eine Aufnahme von K^+ folgt, wenn das osmotische Gleichgewicht aufrechterhalten bleiben soll. Maizel wies durch Hemmungsexperimente weiterhin nach, daß die Energie durch Glykolyse gewonnen wird, was insofern wichtig ist, als Säugererythrozyten Energie nur aus der Glykolyse zur Verfügung haben.

Nach Altmann (1955) ist es außerdem typisch für ernergetisch gestörte Zellen, daß sie zunächst schrumpfen und später schwellen. Dieser Effekt ist zwar noch nicht zu erklären. Er wurde aber auch nach Bestrahlung beobachtet. Ein weiterer Hinweis also, daß hier energieabhängige Prozesse geschädigt sind (Williams, 1925; Buchsbaum u. Zirkle, 1949; Parsons, 1962).

Der Ausgleich des K^+-Na^+-Ungleichgewichtes infolge Bestrahlung wurde noch von zahlreichen Autoren beschrieben, sowohl an Erythrozyten als auch an anderen Zellen. An Erythrozyten fanden Bühlmann u. Mitarb. (1942) und Morzek (1955) gesteigerte K^+-Abgabe, außerdem Rothstein u. Bruce (1958) und Rothstein (1959) das gleiche an Hefen, Ellinwood u. Mitarb. (1957) an Kaninchen- und Hundeherzen und Bergeder (1958) und Darden (1960) an quergestreifter Muskulatur. Neuerdings konnte die K^+-Abgabe auch noch indirekt nachgewiesen werden. Bergeder (1961) und offenbar auch Bohomolets (1961) gelang es an Froschmuskeln, nach Bestrahlung einen Ausgleich der Potentialdifferenz festzustellen, die durch den K^+-Überschuß in der Zelle zustande kommt.

Es erhebt sich nun die Frage nach dem Ort der primären Schädigung dieser energieabhängigen Permeation. In 2 Arbeiten mit Erythrozytenmembranen, „ghosts" genannt, die durch hypotonische Glykolyse gewonnen wurden, zeigen die ghosts noch die volle Funktion des Stofftransportes (Hoffmann, 1962).

Man muß im Hinblick auf die Signifikanz dieser Versuche allerdings die Einschränkung machen, daß nicht mit Sicherheit zu entscheiden ist, ob die ghosts wirklich nur aus der

Membran bestehen oder ob Plasmareste erhalten bleiben, an die die energetischen Prozesse gebunden sein könnten. Die endgültige Entscheidung über den Ort der primären Schädigung muß also noch offen bleiben.

Unabhängig davon, ob die primäre Schädigung tatsächlich in der Membran erfolgt oder ob die hier auftretenden Änderungen bereits sekundär sind, müssen wir weiter fragen, ob spezifische Moleküle der Membran betroffen sind — etwa die Carrier-Moleküle oder Enzyme — oder ob die Gesamtstruktur der Plasmamembran gestört ist, zu deren Erhaltung ebenfalls Energie nötig ist.

Wenn spezifische Einzelmoleküle angegriffen werden, sollte man annehmen, daß auch die Aufnahme oder Abgabe spezieller Stoffe beeinflußt wird. Das ist nun offenbar der Fall bei dem K^+-Na^+-Austausch. Der verminderte K^+-Gehalt und ebenso womöglich die durch die Na^+-Aufnahme bedingte Wasserzufuhr würden dann die weiteren physiologischen Schäden möglicherweise nur zur Folge haben. So schieben DOSE u. BRESCIANI (1959) den völligen Zusammenbruch des Energiestoffwechsels bei Rattendiaphragmen und Froschherzventrikeln nach Röntgenbestrahlung auf den K^+-Verlust. Es ist aber bis jetzt nicht gelungen abzuklären, ob die nach Bestrahlung erhöhte Permeabilität für Wasser und Anelektrolyte tatsächlich nur eine solche Folgeerscheinung ist, oder ob sie unabhängig als Parallelreaktion auftritt. Das würde dann für einen primären allgemeinen Zusammenbruch der Membranstruktur sprechen.

TING u. ZIRKLE (1940) beobachteten, daß Erythrozyten Wasser, Thioharnstoff und Äthylenglycol nach Bestrahlung verstärkt aufnahmen, und zwar nach Applikation der gleichen Strahlendosis, die auch die K^+-Abgabe verstärkte. Vor allem die Wasseraufnahme war um 20 % heraufgesetzt. Ähnliche Beobachtungen machte BIEBL (1941). Umgekehrt wurde oft verstärkte Stoffabgabe aus den Zellen beobachtet, so von WEIJER an *Neurospora*-Konidien und von MAGATH (1930) an Rattenleberschnitten, deren Phosphatabgabe gesteigert war. BILLEN u. Mitarb. (1957) fanden ebenfalls erhöhte Stoffabgaben, und zwar ATP, Aminosäurefragmente und freie Basen. Da zumindest die ATP-Abgabe bei BILLEN nur unter Bedingungen auftrat, die einen ATP-Umsatz zuließen, könnte hier auch eine Entkoppelung in den energieübertragenden Prozessen vorliegen, in deren Folge mehr ungebundenes ATP anfällt, das dann in verstärktem Maße aus der Zelle austritt. Womöglich beruht die Störung der energieabhängigen Permeationsvorgänge sogar auf einer solchen Entkoppelung, und nicht auf der Störung der primären energieliefernden Prozesse. Diese Annahme wird von dem Befund GREENS (1956) gestützt, der feststellte, daß der energieliefernde Prozeß, die Glykolyse, durch Strahlendosen nicht angegriffen wird, die den K^+-Na^+-Austausch bereits stark beschleunigen.

Es erscheint außerdem nicht ausgeschlossen, daß zumindest in Erythrozyten, die Permeabilitätsänderung durch ähnliche Vorgänge zustande kommt wie der Potentialausgleich der Nervenzellen bei Reizung. Allerdings ist noch unsicher, ob die Acetylcholinesterase in Erythrozyten vorkommt. In diesem Zusammenhang scheint es jedenfalls interessant, daß JÄRNEFELT (1961) es für möglich hält, daß der Na^+-Transport an den Acetylcholinkreislauf gebunden ist.

CALI u. VERGA (1960) halten die Depolimerisation der Grundsubstanz für die Ursache der erhöhten Permeabilität von Mesenterienkapillarwänden für Farbstoffe, und auch BERGEDER sieht hierin die primäre oder sekundäre Ursache für den Potentialausgleich der Muskelzellen.

WEIJER (1961) konnte zeigen, daß die Stoffabgabe nach Bestrahlung durch Zusatz von Ca^{++}-Ionen zum Bestrahlungsmedium herabgesetzt ist. Es liegt nahe, daß die Ca^{++}-Wirkung hier die gleiche ist wie bei dem bekannten heilenden Effekt bei mechanischen Membranverletzungen, bei dem zweifellos die Zweiwertigkeit des Ca^{++} eine Rolle spielt. Falls die Hypothese stimmt, daß Viskositätsänderungen des Plasmas z. T. durch Ca-Ionen ausgelöst werden, die von der Membran abgegeben werden, wäre die heilende Wirkung einer ergänzenden Ca^{++}-Versorgung für die Membran besonders gut verständlich. Es wäre aber durchaus verfrüht, hier irgendwelche endgültige Schlüsse zu ziehen.

Bergeder (1963) erwägt, ob etwa strahleninduzierte Membranschäden allgemein für die Strahlenschädigung von Organen und Geweben verantwortlich gemacht werden können. Dies zu entscheiden werden noch zahlreiche Untersuchungen nötig sein.

2. Das endoplasmatische Retikulum (EPR)

Zuerst beschrieben Scherer u. Vogell (1958) strahleninduzierte Veränderungen am endoplasmatischen Retikulum (EPR) in Leber- und Nierenzellen von Mäusen nach Applikation von 100 R. Demnach nimmt das Netzwerk des EPR nach Bestrahlung insge-

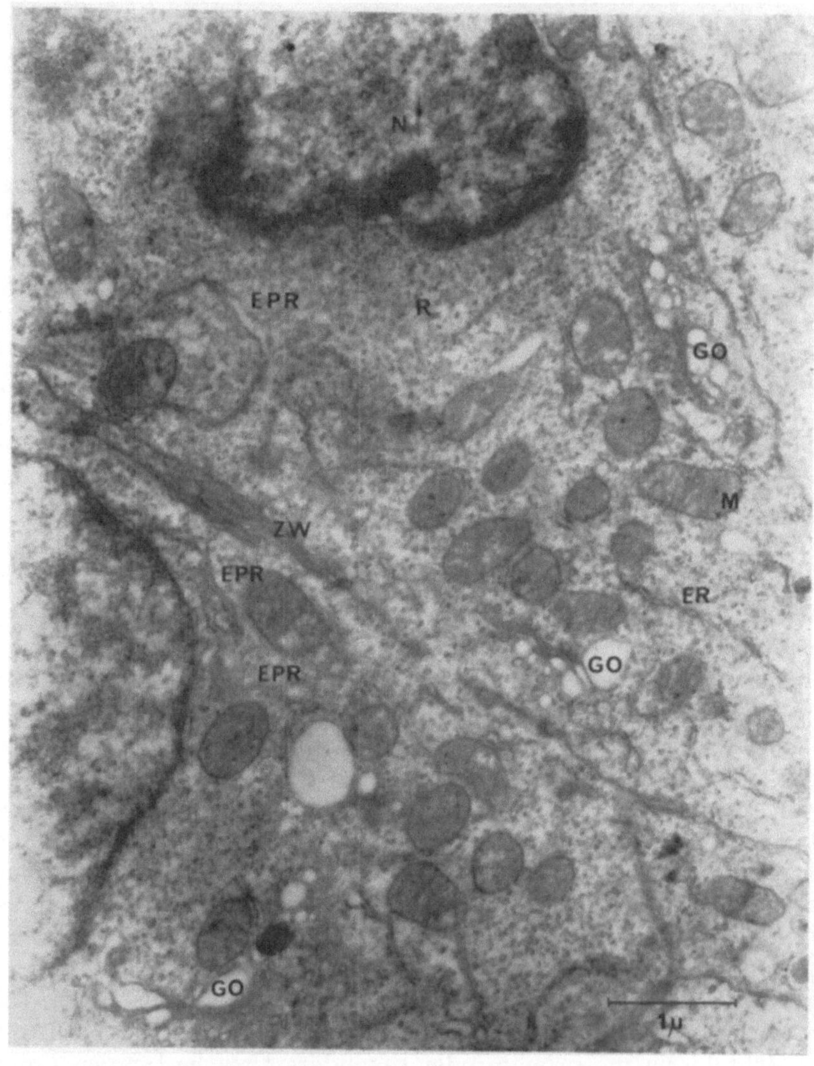

Abb. 9. Dünndarmepithel der Maus, unbestrahlt. Mitochondrien (M), Ribosomen (R), endoplasmatisches Retikulum (EPR), Zellkern (N), Golgikörper (Go), Zellwand (ZW). Vergr. 16800fach. (Nach Braun, H. unveröffentlicht)

samt zu und tritt u. U. stärker hervor. Sie geben allerdings an, daß es in beiden Zellarten längere Zeit nach Bestrahlung (3 Tage) kleinwabig bzw. vakuolig zerrissen ist. Eine Vakuolisation des EPR, bzw. eine Abrundung beschreiben auch McQuade u. Evans (1959) an Schilddrüsen nach 13 min Bestrahlung. Je größer die Dosis war, desto kleiner und zahlreicher wurden die Bläschen. HAMPTON u. QUASTLER (1960) sprechen mehr allgemein von einem desorganisierten EPR, das schließlich fragmentiert bleibt. SCHNEIDER (1961a) fand an Paramaecien mit sehr hohen Dosen, die er wegen der Strahlenresistenz dieser Einzeller anwendete (ca. 200 kR), ebenfalls vermehrtes EPR. Vakuolige Erwei-

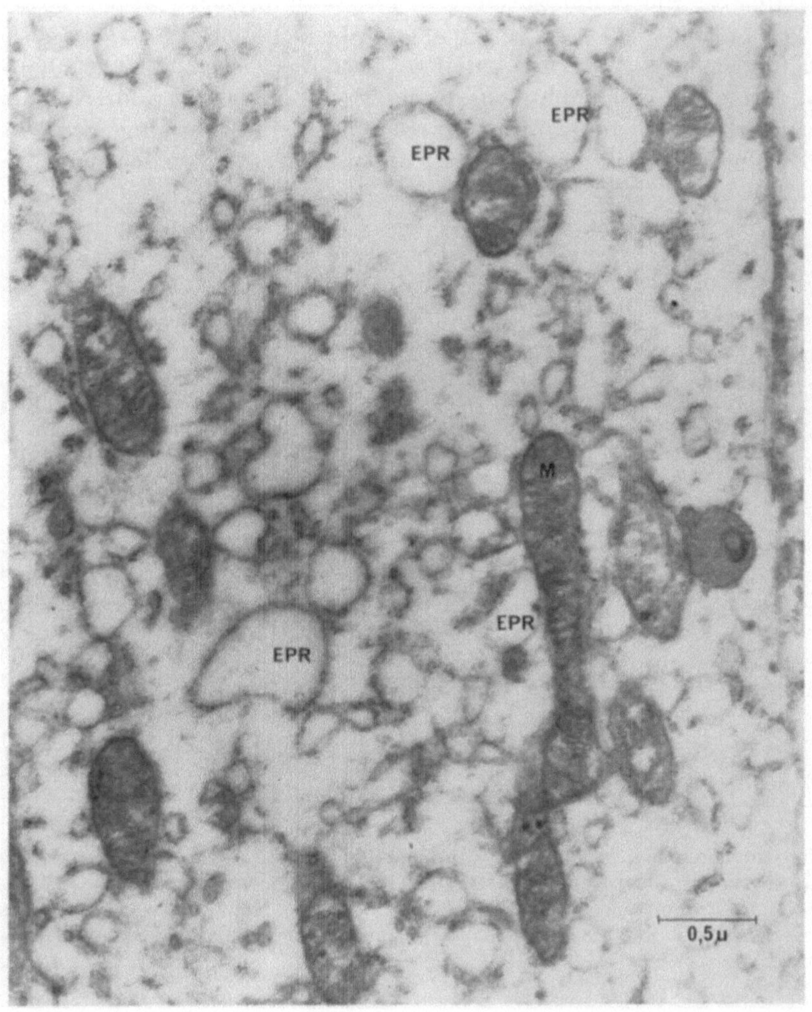

Abb. 10. Dünndarmepithel der Maus. 2 Stunden nach Ganzkörperbestrahlung mit 450 R. Endoplasmatisches Retikulum (EPR), Mitochondrien (M); Vergr. 25 200fach. (Nach BRAUN, H., unveröffentlicht)

terungen des EPR fand auch BRAUN (1960) an Dünndarmepithelzellen von Mäusen 1—2 Stunden nach Bestrahlung mit 450 R (Abb. 9 u. 10). Sie stellte aber, im Gegensatz zu den anderen Autoren, keine Vermehrung des EPR, sondern 6—24 Stunden nach Bestrahlung das fast völlige Verschwinden dieser Membranen fest.

3. Das Ergastoplasma

Beobachtungen über die strahleninduzierten Änderungen des Ergastoplasmas ergeben übereinstimmend, daß diese Strukturen abnehmen und eventuell sogar ganz verschwinden (GLAUSER, 1956; LEVI u. CAFFARATTI, 1960 und BRAUN u. MÜLLER, 1961). Nach GLAUSER, der Ratten mit 1000 R bestrahlte, verschwindet das Ergastoplasma der Leberzellen 3 Tage nach Bestrahlung sogar ganz. BRAUN u. MÜLLER beschreiben ebenfalls an Rattenleberzellen nach Bestrahlung mit 800—9600 R, daß die Reste des Ergastoplasmas mit zunehmender Dosis und zunehmendem Zeitabstand von der Bestrahlung mehr aufgetrieben werden.

4. Der Golgiapparat

Der Golgiapparat wurde nur selten nach Bestrahlung beobachtet. Elektronenoptische Beobachtungen an Maus-Oozyten liegen von Parsons (1962) vor. Er konnte an diesem Objekt keinerlei Änderungen erkennen. Parchwitz (1963) fand dagegen in bestrahlten Tumorzellen vermehrte Golgikomplexe im elektronenoptischen Bild (Abb. 11).

Fogg u. Mitarb. (1937) bestrahlten Walker-Carcinom-Zellen und fanden im lichtoptischen Bild zu bis 1 Stunde nach dem Strahleninsult keine Änderungen des Golgiappa-

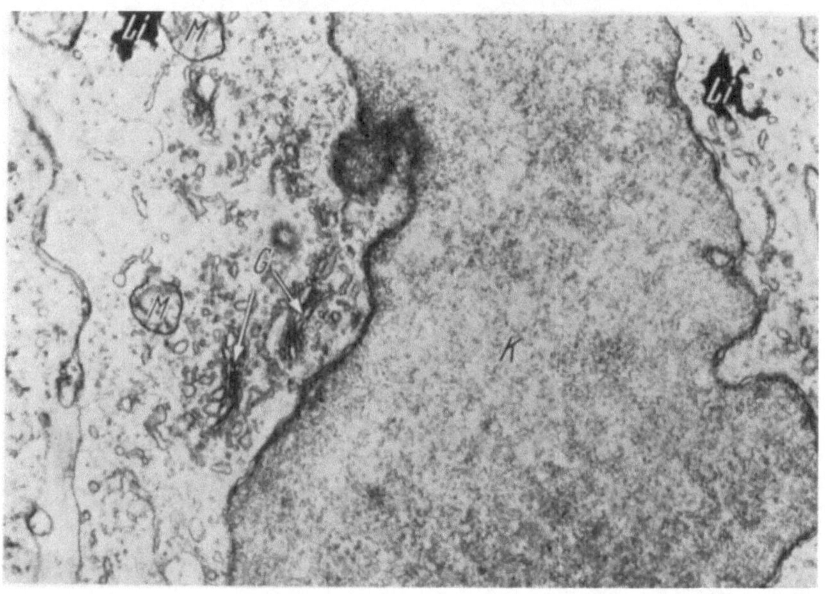

Abb. 11. Walker-Carcinomzelle 4 Tage nach Bestrahlung (5000 R HD); hochgradige Vergrößerung des Kerns (K); starke Vermehrung der Golgi-Komplexe (G); gequollene, deformierte Mitochondrien (M); fortgeschrittene Entdifferenzierung des Cytoplasmas: Lipoidanhäufung (Li); E.O. 6100:1; E.V. 12000:1. Aus: Parchwitz, in: Scherer u. Stender, Strahlenpathologie der Zelle (G. Thieme, Stuttgart 1963)

rates. Danach löste sich der Komplex aber vom Centrosomenbereich ab, vergrößerte sich und wurde massig, wobei er seinen Netzcharakter verlor. Schließlich fragmentierte er, hatte sich aber nach 24 Stunden wieder zu einem normalen Netz reorganisiert.

Zu diesem Zeitpunkt gewannen die Zellen auch ihre Teilungsfähigkeit wieder. Diese Beoachtungen wurden im wesentlichen von Warren u. Mitarb. (1951) an Zellen der verschiedensten Rattenorgane bestätigt. Gatenby u. Mitarb. (1929—30) verfolgten die Strahlenwirkung auf den Golgiapparat bei der Spermiogenese von *Abraxus* und gaben als wesentliche Reaktion an, daß er fortlaufend abortive Acroblasten bildet, bis er sich etwa 2 Tage nach Bestrahlung wieder normalisiert. Strukturänderungen beschreiben sie nicht.

5. Unbekannte Membranstruktur

Schneider (1961a) zeigt einen dichten, geordneten Membrankomplex (Abb. 12a) in *Paramaecium*, über dessen Funktion nichts bekannt zu sein scheint und der auch sonst nicht beschrieben wird. Dieser Komplex wird nach Bestrahlung mit letalen Dosen (über 200 kR) stark reduziert und läßt keine Ordnung mehr erkennen (Abb. 12b).

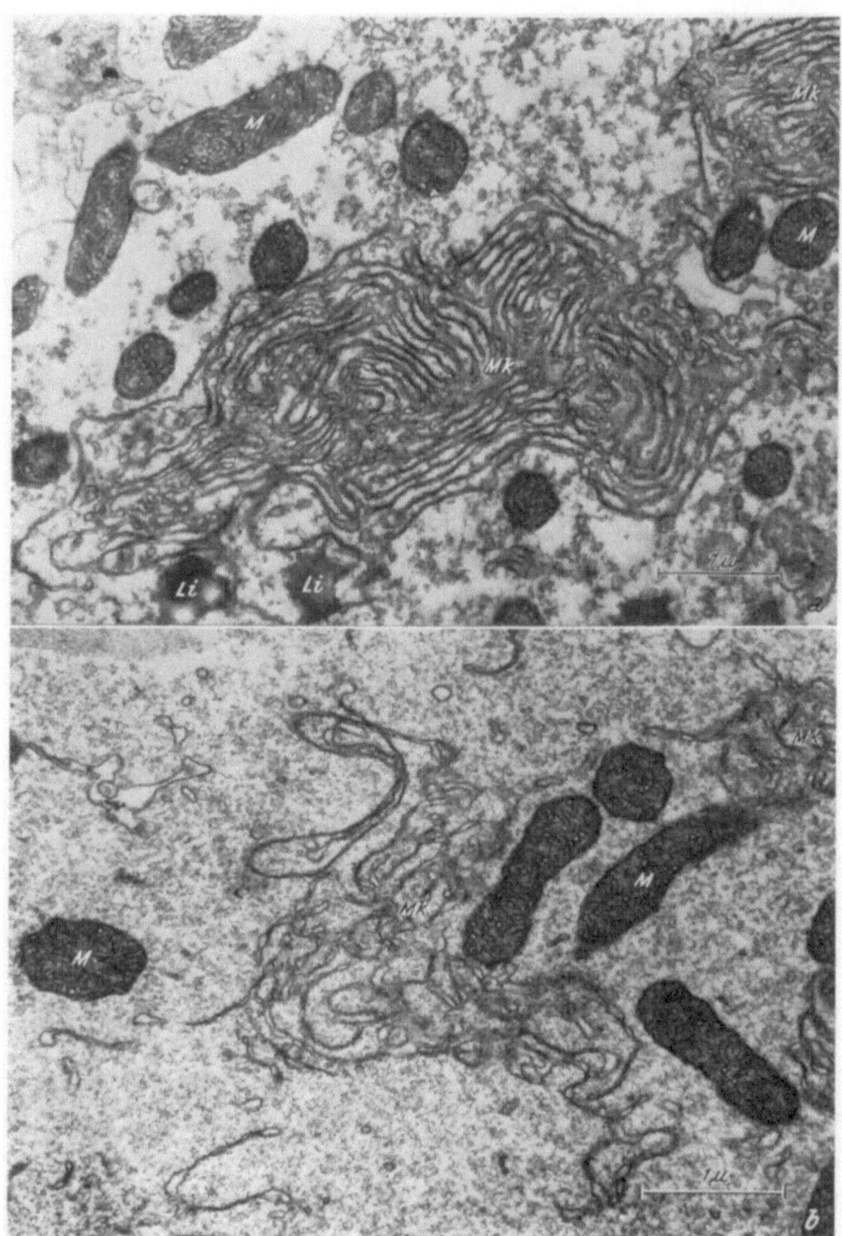

Abb. 12a. Im „normalen", unbestrahlten Cytoplasma vorkommende „geordnete" Membrankomplexe (MK);
Li: Lipoidtropfen; M: Mitochondrien. Fixationsgemisch pH 7,08. E.O. 6800:1; E.V. 16800:1

b. Membrankomponente (MK) nach Einwirkung einer letalen Röntgendosis von 200000 R (= 50 min
Bestrahlungsdauer). Es kann keine „Ordnung" mehr festgestellt werden. M: Mitochondrien. Fixationsgemisch
pH 7,1. E.O. 6800:1; E.V. 19120:1. Aus: SCHNEIDER, Protoplasma **53**, 530 (1961a)

6. Neu auftretende Membranstrukturen

a) Bläschenreihen

Insgesamt scheinen die Membranstrukturen am Plasma infolge Bestrahlung zuzunehmen. Vor allem in *Paramaecium* werden von WOHLFAHRT-BOTTERMANN (1959) und SCHNEIDER (1960, 1961) einige bisher noch nicht oder kaum beobachtete Strukturen beschrieben. Ob sie nur nach den extrem hohen Dosen, die bei Paramaecien angewandt wer-

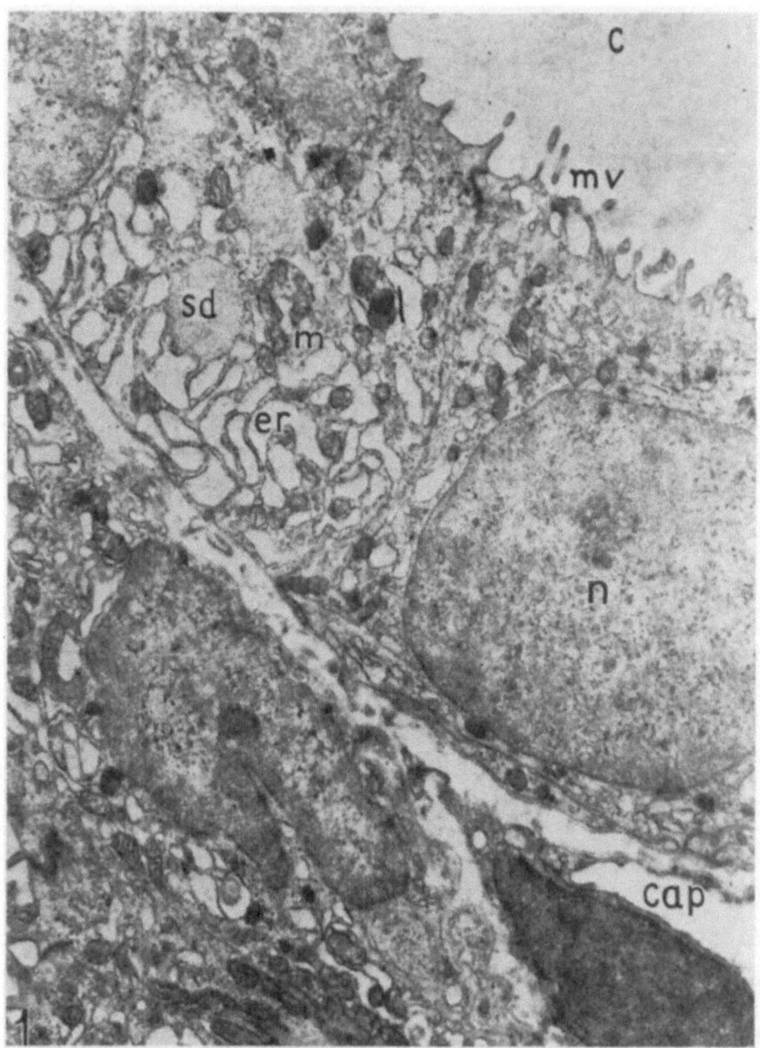

Abb. 13. Follikel-Epithelzellen von Ratten-Schilddrüsen, unbestrahlt. Kolloidale Substanz (C), Microvilli (MV)-
Mitochondrien (M), Endoplasmatisches Retikulum (ER), Lipidgranulae (l), Kern (N), Kapillare (cap), Sekret-
tropfen (sd). Vergr. 14800fach. Aus: McQuade u. Evans, Radiat. Res. **11**, 520 (1959)

den, entstehen, oder bislang in anderen Zellen lediglich übersehen wurden, läßt sich noch
nicht entscheiden. Bei Besprechung der Strahlenwirkung auf das Grundplasma erwähnten wir bereits die Bläschenreihen, die mit dem Elektronenmikroskop sofort nach Bestrahlung zu beobachten sind. Nach Wohlfahrt-Bottermann (1959) liegen diese Bläschenreihen jeweils entlang einer Doppelmembranstruktur (Abb. 5). Zudem scheint auch
jedes einzelne Bläschen von einer Doppelmembran umgeben, deren Entstehung aus gra-
nulärfädigen cytoplasmatischen Grundeinheiten Schneider (1961a) beschreibt.

b) Plasmakapseln

Ebenfalls bereits erwähnt wurden die Plasmakapseln in *Paramaecium*, die z.T. sofort
nach Bestrahlung, verstärkt etwa 1 Stunde später auftreten und jeweils von einer Membran
umgeben sind (Abb. 7). Schneider (1961 a u. b) beschreibt diese Membranen als sehr
kontrastreiche Doppel- bis Mehrfachlamellen. Er nimmt an, daß diese Abkapselungen von
der Zelle vorgenommen werden, um irreversibel geschädigte Plasmaareale auszuscheiden.
Die andere Möglichkeit, daß die vermehrte Doppelmembranbildung des Plasmas als Zu-

fallsprodukt zur Abkapselung derartiger Areale führt, die in der Folge absterben, hält er für sehr unwahrscheinlich. Es ist zu fragen, ob diesen Kapseln Erscheinungen in der Leberzelle entsprechen, die bislang nur lichtoptisch beschrieben wurden. Nach Bestrahlung treten dort stark vakuolisierte, ziemlich scharf umschriebene Bezirke in der Zelle auf.

c) Membrankomplexe

Schließlich wurden ebenfalls von SCHNEIDER (1959) an *Paramaecium* noch membranöse Strukturen beobachtet, die hin und wieder auch in normalen Tieren auftreten sollen, aber bedeutend seltener. Es handelt sich um jeweils mehrere Lamellenpaare, die langgestreckt oder geknäult sein können und anscheinend regellos im Plasma verstreut sind. Den Abstand der Lamellen voneinander gibt er mit 150—200 Å an. Die Enden sollen zu Ösen geschlossen sein. Ähnliche Strukturen fand auch NICKEL (1961) an Paramaecien. — In Schilddrüsenzellen von Ratten sahen McQUADE u. EVANS bereits 1959 Strukturen, die den eben beschriebenen zu entsprechen scheinen. Sie schreiben von ,,curious membrane like struktures which did not seem to be associated with the ER'' (= EPR), (Abb. 13 u. 14).

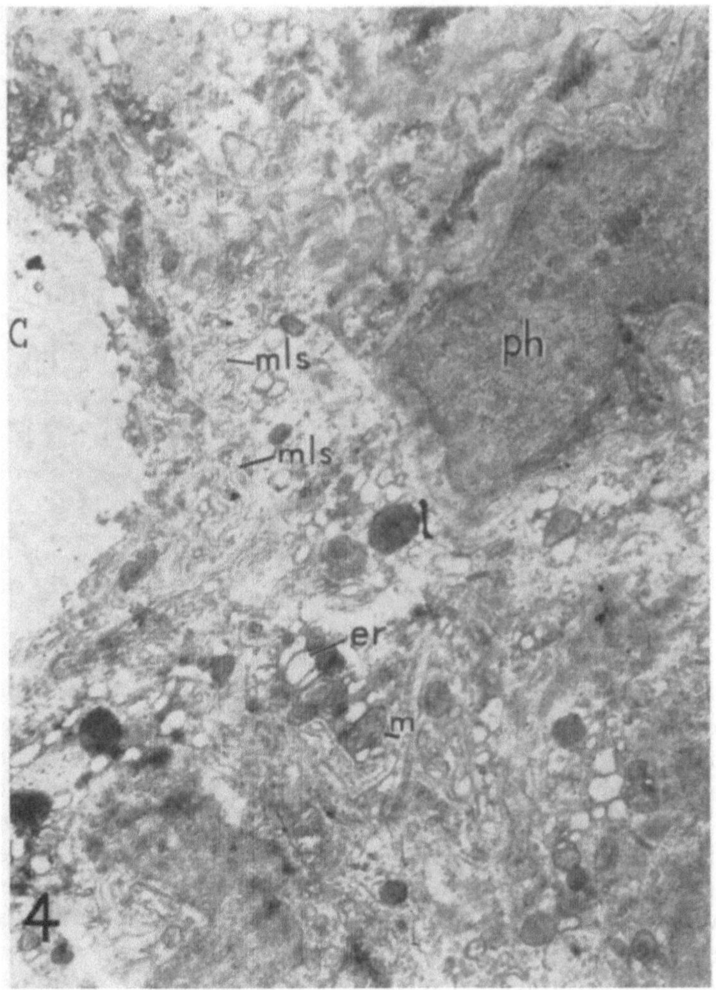

Abb. 14. Follikel-Epithelzellen von Ratten-Schilddrüsen, 3 Tage nach Behandlung mit ^{131}I, geschätzte Dosis 41 500 rad. — Membranöse Strukturen (mls), Kolloidale Substanz (C), Lipoid-Granulae (l), Mitochondrien (M), Endoplasmatisches Retikulum (er), Phagozyte (ph). Vergr. 15 200fach. Aus: McQUADE u. EVANS, Radiat. Res. **11**, 520 (1959)

IV. Geschlossene Zellorganellen mit lamellärem Aufbau

1. Mitochondrien

Genau genommen müßten wir die Mitochondrien, die völlig aus doppellamellären Membranen aufgebaut sind, auch unter den Membranstrukturen aufführen. Da sie aber als in sich geschlossene Körper erscheinen, die als solche bereits seit langem im Lichtmikroskop bekannt waren, ehe man etwas von ihrer Membranstruktur wußte, behandeln wir sie hier getrennt.

a) Volumen und Feinstrukturänderungen

Strahleninduzierte Schädigungen an Mitochondrien sind häufig beschrieben und sehr vielfältig. Kompliziert werden die Verhältnisse noch dadurch, daß die Reaktion der Mitochondrien sogar innerhalb einer Zelle sehr verschieden sein kann. Tatsächlich unterscheiden sich schon in normalen Zellen nicht nur die Mitochondrien verschiedener Spezies, z.B. der Hefe *Saccharomyces cerevisiae*, sondern darüber hinaus findet man innerhalb einer normalen Zelle bereits morphologische Unterschiede der Mitochondrien (Marquardt, 1962a u. b). Entsprechend werden dann auch nach Bestrahlung innerhalb ein und derselben Zelle Schädigungsformen der Mitochondrien beschrieben, die bis zur völligen Auflösung führen können, während gleichzeitig vollkommen ungeschädigte Mitochondrien beobachtet werden. Über die physiologische Bedeutung dieser Unterschiede ist nichts bekannt. Nach

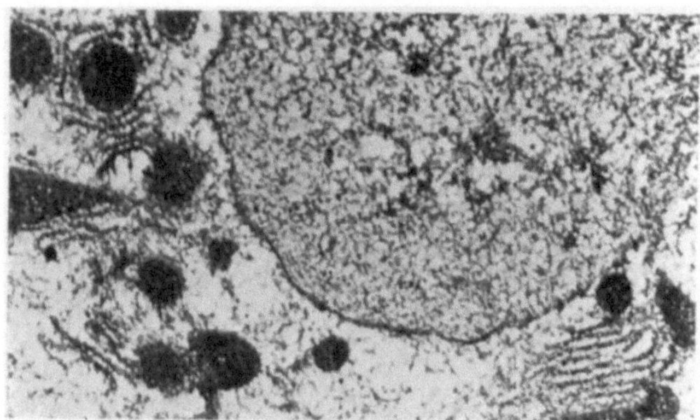

Abb. 15. Normale Rattenleber. Doppeltkonturierte Kernmembran. Mitochondrien stellenweise von osmiophilen Lamellen umgeben. OsO₄-Fixation. Vergr. 8000fach. Aus: Glauser, Schweiz. Z. allg. Path. Bakt. **19**, 150 (1956)

Glauser scheint der Zustand der Mitochondrien in hohem Maße vom umgebenden Plasma abhängig, indem in stark vakuolisiertem Plasma auch die Mitochondrien verändert erscheinen, während in der gleichen Zelle in normal erscheinenden Plasmaarealen auch normale Mitochondrien liegen. Die Schädigungsformen nach Bestrahlung sind insgesamt durchaus unspezifisch und entsprechen völlig den Bildern bei anderen pathologischen Zuständen. Einen guten Eindruck von der unterschiedlichen Reaktion auf ionisierende Strahlen, z.B. in verschiedenen Organen des gleichen Organismus, gibt die Tabelle 1.

Eine der am häufigsten beschriebenen pathologischen Veränderungen nach Bestrahlung ist das Anschwellen der Mitochondrien. Dabei sind 2 Formen der Schwellung zu unterscheiden. In einem Fall vergrößern sich die Mitochondrien lediglich und erscheinen eventuell lichtoptisch im Innern etwas aufgehellt (Ritchie, 1953). Elektronenoptisch erscheinen in diesem Zustand die Cristae bzw. Tubuli weiter auseinandergedrängt (Wohlfahrt-Bottermann, 1960). Im anderen Fall bilden sich Vakuolen innerhalb der Mitochondrien aus, die vesikuläre Form (Nadson u. Rochlin-Gleichgewicht, 1926; Milo-

VIDOV, 1929; GLAUSER, 1956; SCHERER u. VOGELL, 1958), (Abb. 15 u. 16). Da das Plasma durch die geschwollenen Mitochondrien im Lichtmikroskop trübe erscheint, wird dieser Zustand auch als „trübe Schwellung" bezeichnet. Diese Formänderungen der Mitochondrien sind sehr weitgehend reversibel. BRAUN (1960) beschreibt aufgrund elektronenmikroskopischer Untersuchungen, daß bei Maus-Leberzellen die Schädigung erst dann irreversibel ist, wenn im Innern der Mitochondrien keine Doppelmembranen mehr zu erkennen sind, sondern nur noch ein retikuläres Gerüst. Zu diesem Zeitpunkt beobachtete sie auch eine stark verdickte Außenmembran.

Sofern die Schädigung nicht so weit geht, ist also eine Regeneration möglich, deren Verlauf ebenfalls von BRAUN beschrieben wird. Mit zunehmendem zeitlichen Abstand von der Bestrahlung fand sie Mitochondrien mit einem bedeutend dichteren Doppelmembransystem in Innern. Gleichzeitig war die äußere Membran intensiver gefärbt. Dafür, daß es sich dabei um Regenerationsformen handelt, spricht auch, daß von außen endoplasmatischen Lamellen unmittelbar an die Mitochondrien angelagert sind (Abb. 17).

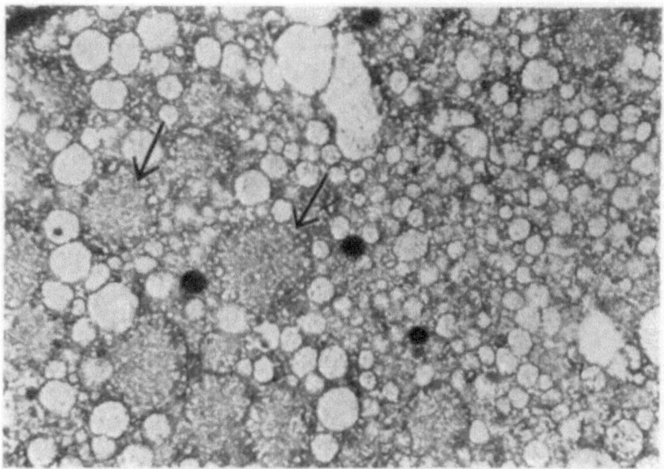

Abb. 16. Rattenleber, 3 Tage nach 1000 R. Mitochondrien hauptsächlich links im Bilde noch erhalten mit feinen Vakuolen unter der Membran. Geringe Osmiophilie. Rechts Vakuolen in der Zellmembran. Stark osmiophile Fettropfen. OsO_4-Fixation. Vergr. 8000fach. Aus: GLAUSER, Schweiz. Z. allg. Path. Bakt. **19**, 150 (1956)

WOHLFAHRT-BOTTERMANN u. SCHNEIDER (1961) scheinen bei Paramaecien die Degeneration der Mitochondrien innerhalb des abgekapselten Plasmabereichs, der dann stark vakuolisiert, für normal zu halten. Ein entsprechendes Bild wurde allerdings von keinem anderen Objekt beschrieben. Eine gewisse Übereinstimmung scheint nur mit GLAUSERs Beobachtung an Rattenleber zu bestehen, da er degenerierende Mitochondrien nur in vakuolisierten Plasmabereichen fand.

Die Frage nach dem zeitlichen Ablauf dieser Strukturänderungen, speziell der Schwellung, wirft noch ein besonderes Problem auf. Offenbar hängt die Geschwindigkeit, mit der geschwollene Mitochondrien auftreten, von der applizierten Strahlendosis ab, indem nach hohen Dosen sehr viel schneller als nach niederen Dosen geschwollene Mitochondrien beobachtet werden. Sehr schön kommt das in einer Arbeit von SCHERER u. WICHMANN (1954) zum Ausdruck, die Mäuse bestrahlten und nach Applikation von 800 R in Milzzellen bereits nach 1 Stunde vergrößerte Mitochondrien fanden, nach 600 R erst nach 3 Stunden und nach 200 R schließlich erst nach 12 Stunden. Auch beim Vergleich verschiedener Arbeiten an verschiedenen Organismen wird dieses System immer wieder deutlich, trotz der unterschiedlichen Strahlempfindlichkeit der Organismen und Organe. Auf diesen Befund wirft die Arbeit von BRAUN u. MÜLLER (1961) etwas Licht. Sie beschreiben, daß sie bei Mauslebern nach Bestrahlung mit 800 R zunächst nach 6—12 Stunden eine Volumenabnahme der

Mitochondrien fanden und daß erst nach 24 Stunden geschwollene Mitochondrien auftraten. Nach Applikation von 6400 R waren die Mitochondrien dagegen bereits 30 min nach Bestrahlung geschwollen. Neuerdings konnte Parson (1962) diesen Befund mit sehr geringen Dosen (7—200 R), an den empfindlichen Maus-Oozyten (Phase I u. II) bestätigen. Er beobachtete allerdings zunächst während weniger Minuten eine zahlenmäßige Abnahme, dann

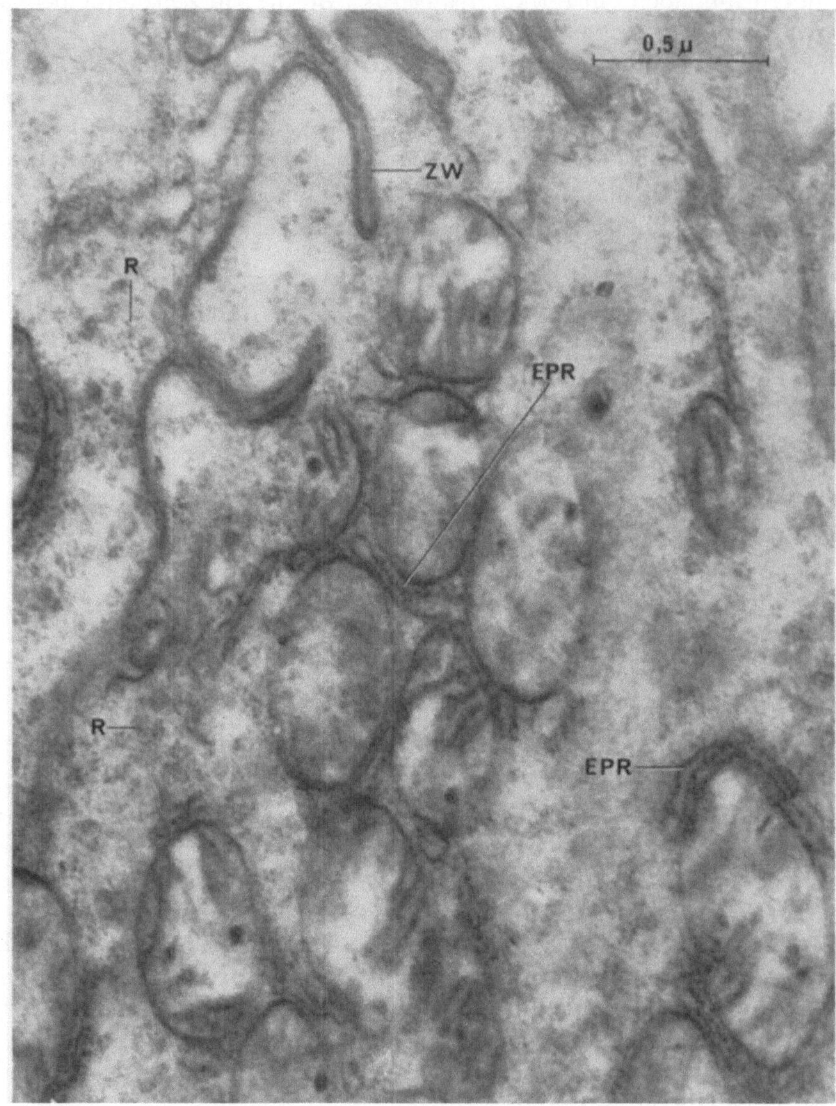

Abb. 17. Dünndarmepithel der Maus, 3 Tage nach Ganzkörperbestrahlung mit 450 R. Mitochondrien in der Regenerationsphase von endoplasmatischen Lamellen umgeben. Endoplasmatisches Retikulum (EPR), Ribosomen (R), Zellwand (ZW). Vergr. 46080fach. Aus: Braun, Exp. Cell Res. **20**, 267 (1960)

normalisierte sich die Zahl, aber die Mitochondrien schrumpften nach 7 R über 2 Stunden, während sie nach 200 R nach anfänglicher Schrumpfung nach 2 Stunden geschwollen waren. Scherer (1956), der isolierte Mitochondrien der Mausleber untersuchte, fand nach 1000 R ebenfalls geschrumpfte und verdichtete Formen. Diese Reaktion könnte also einer Permeabilitätsänderung infolge energetischer Insuffizienz entsprechen, wie wir sie im Kapitel über die Zellmembran bereits besprachen.

Die Frage nach der primären Ursache für die Permeabilitätsänderung ist genau so schwer zu beantworten wie bei der äußeren Plasmamembran. Es ist wieder möglich, daß Änderungen in der Gesamtstruktur der äußeren Membran induziert werden. — Es kann aber ebensogut sein, daß primär Einzelmoleküle, etwa Enzyme des Energiestoffwechsels, geschädigt wurden, ohne welche die Struktur nicht länger aufrecht zu erhalten ist. ALTMANN (1955) hält derartige Schädigungen in den Mitochondrien sogar für die Primärreaktion der meisten pathologischen Zellzustände, da von den Enzymen der Energiehaushalt der Zelle weitgehend abhängig ist. Diese Ansicht würde mit den Befunden von GOLDFEDER und von DANIELS u. ROTH übereinstimmen, die den Mitochondrien eine Schlüsselstellung bei der Strahlenschädigung, bzw. bei der Heilung von Strahlenschäden, zuschreiben. Wir sahen aber bereits, daß in Zellen mit reiner Glykolyse, die nicht in den Mitochondrien lokalisiert ist, die gleichen Schäden auftreten, und weiterhin erörterten wir, daß die Energielieferung nicht unbedingt auszufallen braucht, sondern daß möglicherweise lediglich die Energieübertragung entkoppelt ist. Aus diesem Grunde möchten wir noch keine Schlußfolgerungen über die Primärwirkung der Strahlen ziehen. Daß die Enzymaktivität der Mitochondrien gehemmt ist, wurde zwar mehrfach beschrieben. Es kann sich dabei aber auch um einen Sekundäreffekt infolge des Eindringens von Wasser oder um eine Störung der enzymtragenden Strukturen handeln.

BRAUN u. MÜLLER fanden neben den geschwollenen Mitochondrien, die noch Strukturen im Inneren hatten, auch Mitochondrien normaler Größe, die im Inneren strukturlos waren. Plumpe strukturlose Mitochondrien beschreiben auch SCHERER und VOGELL. Daß an der äußeren Mitochondrien-Membran durch Bestrahlung Änderungen hervorgerufen werden, geht auch daraus hervor, daß häufig Bilder zu beobachten sind mit verklumpten oder verklebten Mitochondrien (NÜRNBERGER, 1923; McCARDLE u. CONGDON, 1955; BRAUN u. MÜLLER, 1961). Auf veränderte Oberflächenstruktur schließen auch SCHERER u. VÖLKER (1960) aus dem veränderten Farbbindungsvermögen von in vivo und in vitro bestrahlten Rattenleber-Mitochondrien.

Nach WOHLFAHRT-BOTTERMANN u. SCHNEIDER (1961) folgt auf die Aufhellung der Mitochondrien im Inneren die völlige Auflösung der äußeren Hüllmembran. BRAUN u. MÜLLER (1961) geben an, daß sie Löcher in der äußeren Mitochondrienmembran beobachteten und OKADA u. PEECHY (1957) sprechen von Brüchen in der Membran. In diesen Fällen dürfte sich jede weitere Frage nach der Ursache der Permeabilitätsänderung erübrigen. Sie scheinen aber recht selten zu sein.

b) Mitochondrien-Zerfall

Weiterhin stellt sich die Mitochondrien-Schädigung auch in einem Zerfall dar. Offenbar beruht auf solch einem Zerfall die Mitochondrien-Vermehrung, die häufig beschrieben wurde, immer mit dem Zusatz, daß die Mitochondrien sehr klein sind. Meist liegen sie dabei in Gruppen zusammen (TSCHASSOWNIKOW, 1928; HIRSCH, 1931; SCHERER u. WICHMANN, 1954; McCARDLE u. CONGDON, 1955). Es kann sich in diesen Fällen nicht etwa um die geschrumpften Mitochondrien von BRAUN u. MÜLLER handeln, da sie die Vermehrung nicht erklären würden. Häufig scheinen auch die vakuolisierten Mitochondrien zu zerfallen (NADSON u. ROCHLIN-GLEICHGEWICHT, 1926; PARCHWITZ, 1957). Es scheint allerdings auch möglich, daß erst die Mitochondrien-Bruchstücke vakuolisieren. Daß es sich jedenfalls um einen Zerfall vakuolisierter Mitochondrien handeln kann, scheint der Befund GLAUSERs (1956) zu zeigen, der mehrere solcher vakuolisierter Teilstücke noch perlschnurartig miteinander verbunden fand, ein Bild, das auch sonst von pathologischen Zellzuständen bekannt ist. Nach ALTMANN zerfallen im allgemeinen die langsam geschwollenen Mitochondrien leichter. Das scheint auch auf die bestrahlten Mitochondrien zuzutreffen, da der Zerfall vor allem nach niederen Dosen gefunden wird, selten nach höheren. Dabei scheinen die Mitochondrien zunächst in vorgebildete Untereinheiten, später aber eventuell noch weiter zu zerfallen. In manchen Fällen wird regelrecht von „Zerstäuben" gesprochen, das bis zum völligen Verschwinden gehen kann. Insgesamt sind die Erscheinungen am besten unter dem Begriff „granulärer Zerfall" zusammenzufassen.

Laudahn (1959) hält diesen Zerfall für nötig, da er die Mitochondrien-Oberfläche vergrößert, und daher die Regenerationsvorgänge in der Zelle fördert.

c) Lipophanerose

Eine weitere Erscheinungsform des Strahlenschadens an Mitochondrien ist die Lipophanerose, die Entwicklung von Fettropfen in den Mitochondrien.

Sie wurde lichtoptisch von Nadson u. Rochlin-Gleichgewicht beschrieben. Wohlfahrt-Bottermann u. Schneider (1961) konnten im elektronenoptischen Bild zeigen, daß die Fettropfen bei starker, irreversibler Schädigung tatsächlich im Innern der Mitochondrien auftreten (Abb. 8). Nach diesen Autoren kann das Fett, das in den Mitochondrien angesammelt wurde, ans Plasma abgegeben werden. Die wahrscheinlichste Erklärung der Lipophanerose dürfte der gestörte Fettabbau sein, der in den Mitochondrien lokalisiert ist. Es ist natürlich auch möglich, daß das Fett infolge von Entmischungen auftritt, die sich aus der Strukturauflösung der Molekülverbände ergeben. Altmann und ebenso Wohlfahrt-Bottermann u. Schneider (1961) halten dies sogar für die einzige Ursache der Lipophanerose.

d) Mitochondrienzahländerungen

Aus der Degeneration der Mitochondrien einerseits und dem Zerfall in Teilstücke andererseits, ergeben sich die unterschiedlichsten Effekte auf die Mitochondrienzahländerungen. So ergibt der Zerfall zunächst eine starke Vermehrung, kann aber letzten Endes zum völligen Verschwinden der Mitochondrien führen (Nadson u. Rochlin-Gleichgewicht, 1926; Nadson u. Rochlin, 1934; Noyes u. Smith, 1959). In anderen Fällen waren keine Mitochondrien mehr zu beobachten, ohne daß jedoch ein Zerfall vorausgegangen war. Meistens traten dabei aber später wieder normale Mitochondrien auf. Der zeitliche Verlauf von Zerfall und Regeneration kann offenbar sehr unterschiedlich sein. Parson (1962) fand an den sehr empfindlichen Maus-Oozyten nach 200 R bereits 2 min nach Bestrahlung weniger Mitochondrien als in den Kontrollen. Schjeide u. Mitarb. (1960) schließen aus Versuchen mit Hühnerembryonen, in denen die Mitochondrienzahl frühestens nach 24 Stunden abnahm, daß nur sekundär die Vermehrung der Mitochondrien gehemmt wird. Dieser Befund deckt sich aber mit keinem anderen vorliegenden. Falls die Untersuchungen wie von Scherer u. Ringleb (1954) mit Janusgrün durchgeführt wurden, beruht das Verschwinden möglicherweise auf einem vorübergehenden Verlust der Färbbarkeit durch Inaktivierung der Enzyme der Atmungskette. In anderen Fällen scheint lediglich der Phasenunterschied zum Plasma vorübergehend aufgehoben. Dieser Vorgang wird als Verdämmern bezeichnet. Im Elektronenmikroskop wurden auch Fälle beobachtet, in denen offenbar nur die Osmophilie der Membranen vorübergehend abnimmt (Glauser, 1956).

e) Verlagerung

Schließlich bleibt noch auf die räumliche Verlagerung der Mitochondrien in den Zellen nach Bestrahlung hinzuweisen. Wiederholt wird beschrieben, daß sie sich dicht um den Kern lagern (Scherer u. Wichmann, 1954; Parchwitz, 1957; Scherer u. Vogell, 1958; Pomerat, 1958). Nach Parchwitz und nach Pomerat werden sie dabei fadenförmig. Scherer u. Vogell fanden geklumpte Mitochondrien um den Kern. Die Verlagerung um den Kern deutet auf eine Schutzfunktion hin. Bei starker Bestrahlung geht in der Folge das äußere Plasma zugrunde. Es kann aber später wieder regeneriert werden. — In manchen Untersuchungen verlagerten sich die Mitochondrien aber auch an den Zellrand. McCardle u. Congdon (1954) beschreiben, daß bei schwacher Bestrahlung die Mitochondrien der Leberzellen sich zu den Blutgefäßen hin bewegen (Abb. 18 u. 19). Bei starker

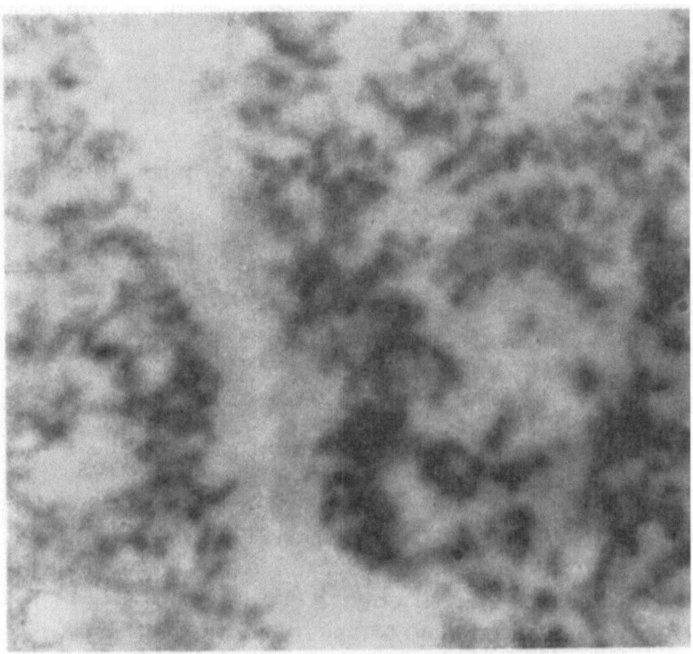

Abb. 18. Leber einer gefütterten, erwachsenen, männlichen Maus, unbestrahlt. Mitochondrien von Leberzellen der mittleren Leberlappenzone. Die Mitochondrien sind in Linien senkrecht zu den Blutgefäßen in den Zellen angeordnet. Färbung mit Hämatoxylin nach REGAUD. 4 μ Schnittdicke, Vergr. ca. 4600 fach. Aus: MCCARDLE u. CONGDON. Amer. J. Pathol. **31**, 725 (1955)

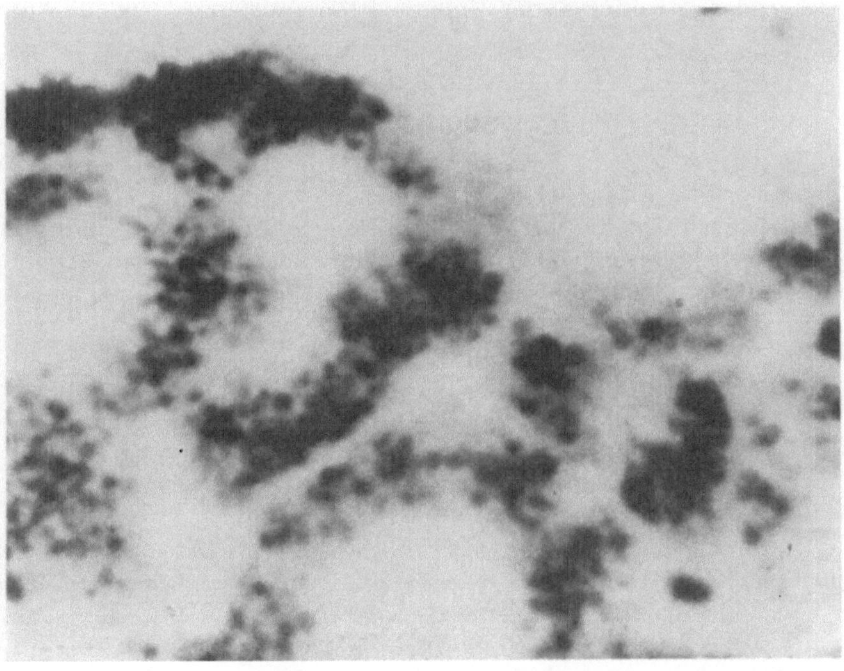

Abb. 19. Leber einer gefütterten, erwachsenen, männlichen Maus, 72 Stunden nach Bestrahlung mit 1200 R. Mitochondrien in Zellen der mittleren Leberlappenzone verklebt als kleine Tropfen sichtbar und vakuolisiert. Das periphere Cytoplasma ist reich an Mitochondrien, während sie im perinuklearen Plasma fehlen. Färbung mit Hämatoxylin nach REGAUD. 4 μ Schnittdicke, Vergr. ca. 4600 fach. Aus: MCCARDLE u. CONGDON, Amer. J. Pathol. **31**, 725 (1955)

Bestrahlung sollen sie sich aber auch um den Kern lagern. Braun u. Müller geben dagegen gerade nach höheren Dosen an, daß die Mitochondrien sich an die Zellwände verlagern. In beiden Fällen wurden Mauslebern bestrahlt. Allerdings waren die von Braun u. Müller angewendeten Dosen noch wesentlich höher als die von McCardle u. Congdon applizierten. Ritchie, der an dem Pilz *Allomyces javanicus* mit extrem hohen Dosen arbeiten konnte, fand auch die Mitochondrien an der Peripherie der Zellen.

2. Plastiden

In den Chloroplasten grüner Pflanzen äußert sich der Strahlenschaden praktisch in den gleichen Formen wie in den Mitochondrien. Eine ausführliche Beschreibung gibt nur Biebl (1935) an Moosblättchen. Nach schwacher Bestrahlung, die nach $^1/_2$—24 Stunden zum Tode führte, nahm das Volumen der Chloroplasten ab. Bei stärkeren Dosen, bei denen der Tod nach 2—5 Stunden eintrat, nahm es dagegen zu. Das entspricht also völlig dem Verlauf von Schrumpfung und Quellung bei Mitochondrien. — In länger lebenden Zellen, die nur schwach bestrahlt waren, rundeten die Chloroplasten sich zunächst ab, konnten dann aber im Verlauf von Tagen anschwellen, eventuell bis sie die ganze Zelle ausfüllten. Amoeboide Riesenplastiden beschreibt auch Hruby (1935) in *Equisetum*-Sporen. Er nimmt an, daß die großen Plastiden außer durch Schwellung durch Verkleben und gehemmte Teilung entstanden sind. Verklebte Chloroplasten fanden auch Biebl und ebenso Zirkle (1932) in bestrahlten Farnsporen. Nach Hruby können die großen, aber auch kleine Chloroplasten nach Bestrahlung vakuolisiert sein. In den Chloroplasten können zusätzlich noch Farbänderungen auftreten. Nach Biebl werden sie nach starken Dosen braun. Biebl beschreibt außerdem, daß Chloroplasten sich auch wie die Mitochondrien in den Zellen verlagern.

Bestrahlungsversuche isolierter Chloroplasten von Füchtbauer u. Simonis (1962) wurden vor allem im Hinblick auf die Fermentaktivität durchgeführt. Sie ergeben, daß die fermenttragenden Strukturen der Chloroplasten resistenter sind als die Fermente selbst.

V. Zelleinschlüsse

1. Cytosomen

Wendt (1961) beschreibt die Wirkung ionisierender Strahlen auf die Cytosomen. Er arbeitete mit Gewebekulturen von Hühnerherzfibroblasten und mit Amnion-Epithelzellen. Nach Applikation von 600—800 R zog sich die äußere Hüllschicht oder Externa

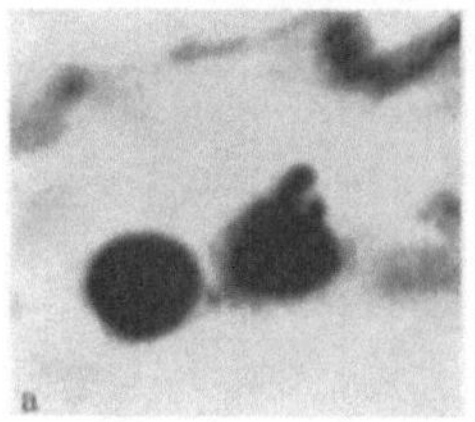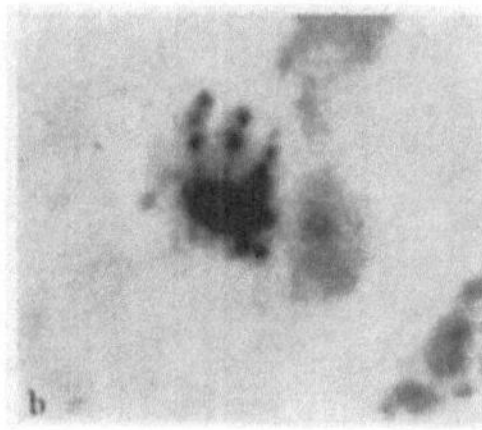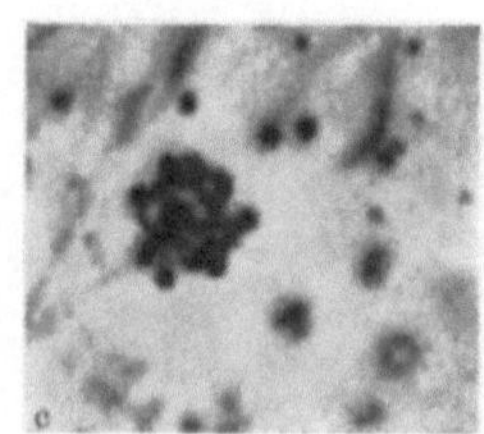

Abb. 20. Durch Strahlenwirkung zerfallende Cytosomen (ca. 1200 R, Lebendaufnahmen, Phasenkontrast, Vergr. 1660fach. Aus: Wendt, Z. Zellforsch. **53**, 172 (1961)

der Cytosomen häufig zusammen und legte den Innenkörper, die Interna, frei. Wurden unreife Cytosomen bestrahlt, so wurde der Reifungsprozeß gefördert, d. h. die Interna teilte sich rascher in Unterkugeln auf. Wurden hohe Dosen appliziert (1000—1500 R), so zerfielen die Cytosomen rasch, die zahlreichen kleinen Teilstücke verteilten sich über das Plasma und wuchsen wieder zu normalen Cytosomen heran (Abb. 20).

2. Neuauftretende Zelleinschlüsse

KOEHLER (1962) beschreibt in HeLa-Giant-Zellen nach Bestrahlung mit 500—1000 R Röntgenstrahlen neuauftretende Zelleinschlüsse von stark lipophilem Charakter. Er vermutet, daß es mitochondriale oder mikrosomale Zerfallsprodukte sind.

VI. Der Zellteilungsapparat

1. Centrosomen und Spindel

Bei lokaler Bestrahlung mit α-Strahlen konnten ZIRKLE u. BLOOM (1953) und BLOOM, ZIRKLE u. URETZ (1955) auch mit hohen Dosen keinerlei sichtbaren Effekt am Centrosom oder an der Spindel erzielen. TAHMISIAN (1961), der Heuschrecken-Spermatozyten bestrahlte, fand allerdings in der Folge eine erhöhte Anzahl von Centrosomen. RUSTAD (1959) fand nach Bestrahlung von Seeigel-Spermien multipolare Spindeln. Die gleichzeitig auftretende Teilungshemmung schiebt er daher auf eine Störung der Centrosomen oder auf den Auslöser der Centrosomenteilung im Kern. In diesem Zusammenhang muß an die abnorm stark und lang gesteigerte Viskosität nach Bestrahlung erinnert werden, die auch zur Teilungsverzögerung führt (S. 188). Der primäre Effekt ist auch hier nicht zu erkennen. LEVIS u. MARIN (1963) beobachteten multipolare Spindeln in Gewebekulturzellen nach Bestrahlung mit 200—400 R Röntgenstrahlen und schlossen auf Schädigungen des Centriols, wobei die Untereinheiten getrennt geschädigt würden. Sie halten es allerdings auch für möglich, daß eine Teilungsverzögerung des Kerns Mehrfachteilungen des Centriols zur Folge hat. ZIRKLE (1932) und FEICHTINGER (1933) fanden nach Bestrahlung von Farnsporen häufig Zwillingskeimlinge, FEICHTINGER auch, wenn er den Kern nicht mitbestrahlte. Offenbar wird die Teilungsebene, d.h. aber die Spindel, hier so verlagert, daß 2 gleichwertige Zellen entstehen.

VII. Erbliche Änderungen an nicht näher bestimmten cytoplasmatischen Einheiten

Es ist seit langem bekannt, daß Mutationen auch außerhalb der Chromosomen und wahrscheinlich auch außerhalb des Kernes vorkommen können. Zahlreiche Versuche wurden unternommen, um die Auslösung solch extrachromosomaler Mutationen durch ionisierende Strahlen nachzuweisen. Sie führten aber fast alle zu keinem sicheren Ergebnis.

Beobachtungen MALYS (1951), daß Farn-Chloroplasten nach Röntgen- und γ-Bestrahlung von Sporen über zahlreiche Prothalliengenerationen konstant verändert waren, lassen keinen sicheren Schluß zu, daß es sich wirklich um erbliche Änderungen handelt. MICHAELIS (1958 u. 1962) konnte an *Epilobium* mit Röntgenstrahlen keine Vermehrung von Plastidenmutanten feststellen. Behandlung mit ^{35}S oder ^{32}P führte zwar zu einer erheblichen Zunahme gescheckter Pflanzen, die auf Plastiden- oder Plasmonmutationen beruhen könnten. Es scheint in diesen Versuchen aber unklar, ob es sich um Straheneffekte oder um Schädigungen durch Umwandlung des eingebauten ^{35}S bzw. ^{32}P in Cl bzw. S handelt.

Erst RÖBBELEN (1962) gelang es, mit Röntgenstrahlen Blattfarbmutationen zu induzieren, die offenbar auf erblichen Änderungen in den Plastiden beruhen. Nach Applikation von ca. 2—20 kR konnte er in der Crucifere *Arabidopsis* die Mutationsrate für Chlorophyllausbildung von spontan $0{,}07\,^0/_{00}$ bzw. $1{,}95\,^0/_{00}$ heraufsetzen, je nachdem, ob er Samen oder Zygoten bestrahlte.

Außerdem beschrieben GECKLER u. KIMBALL bereits 1953 den Verlust von Kappapartikeln in *Paramaecium aurelia* nach Bestrahlung mit 7 kR Röntgenstrahlen. Diese virenartigen Partikel werden auch als cytoplasmatische Erbeinheiten angesehen.

Literatur

Altmann, H.-W.: Allgemeine morphologische Pathologie des Cytoplasmas. Die Pathobiosen. Büchner, F., Hb. allg. Pathol. II, 419–612, Berlin: Springer 1955.

Astaurov, B, L.: Direct evidence that biological effects of X-rays are nuclear and that final X-ray effects do not depend on initial changes in cytoplasm. Ž. obščei Biol. 8, 421 (1947); ref. Chem. Abstr. 42, 8233 (1948).

Bacq, Z. M., Vanderhaegh, F., Damblou, J., Errera, M.: Effet des rayons X sur Acetabularia mediterranea. Exper. Cell. Res. 12, 639–648 (1957).

Bergeder, H.-D.: Kaliumverluste von Kaltblütermuskeln nach Röntgenbestrahlung. Naturwiss. 45, 61 (1958).

— Untersuchungen zum Einfluß ionisierender Strahlen auf Zellmembranen. II. Änderungen von Membranpotential und Kaliumgehalt des Muskels unter Einwirkung von Röntgenstahlen. Strahlentherapie 115, 90–104 (1961).

— Strahlenwirkungen auf Einzelformationen der Zelle. d) Grenzflächen. Scherer-Stender, Strahlenpathologie, Stuttgart: G. Thieme 1963.

Biebl, R.: Die Wirkung der α-Bestrahlung auf Protoplasma und Chloroplasten. Protoplasma 24, 225–257 (1935).

— Weitere Untersuchungen über die Wirkung der α-Strahlen auf die Pflanzenzelle. Protoplasma 35, 187–236 (1941).

Billen, D., Strehler, B. L., Stapleton, G. E., Brigham, E.: Post-irradiation release of adenosine triphosphate from Escherichia coli B/r¹. Arch. Biochem. Biophys. 43, 1–10 (1953).

Bloom, W.: Cellular responses. Oucley, J. L., Biophysical Science, p. 21–29. New York: Wiley 1959.

— Bloom, M. A.: Histological changes after irradiation. Rad. Biol. I, Part. 2, 1091–1143 (1954).

— Zirkle, R. E., Uretz, R. B.: Irradiation of parts of individual cells. III. Effects of chromosomal and extrachromosomal irradiation on chromosome movement. Ann. N. Y. Acad. Sci. 59, 503 (1955).

Bohomolets, V. I.: The effect of X-ray irradiation on the membrane potential and the concentration of K and Na in muscle fibres of the frog. Fiziol. Žur. 7, 214–220 (1961); ref. Biol. Abstr. 38, 17150 (1962).

Bojansky, R.: Quantenphysik und Biologie. Verhandl. Naturf. Ges. Brünn 73, 8–10 (1942).

Bonnier, G.: Indirect effects of X-rays on chromosomes. Brit. J. Radiol. 25, 180–182 (1952).

— Lüning, K. G.: Spontaneous and X-ray induced gynandromorphs in Drosophila melanogaster. Hereditas 37, 469–487 (1951).

— — Arnberg, B.: On an possible mutagenic effect of X-rayed egg cytoplasm. Hereditas 38, 109–112 (1952).

Braun, H.: Elektronenoptische Untersuchungen an Zellen des Dünndarmepithels nach Röntgenbestrahlung. Exper. Cell Res. 20, 267–276 (1960).

— Müller, J.: Einfluß von Röntgenstrahlen auf Leberzellen. Naturwiss. 48, 679 (1961).

Bresciani, F., u. Mitarb.: A biochemical study of the x-radiation-induced inhibition of sodium transport (Na pump) in human erythrocytes. Rad. Res. 22, 463–477 (1964).

Buchsbaum, R., Zirkle, R. E.: Shrinking and swelling after α-irradiation of various parts of large erythrocytes. Proc. Soc. Exper. Biol. Med. 72, 27–29 (1949).

Bühlmann, A., Liechti, A., Wilbrandt, W.: Untersuchungen über Strahlenhämolyse. II. Weitere Versuche über Röntgenhämolyse. Strahlentherapie 71, 285–308 (1942).

Cali, A., Verga, V.: Über die Wirkung der Röntgenstrahlen auf die Permeabilität der Kapillaren. Strahlentherapie 112, 604–607 (1960).

Daniels, E. W.: Studies on the effect of X-irradiation upon Pelomyxa carolinensis with special reference to nuclear division and plasmotomy. J. Exp. Zool. 117, 189–209 (1951).

— Some effects on the cell division in Pelomyxa carolinensis following X-irradiation, treatment with bis-(β-chloroethyl)-methylamine and experimental plasmogamy (fusion). J. Exper. Zool. 120, 509–523 (1952a).

— Cell division in the giant amoeba, Pelomyxa carolinensis, following X-irradiation. 1. Therapeutic effects after fusion with either nonirradiated light or heavy halves of centrifuged amoeba immediately following exposure. J. Exp. Zool. 120, 525–545 (1952b).

— Cell division in the giant amoeba, Pelomyxa carolinensis, following X-irradiation. II. Analysis of therapeutic effects after fusion with nonirradiated cell portions. J. Exp. Zool. 127, 427–461 (1954).

— Breyer, E. P.: Radiorestoration of Amoeba after injection of unirradiated Protoplasm. Rad. Res. 27, 181 (1966).

— Roth, L. E.: X-Irradiation of the giant amoeba, Pelomyxa illinoisensis. III. Electron microscopy of centrifuged organisms. Rad. Res. 14, 66–82 (1961).

Darden, E. B.: Changes in membrane potentials, K content, and fiber structure in irradiated frog sartorius muscle. Amer. J. Physiol. 198, 709–714 (1960).

Dose, K., Bresciani, F.: Über die Wirkung von Röntgenstrahlen auf den Zellstoffwechsel. II. Die Beeinflussung des Phosphor- und Energiestoffwechsels von isoliertem Gewebe durch Röntgenstrahlen. Biochem. Z. 331, 172–186 (1959).

Detrick, C. E., u. Mitarb.: Pyridoxine absorption from the small intestine of x-irradiated rat. Rad. Res. 21, 186–194 (1964).

Duryee, W. R.: The nature of radiation injury to amphibian cell nuclei. J. Natl. Cancer Inst. 10, 735–795 (1949–50).

Ellinwood, L. E., Wilson, J. E., Coon, J. M.: Release of potassium from the X-irradiated mammalian heart. Proc. Soc. Exper. Biol. Med. 94, 129–133 (1957).

Feichtinger, N.: Über die Einwirkung der α- und β-Strahlen auf das Protoplasma. II. Mitt. Protoplasma 14, 36–51 (1932).

FEICHTINGER, N.: Viskositätsänderung des Protoplasmas als Folge radioaktiver Bestrahlung. Naturwiss. **21**, 569–575 (1933).

FOGG, L. C., SHIELDS-WARREN: A comparison of the cytoplasmic changes induced in the Walker rat carcinoma 256 by different types and dosages of radiation. I. Golgi apparatus. II. Mitochondria. Amer. J. Cancer **31**, 567–577 u. 578–585 (1937).

FORBES, A., THACHER, C.: Changes in the protoplasm of Nereis eggs induced by β-radiation. Amer. J. Physiol. **74**, 567–578 (1925).

GATENBY, J. B., MUKERJI, R. N., WIGODER, S. B.: The effect of X-radiation on the spermatogenesis of Abrascus grossulariata. Proc. Roy. Soc. London Series B, **105**, 446–449 (1929–30).

GECKLER, R. P., KIMBALL, R. F.: The effect of hypoxia on X-ray destruction of kappa in Paramaecium aurelia. Genetics **38**, 663–664 (1953).

GILLET, C.: Perméabilité des menbranes cellulaires et modification du courant cytoplasmique de Nitella flexilis après irradiation. Int. J. Rad. Biol. **8**, 533–539 (1964).

GIAUSER, O.: Elektronenmikroskopische Untersuchungen an Rattenlebern nach Röntgenbestrahlung. Schweiz. Z. allgem. Pathol. Bakteriol. **19**, 150–161 (1956).

GOLDFEDER, A.: Radiosensitivity and metabolic properties of two tumor types indigenous to the same host. I. A correlation of cellular structure and radiosensitivity. Int. J. Rad. Biol. **3**, 155–172 (1961).

— Studies on cytoplasmic ultrastructures following irradiation. Rad. Res. **27**, 190 (1966).

GREEN, J. W.: The separation on Ca ion exchange and glycolysis in human red blood cells exposed to non-ionizing radiations. J. Cell. Comp. Physiol. **47**, 125 (1956).

GUTTMAN, P. H.: Ultrastructural studies of delayed changes in the kidney of the mouse irradiated at birth. Rad. Res. **27**, 652–668 (1966).

HAMPTON, J. C.: A comparison of the effects of x-irradiation and colchicine on the intestinal mucosa of the mouse. Rad. Res. **28**, 37–59 (1966).

— Effects of ionizing radiation on the fine structure of paneth cells of the mouse. Rad. Res. **28**, 71–83 (1966).

— QUASTLER, H.: Some observations on radiation damage in epithelial cells of the mouse intestine. 4th Internatl. Conf. Electron Microscopy Berlin 1958, **2**, 480 (1960).

HARRIS, J. W.: Response of isolated leucocyte lysosomes to gamma irradiation. Rad. Res. **28**, 766–778 (1966).

HELANDER, H. F.: Early effects of x-irradiation on the ultrastructure of gastric fundus glands. Rad. Res. **26**, 244–262 (1965).

HEILBRUNN, L. V.: The viscosity of protoplasm. Protoplasmatologia **2** C 1, 1 (1958).

HENSHAW, P. S.: The action of X-rays on nucleated and non-nucleated egg fragments. Amer. J. Cancer **33**, 258–264 (1938).

HERČIK, F.: Über eine durch α-Strahlen verursachte progressive Nekrose in der Pflanzenzelle. Protoplasma **29**, 172–179 (1938 a).

HERČIK, F.: Über morphologische Veränderungen in Allium-Zellen nach α-Bestrahlung. Protoplasma **31**, 228–233 (1938 b).

— Fluoreszenzmikroskopische Analyse der α-Strahlenwirkung. Protoplasma **32**, 527–535 (1939).

HERTWIG, G.: Das Schicksal des mit Radium bestrahlten Spermachromatins im Seeigelei. Arch. Mikroskop. Anat. **79**, Abtl. 2, 201–241 (1916).

HIRSCH, G. C.: Pankreas II. Analyse der Restitution des Sekretmaterials mittels Röntgenstrahlen, Beobachtungen an lebenden Zellen. Roux' Arch. Entwicklungsmechanik **123**, 792–821 (1931).

HODGKIN, A. C.: The effect of potassium on the surface membrane on an isolated axon. J. Physiol. **106**, 319–340 (1947).

HOFFMANN, J. F.: On the reproducibility in the observed ultrastructure of the normal mammalian red cell plasma membrane. J. Cell Comp. Physiol. **47**, 261–287 (1956).

— The active transport of sodium by ghosts of human red blood cells. J. gen. Physiol. **45**, 837–859 (1962).

HOLTHUSEN, H.: Blutveränderungen durch Röntgenbestrahlung und deren Sensibilisierung. Strahlentherapie **14**, 561–570 (1923).

HORIKAWA, M., et al.: Reactivation of x-irradiated mouse L-cells by means of cellular fractions and highly polymerized deoxyribonucleic acid. Exp. Cell. Res. **34**, 198–200 (1964).

HUGON, J., et al.: Changes in ultrastructure of duodenal crypts in x-irradiated mice. Rad. Res. **25**, 489–502 (1965).

— Delayed ultrastructural changes in duodenal crypts of x-irradiated mice. Int. J. Rad. Biol. **10**, 113–122 (1966).

HRUBY, K.: Durch X-Strahlen hervorgerufene abnorme Plastiden. Vestnik. kral. Česk. spol. nauk **XV**, 11 (1935).

JAMES, A. P.: The nature of lethal sectoring in the vegetative progeny of x-irradiated yeast cells. Rad. Res. **27**, 493–494 (1966).

— WERNER, M. M.: Radiation-induced lethal sectoring in yeast. Rad. Res. **29**, 523–536 (1966).

JÄRNEFELT, J.: Mechanism of sodium transport in cellular membranes. Nature **190**, 694–697 (1961).

KOEHLER, J. K.: Electron microscope observations of radiation-induced HeLa giant cells. Protoplasma **54**, 493–503 (1962).

KOLLMANN, G., et al.: The mechanism of radiation hemolysis in human erythrocytes. Rad. Res. **37**, 555–566 (1969).

KUĆAN, Ž.: Inactivation of isolated Escherichia coli ribosomes by gamma irradiation. Rad. Res. **27**, 229–236 (1966).

LAUDAHN, G.: Morphologie, Biologie und Pathophysiologie der Mitochondrien. Arzneimittelforsch. 9. Beih. (1959).

LEFEVRE, P. G.: Persistence in erythrocyte ghosts of mediated sugar transport. Nature **191**, 970–972 (1961).

LEHMANN, F., WELS, P.: Die Wirkung der Röntgenstrahlen auf die Durchlässigkeit der roten Blutkörperchen für Elektrolyte. Pflügers Arch. ges. Physiol. **213**, 628–641 (1926).

LESSLER, M. A.: Low level X-ray damage to amphibian erythrocytes. Science **129**, 1551–1553 (1959).

Lessler, M. A., Herrera, F. M.: Electron-microscope studies of X-ray damage to frog blood cells. Rad. Res. **17**, 111–117 (1962).

Levi, A. C., Caffaratti, E.: Ergastoplasma ed acidi nucleici nelle cellule della glandula parotide di Epimys norvegicus var. albino (Erl.) sottoposta a radiazione roentgen e stimulata con pilocarpina. Sperimentale **110**, 161–176 (1960); ref. Biol. Abstr. **36**, 36107 (1961).

Levine, M.: Cytological studies on irradiated tissues I. The influence of radium emanation on the microsporogensis of the lily. Proc. internatl. Congr. Plant Sci. Ithaca, N. Y. **1**, 271–297 (1926).

Levinson, W.: Toxic effect of x-irradiated medium on chick embryo cells.Exp.Cell.Res.**43**,398–413(1669).

Levis, A. G., Marin, G.: Induction of multipolar spindles in mammalian cells in vitro. Exper. Cell Res. **31**, 448–451 (1963).

Lopriore, G.: Azione dei raggi X sul protoplasma della cellula vegetale vivente. Nuova Rassegna 1897.

Magath, M.: Änderungen der Zellpermeabilität durch Röntgenbestrahlung, gemessen an der Phosphatausscheidung überlebender Tumor- und Leberschnitte. Z. Krebsforsch. **31**, 95–104 (1930).

Maizel, M.: Factors in the active transport of cations. J. Physiol. **112**, 59–83 (1951).

Maly, R.: Cytomorphologische Studien an strahleninduzierten, konstant abweichenden Plastidenformen bei Farnprothallien.Z.f. ind. Abst.- u. Vererbungslehre **83**, 447–478 (1951).

Marin, G., Bender, M. A.: Radiation-induced mammalian cell death: Lapse-time cinemicrographic observations. Exp. Cell Res. **43**, 413–423 (1966).

Marquardt, H.: Der Feinbau von Hefezellen im Elektronenmikroskop. I. Rhodotorula rubra. Z. Naturforsch. **17b**, 42–48 (1962a).

— Der Feinbau von Hefezellen im Elektronenmikroskop. II. Saccharomyces cerevisiae-Stämme. Z. Naturforsch. **17b**, 689–695 (1962b).

Masurovsky, E. B., Bunge, R. P.: Correlative studies of radiation protection and ultrastructural localization of AET derivatives in organotypic mammalian peripheral nervous tissue cultures. Rad. Res. **25**, 216–217 (1965).

— — Cytological changes in neutron-irradiated mammalian peripheral nervous tissue cultures. Rad. Res. **31**, 574 (1967).

McCardle, R. C., Congdon, C. C.: Mitochondrial changes in hepatic cells of X-irradiated mice. Amer. J. Pathol. **31**, 725–746 (1955).

Merrick, T. P., Bruce, A. K.: Radiation response of potassium efflux in Micrococcus radiodurans and Sarcina lutea. Rad. Res. **24**, 612–618 (1965).

McQuade, H. A., Evans, T. C.: The electron microscopy of the response of follicular epithelium cells of rat thyroid to autolysis, ligation, and irradiation by iodine-131. Rad. Res. **11**, 520–534 (1959).

Michaelis, P.: Untersuchungen zur Mutation plasmatischer Erbträger, besonders der Plastiden. 1. Teil. Planta **51**, 600–634 (1958).

— Über gehäufte Plastidenabänderungen. I. Biologisches Zentralblatt **81**, 91–128 (1962).

Milovidov, P. F.: Influence du sodium sur le chondriome des cellules végétales. C. r. Soc. Biol. Paris **101**, 676–678 (1929).

Miwa, M., Yamashita, H., Mori, K.: The action of ionizing rays on sea-urchin IV. The effects of α-rays upon fertilized eggs. Gann. **33**, 323–331 (1939).

Morczek, A.: Untersuchungen über den Kalium-Natrium-Austausch von Erythrozyten durch die Einwirkung ionisierender Strahlen. Strahlentherapie **96**, 618–624 (1955).

Munro, T. R.: α-Irradiation of parts of single cells in tissue culture. III. Irradiation of chick fibroblaste during metaphase and anaphase. Exper. Cell Res. **18**, 76–99 (1959).

Myers, D. K., Bide, R. W.: Biochemical effects of x-irradiation on erythrocytes. Rad. Res. **27**, 250–263 (1966).

— Slade, D. E.: Radiosensitizing action of iodoacetamide. Rad. Res. **27**, 498 (1966).

Nadson, G. A.: Über die Primärwirkung der Radiumstrahlen auf die lebendige Substanz. Biochem. Z. **155**, 381–386 (1925).

— Rochlin-Gleichgewicht, E. J.: Le chondriome est la partie de la cellule la plus sensible aux rayons-X. C. r. Soc. Biol. Paris **95**, 378–380 (1926).

— Rochlin, E. J.: L'effet des rayons-X sur le protoplasme, le noyeau et le chondriome de la cellule végétale d'après les observations sur le vivant. Protoplasma **20**, 31–41 (1934).

Nakao, Y.: Action of irradiated cytoplasm on untreated chromosomes of the silkworm. Nature **172**, 625–626 (1953).

Nickel, E.: Änderungen von Morphologie und Stoffwechsel von Paramaecium caudatum durch Röntgenstrahlen. Z. Naturforsch. **16b**, 538–543 (1961).

Northen, H. T., McVicar, R.: Effects of X-rays on the structural viscosity of protoplasm. Biodynamica **3**, 28–32 (1940).

Noyes, P. P., Smith, R. E.: Quantitative changes in rat liver mitochondria following whole body irradiation. Exper. Cell Res. **16**, 15–23 (1959).

Nürnberger: Histologische Untersuchungen über die Einwirkung der Röntgenstrahlen auf das Zellprotoplasma. Zugleich ein Beitrag zur Kenntnis der Plastosomen. Virchow's Arch. Pathol. Anat. Physiol. **246**, 239–252 (1923).

Okada, S., Peechey, L. D.: Effect of γ-irradiation on the deoxyribonuclease. II. Activity of isolated mitochondria. J. Biophys. Biochem. Cytol. **3**, 239–247 (1957).

Ord, M. J., Danielli, J. F.: The site of damage on amoebae exposed to X-rays. Quart. J. Microscop. Sci. **97**, 29–37 (1956).

Packard, C.: The effect of radium radiations on the development of Chaetopterus. Biol. Bull. **35**, 50–67 (1918).

Pantić, V., et al.: Ultrastructural changes of thyroid intraocular grafts x-irradiated in vitro before transplantation. Int. J. Rad. Biol. **12**, 305–316 (1967).

Parchwitz, H. K.: Morphologische Untersuchungen an extranukleären Zellbestandteilen des Walker-Carcinoms nach einzeitiger Röntgenbestrahlung. Strahlentherapie **104**, 21–28 (1957).

— Strahlenwirkung auf Tumorzellen. Scherer, E., Stender, N. S., Strahlenpathologie der Zelle. Stuttgart: G. Thieme 1963.

PARCHWITZ, H. K., WITTEKINDT, E.: Photometrische Untersuchungen über das Verhalten der Ribonucleoproteide in der Walker-Carcinom-Zelle nach einzeitiger lokaler Röntgenbestrahlung. Strahlentherapie **106**, 282–288 (1958).

PARSONS, D. F.: An electron microscope study of radiation damage in the mouse oocyte. J. Cell Biol. **14**, 31–48 (1962).

PATTERSON, J. T.: The production of gynandromorphs in Drosophila melanogaster by X-rays. J. Exper. Zool. **60**, 173–211 (1931).

PETROVA, J.: Über den Vergleich von α-Strahlenempfindlichkeit von Kern und Plasma. Ber. Dtsch. Botan. Ges. **60**, 148–151 (1942a).

— Über die verschiedene Wirkung von α-Strahlen auf Kern und Plasma der Zelle. Botan. Cbl. Beih. A **61**, 399–430 (1942b).

PERRIS, A. D.: Whole-body irradiation and active transport in the rat small intestine in vitro. Rad. Res. **29**, 597–607 (1966).

POMERAT, C. M.: Cellular changes induced by radiation. Ann. N. Y. Acad. Sci. **71**, 1143–1155 (1958).

RAJEWSKY, B.: Weitere Untersuchungen an der Strahlenreaktion des Eiweißes. Strahlentherapie **33**, 362–374 (1929).

RIESER, P.: The effect of roentgen rays on the colloidal properties of the starfish egg. Biol. Bull. **109**, 108–112 (1955).

— KAYE, A. M.: Release of an anticoagulant from irradiated Spisula eggs. Biol. Bull. **105**, 380 (1953).

RITCHIE, D.: Cytoplasmic damage caused by γ-radiation in Allomyces javanicus. Botan. Gaz. **115**, 138–146 (1953).

RIXON, R. H.: Cytological manifestations of radiation-induced death in living lymphocytes from rat thymus. Rad. Res. **25**, 233 (1965).

RÖBBELEN, G.: Plastommutationen nach Röntgenbestrahlung von Arabidopsis Thaliana (L) Heynh. Z. Vererbungsl. **93**, 25–34 (1962).

ROCHLIN-GLEICHGEWICHT, E.: Effect of radon on chlorophyll containing cells. Vestnik Roentgen i Radio **8**, 387–407 (1930).

ROMANI, R. J., et al.: Mitochondria: Increase in oxidative capacity and quantitative recovery after massive doses of ionizing radiation. Rad. Res. **28**, 257–265 (1966).

ROTHSTEIN, A.: Biochemical and physiological changes in irradiated yeast. Rad. Res. Suppl. **1**, 357 (1959).

— BRUCE, M.: The potassium efflux and influx in yeast at different potassium concentrations. J. Cell. Comp. Physiol. **51**, 145–159 (1958).

RUSTAD, R. C.: Centriol damage: a possible explanation of radiation-induced mitotic delay. Rad. Res. **11**, 465 (1959).

— Cytoplasmic effects in radiation induced mitotic delay. Rad. Res. **25**, 234 (1965).

SCAIFE, J. F., ALEXANDER, P.: Inability of X-rays to alter the permeability of mitochondria. Rad. Res. **15**, 658–674 (1961).

SCHERER, E.: Morphologische und Fermenthistochemische Studien zur Strahlenwirkung auf den Organismus. I. Untersuchungen an isolierten Mitochondrien der Maus. Strahlentherapie **99**, 230–241 (1956).

SCHERER, E., RINGLEB, D.: Beobachtungen an den Mitochondrien der Mäuseascites-Tumorzellen unter der Einwirkung von Röntgenstrahlen. Strahlentherapie **90**, 34–40 (1953).

— STOLLE, F.: Das Verhalten der Zellmitochondrien in der Mäusemilz unter Einwirkung einer Röntgentotalbestrahlung. Strahlentherapie **93**, 317–320 (1954).

— VOGELL, W.: Elektronenoptische Untersuchungen zur Strahlenwirkung auf Leber, Milz und Niere. Strahlentherapie **106**, 202–211 (1958).

— VÖLKER, K.: Das Farbstoffbindungsvermögen isolierter Lebermitochondrien nach Röntgenbestrahlung in vitro und in vivo. Strahlentherapie **111**, 237–293 (1960).

— WICHMANN, K. O.: Beobachtungen über den Ablauf der Strahlenreaktion im Milzgewebe der Maus bei Anwendung der Phasenkontrastmikroskopie. Strahlentherapie **95**, 195–208 (1954).

SCHJEIDE, O. A., MEAD, J. F., MYERS, L. S., JR.: Notions on sensitivity of cells to radiation. Science **123**, 1020–1022 (1956).

— RAGAU, N., McCAUDLESS, R. C., BISHOP, F. C.: Effect of X-irradiation on cellular inclusions in chicken embryo livers. Rad. Res. **13**, 205–213 (1960).

SCHNEIDER, L.: Elektronenmikroskopische Analyse von Strahlenschäden im Cytoplasma. 4. Internatl. Congr. für Elektronenmikroskopie Berlin 1958, Bd. II, 477–479, 1960.

— Elektronenmikroskopische Untersuchungen über die Wirkung von Strahlen auf das Cytoplasma. 1. Die Frühwirkungen von Röntgenstrahlen auf das Cytoplasma von Paramaecium. Protoplasma **53**, 530–553 (1961a).

— Elektronenmikroskopische Untersuchungen über die Wirkung von Strahlen auf das Cytoplasma. 2. Die Spätwirkung von Röntgenstrahlen auf das Cytoplasma von Paramaecium. Protoplasma **53**, 554–574 (1961b).

SEIFRIZ, W.: Reaction of protoplasm to radium radiation. Protoplasma **25**, 196–200 (1936).

SHAPIRO, B., et al.: Mechanism of the effect of ionizing radiation on sodium uptake by human erythrocytes. Rad. Res. **27**, 139–158 (1966).

— KOLLMANN, G.: The nature of the membrane injury in irradiated human erythrocytes. Rad. Res. **34**, 335–346 (1968).

SHEPPARD, C. W., BEYL, G. E.: Cation exchange in mammalian erythrocytes. III. The prolytic effect of X-rays in human cells. J. gen. Physiol. **34**, 691–704 (1951).

— STEWARD, M.: The direct effects of radiation on erythrocytes. J. Cell. Comp. Physiol. **39**, Suppl. 2, 189–215 (1952).

SHIVELY, J. N., EPLING, G. P.: Early changes in the fine structure of the thyroid of midlethally irradiated dogs. Rad. Res. **34**, 71–82 (1969).

SIX, E.: Die Wirkung von Strahlen auf Acetabularia. II. Die Wirkung von Röntgenstrahlen auf kernlose Teile von Acetabularia mediterranea. Z. Naturforsch. **11b**, 598–603 (1956).

STRUGGER, S. P., KREBS, A. T., GIERLACH, Z. S.: Investigations into the first effects of Roentgen rays on living protoplasm as studied with modern fluorochromes. Amer. J. Roentgenol. **70**, 365–375 (1953).

Škreb, Y., Horvat, D.: Influence of gamma-radiation on the incorporation of 14 C-Adenine and 14 C-Phenylalanine into whole Amoeba and nucleate and anucleate Amoeba fragments. Exp. Cell Res. **43**, 639–644 (1966).

Spoerl, E., et al.: Permeability changes in yeast cells after x-irradiation and starvation. Rad. Res. **21**, 86–90 (1964).

Srb, V.: Immediate and short-term changes in cell permeability after x-irradiation. Rad. Res. 308–313 (1964).

— Dauerhafter Einfluß der Röntgenstrahlen auf Zellpermeabilität. Exp. Cell Res. **34**, 318–324 (1964).

— Effect of storage of x-irradiated onions Allium cepa L. on changes in cell permeability. Exp. Cell Res. **36**, 270–274 (1964).

Sutherland, R. M., et al.: Evidence for a key role of sulfhydril groups in radiation damage to the erythrocyte membrane. Rad. Res. **27**, 497–498 (1966).

— Pihl, A.: Repair of radiation damage to erythrocyte membranes: the reduction of radiation-induced disulfide groups. Rad. Res. **34**, 300–314 (1968).

Tahmisian, T. N., Devine, R. L.: The influence of X-rays on organelle induction and differentiation in grasshopper spermatogenesis. J. Biophys. Biochem. Cytol. **9**, 29–45 (1961).

Ting, T. P., Zirkle, R. E.: Nature and cause of hemolysis produced by X-rays. J. Cell. Comp. Physiol. **16**, 189–195 (1940a).

— — The kinetics of the diffusion of salts into and out of X-irradiated erythrocytes. J. Cell. Comp. Physiol. **16**, 197–206 (1940b).

Tschassownikow, N.: Über die Wirkung von Röntgenstrahlen auf den feinen Bau der Leberzellen beim Frosch. Virchow's Arch. Path. Anat. **269**, 166–177 (1928).

Ulrich, H.: Ergebnisse strahlengenetischer Untersuchungen an Drosophila-Zygoten. Schriftenreihe d. Bundesministers für Atomkernenergie u. Wasserwirtschaft. Strahlenschutz **17**, 10–17 (1959).

Vintemberger, P.: Sur le résultat de l'application d'une dose forte de rayons X à une région de la cellule ne renfermant pas le noyeau. C. r. Soc. Biol. **99**, 1965–1967 (1928a).

— Sur les effets d'applications des rayons-X localisées soit au protoplasm, soit à la région nucléaire de la cellule. C. r. Soc. Biol. **99**, 1968–1971 (1928b).

Virgin, H. I., Ehrenberg, L.: Effects of β- and γ-rays on the protoplasmic viscosity of Helodea cells. Physiol. Plantarum **6**, 159–165 (1953).

Warren, S., Holt, M. W., Sommers, S. C.: Some early nuclear effects of ionizing radiation. Proc. Soc. Exper. Biol. Med. **77**, 288–291 (1951).

Weber, F.: Röntgenstrahlenwirkung und Protoplasmaviskosität. Arch. ges. Physiol. **198**, 644–647 (1923).

Weijer, J.: Protective action of calcium gluconate against after-effects of X-irradiation on conidia of Neurospora crassa. Nature **189**, 760 (1961).

Wendt, E.: Die Wirkung von Röntgenstrahlen auf das Centroplasma und die Cytosomen von Gewebekulturzellen. Z. f. Zellforschung **53**, 172–184 (1961).

Whiting, A. R.: Androgenesis, a differentiator of cytoplasmic injury induced by X-rays in Habrobracon eggs. Biol. Bull. **97**, 210–220 (1949).

— The non-induction of mutations by X-rayed cyptolasm. Genetics **35**, 139 (1950a).

— Absence of mutagenic action on X-rayed cytoplasm in Habroboacon. Proc. Natl. Acad. Sci. Wash. **36**, 368–372 (1950b).

— Androgenesis as evidence for the nature of X-ray induced injury. Rad. Res. **2**, 71–78 (1955).

Wichterman, R., Figge, E. H. J.: Lethality and biological effects of X-rays in Paramaecium. Radiation resistance and its variability. Biol. Bull. **106**, 253 (1954).

Wilbur, K. M., Recknagel, R. O.: The radiosensitivity of eggs of Arbacia punctulata in various salt solutions. Biol. Bull. **85**, 193–200 (1943).

Williams, M.: Observations on the action of X-rays on plant cells. Ann. Botany **37**, 217–223 (1923).

— Some observations on the action of radium on certain plant cells. Ann. Botany **39**, 547–562 (1925).

Wilson, W. L.: The effect of roentgen-rays on protoplasmic viscosity during mitosis. Protoplasma **39**, 305–317 (1950).

Wohlfahrt-Bottermann, K. E.: Cytologische Studien V. Feinstrukturveränderungen des Cytoplasmas und der Mitochondrien von Paramaecium nach Einwirkung letaler Temperaturen und Röntgendosen. Protoplasma **50**, 82–92 (1959).

— Schneider, L.: Strahlenwirkungen an Mitochondrien. Strahlentherapie **116**, 25–38 (1961).

Zacek, J., Rosenberg, R.: Action des rayons X sur la membrane des globules rouges. C. r. Soc. Biol. **144**, 462–464 (1950).

Zirkle, R. E.: Some effects of α-irradiation upon plant cells. J. Cell. Comp. Physiol. **2**, 251–278 (1932).

— Bloom, W.: Irradiation of parts of individual cells. Science **117**, 487–493 (1953).

Zuelzer, M., Philipp, E.: Beeinflussung des kolloidalen Zustands des Zellinhalts von Protozoen durch Radiumstrahlen. Strahlentherapie **20**, 737–770 (1925).

E. Irradiation of generative organs*

E. F. Oakberg and Evelyn C. Lorenz

With 5 figures

Our understanding of radiation response of the gonads is dependent on our knowledge of the origin of the germ cells, their subsequent development during uterine and prepubertal life, and gametogenesis in the adult. Whereas a general radiation response of the testis of mammals can be formulated, species have their characteristic variations within this general framework. In the case of the ovary, species differences are so great that no general response can as yet be delineated. Data on the human have been used wherever possible, but it is necessary to rely primarily upon studies of experimental animals in this discussion.

I. Gametogenesis

1. Prenatal and neonatal

Migration of primordial germ cells from an extragonadal origin to the germinal ridges was first described by WITSCHI (1948) in human embryos. Later, CHIQUOINE (1954), demonstrated selective alkaline phosphate positive staining of the primordial germ cells of the mouse, and by this technique, was able to trace their migration from their origin in the region of the caudal end of the primitive streak, root of the allantoic mesoderm, and yolk sac splanchnopleure in the 8-day mouse embryo, to the germinal ridges of the 12-day embryo. The demonstration by MINTZ (1960) that sterility and reduced fertility associated with certain genotypes of the mouse can be correlated with a reduced number of primordial germ cells is conclusive evidence that these are the stem cells of the definitive gametes. Oocyte counts in rat embryos have led to the same conclusion (BEAUMONT and MANDL, 1962). Mitotic division occurs both during migration of the primordial germ cells and in the germinal ridge. Primordial germ cells transform directly into oocytes in the female (BRAMBELL, 1927; BEAUMONT and MANDL, 1962; MINTZ, 1960; BAKER, 1963). In males, they give rise to type A spermatogonia soon after birth in the rat (CLERMONT and PEREY, 1957; HUCKINS, 1965) and by 10 years in man (CHARNY, CONSTON, and MERANZE, 1952). The human testis has not been studied as thoroughly as that of rodents, and whereas the general mechanism of establishment of the adult seminiferous epithelium is the same, precise comparisons with experimental animals are not yet feasible.

2. Female

The most distinctive feature of oogenesis in mammals is that the definitive number of oocytes is determined before, or at the latest, soon after birth, and that the only germ cell stage present thereafter is the oocyte. (For a comprehensive review, see FRANCHI, MANDL and ZUCKERMAN, 1962.) The number of oocytes decreases steadily with age, primarily by follicular atresia (ZUCKERMAN, 1951; OAKBERG, 1966). Study of the nuclear cytology of the mammalian oocyte is difficult, and insufficient work has been done in this field, but development usually is arrested in diplotene. The degree of chromosme conden-

---

* Research sponsored by the U. S. Atomic Energy Commission under contract with the Union Carbide Corporation.

sation in diplotene of the oocyte, however, varies widely between species. For example, a "typical" diplotene is characteristic of the "arrested" oocyte in the human, goat, and dog, but a synizesis-like nucleus is characteristic of the guinea pig, and the diffuse, interphase-like dictyate stage is typical for mouse and rat (Oakberg and Clark, 1964). In all species, the chromosomes become more diffuse and oxyphylic during growth of the follicle. An active RNA synthesis, as measured by ^{3}H-uridine uptake, occurs in the growing follicle, but ceases at the time of antrum formation (Oakberg, 1968). The first meiotic division occurs in the ovary; ovulation occurs with the chromosomes in metaphase of the second meiotic division (Sobotta, 1895; Austin and Amoroso, 1959). Although the basic mechanisms involved in radiation damage still are not known, sensitivity to cell death and chromosome breakage is closely correlated with meiotic prophase stage in both plants and animals (Sparrow, Moses, and Dubow, 1952; Mitra, 1958; Whiting, 1940; L. B. Russell and W. L. Russell, 1956; Oakberg and DiMinno, 1960). Differences in nuclear structure of the "arrested" stage probably are related to differences in metabolic activity and other factors which could lead to widely different effects between species.

3. Male

Our understanding of normal spermatogenesis has advanced markedly in recent years owing to the accurate identification of cells and developmental sequences made possible by the periodic acid-Schiff technique (Leblond and Clermont, 1952; Clermont, 1962; Oakberg, 1956a). In rodents, stages of the cycle of the seminiferous epithelium occupy relatively large areas of the tubule, and a given tubule cross section usually shows a single stage. In man, however, an average of three different stages appears in a single cross section, and while analysis of the cycle of the seminiferous epithelium is therefore very difficult, it has been shown to be fundamentally the same as that observed in other species (Clermont, 1963; Heller and Clermont, 1964).

It long has been recognized that the stem cell of the mammalian testis is a type A spermatogonium (see review by Roosen-Runge, 1962), and that by the process of stem cell renewal, these cells maintain a steady state population, yet give rise to unlimited numbers of differentiating cells. The precise mechanism of stem cell renewal still is not completely resolved, but important contributions have recently been made by Leblond and Clermont (1952); Clermont (1963); Clermont and Bustos-Obregon (1968); Hilscher (1968); Hilscher and Makoski (1968); de Rooij and Kramer (1968); de Rooij (1969); Hochereau-de Reviers (1970); Huckins (1971); and Oakberg (1971). In the model of Huckins (1971a), for the rat and of Oakberg (1971a), for the mouse, isolated A spermatogonia with oval, darkly staining, granular nuclei are considered to be the stem cells and have been designated A_s. At division of A_s spermatogonia, the daughter nuclei either move apart to form two isolated cells, or remain close together as a "pair". The "pair" then divides to form a chain of 4, 8, and 16 spermatogonia with morphology similar to that of the A_s. These "chains" then transform into spermatogonia A_1, divide, and form type A_2 cells. Division of the A_2 leads to formation of A_3, of the A_3 to form A_4 which form In (intermediate) spermatogonia. In agreement with Monesi (1962a), there is no evidence for the formation of anything but the In from the type A_4 spermatogonia. Evidence from both whole mounts and conventional sections suggest that members of the pairs and chains are joined by intercellular bridges, and that this is a factor in maintenance of synchrony among members of the group (Oakberg, 1971a; Huckins and Oakberg, 1971). Observations with the electron microscope have, indeed, confirmed the presence of such bridges between spermatogonia (Dym and Fawcett, 1971; Rowley et al., 1971; Gondos and Zemjanis, 1970). Furthermore, morphology of the A_L spermatogonium of man (Rowley et al., 1971) is extremely close to that of A_s cells of mouse and rat, and homology of these cells appears likely. If true, this could be an important factor in the slow depletion and slow recovery of spermatogonia in the irradiated human testis.

The time required for development of spermatozoa from type A_1 spermatogonia is about 35 days in the mouse (Oakberg, 1956b), 52 days in the rat (Clermont and Harvey, 1965), and from A_d, about 72—74 days in man (Heller and Clermont, 1964). Study of the cellular associations following low doses of radiation (Oakberg, 1956b), progression of ^{3}H-thymidine labeled cells in irradiated testes (Edwards and Sirlin, 1958), and endocrinological studies (Ortavant and Courot, 1963) suggest that the duration of spermatogenesis is a biological constant for each species. Sperm transport takes 7—8 days in the mouse, 14 days in the rat, and is quite variable in man. Since the time required for development of all stages later than type A_s is short in relation to reproductive life-span in mammals, the type A_s spermatogonium is the most important cell in terms of both long-term fertility and genetic effects in irradiated males.

II. Radiation response, males

1. Prenatal and neonatal stages

Two periods of high sensitivity to radiation-induced sterility have been observed in the immature rat testis. The first, in the 13.5- to 17.5-day embryo, is associated with high mitotic activity of the primordial germ cells. The second and most sensitive period occurs around the time of birth (19-day fetus to 2 days postpartum), when primordial germ cells are giving rise to type A spermatogonia (Beaumont, 1960). A similar pattern, but at slightly younger ages, occurs in the mouse, and probably is common to most species (Rugh and Jackson, 1958; Russell, Badgett, and Saylors, 1959). Leonard, Imbaud, and Maisin (1964) observed that sensitivity of the rat testis at 17 days after birth was higher than at 8 days. The radiation effect in both the rat and mouse can be attributed to killing of germ cells and subsequent deficiency in type A spermatogonia in the adult. Time sequences in human testicular development are not as well known (Charny et al., 1952), but comparable stages in germ cell development to those studied above may be expected.

2. Adult

After an acute radiation dose of 100 to 300 R, depending on species and genetic strain, male animals are initially fertile owing to continued development of cells irradiated as spermatozoa, spermatids, and possibly spermatocytes. A temporary sterile period, the

Table 1. *Duration of initial fertile and sterile periods following irradiation of males*

Species	Dose (R)	Duration (weeks)		Reference
		Presterile period	Sterile period	
Mouse	300	6	2	Craig et al. (1961)
	500	3	10	Bateman, A. J. (1958)
	600	4	$4^1/_2$	Russell, W. L. (1954)
	800	$2^1/_2$	10	Snell, G. D. (1933)
	800	3	11	Hertwig, P. (1938)
	800	2	10	Russell, W. L. (1954)
	1000	2	11	Russell, W. L. (1954)
Rat	300	9	2	Craig et al. (1961)
	500	6	12	Craig et al. (1961)
Guinea pig	173–864	8	3	Strandskov, H. H. (1932)
	1296	4	24	Strandskov, H. H. (1932)
	1728	2	24	Strandskov, H. H. (1932)

duration of which is dependent upon dose and species (Table 1), then occurs as a result of spermatogonial killing. With high doses, killing of significant numbers of spermatocytes results in an earlier onset of the sterile period, and a prolongation occurs owing to slow repopulation of the seminiferous epithelium when spermatogonial survival is low. Eventually the seminiferous epithelium is repopulated from surviving type A_s spermatogonia, and fertility returns (Oakberg, 1971b).

3. Spermatids and spermatozoa

Morphology and spermiogenesis of cells irradiated as spermatids and spermatozoa are unaffected by doses of 1500 R in the mouse; exposure to 32000 R or more is required to affect motility of human sperm (Gerber, 1955) and fertilizing capacity (Chang, Hunt, and Romanoff, 1957) of mature rabbit spermatozoa was normal after 60000 R. No viable zygotes are formed after such doses owing to extensive chromosomal damage. Many abnormal spermatids and spermatozoa can be seen after doses of 100 R or more, but these have developed from cells which were spermatocytes at the time of irradiation (Oakberg and Di Minno, 1960). Genetic effects ranging from presumed point mutations to deficiencies and chromosome rearrangements are induced with high frequency, however, especially in early spermatids (Russell and Saylors, 1963).

4. Spermatocytes

Spermatocytes follow a pattern of radiation response which is typical for meiotic prophase stages in general (Oakberg and Di Minno, 1960). Chromosome breakage, scored as abnormal anaphases during meiotic division, is highest for diakinesis-metaphase I and lowest for leptotene and preleptotene (Table 2). Cells urvival is highest for diplotene and diakinesis, intermediate for pachytene, and lowest for preleptotene. Whereas probability of elimination of cells with specific types of chromosomal damage may differ with prophase stage irradiated, materials where this factor can be excluded have given results comparable to the mouse (Sparrow, Moses, and Dubow, 1952; Mitra, 1958). As a result of killing of spermatocytes, and chromosome breakage which results in abnormal spermatozoa (Oakberg and Di Minno, 1960), onset of the sterile period is earlier for radiation doses of 800 R or more. There apparently is a strain effect in this response (Bateman, 1958), but this

Table 2. *Effect of meiotic prophase stage on survival and on chromosome breakage in primary spermatocytes of the mouse. (From* Oakberg *and* Di Minno, *1960)*

Meiotic prophase stage	Survival data			Chromosome breakage D_{50}	
	Point estimate LD_{50} (R)	95% confidence limits		Anaphase I	Anaphase II
		Lower	Upper		
Preleptotene	205	175	233	612 ± 93	
Leptotene	492	273	719	1443 ± 182	
Zygotene	520	413	637	411	
Pachytene (early)	404	329	470	242	
Pachytene (mid)	382	301	452	265	
Pachytene (late)	664	601	733	321	
Diplotene	564	365	771	275	
Diakinesis — Metaphase I	837	679	1161		
Diakinesis				204	
Metaphase I					138 ± 6

probably reflects differences in normal sperm numbers rather than differential cell response. Radiation sensitivity of spermatocytes has been claimed to be higher in the monkey than in the mouse (ARSENIEVA and BOCHKOV, 1963), with the implication that sensitivity in man may be closer to that of the monkey.

5. Spermatogonia

The primary radiation response of spermatogonia is cell death, which occurs prior to cell division (OAKBERG, 1955; MONESI, 1962b; BAKULINA and ORLOVA, 1963). As a result of spermatogonial killing, sperm production is interrupted after radiation exposure, and if the dose is high enough a period of oligospermia and infertility occurs (Table 1). The relative frequencies of degenerating type A spermatogonia of the mouse are shown for different times and doses in Fig. 1. Return to control levels occurs by 2 days for doses of 20 to 300 R; the high values for 600 R at 2—8 days are based on very small cell populations and represent an *absolute* number of necrotic cells which is actually lower than control. Intermediate, type B, and late type A spermatogonia of the mouse are uniformly sensitive

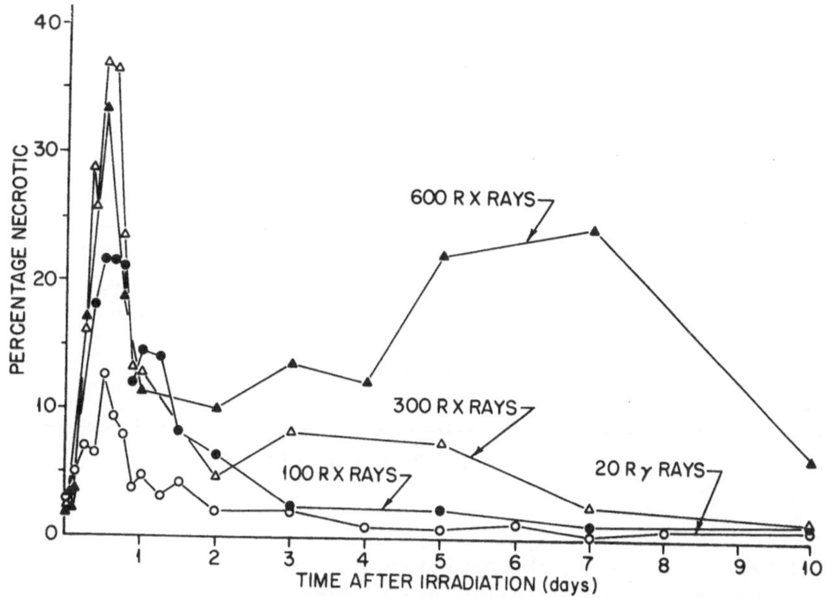

Fig. 1. Percentage of necrotic type A spermatogonia 1 hr to 10 days after irradiation of the male mouse. (From OAKBERG, 1959)

to cell killing, with LD_{50}s in the range of 20—24 R for 60 Co γ rays (OAKBERG, 1957), and the effect of any acute dose above 2 rads can be detected (OAKBERG, 1962a). It should be pointed out, however, that the most sensitive spermatogonia occur among the type A population. This is demonstrated by the fact that survival of the total A population at doses below 25 R is the same as survival of A_4-In and In-B spermatogonia (OAKBERG, 1957). This occurs in spite of the fact that about 40 % of the type A population is more resistant, with linear survival kinetics over the 100—1000 R dose range (OAKBERG, 1964). A possible factor in the high sensitivity of some A spermatogonia is provided by the studies of HUCKINS and OAKBERG (1971) on tubule whole mounts of mouse, and of OAKBERG (1971a) on sections of mouse testis, which reveal cytoplasmic connection between the "paired" and "aligned" spermatogonia. This may be an important factor in radiation response, for it can be demonstrated that entire chains either degenerate or survive (HUCKINS, unpublished data).

The duration of the temporary period of infertility increases at high doses within species owing both to lower numbers of surviving spermatogonia and hence slower recovery, and to killing of spermatocytes, which leads to an earlier onset of infertility (Table 1). The variations between species shown in Table 1 arise primarily from differences in duration of spermatogenesis. The type A population, however, is of heterogeneous radiation sensitivity, and only a few survivors are required for regeneration of the seminiferous epithelium (Fig. 2; Oakberg, 1955). In addition to different rates of recovery shown for doses given in Fig. 2, it is clear that the time required for maximum depression of cell numbers is greater with high doses. This results from concurrence of cell degeneration and cell repopulation, with the interaction between these factors specific for each dose. Thus there is no *one* optimum time for comparison of the effect of dose on spermatogonial survival. The mechanisms involved in radiation-induced death of spermatogonia are not known, but there is some indication that G_1, S, and G_2 phases of the cell cycle differ

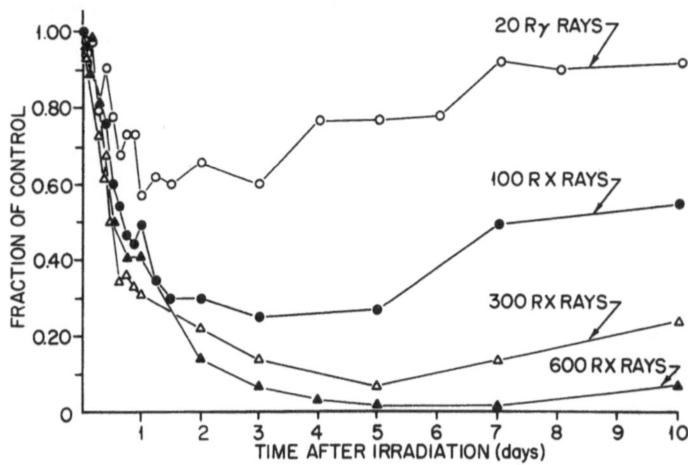

Fig. 2. Experimental/control ratios for "normal" type A spermatogonia 1 hr to 10 days after irradiation of the male mouse. (From Oakberg, 1959)

in radiation sensitivity (Monesi, 1962b; Oakberg, 1964). Recently, Monesi (1964) has observed that "dormant" type A spermatogonia synthesize very little RNA, which may indicate low metabolic activity for these cells, and which could possibly be related to radiation response. Another promising approach to the problem of differential radiation response of spermatogonia is the use of chemicals which affect specific metabolic processes (Partington, Fox, and Jackson, 1964).

Recent data on stem cell renewal have revealed complications in the study of mitotic inhibition in the irradiated testis which may also apply to other germinative tissues. Monesi (1962b) observed a delay of about 2 hours in spermatogonial divisions after 100 R; a response comparable to that observed in other tissues. Previously, we had pointed out that it is difficult to do studies of this nature owing to the fact that division of surviving cells began before cell degeneration had returned to control levels, and that this degeneration occured prior to mitosis (Oakberg, 1959). It is now clear that greater survival of A_s spermatogonia, which inherently have a low mitotic index, is an important factor. It is possible that the mitotic rate of A_s cells may even be enhanced as they begin repopulation of the seminiferous epithelium. It has been claimed by Dym and Clermont (1970) that cells they classified as A_0 abandoned their "reserve stem-cell" role to regenerate the A_1 population. However, it already had been observed by Oakberg (1964) that some type A spermatogonia labeled with ^{3}H-thymidine survived high radiation exposures. It now is almost certain that these were isolated A_s cells (OAKBERG, 1971), and indicates that these cells were mitotically active prior to irradiation, and not stimulated into activity as proposed by DYM and CLERMONT (1970). This is further evidence for the model of stem-cell renewal proposed by HUCKINS (1971a) and OAKBERG (1971a). The basis of the high labeling index observed at certain intervals after X-ray (OAKBERG, 1964) has not been explained, but acceleration of division of A_s cells may be achieved by shortening the cell cycle, or by decrease in the frequency of cells with the longer cycle times. In either case, S would be longer than for A_2—A_4 spermatogonia (HUCKINS, 1971) previously used as a basis of comparison.

The A_s spermatogonia are the most important cells of the mammalian testis, both in terms of effects on fertility and genetic damage (OAKBERG, 1971b). If sufficient numbers survive radiation exposure, they will repopulate the seminiferous epithelium and fertility will return. Any genetic damage which does not result in cell lethality will be manifest throughout the remaining reproductive life of the individual.

6. Dose rate

Cells have the capacity to repair and/or prevent certain types of primary radiation damage provided the events are sufficiently distributed in space and time. As a result, higher doses often can be tolerated than if given in an acute exposure. The degree of effect, however, will depend upon the cell, the tissue, and the response being observed. No effect of dose rate on spermatogonial killing in the mouse has been observed over the range of 93 to 0.8 R/min (OAKBERG and CLARK, 1961). A marginal response was observed at 0.009 R/min. These results are in agreement with the observation that fertility of adult male mammals is not impaired by either acute or continuous X- and γ-ray exposures until the level exceeds 2 R/day (LANGENDORFF and LANGENDORFF, 1957; ESCHENBRENNER, MILLER, and LORENZ, 1948; BROWN et al., 1964).

In studies of mutation frequency in males, RUSSELL et al. (1959) and RUSSELL (1963) have observed that reduction of the dose rate from 90 to either 0.8 or 0.009 R/min reduced the number of mutations by a factor of about 3.2. An intermediate frequency was observed at 9 R/min (RUSSELL, 1963). Thus the full range of dose-rate effect on mutation frequency occurred within the range shown to have no effect on cell survival. This is a strong argument for independence of the mechanisms leading to cell killing from those concerned in production of mutations recovered by the specific locus method (OAKBERG and CLARK, 1961).

7. Dose fractionation

Conflicting results have been obtained in attempts to verify the conclusion of REGAUD and NOGIER (1911) that sterility is more readily induced by fractionated than by single exposures. However, this effect should be a function both of the dose of each fraction and of the interval between fractions, and schedules effective in one species may not be generally applicable owing to differences in rates of gametogenesis. Furthermore, criteria of measurement must be properly chosen. Thus, failure of KOHN and KALLMAN (1955) and SILINI, HORNSEY, and BEWLEY (1963) to observe a fractionation effect with intervals of less than 4—7 days between exposures may be explained by use of testis weight as the measure of response. This is made even more likely by the observation of W. L. RUSSELL (1963) that five daily 200 R fractions gave the longest, two 500 R exposures 24 hr apart the second longest, and a single 1000 R exposure the shortest sterile period. Our observations on cell survival confirm the results of W. L. RUSSELL (1963), (Table 3), yet it is doubtful that recovery after these treatments would be detectable by testis weight differences at 28 days. Thus, divided doses can be more effective when the proper doses, fractionation schedules, and criteria of measurement are used.

Table 3. *Experimental control ratios for type A spermatogonia of the mouse after irradiation at different dose rates.* (From Oakberg and Clark, 1961)

| Dose | Postirradiation interval | Dose rates, R/min | | | | |
| | | X-rays | | ^{137}Cs γ-rays | | |
(R)	(days)	86	9.3	0.8	0.009	0.001
5	3			0.856	0.933	
11	3	0.810	0.825	0.758	0.783	
21	3	0.611	0.710	0.570		
100	3	0.220	0.260	0.190		0.796
300	3	0.119	0.134	0.152		
					0.372*	0.846*
300	5	0.075	0.083	0.104		
600	3	0.075	0.086	0.095		
					0.061*	
600	5	0.026	0.028	0.042		

* Combined values for 6, 12, 18 hr after end of irradiation.

8. Radiation quality

The effectiveness of different radiations is of increasing interest in relation to exposure from use of nuclear energy, space travel, and medical procedures. The relative biological effectiveness (RBE) is most easily interpreted in terms of linear energy transfer (LET).

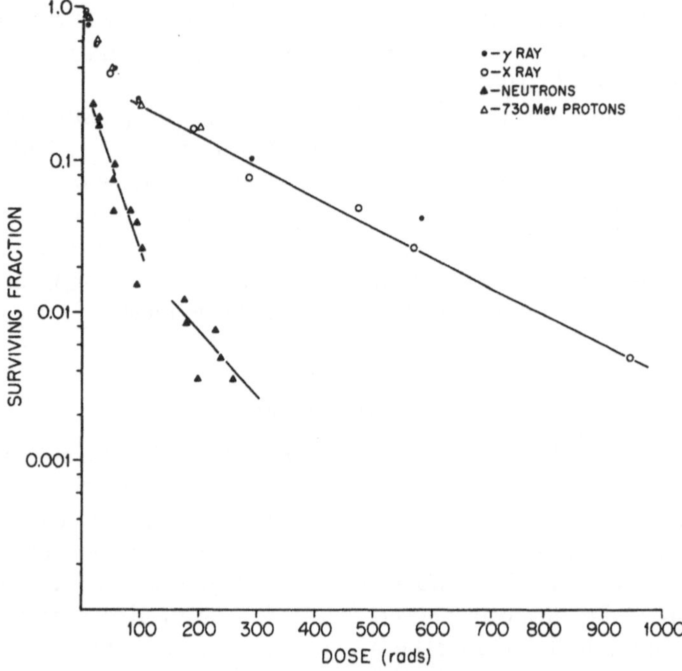

Fig. 3. Relative biological effectiveness of γ-rays, X-rays, 730 MeV protons, and fission neutrons (average energy 1–2 MeV) as estimated by spermatogonial survival in the mouse. (From Oakberg, 1964)

^{137}Cs γ-rays, X-rays, and 730 MeV protons are about equally effective in killing spermatogonia of the mouse (Fig. 3). Both 2.5 and 14.1 MeV neutrons have given an RBE of about 2 when compared to ^{60}Co γ-rays (Oakberg and Clark, 1961; Oakberg, 1962a). Recently, studies with fission neutrons with an average energy of 1—2 MeV have given an RBE of

6.5 for doses of 18—101 rads, and 4.6 for doses of 175—260 rads. These results, in comparison with those for 2.5 MeV neutrons, raise the possibility of very high effectiveness of certain components of the fission neutron spectrum. In general, in terms of absorbed energy, exposure to neutrons is far more damaging to the testis than comparable X- or gamma-ray exposures.

9. Endocrine system

No effect of irradiation on Leydig cell function has been observed. The apparent increase in interstitial tissue in the irradiated testis is relative; volume remains constant if correction is made for testis shrinkage (ESCHENBRENNER, MILLER, and LORENZ, 1948). Likewise, the increase in number of Sertoli cells per tubule cross section is the result of shrinkage in tubule length (OAKBERG, 1959). Any effects on libido result from general radiation sickness and not from direct testicular effects.

10. Response of the human testis

The above discussions have been based primarily on experiments with mice, but the general response of the testis is the same for all organisms studied, including man. The inability to sterilize men permanently by radiation (GOUYGOU, 1960), the recovery of fertility after accidental exposure (OAKES and LUSHBAUGH, 1952), and the histological response of irradiated testes (SCHINZ and SLOTOPOLSKY, 1925; HELLER *et al.*, 1968) all indicate that these general concepts apply to man. It must be emphasized, in making general application of these data, that comparisons must be based on comparable cell types and correction must be made for differences in the dynamics of spermatogenesis (OAKBERG and CLARK, 1964). These adjustments, however, are not always straightforward. For example, the duration of spermatogenesis from A_1 spermatogonia to mature spermatids is 35 days in the mouse (OAKBERG, 1956b) and 72—74 days from A_{dark} to mature spermatids in man (HELLER and CLERMONT, 1964). Yet, intermitotic time for type A_1—A_4 spermatogonia is 26—28 hr in the mouse (MONESI, 1962a) and *16 days* for Ad gonia in man (HELLER and CLERMONT, 1964). As a result, both initial depletion and subsequent recovery of type A cells may be expected to be much slower in man. Slow recovery in man has, indeed, been observed (OAKES and LUSHBAUGH, 1952; MACLEOD, HOTHCISS, and SITTERSON, 1964).

That the slow recovery in man is a function of long mitotic cycles is made even more likely by the observation in man (ROWLEY *et al.*, 1971) of a cell (A_L) comparable to the A_s in mouse (OAKBERG, 1971a) and rat (HUCKINS, 1971a). In the rat, HUCKINS (1971b) has measured the cell cycle of A_2—B spermatogonia as 41—42.5 hr, and in the mouse the total cycle for comparable cells is 26—28 hr (MONESI, 1962). The A_s spermatogonia of the rat have a variable cycle time which is greater than 60 hr (HUCKINS, 1971c), and some stem cells have a much longer cell cycle, dividing at the most only once each cycle of the seminiferous epithelium (13 days), (HUCKINS, 1971c). A similar observation has been made by OAKBERG (1971a) for the mouse. It is logical to expect similar stem cell behaviour in man, and the magnitude of the effect of stem cell kinetics on both cell depletion and recovery may be much greater than anticipated on the basis of estimates of duration of spermatogenesis given above, for these estimates ignore the time required for the stem cell divisions leading to the differentiating spermatogonia used as time zero for such estimates.

III. Radiation response of females

1. Prenatal and neonatal stages

The most comprehensive studies of ovarian response during prenatal development are those of BEAUMONT (1961) on the rat. A period of relatively high sensitivity occurs during the final primordial germ cell divisions, just as in the male. Meiotic prophase stages intervening between the primordial germ cells and late pachytene or dictyate are relatively radioresistant. On the basis of histological studies, however, Peters and Borum (1961) conclude that pachytene is the most sensitive stage in the new-born mouse, but this is difficult to reconcile with the highly sensitive period observed during the early dictyate stage (Russell *et al.*, 1959; Oakberg, 1962b; Peters and Levy, 1963, 1964). An LD_{50} of only 8.4 R has been observed for early dictyate oocyte stages (Oakberg, 1962b). In the rat ovary also, sensitivity to radiation is greater at 8 than at 17 days after birth (Leonard and Maisin, 1963). Sensitivity typical of the adult 101 X C3H mouse is established by 3 weeks

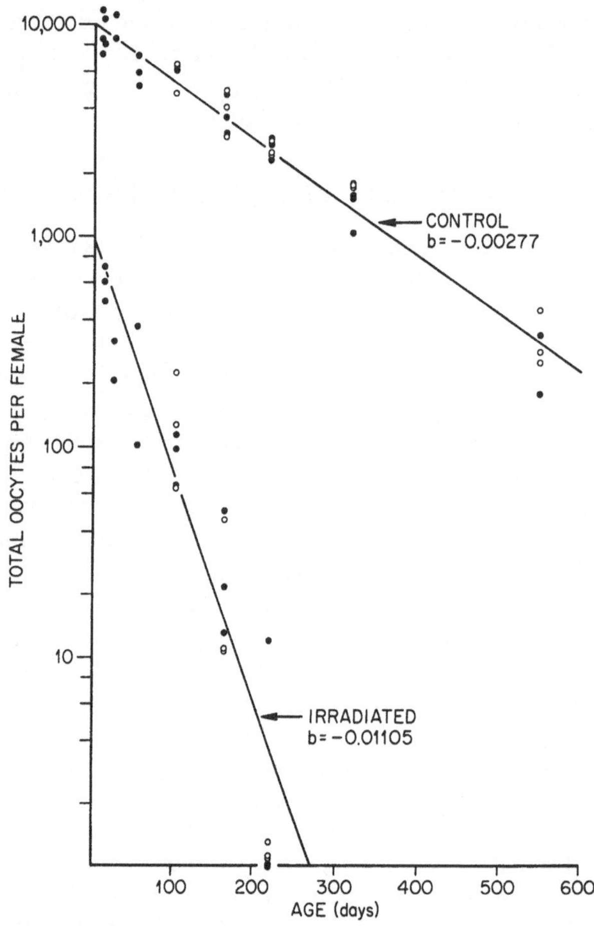

Fig. 4. The effect of 25 R X-rays at 10 days of age on decrease in oocyte number with age in 101 X C3H mice. (From Oakberg, 1966)

of age (W. L. Russell *et al.*, 1959). Peters and Levy (1963) have confirmed these results, but also have observed that the period of peak sensitivity is shifted by about a week in different strains.

The number of young produced by females irradiated during this sensitive period, however, is much greater than would be predicted on the basis of oocyte survival (Oakberg, 1966). 25 R at 10 days of age reduced total oocyte numbers to 3.9 % of control at 56 days, yet these females produced an average of 36.5 young compared to 104.9 for controls (Oakberg, 1966). It was thought that less degeneration may occur in the irradiated female, but the opposite was found to be true (Fig. 4). Study of the reproductive behavior revealed that irradiated females had only about 2 mice per litter less than control during the early reproductive period, but were sterile by 250 days. Control females, albeit the later litters were small, continued to breed until 524 days. Sterility resulted from depletion of oocytes in irradiated females, but for physiological reasons in controls, since control females became sterile with normal appearing oocytes in the ovary (Fig. 4). Thus the unexpected performance of the irradiated females is attributable to ovulation primarily during the age at which peak reproductive performance normally occurs.

It is possible that highly sensitive stages occur during prenatal and pre-adult stages in the developing human ovary. BAKER (1963), however, has suggested that the dictyate stage does not occur in the human. Also, our work with guinea pigs has not shown the high postnatal sensitivity of oocytes typical of the mouse. Therefore, results of experiments on mouse and rat may not be generally applicable, but caution in exposure of fetal and pre-pubertal stages in the human female is urged in view of lack of more precise information on germ cell development.

2. Adult

The adult ovary contains a finite number of oocytes, the majority of which are "arrested" in some stage of diplotene and are contained in small follicles of only a few cells. All stages of follicular development, up to and including large Graafian follicles ready for ovulation, also occur. The number of small follicles gradually decreases as a result of growth and atresia, and only a few complete development and are ovulated. Since no new oocytes are formed, the ovary is gradually depleted with age (ZUCKERMAN, 1951; OAKBERG, 1966; Table 4).

Table 4. *Survival of Stage 1 oocytes in adult and young mice.* (From OAKBERG and CLARK, 1961)

Age at exposure* (days)	Number of mice	Dose (R)	Radiation	R/h	Number of cells per mouse	Exp./control
10	1	0	–	–	4192	
10	1	25	^{60}Co γ	171	82	0.020
10–12	1	0	–	–	5090	
10–12	1	26	^{137}Cs γ	0.543	672	0.132
7–14	1	0	–	–	4819	
7–14	1	91	^{137}Cs γ	0.543	2	0.0004
70	3	0	–	–	3040	
59	3	50	X rays**	5220	4	0.0013
137	1	0	–	–	1303	
133–136	1	44	^{137}Cs γ	0.543	407	0.312
125–131	1	87	–	0.543	364	0.279
119–132	1	164	–	0.543	24	0.074

* All mice killed 72 hs after termination of radiation exposure.
** Head shielded with lead during irradiation.

In the mouse and rat the "arrested" dictyate stage of small oocytes is sensitive to radiation, and degeneration occurs within the first 24 hr after irradiation in the mouse (Fig. 5a). This is surprising, since no cell division occurs and the cells are in meiotic prophase, which usually is radiation resistant. Radiation sensitivity of the oocyte decreases with growth of the follicle (Fig. 5b), and those in mature follicles are not killed by doses of several hundred roentgens. As a result of the killing of early oocytes, permanent sterility occurs after the older, more resistant follicle stages are depleted by ovulation (BRAMBELL, 1927; SCHUGT, 1928; MURRAY, 1931). In the mouse, one normal-sized and a second small litter are obtained after 300 R; reduction of the dose to 50 R increases the number of litters to only four (RUSSELL, STELZNER and RUSSELL, 1959). A similar response is observed in the rat (Mandl, 1959), but higher doses are required to produce comparable effects. Caution must be used in interpreting such species differences, however, since Ehling (1964) has observed highly significant strain differences in fertility of irradiated female mice.

Our experiments have shown a quite different response in the guinea pig, where about 30 % of the "arrested" oocytes survive a radiation dose of 200 R (Table 5). Furthermore, whereas follicles with an antrum are resistant in the mouse, they are destroyed in the guinea pig (Genther, 1931; Oakberg and Clark, 1961) and are replaced from surviving early

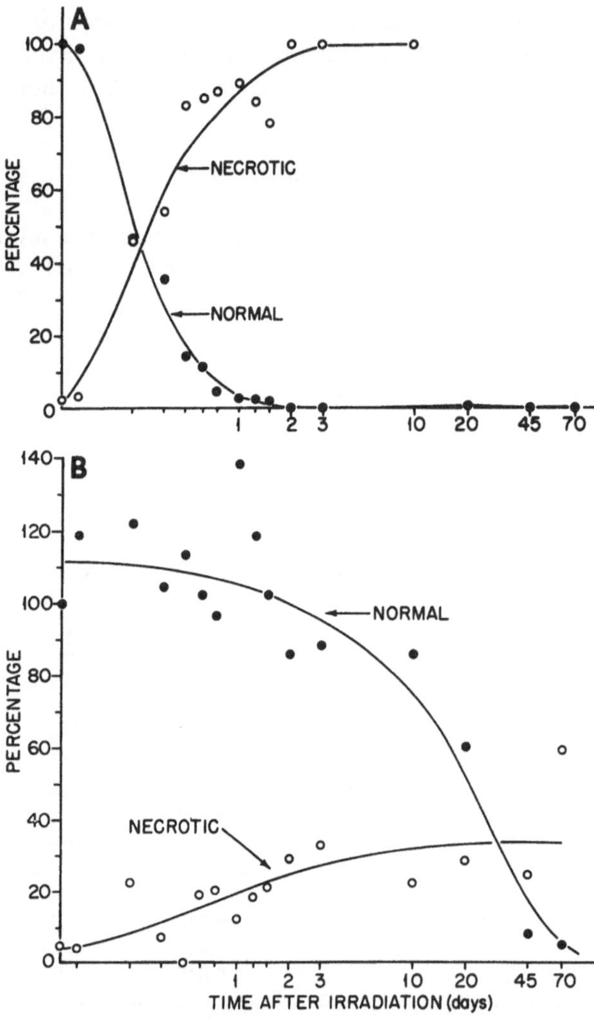

Fig. 5. Frequencies of normal and necrotic oocytes in the mouse ovary at different times after 50 R X-rays. A: Earliest follicle stages. B: Follicles with an antrum

stages (Oakberg and Clark, 1961). A similar situation obtains in the rabbit, where La-cassagne and Gricouroff (1958) observed survival of some early oocyte stages after high radiation doses. After several months these few oocytes developed into Graafian follicles and were ovulated; then permanent sterility ensued. No effect on fertility of adult beagles has been observed after an exposure of 300 R (Andersen, Shultz, and Hage, 1961), suggesting a response similar to that in the guinea pig and rabbit. Our cytological obser-vations on normal dog ovaries reveal "arrest" in a stage close to a "classical" diplotene, and the similar nuclear morphology of the arrrested oocyte (Baker, 1963; Baker and Franchi, 1967) are associated with similar radiation response of the human female. Thus Baker (1969) has shown that in organ culture, the majority of rat oocytes were destroyed by

700 R, those of the monkey by 2000 R, and those of the human female were the most resistant of all, requiring 4000 R. BAKER (1969) observed that sensitivity *in vitro*, however, was higher than *in vivo*, suggesting that comparative sensitivities of oocytes of these species is more reliable than the absolute values observed.

Initial ovulation, a period of amenorrhea, and resumption of ovulation some months later is characteristic of women exposed to radiation doses up to 300 R (PECK *et al.*, 1940). The dose required to produce permanent sterility is not known, but the data of BAKER (1969) on organ cultures are compatible with the observation that in young women, 1740—2000 R has only a temporary effect on fertility (GANS *et al.*, 1963; VUKSANOVIC, 1966). These conclusions are confirmed by other cases in the literature, where conception occurred and apparently normal children have been born after the period of amenorrhea

Table 5. *Mean numbers of oocytes surviving 50 R in the mouse and 200 R in the guinea pig.*
(From OAKBERG and CLARK, 1964)

| Time after irradiation (days) | Early follicles | | | | Late follicles | | | |
| | Mice (50 R) | | Guinea pigs (200 R) | | Mice (50 R) | | Guinea pigs (200 R) | |
	No. cells *	Exptl./ Control	No. cells	Exptl./ Control	No. cells *	Exptl./ Control	No. cells	Exptl./ Control
Control	3 549		33 720**		46		35**	
1	959	0.270	37 780	1.120	48	1.043	15	0.429
2	27	0.008	21 020	0.623	55	1.196	3	0.086
3	35	0.010	17 580	0.521	61	1.326	0	0.000
7			15 420	0.457			2	0.057
10	24	0.007	13 300	0.394	65	1.413	0	0.000
14			11 560	0.343			41	1.171
20	10	0.003			71	1.543		
21			18 440	0.547			49	1.400
42			10 500	0.311			19	0.543
45	3	0.001			10	0.217		

* All means for mice based on three animals per group.
** Means for guinea pigs based on three controls; data based on one animal for each time after irradiation.

following irradiation (MARKOVITS, 1922; JACOX, 1939; ZIMMER, 1953). These children would be expected to be normal by usual criteria; however, they may have a significant amount of radiation-induced genetic damage.

Protraction of the radiation dose, either by fractionation or by reduction of the dose rate, greatly improves fertility (RUSSELL, STELZNER, and RUSSELL, 1959). Cell survival also is improved by reduction of the dose rate (OAKBERG and CLARK, 1961; Table 4). The change in slope of the survival curve at doses above 10 R (OAKBERG, 1962a) indicates that in order for fractionation to be significantly less effective, size of the fractions should be 10 R or less. The improved oocyte survival with low dose rate and fractionated exposure, as yet observed only in the mouse, constitutes conclusive evidence for intracellular repair of radiation damage, since fertility and cell survival are enhanced in a fixed population of nondividing oocytes.

Superovulation, which can be observed as early as 2 days and reaches a peak 7—10 days after irradiation of the mouse, can mask radiation damage to oocytes when litter size is the only criterion measured (RUSSELL and RUSSELL, 1956). As expected, the increase in the number of mature follicles necessary for superovulation can be detected histologically (Table 5); but the bases for accelerated development of follicles approaching maturation are not known. Even though it occurs with the pituitary shielded, one cannot completely exclude the endocrine system from this effect, since the ovary itself must be irradiated.

During the initial postirradiation period, endocrine function appears relatively normal, with the possible exception of changes involved in superovulation. As the period of amenorrhea is reached in the human, symptoms typical of the menopause appear, but regress with resumption of ovulation and menstruation (Jacox, 1939). In the mouse and rat, cycles continue long after all oocytes are gone from the ovary, but intervals between estrus and duration of estrus vary greatly (Brambell and Parkes, 1927; Brambell, Parkes, and Fielding, 1927; Mandl, 1964). Animal variation also is high, and in some cases permanent estrus occurs.

In certain strains of mice, ovarian tumors develop in almost all animals given a radiation dose sufficient to destroy the early oocytes. It appears that all oocytes must be lost in order for this process to begin, and after many months, tumors comprised of granulosa cells, lutein cells, in fact any cell except oocytes, may occur (Peters, 1969). Treatments such as the administration of estrogens of the shielding of one ovary will prevent tumor induction (Kirschbaum, 1957). A sufficient time must be available for tumors to develop after disappearance of all oocytes; i.e. irradiation late in life, or with small doses which decrease reproductive life only slightly, are not effective. Generality of this response is not known, and the mouse may be unique, but sterilization of women by radiological procedures may involve risks of subsequent tumor development.

In female mammals, effect of radiation on fertility will be influenced by basic radiation sensitivity, by cytological stage of the "arrested" oocyte, by reproductive life span, by relative frequencies of follicle stages with different sensitivities, by spontaneous rates of atresia, and by rates of development and utilization of the oocyte pool (Oakberg, 1966). Wide species differences exist in ovarian response, and extrapolation of results must be made with caution. However, one must be especially cautious in exposing the fetal or prepubertal ovary lest particularly sensitive oocyte stages be destroyed. They can never be replaced.

Resolution of the precise radiation response of the ovary will be possible only when the chronological history of all stages from primordial germ cells to the fertilized ovum is known. At present, this information is available only for the mouse and rat, where marked differences in radiation sensitivity have been demonstrated for primordial germ cells, early meiotic prophase stages, and for the dictyate oocyte in follicles at different stages of growth. Oocyte response in the guinea pig and rabbit and fertility of irradiated dogs and the human female indicate that the model worked out for the rat and mouse does not apply to all species. At present, it is known that the diplotene stage of the "arrested" oocyte is characteristic for a species, and this may be an important factor in radiation response. However the relative duration of gametogenic stages, the rate of follicular development, and normal rate of depletion of the oocyte pool will have to be known in order to make a comprehensive evaluation of radiation response of the ovary.

References

Andersen, A. C., Shultz, F. T., Hage, T. J.: The effect of total-body x-irradiation on reproduction of the female beagle to 4 years of age. Radiat. Res. 15, 745–753 (1961).

Arsenieva, M. A., Bochkov, N. P.: Cytogenic radiosensitivity of certain stages of meiosis in monkeys and mice. Radiobiol., USSR (Eng. trans.) 3 (4), 107–116 (1963).

Austin, C. R., Amoroso, E. C.: The mammalian egg. Endeavor 18, 130–143 (1959).

Baker, T. G.: A quantitative and cytological study of germ cells in human ovaries. Proc. Roy. Soc. (London) Ser. B. 158, 417–433 (1963).

Baker, T. G.: The sensitivity of rat, monkey, and human oocytes to X irradiation in organ culture. Radiation Biology of the Fetal and Juvenile Mammal, ed., Sikov, M. R., Mahlum, D. D., USAEC Div. Tech. Inf. CONF-690501, pp. 655–661 (1969).

— Franchi, L. L.: The fine structure of oogonia and oocytes in human ovaries. J. Cell. Sci. 2, 213–224 (1967).

BAKULINA, E. D., ORLOVA, N. N.: Comparative analysis of the radiosensitivity of spermatogonia of various types in *Macaca mulatta*. Radiobiol., USSR (Eng. trans.) **3** (4), 117–125 (1963).

BATEMAN, A. J.: Mutagenic sensitivity of maturing germ cells in the male mouse. Heredity **12**, 213–232 (1958).

BEAUMONT, H. M.: Changes in the radiosensitivity of the testis during foetal development. Int. J. Rad. Biol. **2**, 247–256 (1960).

— Radiosensitivity of oogonia and oocytes in the foetal rat. Int. J. Rad. Biol. **3**, 59–72 (1961).

— MANDL, A. M.: A quantitative and cytological study of oogonia and oocytes in the foetal and neonatal rat. Proc. Roy. Soc. (London) Ser. B **155**, 557–579 (1962).

BRAMBELL, F. W. R.: The development and morphology of the gonads of the mouse. I. The morphogenesis of the indifferent gonad and of the ovary. Proc. Roy. Soc. (London) Ser. B **101**, 391–408 (1927).

— PARKES, A. S.: Changes in the ovary of the mouse following exposure to X-rays. Part III. Irradiation of the non-parous adult. Proc. Roy. Soc. (London) Ser. B **101**, 316–328 (1927).

— — FIELDING, U.: Changes in the ovary of the mouse following exposure to X-rays. Part I. Irradiation at three weeks old. Proc. Roy. Soc. (London) Ser. B **101**, 29–56 (1927).

BROWN, S. O., KRISE, G. M., PACE, H. B., DE BOER, J.: Effect of continuous radiation on reproductive capacity and fertility of the albino rat and mouse. Effects of Ionizing Radiation on the Reproductive System, ed., CARLSON, W. D., GASSNER, F. X. Oxford: Pergamon Press, pp. 103–110 (1964).

CHANG, M. C., HUNT, D. M., ROMANOFF, E. B.: Effects of radiocobalt irradiation of rabbit spermatozoa *in vitro* on fertilization and early development. Anat. Rec. **129**, 211–229 (1957).

CHARNY, C. W., CONSTON, A. S., MERANZE, D. R.: Development of the testis. A histologic study from birth to maturity with some notes on abnormal variations. Fertility Sterility **3**, 461–479 (1952).

CHIQUOINE, A. D.: The identification, origin, and migration of the primordial germ cells in the mouse embryo. Anat. Rec. **118**, 135–146 (1954).

CLERMONT, Y.: Quantitative analysis of spermatogenesis of the rat: A revised model for the renewal of spermatogonia. Am. J. Anat. **111**, 111–129 (1962).

— The cycle of the seminiferous epithelium in man. Am. J. Anat. **112**, 35–51 (1963).

— BUSTOS-OBREGON, E.: Re-examination of spermatogonial renewal in the rat by means of seminiferous tubules mounted "in toto". Am. J. Anat. **122**, 237–248 (1968).

— HARVEY, S. C.: Duration of the cycle of the seminiferous epithelium of normal, hypophysectomized and hypophysectomized hormone treated albino rats. Endocrinology **76**, 80–89 (1965).

— PEREY, B.: Quantitative study of the cell population of the seminiferous tubules in immature rats. Am. J. Anat. **100**, 241–268 (1957).

CRAIG, A. W., FOX, B. W., JACKSON, H.: Effect of radiation on male mouse and rat fertility. J. Reprod. Fertility **2**, 466–472 (1961).

DYM, M., CLERMONT, Y.: Role of spermatogonia in the repair of the seminiferous epithelium following x-irradiation of the rat testis. Am. J. Anat. **128**, 265–282 (1970).

— FAWCETT, D. W.: Spermatogonial intercellular bridges. Anat. Rec. **169**, 309 (1971).

EDWARDS, R. G., SIRLIN, J. L.: The effect of 200 r of X-rays on the rate of spermatogenesis and spermiogenesis in the mouse. Exptl. Cell Res. **15**, 522–528 (1958).

EHLING, U. H.: Strain variation in reproductive capacity and radiation response of female mice. Radiation Res. **23**, 603–610 (1964).

ESCHENBRENNER, A. B., MILLER, E., LORENZ, E.: Quantitative histologic analysis of the effect of chronic whole-body irradiation with gamma rays on the spermatogenic elements and the interstitial tissue of the testes of mice. J. Natl. Cancer Inst. **9**, 133–147 (1948).

FRANCHI, L. L., MANDL, A. M., ZUCKERMAN, S.: The development of the ovary and the process of oogenesis. The Ovary. Vol. 1, ed., ZUCKERMAN, S. London: Academic Press, pp. 1–88 (1962).

GANS, B., BAHARY, C., LEVIE, B.: Ovarian regeneration and pregnancy following massive radiotherapy for dysgerminoma. Obst. & Gynecol. **22**, 596–600 (1963).

GENTHER, I. T.: Irradiation of the ovaries of guinea-pigs and its effect on the oestrous cycle. Am. J. Anat. **48**, 99–137 (1931).

GERBER, G.: Beweglichkeit und Morphologie menschlicher Spermien nach Einwirkung langwelliger Röntgenstrahlen. Strahlentherapie **99**, 632–636 (1955).

GONDOS, B., ZEMJANIS, R.: Fine structure of spermatogonia and intercellular bridges in *Macaca nemestrina*. J. Morphol. **131**, 431–446 (1970).

GOUYGOU, C.: Action des radiations ionisantes sur la gametogenese et la glande interstitielle. Lésions Provoqués par les Radiations Ionisantes, ed., LACASSAGNE, A., *et al.* Paris: Masson et cie., pp. 175–205 (1960).

HELLER, C. G., CLERMONT, Y.: Kinetics of the germinal epithelium in man. Recent Progr. Hormone Res. **20**, 545–575 (1964).

— HELLER, G. V., WARNER, G. A., ROWLEY, M. J.: Effects of graded doses of ionizing radiation on testicular cytology and sperm count in man. Radiat. Res. **35**, 493 (1968).

HERTWIG, P.: Unterschiede in der Entwicklungsfähigkeit von F_1-Mäusen nach Röntgenbestrahlung von Spermatogonien, fertigen und unfertigen Spermatozoen. Biol. Zentr. **58**, 273–301 (1938).

HILCHER, W.: DNA synthesis: Proliferation and regeneration of the spermatogonia in the rat. Arch. Anat. Microscop. Morphol. Exp. **56**, Suppl. No. 3–4, 75–84 (1968).

— MAKOSKI, H. B.: Histologische und autoradiographische Untersuchungen zur „Präspermatogenese" und „Spermatogenese" der Ratte. Z. Zellforsch. **86**, 327–350 (1968).

Hochereau-de Reviers, M. T.: Études des Divisions Spermatogoniales et de Renouvellement de la Spermatogonie Souche chez le Taureau. Thèse de Doctorat D'État Ès-Sciences Naturelles N° d'enregistrement au C.N.R.S. AO 3976. 134 pp., 1970.

Huckins, C.: The initiation of spermatogenesis in the testis of the Wistar albino rat. Ph. D. Thesis, McGill University, Montreal, 1965.

— The spermatogonial stem cell population in adult rats I. Their morphology, proliferation and maturation. Anat. Rec. **169**, 533–558 (1971a).

— Cell cycle properties of differentiating spermatogonia in adult Sprague-Dawley rats. Cell. Tissue Kinet. **4**, 139–154 (1971b).

— The spermatogonial stem cell population in adult rats II. A radioautographic analysis of their cell cycle properties. Cell Tissue Kinet. **4**, 313–334 (1971c).

— Oakberg, E. F.: Cytoplasmic connections between spermatogonia seen in whole mounted seminiferous tubules from normal and irradiated mouse testes. Anat. Rec. **169**, 344 (1971).

Jacox, H. W.: Recovery following human ovarian irradiation. Radiology **32**, 538–545 (1939).

Kirschbaum, A.: The role of hormones in cancer: Laboratory animals. Cancer Res. **17**, 432–453 (1957).

Kohn, H. I., Kallman, R. F.: The effect of fractionated x-ray dosage upon the mouse testis. I. Maximum weight loss following 80 to 240 R given in 2 to 5 fractions during 1 to 4 days. J. Natl. Cancer Inst. **15**, 891–899 (1955).

Lacassagne, A., Gricouroff, G.: Action of radiation on tissues: Introduction to Radiotherapy. New York: Grune and Stratton, Inc. 1958.

Lagendorff, H., Langendorff, M.: The effect of repeated small doses on the fertility of the white mouse. Advances in Radiobiology, ed., de Henesy, G. E., et al. Edinburgh: Oliver and Boyd, pp. 257–260, 1957.

Leblond, C. P., Clermont, Y. Spermiogenesis of rat, mouse, hamster and guinea pig as revealed by the "periodic acid-fuchsin sulfurous acid" technique. Am. J. Anat. **90**, 167–215 (1952).

Léonard, A., Maisin, J. R.: Influence des rayons x sur la fertilité de jeunes rats irradies 8 ou 17 jours après la naissance. Compt. Rend. Soc. Biol. **157**, 1529–1533 (1963).

— Imbaud, F., Maisin, J. R.: Testicular injury in rats irradiated during infancy. Brit. J. Radiol. **37**, 764–768 (1964).

MacLeod, J., Hotchkiss, R. S., Sitterson, B. W.: Recovery of male fertility after sterilization by nuclear radiation. J. Am. Med. Assoc. **187**, 637–641 (1964).

Mandl, A. M.: A quantitative study of the sensitivity of oocytes to x-irradiation. Proc. Roy. Soc. (London) Ser. B **150**, 53–71 (1959).

— The radiosensitivity of germ cells. Biol. Rev. **39**, 288–371 (1964).

Markovits, E.: Temporäre Sterilisation von Mann und Frau in wechselnder Folge mittels Röntgenstrahlen. Dtsch. med. Wschr. **48**, 459–460 (1922).

Mintz, B.: Embryological phases of mammalian gametogenesis. J. Cell. Comp. Physiol. **56** (suppl. 1), 31–47 (1960).

Mitra, S.: Effects of x-rays on chromosomes of *Lilium longiflorum* during meiosis. Genetics **43**, 771–789 (1958).

Monesi, V.: Autoradiographic study of DNA synthesis and the cell cycle in spermatogonia and spermatocytes of mouse testis using tritiated thymidine. J. Cell. Biol. **14**, 1–18 (1962a).

— Relation between x-ray sensitivity and stages of the cell cycle in spermatogonia of the mouse. Radiation Res. **17**, 809–838 (1962b).

— Ribonucleic acid synthesis during mitosis and meiosis in the mouse testis. J. Cell. Biol. **22**, 521–532 (1964).

Murray, J. M.: A study of the histological structure of mouse ovaries following exposure to roentgen irradiation. Am. J. Roentgenol. Radium Therapy Nucl. Med. **25**, 1–45 (1931).

Oakberg, E. F.: Sensitivity and time of degeneration of spermatogenic cells irradiated in various stages of maturation in the mouse. Radiat. Res. **2**, 369–391 (1955).

— A description of spermiogenesis in the mouse and its use in analysis of the cycle of the seminiferous epithelium and germ cell renewal. Am. J. Anat. **99**, 391–414 (1956a).

— Duration of spermatogenesis in the mouse and timing of stages of the cycle of the seminiferous epithelium. Am. J. Anat. **99**, 507–516 (1956b).

— Gamma-ray sensitivity of spermatogonia of the mouse. J. Exptl. Zool. **134**, 343–356 (1957).

— Initial depletion and subsequent recovery of spermatogonia of the mouse after 20 R of gamma rays and 100, 300, and 600 R of x-rays. Radiat. Res. **11**, 700–719 (1959).

— The effect of low radiation doses on spermatogonia and oocytes of the mouse. Strahlentherapie, Suppl. No. **51**, 103–111 (1962a).

— Gamma-ray sensitivity of oocytes of immature mice. Proc. Soc. Exptl. Biol. Med. **109**, 763–767 (1962b).

— The effects of dose, dose rate and quality of radiation on the dynamics and survival of the spermatogonial population of the mouse. Japan. J. Genetics (Suppl.) **40**, 119–127 (1964).

— Effects of 25 R of X-rays at 10 days of age on oocyte numbers and fertility of female mice. Radiation and Ageing, ed. Lindop, P. J., Sacher, G. A. Taylor and Francis, Ltd., pp. 293–306, 1966.

— Relationship between stage of follicular development and RNA synthesis in the mouse oocyte. Mutat. Res. **6**, 155–165 (1968).

— Spermatogonial stem-cell renewal in the mouse. Anat. Rec. **169**, 515–532 (1971a).

— A new concept of spermatogonial stem-cell renewal in the mouse and its relationship to genetic effects. Mutat. Res. **11**, 1–7 (1971b).

— Clark, E.: Effect of dose and dose rate on radiation damage to mouse spermatogonia and oocytes as measured by cell survival. J. Cell. Comp. Physiol. **58** (Suppl. 1), 173–182 (1961).

OAKBERG, E. F., CLARK, E.: Species comparisons of radiation response of the gonads. Effects of Ionizing Radiation on the Reproductive System, ed., CARLSON, W. D., GASSNER, F. X. Oxford: Pergamon Press, pp. 11–24, 1964.

— DI MINNO, R. L.: X-ray sensitivity of primary spermatocytes of the mouse. Intern. J. Radiation Biol. 2, 196–209 (1960).

OAKES, W. R., LUSHBAUGH, C. C.: Course of testicular injury following accidental exposure to nuclear radiations. Radiology 59, 737–743 (1952).

ORTAVANT, R., COUROT, M.: Problems concerning the action of gametogenic hormones on the spermatogenesis of mammals. Excerpta Med. Intern. Cong. Ser. 70, 133 (1963).

PARTINGTON, M., FOX, B. W., JACKSON, H.: Comparative action of some methane sulphonic esters on the cell population of the rat testis. Exptl. Cell Res. 33, 78–88 (1964).

PECK, W. S., MCGREER, J. T., KRETZSCHMAR, N. R., BROWN, W. E.: Castration of the female by irradiation. Rad. 34, 176–186 (1940).

PETERS, H.: The effect of radiation in early life on the morphology and reproductive function of the mouse ovary. Advances in Reproductive Physiology, vol. 4, ed., MCLAREN, A. New York: Academic Press, pp. 149–185, 1969.

— BORUM, K.: The development of mouse ovaries after low-dose irradiation at birth. Intern. J. Radiation Biol. 3, 1–16 (1961).

— LEVY, E.: Effect of irradiation in infancy on the fertility of female mice. Radiat. Res. 18, 421–428 (1963).

— — Radiation sensitivity of the mouse ovary: Fertility and oocyte survival. Fertility Sterility 15, 407–418 (1964).

REGAUD, CL., NOGIER, TH.: Stérilisation röntgénienne, totale et définitive, sans radiodermite, des testicules du Bélier adulte. Conditions de sa réalisation. Compt. Rend. Soc. Biol. 70, 202–203 (1911).

DE ROOIJ, D. G.: Further evidence for the proposed way of spermatogonial stem cell renewal in the rat and the mouse. Zeitschr. Zellforsch. 99, 134–138 (1969).

— KRAMER, M. F.: Spermatogonial stem cell renewal in rats and mice. Zeitschr. Zellforsch. 85, 206–209 (1968).

ROOSEN-RUNGE, E. C.: The process of spermatogenesis in mammals. Biol. Rev. 37, 343–377 (1962).

ROWLEY, M. J., BERLIN, J. D., HELLER, C. G.: The ultrastructure of four types of human spermatogonia. Zeitschr. Zellforsch. 112, 139–157 (1971).

RUGH, R., JACKSON, S.: Effect of fetal x-irradiation upon the subsequent fertility of the offspring. J. Exptl. Zool. 138, 209–221 (1958).

RUSSELL, L. B., RUSSELL, W. L.: The sensitivity of different stages in oogenesis to the radiation induction of dominant lethals and other changes in the mouse. Progress in Radiobiology, ed., MITCHEL, J. S., et al. Edinburgh: Oliver and Boyd, pp. 187–192, 1659.

RUSSELL, L. B., SAYLORS, C. L.: The relative sensitivity of various germ cell stages of the mouse to radiation-induced nondisjunction, chromosome losses and deficiences. Repair from Genetic Radiation Damage, ed. SOBELS, F. H. Oxford: Pergamon Press, pp. 313–342, 1963.

— BADGETT, S. K., SAYLORS, C. L.: Comparison of the effects of acute, continuous, and fractionated irradiation during embryonic development. Int. J. Rad. Biol. (Suppl.), 343–359 (1959).

— STELZNER, K. F., RUSSELL, W. L.: Influence of dose rate on radiation effect on fertility of female mice. Proc. Soc. Exptl. Biol. Med. 102, 471–479 (1959).

RUSSEL, W. L.: Genetic effects of radiation in mammals. Radiation Biology, Vol. 1, ed., HOLLAENDER, A. New York: McGraw-Hill, pp. 825–859, 1954.

— The effect of radiation dose rate and fractionation on mutation in mice. Repair from Genetic Radiation Damage, ed., SOBELS, F. H. Oxford: Pergamon Press, pp. 205–217, 1963.

— RUSSELL, L. B., STEELE, M. H., PHIPPS, E. L.: Extreme sensitivity of an immature stage of the mouse ovary to sterilization by irradiation. Science 129, 1288 (1959).

SCHINZ, H. R., SLOTOPOSLKY, B.: Der Röntgenhoden. Ergebn. Med. Strahlenforsch. 1, 443–526 (1925).

SCHUGT, P.: Untersuchungen über die Wirkung abgestufter Dosen von Röntgenstrahlen verschiedener Wellenlänge auf die Struktur und Funktion der Ovarien. Strahlentherapie 27, 603–662 (1928).

SILINI, G., HORNSEY, S., BEWLEY, D. K.: Effects of x-ray and neutron dose fractionation on the mouse testis. Radiat. Res. 19, 50–63 (1963).

SNELL, G. D., X-ray sterility in the male house mouse. J. Exptl. Zool. 65, 421–441 (1933).

SOBOTTA, J.: Die Befruchtung und Furchung des Eies der Maus. Arch. Microskop. Anat. 45, 15–93 (1895).

SPARROW, A. H., MOSES, M. J., DUBOW, R. J.: Relationships between ionizing radiation, chromosome breakage and certain other nuclear disturbances. Exptl. Cell. Res. (Suppl. 2), 245–267 (1952).

STRANDSKOV, H. H.: Effect of X-rays in an inbred strain of guinea-pigs. J. Exptl. Zool. 63, 175–202 (1932).

VUKSANOVIC, M. M.: Pregnancy following ovarian irradiation. Am. J. Roentgenol. Radium Ther. Nucl. Med. 97, 951–956 (1966).

WHITING, ANNA, R.: Sensitivity to x-rays of different meiotic stages in unlaid eggs of Habrobracon. J. Exptl. Zool. 83, 249–269 (1940).

WITSCHI, E.: Migration of the germ cells of human embryos from the yolk sac to the primitive gonadal folds. Contrib. Embryol. Carnegie Inst. 32, 67–80 (1948).

ZIMMER, K.: Röntgenbestrahlung der Ovarien und nachfolgenden Konzeption. Strahlentherapie 92, 117–122 (1953).

ZUCKERMAN, S.: The number of oocytes in the mature ovary. Recent Progr. Hormone Res. 6, 63–109 (1951).

F. Strahlenbedingte Entwicklungsstörungen

Von

Hedi Fritz-Niggli

Mit 42 Abbildungen

I. Einführung

Fehlleitung und Unterbrechung der Entwicklung sind wohl die eindrucksvollsten somatischen Strahleneffekte. Mit einem Minimum an Energie wird ein Maximum an Wirkung erzeugt. In zweifacher Hinsicht interessiert den Mediziner und Forscher die Wirkung energiereicher Strahlen auf das heranwachsende Lebewesen, nämlich zum ersten, um im Experiment Aufschlüsse über noch unbekannte Entwicklungs- und Differenzierungserscheinungen zu gewinnen und zum zweiten, um die Strahlengefährdung des Menschen besonders durch kleine Dosen richtig beurteilen zu können. Sämtliche heranwachsenden Lebewesen, die untersucht wurden, seien sie nun Wirbellose oder Säugetiere, zeichnen sich durch ihre besondere Strahlensensibilität aus. Die Diskrepanz in der Strahlensensibilität adulter und jugendlicher Formen zeigt sich besonders drastisch bei den Insekten, indem die Letaldosis für adulte Taufliegen beispielsweise 500 mal größer sein kann als diejenige für gewisse Embryonalstadien.

Die Strahlenwirkung äußert sich in Wachstumshemmung, Mißbildung, Mehrfachbildung, Auslassung, Funktionsstörung, Aktivitätsverlust usw. und Tod. Die embryonalen und fetalen Entwicklungsprozesse sind komplexer Natur, indem sie sich auf verschiedenen Ebenen abspielen können, nämlich:

1. Intrazellulär

Makromolekulare Vorgänge, wie Übertragung der Gen-Information (Transcription), Bildung bestimmter Proteine (Translation), Veränderung, Aktivitätshemmung und Induktion von „Biomolekülen", Regulationsvorgänge, stehen im Vordergrund, ebenso wie die Bildung der intrazellulären Struktur und besonderer Organellen, Differenzierung von Membranen und Membransystemen.

2. Zellulär

Zellkinetische Faktoren bestimmen, wie Begrenzung und Förderung der mitotischen Aktivität, Vermehrungsgeschwindigkeit, ferner Wachstum, Wanderung der Zellen, Differenzierung bestimmter Zelltypen etc.

3. Interzellulär

Lagerung der Zellen, Induktion und Differenzierung von Zellkomplexen in Abhängigkeit von andern, Bildung und koordinierte Gestaltung übergeordneter Strukturen, Regulationsmechanismen etc.

Energiereiche Strahlen vermögen nun in alle diese komplexen Geschehnisse einzugreifen, indem sie u.a. Transcription und Translation verändern, die Zellteilung unterbrechen, Zellen zerstören oder ihren Stoffwechsel subletal beeinflussen und damit das Gleichgewicht sowie die Sequenz der Entwicklungsabläufe empfindlich stören. Es ist deshalb nicht verwunderlich, daß bereits kleinste Dosen Entwicklungsstörungen provozieren. Ebenso wird aus dem komplexen Geschehen verständlich, daß der Mechanismus der embryonalen Strahlenschädigung schwierig zu deuten ist.

Eine „neutrale" Stammzelle hat bis zur endgültigen Fixierung ihrer Struktur und Funktion etliche Phasen zu durchlaufen, die von ganz unterschiedlichen Ereignissen geprägt werden. Dies hat zur Folge, daß die strahlenbedingte Entwicklungsstörung ausgesprochen stadienabhängig ist. Sowohl das Ausmaß als auch die Art der Schädigung wird durch das Entwicklungsstadium während der Bestrahlung diktiert.

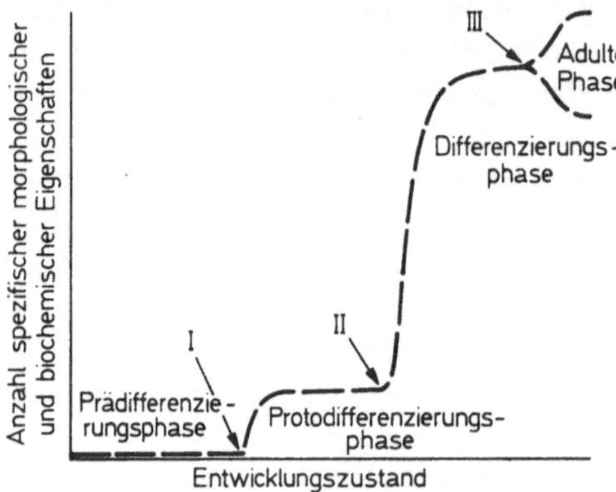

Abb. 1. Cytodifferenzierung, ein Schema aus Experimenten mit Zellen des Pankreas von Ratten (nach Rutter u. Mitarb., 1968 umgezeichnet). I, II, III Regulative Übergänge

Die Entwicklung vom Embryo zum Adulten kann ganz allgemein als eine Bildung von Zellen mit verschiedenem Phänotyp aus Zellen mit einem gleichen Genotyp beschrieben werden.

Verschiedene Stufen werden dabei durchlaufen, die sich hauptsächlich nach makromolekularen Gesichtspunkten folgendermaßen aufteilen (Rutter u. Mitarb., 1968) und beschreiben lassen (siehe auch Abb. 1).

I. Prädetermination; neutrale Stamm- (Urzelle), pluripotent, große Teilungsaktivität.

II. Protodifferenzierung; Transcriptionsvorgänge, Potenz eingeschränkt.

III. Differenzierung; Verlust der mitotischen Aktivität, Spezialisierung, Translationsvorgänge.

Die Reaktion dieser verschiedenen Systeme auf die Bestrahlung muß eine unterschiedliche sein, wobei zusätzlich Regulationsvermögen und Repairfaktoren die Strahlenwirkung modellieren. Es sei versucht, in dieser Darstellung einige der neueren Befunde über strahlenbedingte Entwicklungsstörungen zu zeigen, während frühere Analysen gestreift und auf ältere Übersichtsreferate verwiesen wird.

Die Geschichte der Strahlenembryologie beginnt 1903, als Bohn feststellte, daß eine Radiumbestrahlung besonders Amphibienembryonen schädigt und bei Seeigeleiern zu Monstren und Wachstumsverzögerung führte.

1906 postulierten dann Bergonié u. Tribondeau im Anschluß an andere Arbeiten (Schaper, 1904; Toussey, 1905), daß Röntgenstrahlen um so intensiver auf die Zellen einwirken, je größer ihre Vermehrungstätigkeit sei, je länger ihre karyokinetische Zukunft und je weniger ihre Morphologie und Funktionen fixiert sind. Diese These ist für viele Fälle zutreffend. OTTO HERTWIG hat dann 1911 den Begriff Radiumkrankheit geprägt, um besonders Strahlenschäden an Amphibienembryonen zu charakterisieren (O. HERTWIG, 1911; G. HERTWIG, 1911; Zusammenfassung P. HERTWIG, 1927). Nach Experimenten mit Säugetierembryonen (TOUSSEY, 1905; BURCKHARD, 1905; LENGFELLNER, 1906; FELLNER u. NEUMANN, 1907; FÖRSTERLING, 1907 etc.), beschrieb vermutlich FRIEDRICH (1910) die erste Mißbildung am Menschen, nachdem 1901 BAR u. BOULLE und SCHMIDT (1909) fetale Todesfälle festgestellt hatten. An Säugetieren wieder sind im Anfang der Fünfziger Jahre größere Untersuchungen aufgenommen worden, nachdem hauptsächlich früher mit Amphibien experimentiert worden war. Die heutige Literatur ist so umfangreich geworden, daß sie mit diesem Beitrag lediglich durchstreift werden konnte.

II. Strahlenbedingte Entwicklungsstörungen bei Insekten (Dipteren) als Vertretern der Wirbellosen

Die Hemmung der Entwicklung verschiedenster Insekten ist nicht nur als Problem der Grundlagenforschung, ferner der praktischen Anwendung, wie Vernichtung von Schädlingen, interessant, sondern interessiert auch von der Sicht des Strahlenschutzes. So wurde wiederholt als sogenanntes biologisches Dosimeter für Strahlen der Letalitätstest mit Embryonen von Drosophila melanogaster (Taufliege) vorgeschlagen (PACKARD, 1926; CROWTHER, 1927; SIEVERT u. FORSSBERG, 1931; JÜNGLING u. LANGENDORFF, 1933; GLASSER u. MAUTZ, 1933; LANGENDORFF u. SOMMERMEYER, 1939, 1940; ZIMMER, 1940; GLOCKER, 1949).

In großer Zahl lassen sich Drosophila-Eier sammeln, die Letalitätsteste sind einfach auszuwerten, und vor allem ist die Geometrie des kleinen Objektes für vergleichende Untersuchungen mit verschiedenen Strahlenarten geeignet. In relativ kurzer Zeit läßt sich die biologische Wirksamkeit einer zu testenden Strahlenart schätzen.

In neuerer Zeit versuchte so AMMON (1964) die Wirkung einer radonhaltigen Atmosphäre auf Drosophila-Embryonen zu prüfen. Es zeigte sich, daß die Reduktion der Schlüpfrate in erster Linie auf die α-Strahlung der auf den Eiern und der Unterlage abgelagerten Folgeprodukte des Radon zurückzuführen war.

Zudem bietet besonders die holometabole Ei-Larve-Puppe-Imago-Entwicklung der Dipteren weitere interessante Ansatzpunkte für die experimentelle Strahlenbiologie.

Während der eigentlichen Embryonalentwicklung (Zygote bis schlüpffähiges „Ei") differenzieren hauptsächlich die Primordien der larval funktionellen Organe. Von der Larve übernimmt die Imago (erwachsenes Stadium) lediglich die malpighischen Gefäße und das Herz. Der größte Teil der adulten imaginalen Organe nimmt dagegen seinen Ursprung aus Blastemen, die in der Larve als sogenannte Imaginalscheiben heranwachsen. Die Zellen in diesen Blastemen sind in ihrer Potenz bereits eingeschränkt und dürften sich im Protodifferenzierungsstadium befinden. In einer zweiten Differenzierungsperiode entwickeln sich während der Pupalperiode aus den Imaginalscheiben die imaginalen adulten Organe.

Die Imaginalscheiben stellen demnach örtlich fixierte Zellkomplexe dar, die von der pluripotenten Zelle zur irreversibel differenzierten Zelle verschiedene Stadien durchlaufen.

1. Abhängigkeit der Strahlenreaktion vom Entwicklungsstadium

a) Embryonale Sterblichkeit

Die meisten Untersuchungen sind an Drosophila-Embryonen durchgeführt worden. Als Kriterium der Strahlenschädigung gilt durchweg das Ausschlüpfen des Embryos aus der Eihülle, das bei Drosophila melanogaster bei 25° C 19—20 Std nach der Eiabgabe erfolgt. Es stellte sich heraus, daß das Nichtausschlüpfen aus der Eihülle weitgehend vom Entwicklungszustand während der Bestrahlung abhängt (Abb. 2).

Als das empfindlichste Stadium erwiesen sich Embryonen von $1^3/_4$ h $\pm$ $^1/_4$ h (FRITZ-NIGGLI, 1952a, 1955), indem für sie die Dl 50 % (Dosis letalis 50 %) 160 R beträgt, während bestrahlte 7—8 h-Embryonen eine Dl 50 % von 5000 R aufweisen.

Die Resistenz nimmt nach Abschluß der Blastodermbildung und der komplizierten Vorgänge der Gastrulation (3 Std nach Befruchtung) zu. Nachdem bereits ULRICH (1953) mit einer speziellen Methode das Alter der abgelegten Drosophila-Embryonen auf $\pm$ 5 min einschränkte, untersuchte WÜRGLER (1961, 1962, 1968) frühe Embryonalstadien mit einer Alters-Variabilität von 3 min. Damit wurde es möglich, Strahleneffekte differenziert an Zygoten (SCHNEIDER-MINDER, 1966) in Meiose und verschiedenen Furchungs-, resp. Kern-

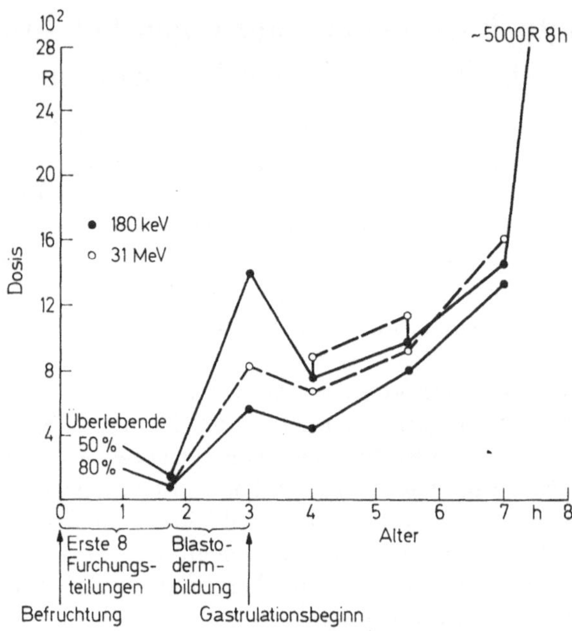

Abb. 2. Abhängigkeit der Strahlensensibilität der Drosophila-Embryonen vom Alter. Eingetragen sind Kurven für 50% Überlebende (dicke Linie) und 80% Überlebende. Die Embryonen sind am strahlenempfindlichsten im Alter von $1^3/_4$ Stunden. (Aus FRITZ-NIGGLI, 1955)

teilungsstadien zu studieren. Es zeigte sich, daß die Strahlensensibilität während des Endes der Anaphase am höchsten und bei Beginn der Prophase am tiefsten war (Diskussion der Ursache der unterschiedlichen Wirksamkeit bei MATTER, 1970). Bei der Analyse der embryonalen Schädigung stellten sich während der Embryonalentwicklung zum mindesten 3 Schädigungskategorien (FRITZ-NIGGLI, 1952a) ein, nämlich

1. die bestrahlten Embryonen entwickelten sich nicht weiter (Frühtod),

2. die Embryonen entwickeln sich weiter, sterben aber vor der Schlüpfreife (Frühtod),

3. die Embryonen wachsen zu annähernd normalen schlüpfreifen Larven, die aber nicht mehr aus der Eihülle schlüpfen (Spättod).

Makroskopisch kann die 3. Kategorie relativ einfach durch ihre Braunfärbung (vermutlich bedingt durch Austritt von Hämolymphe) von den „weißen" Toten unterschieden werden.

Ferner können die geschlüpften Larven während der larvalen oder pupalen Phase sterben oder noch als frühe Imago an der Folge der embryonalen Bestrahlung zugrunde gehen oder Anomalien aufweisen. Diese Modifikationen entsprechen den Mißbildungen der neugeborenen Säugetiere nach Bestrahlung in utero. Sie verschwinden allerdings zahlenmäßig gegenüber den embryonalen, larvalen und pupalen Todesfällen, da die komplizierte holometabole Entwicklungsweise selektiv wirkt und Anomalien frühzeitig ausschaltet.

Die Todesart ist weitgehend vom Bestrahlungsalter und der Dosis abhängig (FRITZ-NIGGLI, 1952a, 1955), bestätigt von WÜRGLER (1968). So überwiegen in frühen Stadien bei niederen Dosen Spättote, während mit großen Dosen die Entwicklung sofort unterbrochen wird. Diese Feststellungen verbieten übrigens treffertheoretische Interpretationen von Dosis-Effektkurven, da diese Kurven lediglich Resultanten von Kurvenscharen darstellen. Äußerlich erkennbare Schädigungen beim Spättod sind hauptsächlich Störungen in der Ausbildung der Muskulatur, des Pharynx und der Hypodermis.

b) Strahlenreaktionen der Puppe

Nach der Bildung des harten Pupariums vollzieht sich im Innern die eigentliche Metamorphose, in deren Verlauf aus den Imaginalscheiben die imaginalen Organe endgültig ausgebildet werden. Wiederum lassen sich bei bestrahlten Puppen verschiedenen Altert erhebliche Sensibilitätsunterschiede feststellen, die anscheinend in strenger Abhängigkeis vom jeweiligen Stadium des lebensnotwendigen Systems stehen. So steigt die Strahlen-

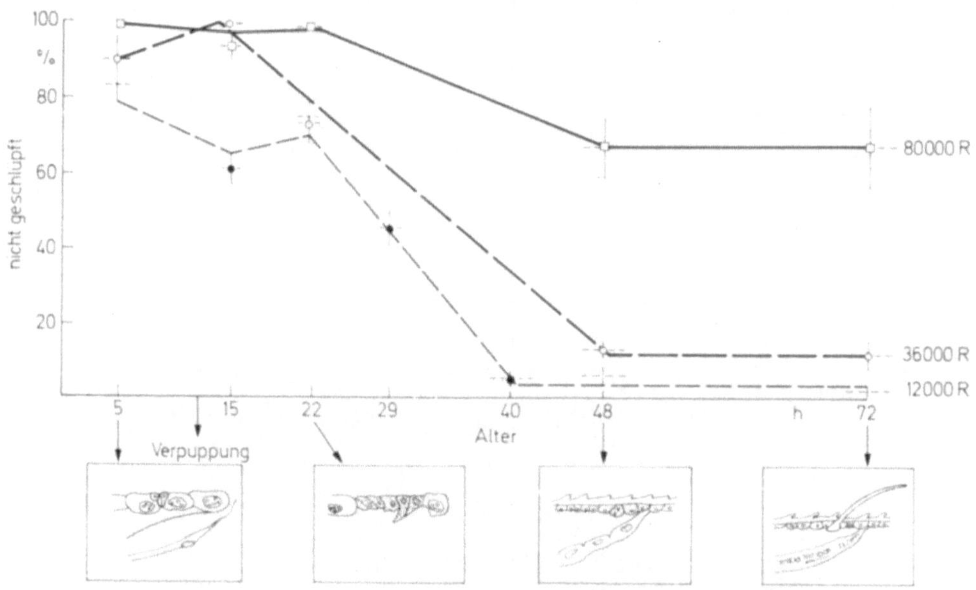

Abb. 3. Abhängigkeit der Strahlensensibilität von Drosophilapuppen vom Alter während der Bestrahlung. Dargestellt unter Abszisse Entwicklungszustand der Hypodermis während der Bestrahlung (aus FRITZ-NIGGLI, 1952b)

resistenz steil an (FRITZ-NIGGLI, 1952b), (Abb. 3), wenn das Puppenalter von 30 Std erreicht wird. Nach 12000 R sterben 5—22stündige Puppen beinahe zu 100 %, während 80000 R 40stündige Puppen nicht einmal zu 80 % töten. Die bestrahlten Puppen entwickeln sich übrigens meistens zur schlüpfreifen Form. Es zeigte sich, daß die pupale strahlenbedingte Letalität zumeist auf einer Fehlentwicklung des Körperinteguments beruht (Abb. 4). Bestimmend für die variable Strahlensensibilität der einzelnen Stadien scheint der Entwicklungszustand der Integuments-Histoblasten zu sein.

2. Abhängigkeit der strahlenbedingten Entwicklungsstörungen von verschiedenen Parametern

Neben der bestimmenden Bedeutung des Entwicklungszustandes für die embryonale und postembryonale Schädigung zeichnen sich noch andere modellierende Faktoren ab:

a) Milieufaktoren

Sowohl die embryonale (Ulrich u. Würgler, 1962; Finsinger, 1964; Havin u. Ofte-dal, 1968) als auch die pupale Sterblichkeit (Fritz-Niggli u. Mitarb., 1963) lassen sich durch den Sauerstoffgehalt während der Bestrahlung beeinflussen. So fanden Havin u. Oftedal (1968) eine OER[1] (Oxygen enhancement ratio) von 2 für 1 h 38 min $\pm$ 5 min und 2 h 38 min $\pm$ 5 min alte Embryonen.

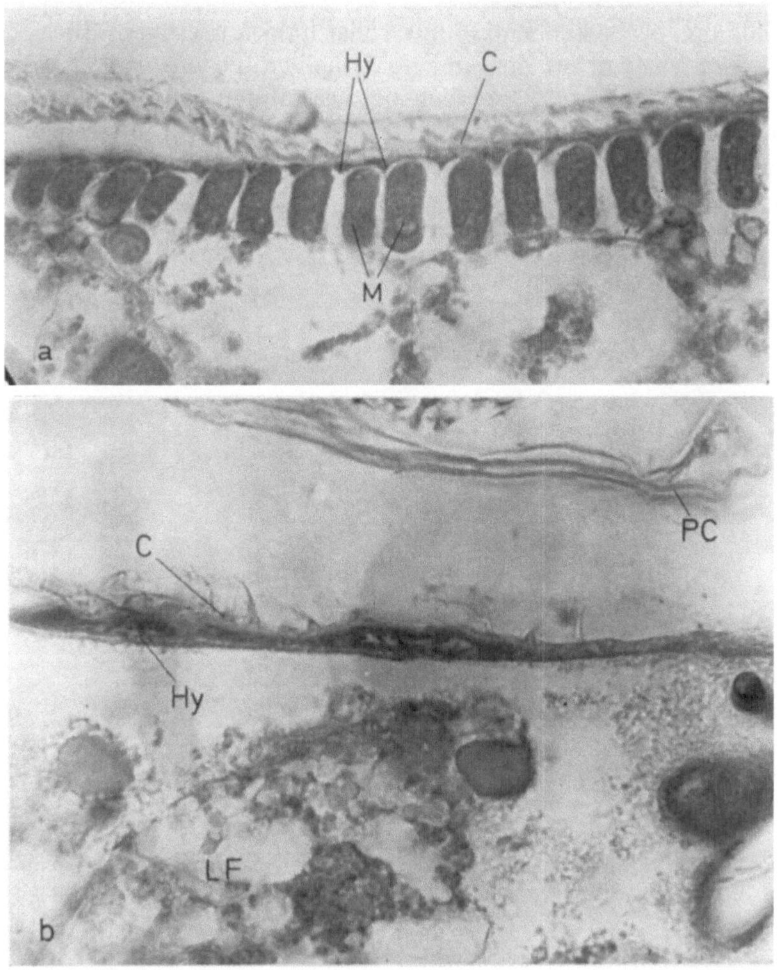

Abb. 4. Entwicklungsstörungen nach Bestrahlung von Vorpuppen (Drosophila melanogaster). a) Normale Aus-bildung der Hypodermis einer schlüpfreifen Puppe. b) Körperwand einer schlüpfreifen Puppe nach Bestrahlung im Alter von 5 h. Die Muskulatur fehlt. C = Cuticula, Hy = Hypodermis, LF = Fettkörper, M = Muskulatur, PC = pupale Cuticula. (Aus Fritz-Niggli, 1952b)

---

1 OER ist das Maß für den Sauerstoffeffekt und drückt das Verhältnis der Dosen aus, die für den gleichen Effekt in anoxischem (oder sauerstoffarmem) und sauerstoffreichem Milieu gebraucht werden.

Für 31 MeV-Photonen und 200 keV-Photonen war der Sauerstoffeffekt nach Puppenbestrahlung annähernd identisch (Abb. 5). Eine Kältebehandlung nach Bestrahlung beeinflußt die pupale Letalität unwesentlich (SCHLEUSS, 1964). Über eine Schutzwirkung von H_2S auf $29 \pm 1{,}5$ min Embryonen berichtet MATTER (1968).

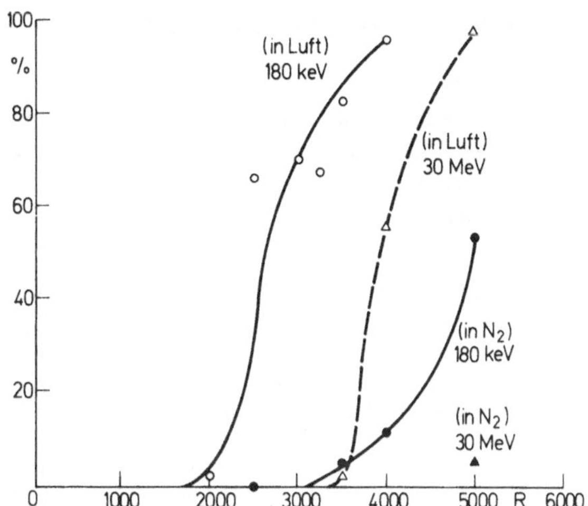

Abb. 5. Erzeugung der Modifikation „gespreizte Flügel" nach Bestrahlung von 5 stündigen Vorpuppen (Drosophila melanogaster) mit 180 keV-Photonen in Luft (leere Kreise) in N_2 (ausgefüllte Kreise) und 30 MeV-Elektronen in Luft (leere Dreiecke) und in N_2 (ausgefüllte Dreiecke). (Aus FRITZ-NIGGLI u. Mitarb., 1963)

b) LET[1] (linear energy transfer) Qualität der Strahlung

Werden verschiedenaltrige Drosophila-Embryonen mit 180 keV-Photonen und 30 MeV-Elektronen, sowie 31 MeV-Photonen bestrahlt, dann zeigt sich bemerkenswerterweise nur für 3-, 4- und 7 stündige Embryonen eine Abhängigkeit von der Strahlenqualität, während 1- und $1^3/_4$ stündige Embryonen eine RBE[1] von 1 aufweisen (Zusammenfassung siehe FRITZ-NIGGLI, 1955, 1958a).

Gleicherweise fanden SCHNEIDER u. Mitarb. (1969) für 0—10 minütige Embryonen nach Bestrahlung mit α-Strahlen (Americium 241) eine RBE von 1. Vermutete Differenzen (WIDERÖE, 1959) in der LET in verschiedenen Tiefen der Transitionskurve ließen sich mit dem Letalitätstest mit 1- und 4 stündigen Embryonen nicht nachweisen (FRITZ-NIGGLI u. SCHINZ, 1961, 1962).

Wie schon mit anderen Objekten zeigt sich eindeutig eine Abhängigkeit der RBE vom Zustand des bestrahlten Reaktionssystems. Es ist durchaus möglich (Diskussion siehe FRITZ-NIGGLI, 1968), daß das Repairsystem verschieden auf die unterschiedliche Energieverteilung anspricht. Während frühere Experimente (MÜLLER, 1939) keinen Unterschied zwischen Gammabestrahlung (Radium) und konventioneller Röntgenbestrahlung von Puppenstadien zeigten, wurde nach 31 MeV-Photonenbestrahlung eine relative biologische Wirksamkeit unter 1 festgestellt, und zwar nicht nur in bezug auf den Strahlentod (FRITZ-NIGGLI, 1954; FRITZ-NIGGLI u. Mitarb., 1963), sondern auch auf Modifikationen, wie gespreizte Flügel (FRITZ-NIGGLI, 1951) und Borstenanomalien (NAVILLE, 1955). Selbst die

---

1 Der LET (lineare Energieübertragung) beschreibt die Strahlenqualität anhand der linearen Energieübertragung (Maß = keV/μm Weglänge) längs des Wegs des ionisierenden Partikels. Mit der RBE wird die relative biologische Wirksamkeit bezogen auf die Wirkung einer Strahlung mit LET von 3,5 keV/μm RBE = 1 beschrieben.

relativ geringen Unterschiede im LET von 100 keV-Photonen und 200 keV-Photonen scheinen ein verschiedenes Ausmaß der Strahlenschädigung zur Folge zu haben (Suter, 1967). Die RBE beträgt etwa im Durchschnitt 1,7 für die 100 keV-Strahlung. Ebenso stellte sich eine erhebliche Abhängigkeit von der Intensität der Strahlung heraus, indem eine verdünnte Bestrahlung weniger wirkt.

3. Strahleneffekte an Blastemen

Die Imaginalscheiben der Drosophila eignen sich vorzüglich zur Untersuchung von Entwicklungsvorgängen (s. Hadorn, 1955, 1963, 1966 etc.). In ihnen befinden sich Zellen in Teilung und Differenzierung. Wenn verschiedene Imaginalscheiben nach Bestrahlung von 80—85 h-Larven in Gewebekultur (Horikawa u. Sughara, 1960) gezüchtet werden, zeigt sich eine unterschiedliche Strahlenempfindlichkeit. Ebenso läßt sich eine Abhängigkeit der Art der Mißbildungen vom Alter der bestrahlten Entwicklungsstadien (resp. Imaginalscheiben) erkennen. Mit bestimmten Methoden lassen sich nun strahleninduzierte Anomalien adulter Gewebe bis zu einem gewissen Grade analysieren.

a) Genitalprimordien

So untersuchte Schweizer (1967, 1969) die Strahlenmodifikation des männlichen Genitalapparates von Drosophila melanogaster (Fritz-Niggli, 1952b), der sich aus zwei Primordien entwickelt, der Genitalimaginalscheibe und den paarigen ellipsoiden Gonaden der Larve.

Während selbst eine lokale Bestrahlung der larvalen Gonaden mit 48000 R zu keiner späteren Mißbildung führt, erweist sich die Genitalscheibe als wesentlich strahlenemp-

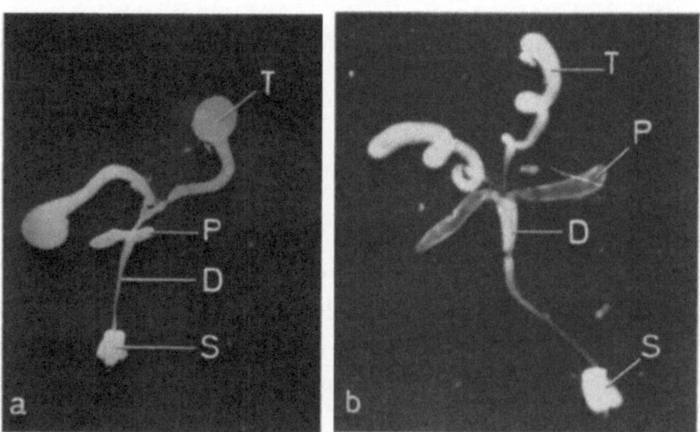

Abb. 6. Unterschiedliche Sensibilität der Primordien des männlichen Genitalapparates von Drosophila melano, gaster. a) Mißbildungen der Gonaden nach lokaler Bestrahlung der Genitalscheibe in 0 h-Vorpuppen mit 3000 R- b) Normale Ausbildung der Gonaden nach Bestrahlung des Gonaden-Blastems in 0 h-Vorpuppen mit 30000 R, D = Ductus ejaculatorius, P = Paragonien, T = Testes, S = Samenpumpe. (Schweizer, unveröffentlicht)

findlicher (Abb. 6). Nach Bestrahlung von 48 h—72 h-Larven, 0 h- und 10 h-Vorpuppen, sowie 30 h-Puppen wurde eine deutliche Abhängigkeit der strahlenbedingten imaginalen Strukturdefekte vom Alter während der Bestrahlung gefunden. So sind beispielsweise Schädigungen der Analplatten und Claspers nach Bestrahlung der Genitalscheibe in 48 h-Larven mit 4000 R selten, in 72 h-Larven häufig. Hingegen wird die Penistragplatte und die Entwicklung der Samenpumpe nach Bestrahlung des Blastems in 48stündigen Larven am meisten geschädigt (Abb. 7).

Die unterschiedliche Empfindlichkeit könnte u.a. auf Unterschiede in der Empfindlichkeit geschädigter Blasteme beruhen. Es ist bekannt, daß Dipteren-Blasteme in proliferativer Regulation vom Restblastem ersetzt werden, ein Vorgang, der naturgemäß eine Funktion der Zeit ist, die zwischen Verletzung und Enddifferenzierung liegt. Tatsächlich lassen sich gewisse embryonale Störungen durch Rücktransplantation (SCHWEIZER 1972) in jüngere Larvenstadien (Abb. 8) durch eine verlängerte Entwicklungszeit aufheben.

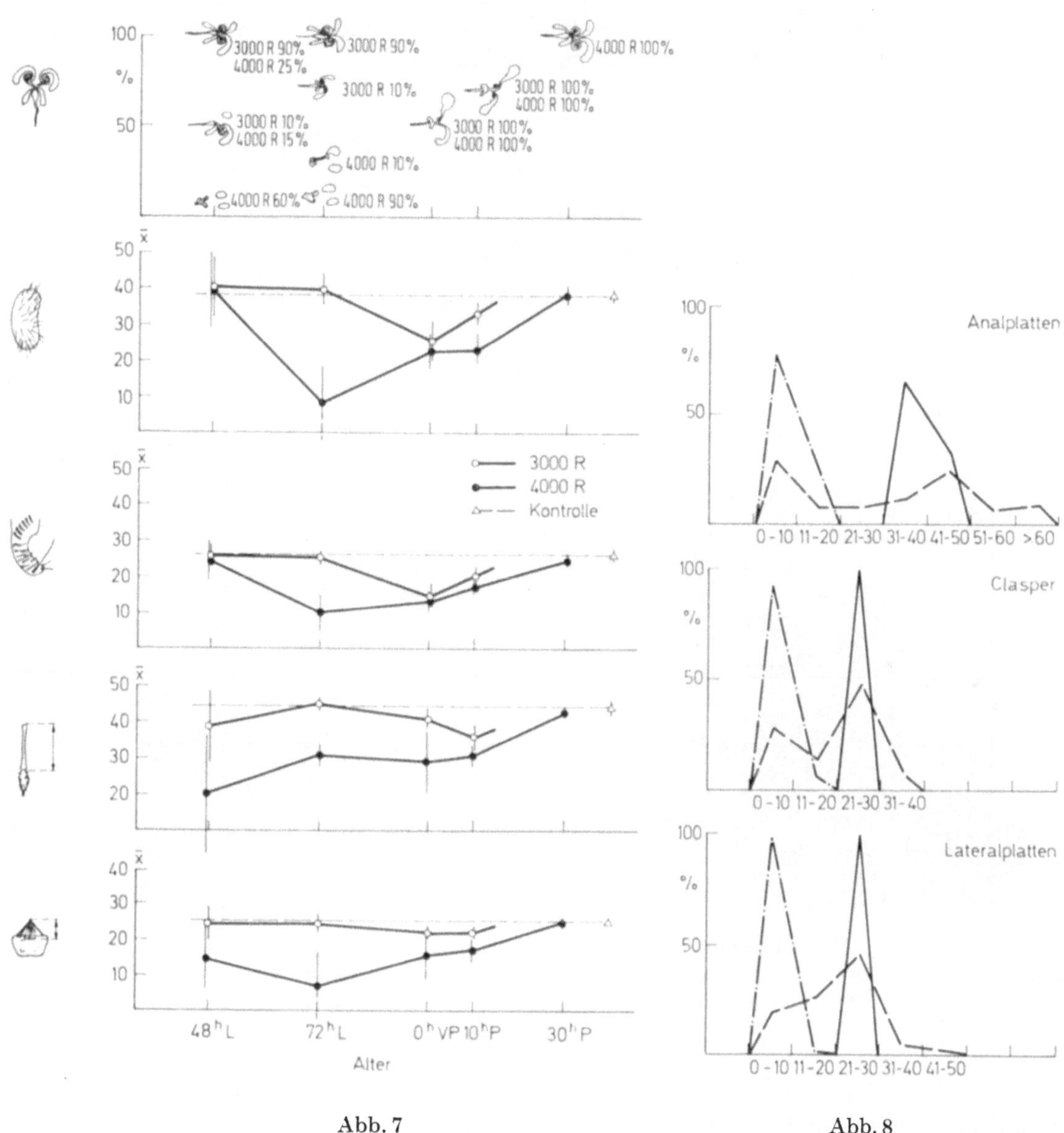

Abb. 7   Abb. 8

Abb. 7. Abhängigkeit der Schädigungsrate der Weichteile und Gonaden, Analplatten, Claspers, Penistragplatten und Samenpumpensklerite von der Dosis und dem Larven- und Puppenalter bei Bestrahlung (Larvenalter in h nach dem Schlüpfen aus der Eihülle. (Aus SCHWEIZER, 1969)

Abb. 8. Vergleich der Entwicklungsleistung, resp. Ausbildung von Borsten, der Genitalscheibe nach Bestrahlung von 72 h-Larven und Entwicklung in situ (— · — · —) sowie nach Rücktransplantation in 48 h-Larven (— — — —) mit der Normalleistung unbestrahlter Genitalscheiben (———). Ordinate: % Strukturen einer Klassengröße. Abszisse: Borstenzahl pro Struktur in der Klasse (Zahl der Untersuchten: Kontrolle = 70; 4000 R in situ = 90, Rücktransplantate = 100). (Nach SCHWEIZER, 1972)

Durch eine Induktion von somatischen Crossing over in heterozygoten Zellen läßt sich der Anteil einer einzelnen Zelle am Endorgan untersuchen (s. S. 268, Diskussion der Mechanismen).

b) Differenzierung männlicher Keimzellen

In larvalen und pupalen Gonaden von Drosophila können Zellen ausgezeichnet in ihrer Entwicklung aus primitiven Vorstufen (Spermatogonien) zu hoch differenzierten Stadien (Spermien), (Abb. 9) verfolgt werden. Nach Meyer (1963, 1969) ist für bestimmte Differenzierungsleistungen die Anwesenheit des Y-Chromosom in den noch diploiden prämeiotischen Keimzellen nötig. Sobald die Geninformationen der Zelle übermittelt werden, scheint die Entwicklung autonom abzulaufen.

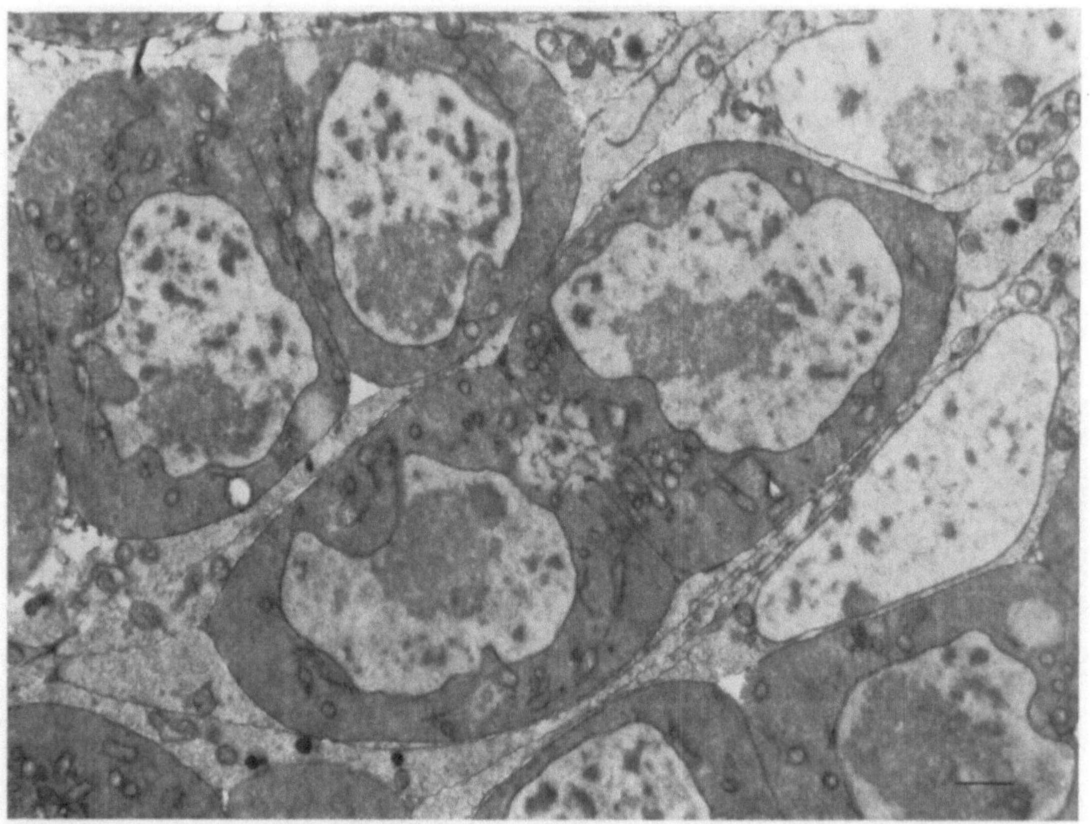

Abb. 9[1]. Verschiedene Entwicklungsstadien männlicher Keimzellen von Drosophila melanogaster. a) Spermatogonien I, b) Spermatozyten, c) Meiose mit Bildung von Lamellen, langgezogene Mitochondrien, d) Zusammenschluß der Mitochondrien in jungen Spermatiden, e) Bildung des „Nebenkerns", Strich = 1 μm

Tatsächlich vollenden mit 2000 R in O_2 bestrahlte Spermatozyten in Prophase die meiotische Teilung und werden zu mehr oder minder normalen Spermatiden. Die Zellen zeichnen sich (Abb. 10, 11, 12, 13) durch eine unterschiedliche Strahlensensibilität aus, wobei einzelne Organellen eine zum Teil große Kapazität zur Erholung besitzen. Als ebenso empfindlich wie erholungsfähig erweisen sich die Mitochondrien, die übrigens auch einer Stickstoffbehandlung gegenüber sehr verletzlich sind (Abb. 12, 13, 14, 15).

1 Sämtliche elektronenoptischen Aufnahmen wurden mit dem Hitachi-Mikroskop Typ HS 6 oder HU-11 E gemacht. Fix. in 3% $KMnO_2$. Herrn T. Suda sei an dieser Stelle für seine ausgezeichnete Mitarbeit herzlich gedankt.

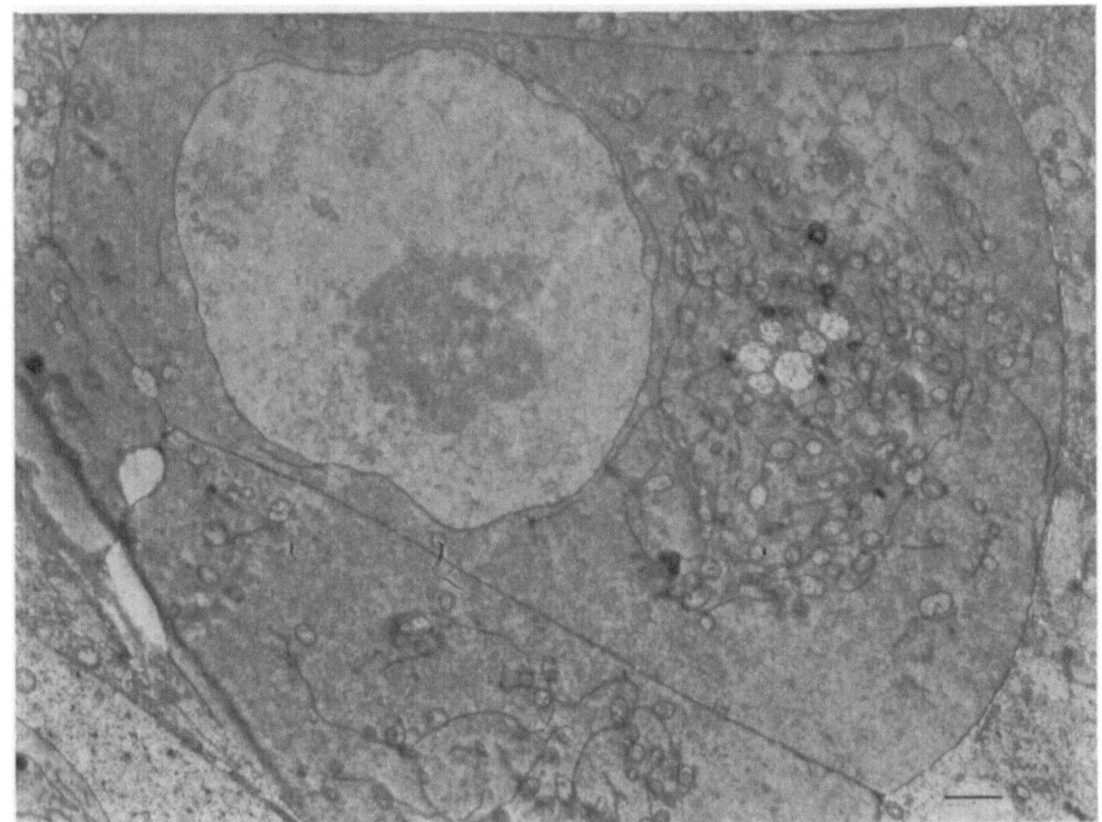

9b

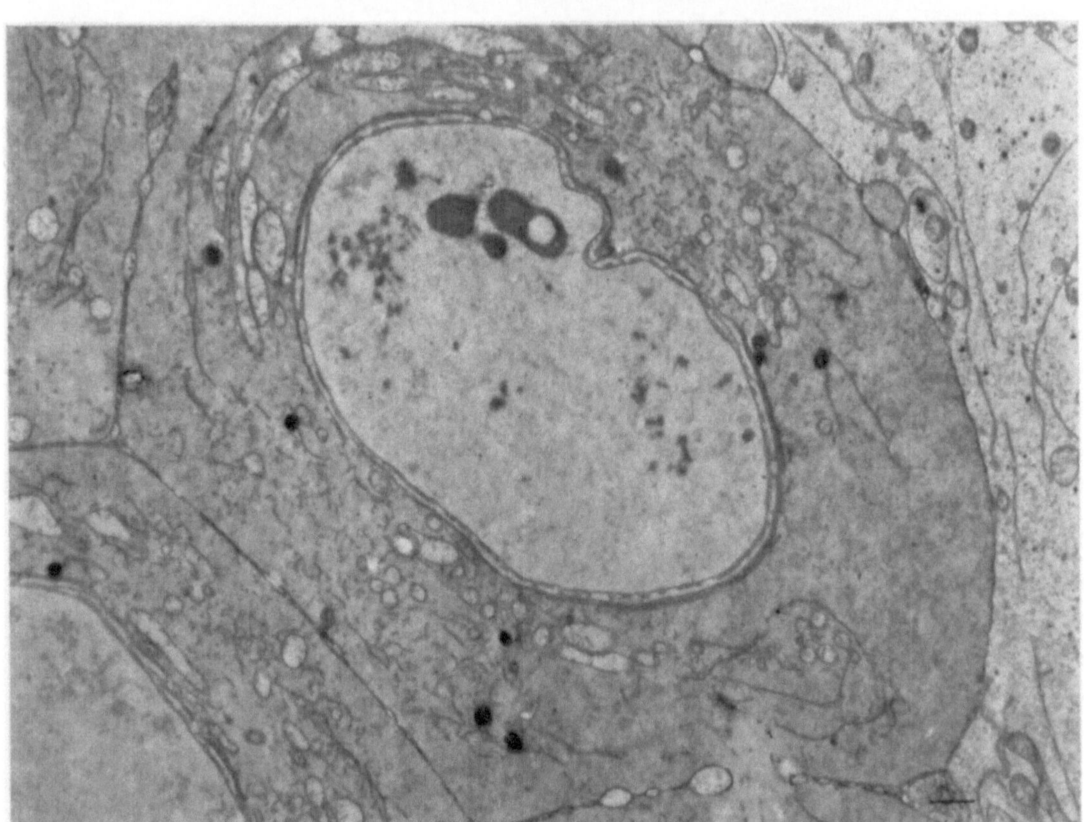

9c

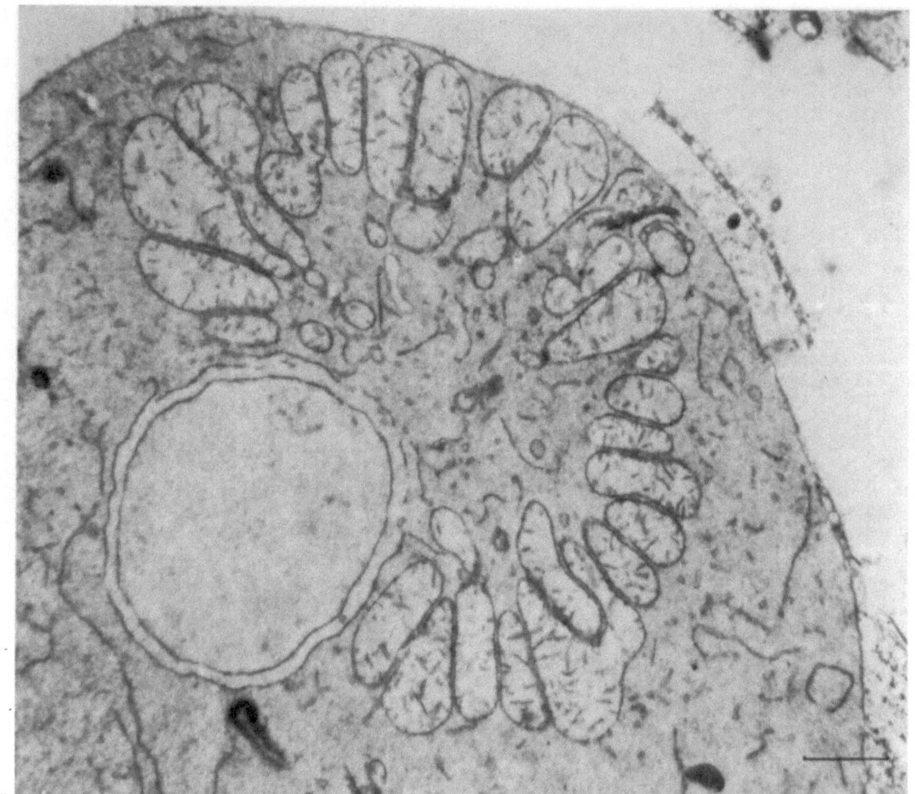

9d

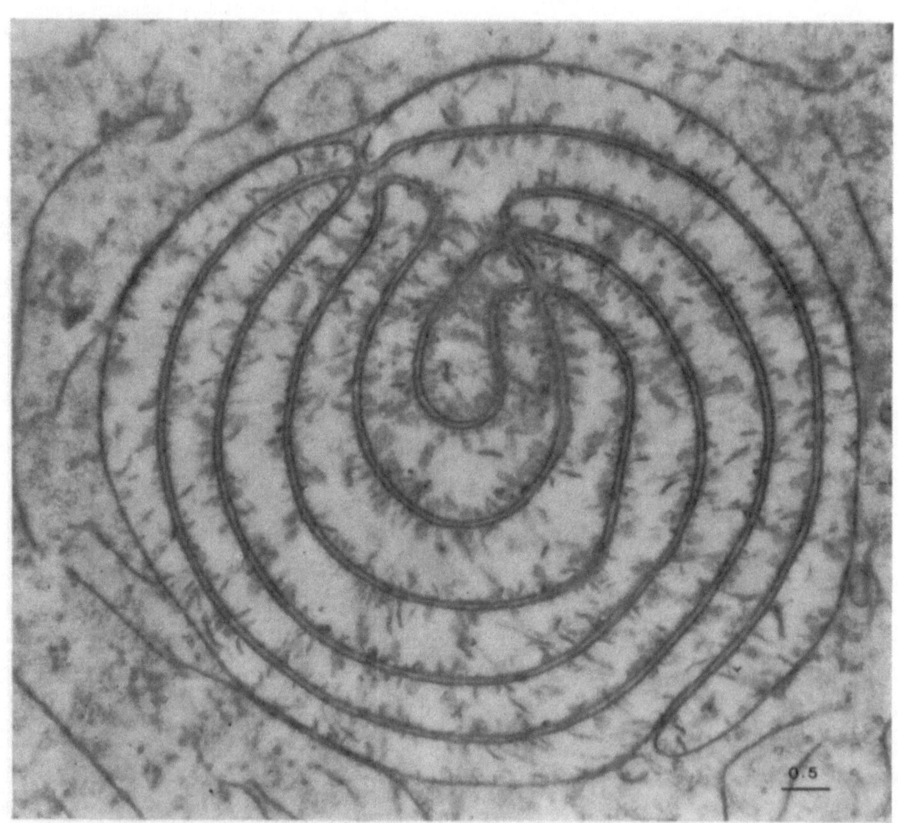

9e

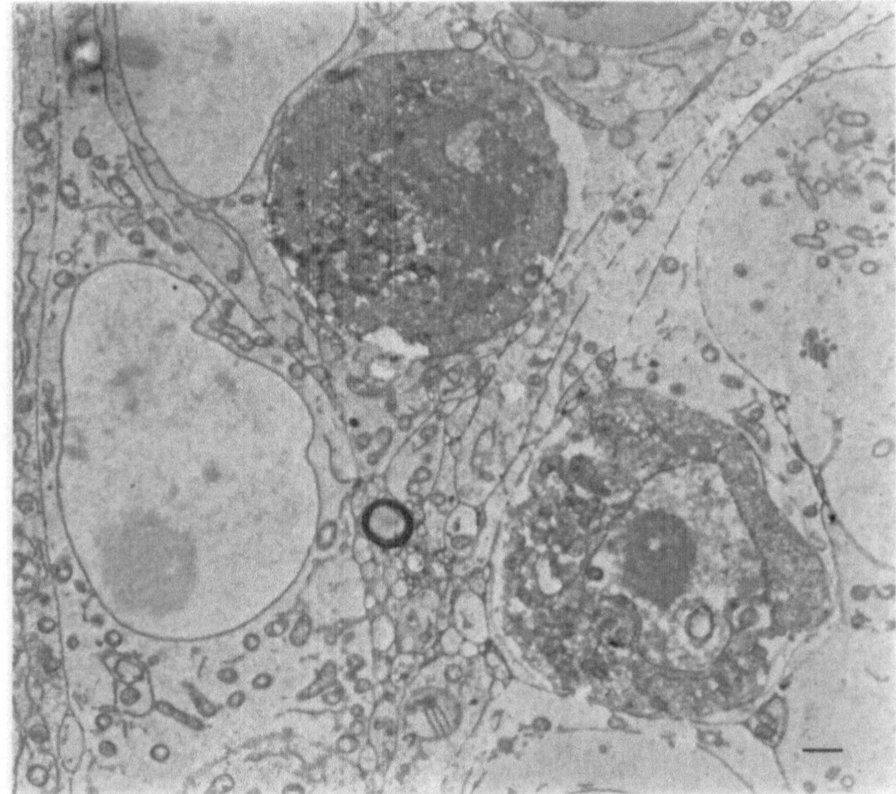

10a

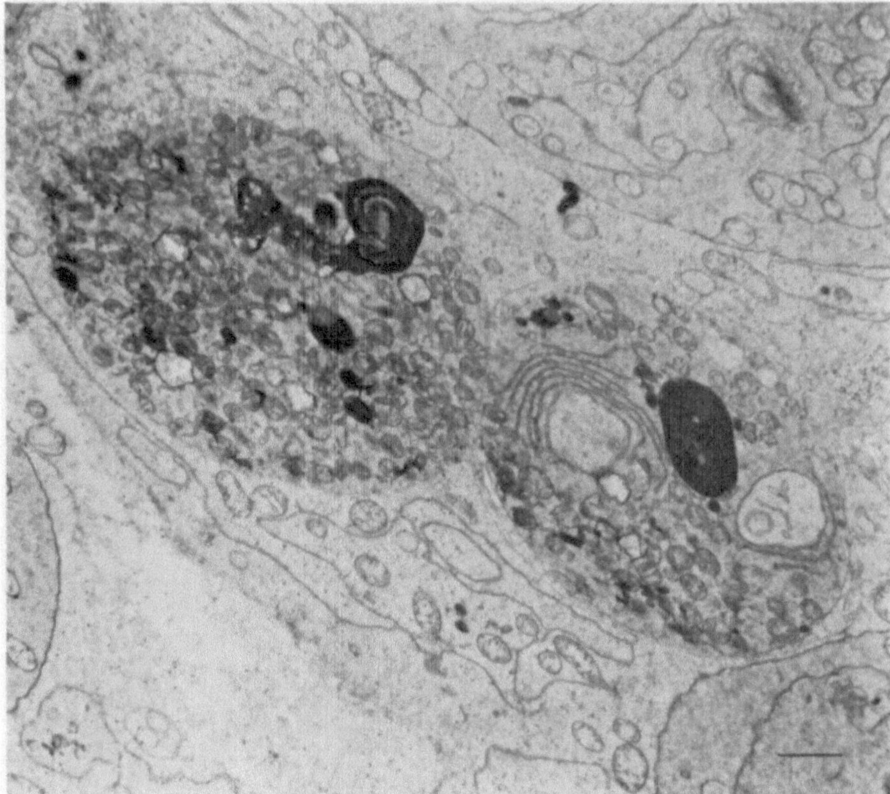

10b

Abb. 10. Geschädigte Spermatogonien nach Bestrahlung von Vorpuppen mit 2000 R in O_2. a) Zwei geschädigte Spermatogonien, links ungeschädigte Interstitialzellen, b) Unmittelbar nach Teilung geschädigter Zellen mit Lysosomen

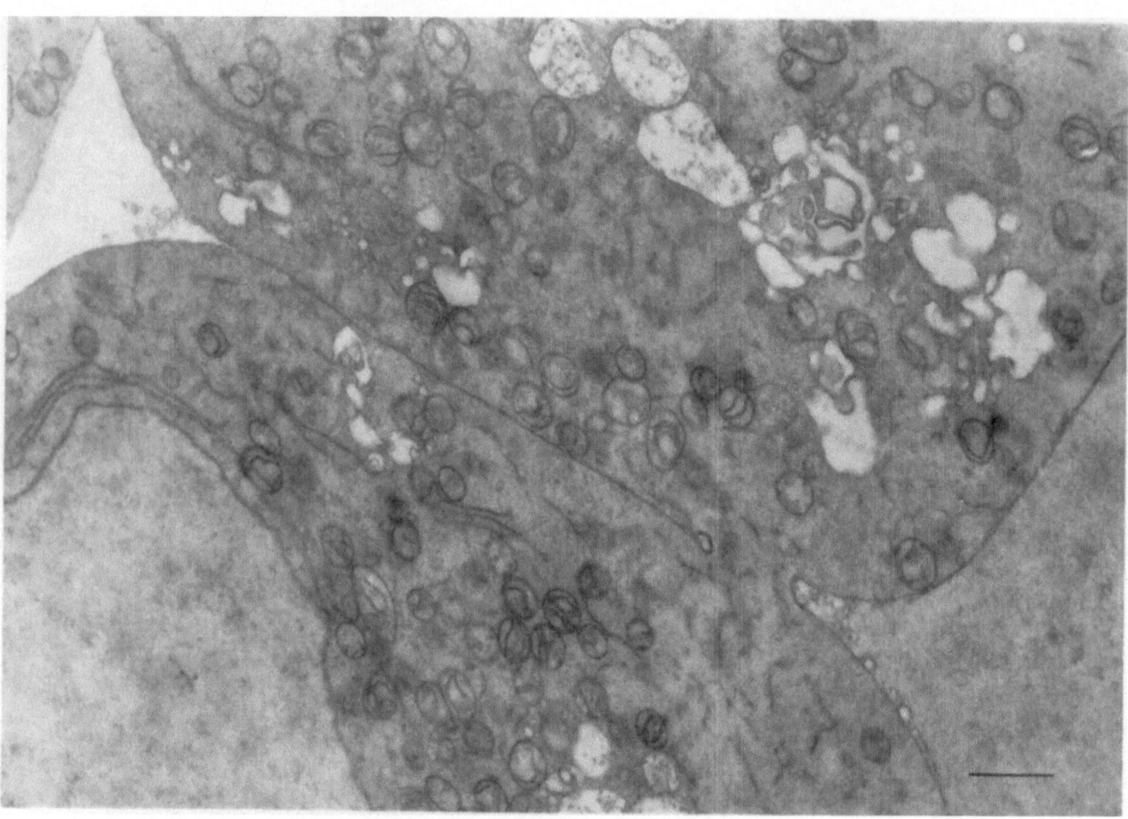

Abb. 11. Zerstörter Golgi-Apparat in Spermatozyten 48 h nach Bestrahlung mit 20000 R in O_2

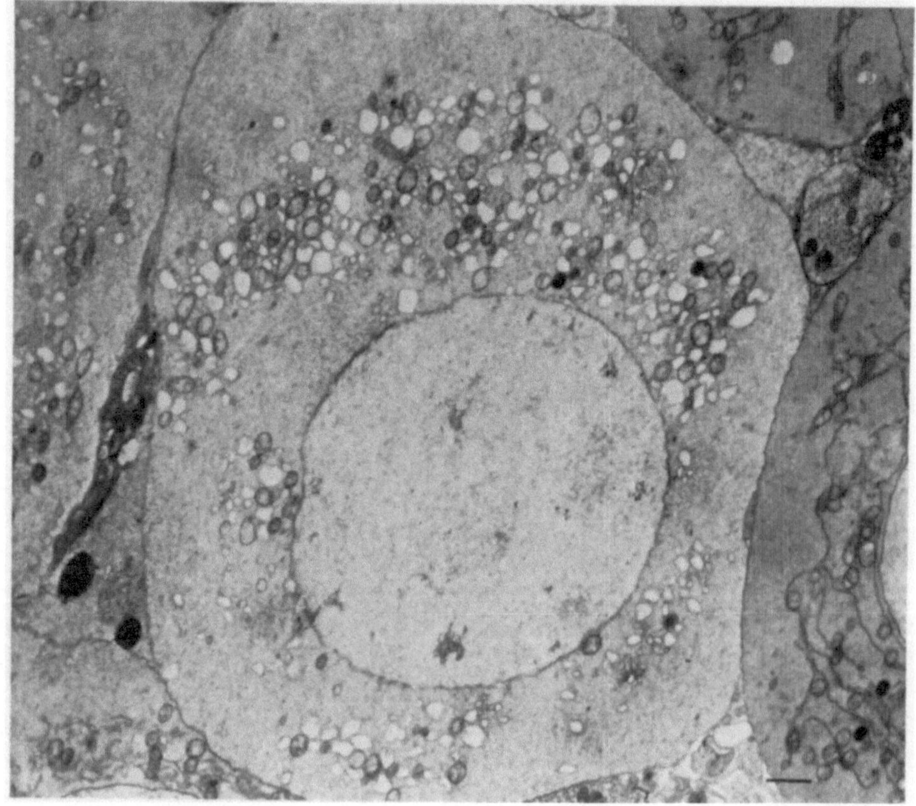

Abb. 12. Spermatozyte mit zahlreichen Vakuolen und veränderten Mitochondrien

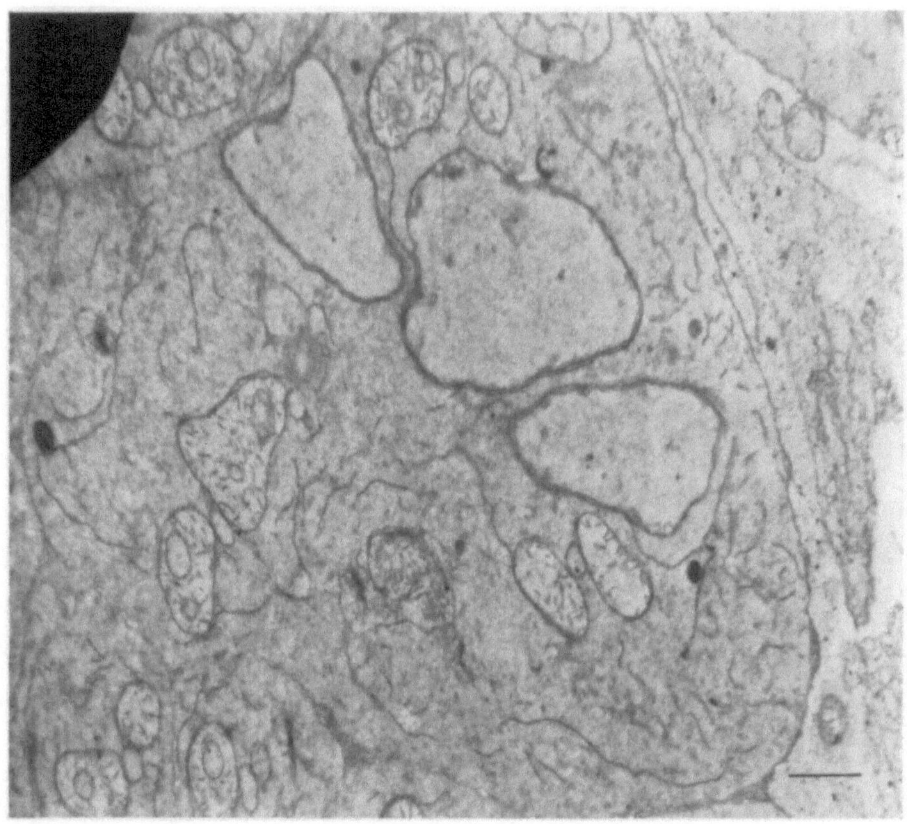

Abb. 13. Dreikernige Spermatide nach Bestrahlung von Spermatozyten in Prophase mit 2000 R in O_2

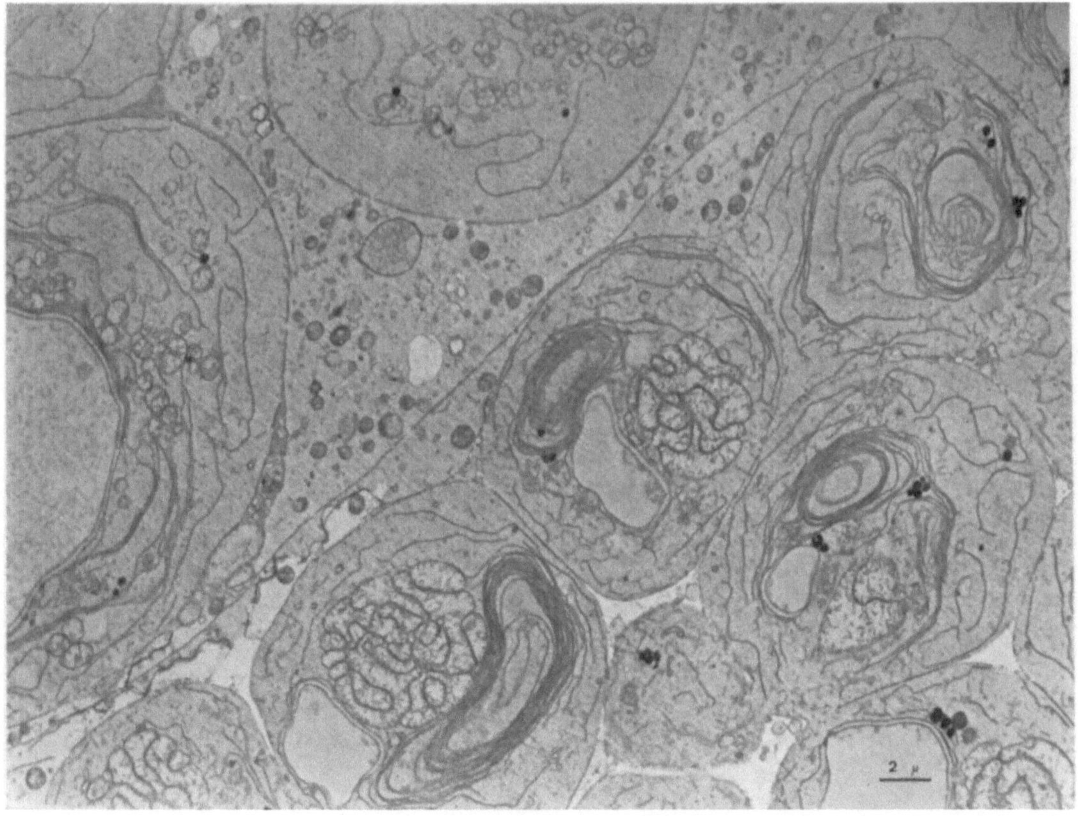

Abb. 14. Anomalien in Spermatiden nach Bestrahlung von Spermatozyten in Prophase mit 20000 R in O_2. a) Mißgebildete „Nebenkerne", Lamellen bleiben bestehen, b) Aufgetriebene Mitochondrien ohne Bildung eines Nebenkerns, komplizierte Lamellen-Struktur

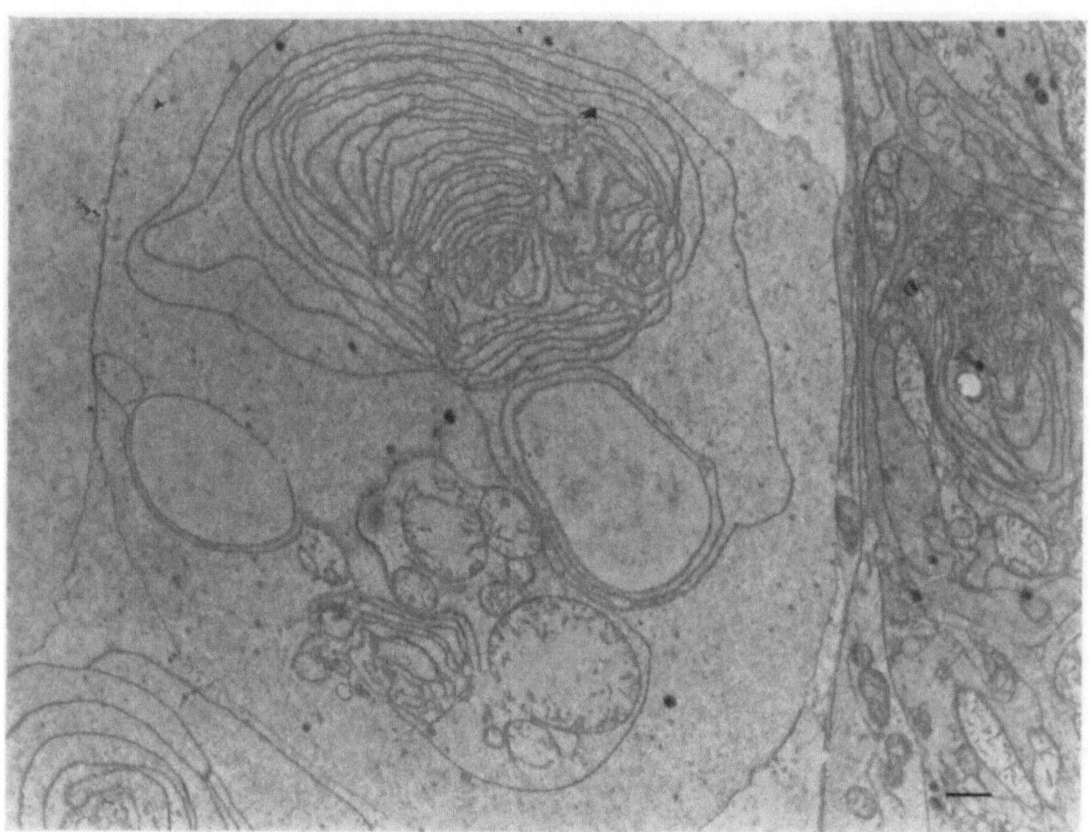

Abb. 14b

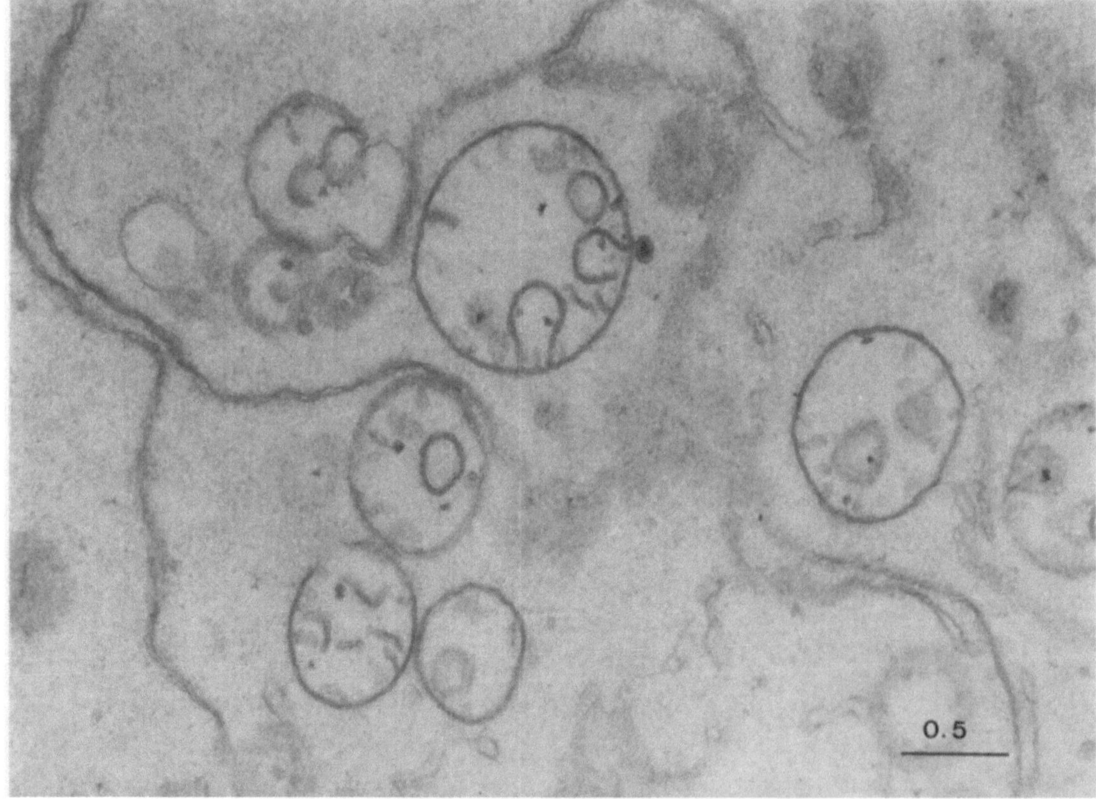

Abb. 15. Veränderte Mitochondrien mit ringförmigen Cristen nach Applikation von N_2 während 12 h an männliche Drosophila-Vorpuppen

III. Strahlenbedingte Entwicklungsstörungen bei Wirbeltieren (Amphibien, Säugetiere und Mensch)[1]

Nachdem in früheren Jahren den Strahleneffekten an Amphibien-Embryonen große Aufmerksamkeit geschenkt wurde, sind in der letzten Zeit vermehrt Experimente mit Säugetieren unternommen worden.

1. Abhängigkeit des Strahleneffektes vom Entwicklungsstadium

Ebenso wie auf andere teratogene Agentien (RIVERS u. Mitarb., 1959) reagieren die verschiedenen Entwicklungsstadien auf ionisierende Strahlen unterschiedlich. Nach der Bestrahlung kann sich Folgendes ereignen:

1. Sofortiger Entwicklungsstillstand (Frühtod).
Bei Säugetieren werden die toten Embryonen entweder resorbiert oder abgestoßen (Abort). Nach der Bestrahlung früher Entwicklungsstadien kann die Resorption vor der Implantation erfolgen (präimplantative Resorption).

2. Weiterentwicklung und später einsetzender Tod als Embryo oder Fetus.
(1. und 2. stellen bei Säugetieren intrauterine Todesfälle dar.)

3. Weiterentwicklung bis zur Geburt, Auftreten von Mißbildungen und Anomalien.

4. Normalentwicklung und Normalgeburt (in 3. und 4. kann die Entwicklung verzögert sein).

Nachdem DE NOBELE u. LAMS bereits 1927 festgestellt hatten, daß der Tod der Frucht um so sicherer eintritt, je frühzeitiger die Bestrahlung stattfindet, haben JOB u. Mitarb. (1935) als erste von sensiblen, resp. kritischen Perioden gesprochen und unterschieden zwischen der Strahlenschädigung der sogenannten Präimplantationsperiode, der Organogenese und der fetalen Entwicklung. Je nach Entwicklungsstadium stellen sich ganz verschiedene Ereignisse ein und ebenso wurde eine Häufung bestimmter Anomalien in Abhängigkeit vom bestrahlten Stadium beobachtet. Sowohl Häufigkeit als auch Eigenart der Anomalien sind demnach an besondere Stadien gebunden.

In Abb. 16 sind nach RUGH die Verteilungen bestimmter Anomalien in Abhängigkeit vom Bestrahlungsalter für die Maus dargestellt.

a) Periode der Blastogenese

Die Periode der Blastogenese, ungenau oft Präimplantationsperiode genannt, umfaßt die Zeit von der Befruchtung bis zur Organogenese. Sie entspricht der Eifurchung, der Differenzierung von Entoderm- und Ektodermzellen der Blastocyste bis zur Scheidung in 3 Keimblätter und dem Einsetzen der Gastrulation. Sie erstreckt sich etwa bei der Maus bis zum 7. d, bei der Ratte bis zum 9. d, beim Menschen bis zum 18. d nach Befruchtung (siehe Tabelle 1).

In bezug auf den *Strahlentod* (Abb. 17) zeigt sich dieses Stadium als äußerst sensibel. Mit relativ großen Strahlendosen (100—400 R), (RUSSELL u. RUSSELL, 1950 a, b; RUSSELL u. RUSSELL, 1954) wird bei der Maus die Zahl der Würfe nach Bestrahlung der Mutter während dieser Periode deutlich reduziert. Das gleiche berichteten RUGH u. WOHLFROMM (1965), wobei aber die Sensibilität innerhalb der ersten 5 Tage beträchtlich zu schwanken scheint, wie es die Dl 50 %-Kurve in Abhängigkeit zum Entwicklungsalter darstellt (Abb. 18). Auch die frühen Furchungsstadien der Maus (RUGH, 1969) zeigen ein besonderes

---

1 Übersichten: BUTLER (1936); FRITZ-NIGGLI (1959, 1960); RUGH (1953, 1959, 1960, 1963 a, b); HICKS u. D'AMATO (1966); RUSSELL (1954); SIKOV u. MAHLUM (1969); BRUNST (1965).

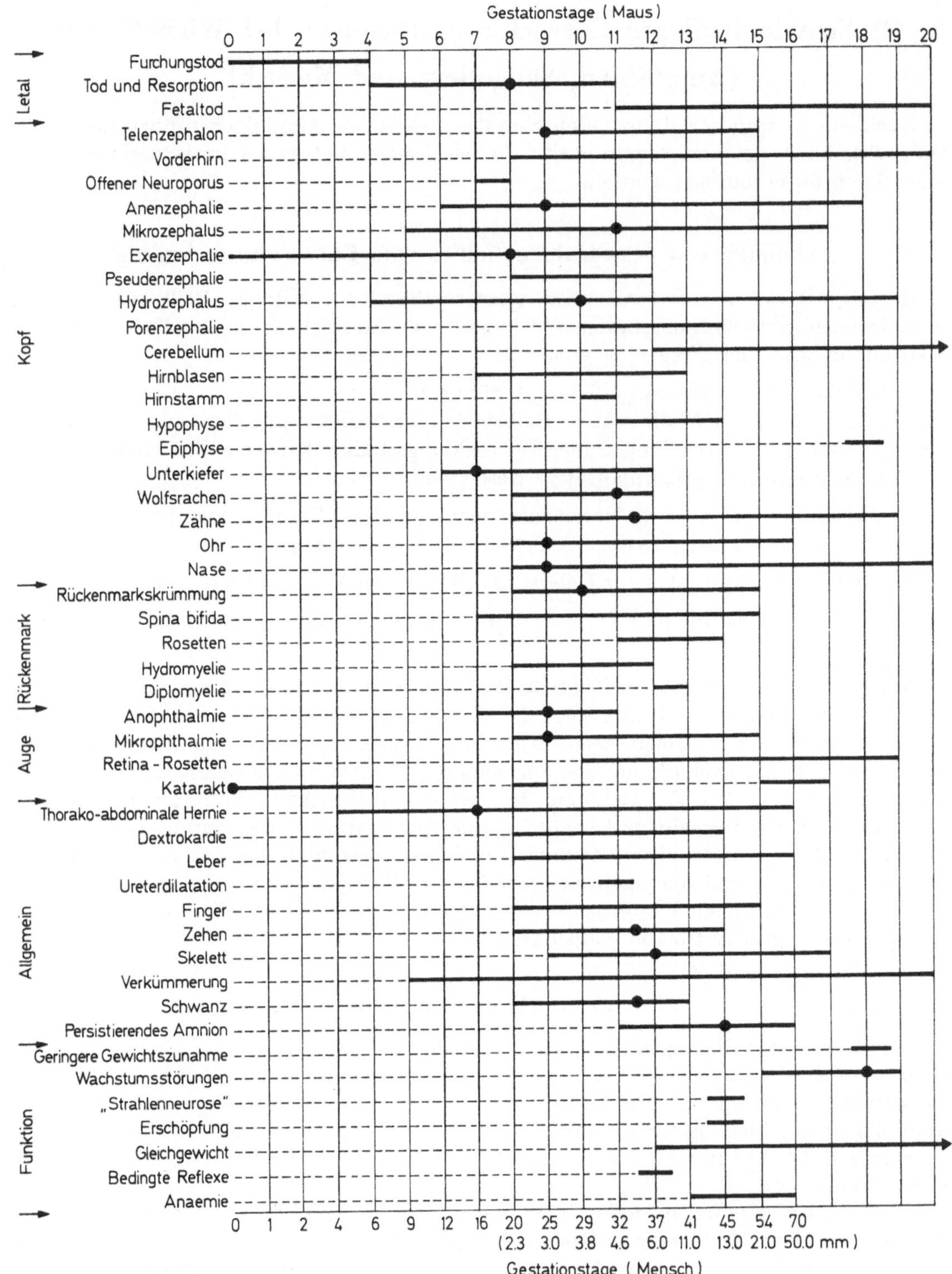

Abb. 16. Strahleninduzierte Anomalien bei der Maus in Abhängigkeit vom Alter. (Nach Rugh, 1964)

Tabelle 1. *Zeittafel der Entwicklung in utero für Maus, Ratte, Mensch.*
(Daten nach HENNEBERG, 1937; SNELL, 1941; RUGH, 1960; HAMILTON u. Mitarb., 1962)

Entwicklungsstadium	*Maus*	*Ratte*	*Mensch*
2 Zell-Stadium	24–38 h	24–48 h	24–36 h
16 Zell-Stadium	60–70 h	96 h	72–96 h
Implantation	4,5–5 d	6–6,5 d	6–6,5 d
frühe Organogenese	7,5 d	9 d	17–18 d
1. Somiten	7,75 d	9,5 d	20–21 d
Beginn der Fetalentwicklung	13 d	14,5 d	38 d
Geburt	17–19 d	19–22 d	240–295 d

Schädigungsmuster mit zwei Sensibilitätsmaxima 7 h und 18 h nach Kopulation (Abb. 19), wobei bereits 10 R schädigen.

Bei der Ratte erscheint ebenfalls in bezug auf den intrauterinen Tod das Stadium der Organogenese ein Sensibilitätsmaximum (WILSON u. KARR, 1951; WILSON, 1954). Verschiedene (wie DE NOBELE u. LAMS, 1925; JOB u. Mitarb., 1935; HICKS, 1954) beobachteten an Ratten, und RUSSELL u. RUSSELL (1950 a, b) an Mäusen, daß nach einer Bestrahlung die Überlebenden meist normal waren. Sie schlossen auf eine erhöhte Regulationsfähigkeit der bestrahlten Keime. TRAUTMANN u. Mitarb. (1967) sahen ebenfalls nach

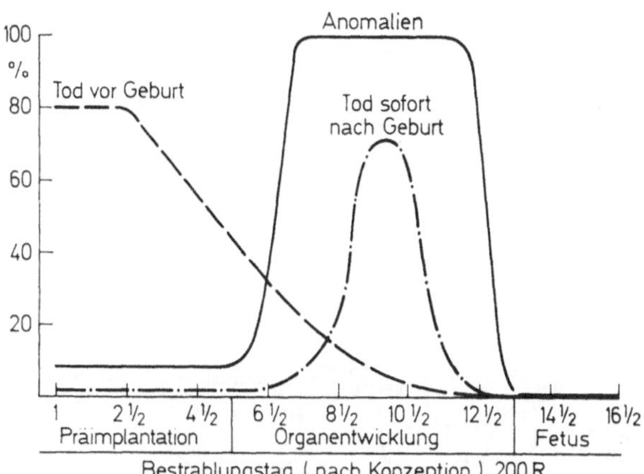

Abb. 17. Häufigkeit von Mißbildungen und Todesfällen nach Bestrahlung verschiedener Entwicklungsstadien von Mäusen mit 200 R. (Nach RUSSELL u. RUSSELL, 1954)

Bestrahlung von Mäuseembryonen während der Blastogenese mit 100 R keine auffallenden Modifikationen.

Bei der Bestrahlung von Zygoten im 2—4 Zell-Stadium mit 200 R und Beobachtung der Feten am 18. Tag traten in 40 % Resorption und lediglich 2 Hirnmißbildungen auf, während die durchschnittliche Wurfgröße von 7,8 auf 6,1 reduziert war.

Hingegen (RUGH, 1963a, b) stellen sich nach einer Bestrahlung des Zweizellstadiums der Maus mit lediglich 10 R Exencephalien und cerebrale Hernien ein. Ebenso wurde die Resorptionsrate um 10 % erhöht. OHZU (1965) beobachtete gleicherweise nach Bestrahlung von 0,5–1,5 tägigen Mäuse-Embryonen mit 5–25 R eine Zunahme der Resorptionen und zum Teil Polydaktylie. Eine Untersuchung von Neugeborenen, die in utero im Alter von 0—5 Tagen bestrahlt worden sind, ergab eine geringe Erhöhung der Zahl weißer Blutkörperchen und eine Erniedrigung der Zahl roter, hingegen keine Skeletmißbildungen (RUGH u. Mitarb., 1966). Wurde am 1. bis 4. Tag nach Befruchtung bestrahlt, stellte sich eine geringe Reduktion des Körpergewichtes ein. Häufig waren Trübungen der Cornea und beginnende Katarakte. Nach Rugh (1962a) kann das befruchtete, aber noch nicht gefurchte Ei (0,5d) der Maus nach einer Bestrahlung mit 5 R in der Entwicklung gehemmt werden. Diese strahlenbedingte Verlangsamung der Furchungen steht in einem gewissen Gegensatz zu den Beobachtungen bei Amphibien. Bestrahlte Amphibien-

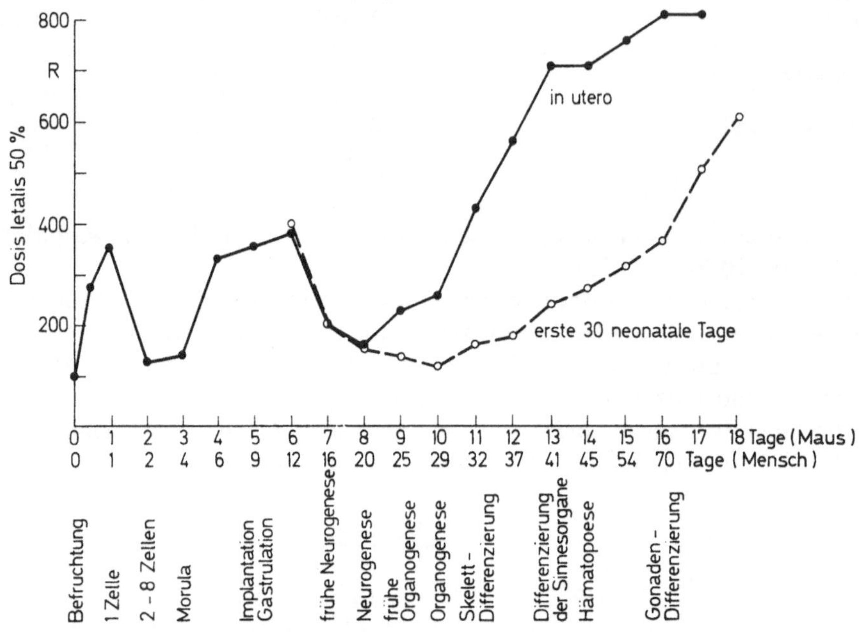

Abb. 18. Intrauterine und neonatale Dosis letalis 50% der Maus in Abhängigkeit vom Bestrahlungsalter. (Nach Rugh u. Wohlfromm, 1965)

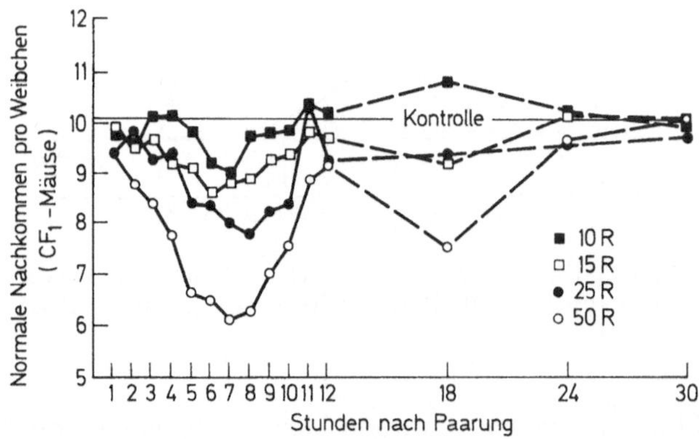

Abb. 19. Zahl (Mittelwert) normaler Nachkommen pro Wurf nach Bestrahlung von Mäusen zu verschiedenen Stunden nach Konzeption. Der Sensibilitätsgipfel 7 h nach Konzeption ist vermutlich durch das Erscheinen der Pronuclei bedingt. (Nach Rugh, 1969)

Zygoten nämlich entwickeln sich selbst nach relativ großen Strahlenmengen normal weiter. Die Furchungen erfolgen synchron, in der gleichen Geschwindigkeit wie bei unbestrahlten Embryonen, sie vermögen allerdings die „Hürden" der Gastrulation nicht zu nehmen und sterben vorzeitig. So wird die Furchung zweigeteilter Amphibien-Eier nach Rugh (1954) durch 300—1500 R nicht gehemmt. Werden 64 und 128 Zellstadien mit 120 R bestrahlt, furchen sich die Keime weiter, vermögen aber nicht das kritische Stadium der Gastrulation zu überbrücken (Schinz u. Fritz-Niggli, 1953). Nach einer Bestrahlung von

12 stündigen noch nicht gefurchten Zygoten der Maus mit 5 R hingegen waren bei den Bestrahlten 6 h nach Bestrahlung 94 % der Zygoten noch nicht gefurcht, gegenüber 85 % bei den Unbestrahlten. 24 h nach Bestrahlung waren bei den Unbehandelten 83 % im Zweizellstadium, bei den Bestrahlten lediglich 50 % und ebenso waren 24 h nach Bestrahlung 20 % Anomalien gegenüber 2,5 % der Kontrolle zu verzeichnen (RUGH, 1962a, b). Wurden die trächtigen Weibchen 18,5 d nach Befruchtung getötet, um die Zahl der Todesfälle in utero festzustellen, dann erhöhten sich bereits durch 5 R auch bei 0,5 tägigen Embryonen die Resorptionen um 11 % gegenüber der Kontrolle, mit 25 R um 38 % (RUGH u. GRUPP, 1959a).

b) Organogenese und Gastrulation

Nach der Bestrahlung von Stadien der Organogenese und der einleitenden Phasen treten in hohem Maße Mißbildungen auf, besonders eindrücklich dargestellt in den Experimenten von WILSON und RUSSELL. Die intrauterinen Todesfälle hingegen nehmen ab. Bei den Amphibien steigt die Strahlenresistenz in bezug auf Letalität ebenfalls mit zunehmendem Alter an, indem bestrahlte Neurulastadien doppelt so hohe Dosen wie Blastula- und Morula-Stadien ertragen. Die strahleninduzierte Mißbildungsrate erreicht mit dem Einsetzen der Organogenese das Maximum, ebenso auch die neonatale Sterblichkeit. Anscheinend ist in diesem Stadium der Embryo zum Mosaiklebewesen mit fixierten Funktionen geworden, und eine Schädigung kann kaum mehr repariert, resp. reguliert werden. Bereits 12,5 R (WILSON u. Mitarb., 1953) hemmen bei 8 tägigen Rattenembryonen das

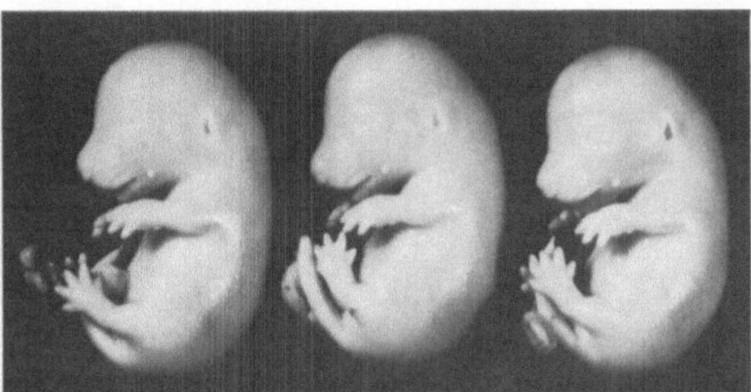

Abb. 20. Augenanomalien bei 17 tägigen Ratten-Feten nach Bestrahlung von 9 tägigen Embryonen mit 50 R. Rechts unbestrahlte Kontrolle. Mitte Mikrophthalmie, links Anophthalmie. (MICHEL, unveröffentlicht)

allgemeine Wachstum. Wird am 9. Tag mit 25 R bestrahlt, dann stellen sich Mikrophthalmien ein. Mit höheren Dosen (50 R) sind schwere Augenmißbildungen, wie Anophthalmien häufig. Nach der Bestrahlung 8–9 tägiger Rattenembryonen treten nach JOB u. Mitarb. (1935) WARKANY u. SCHRAFFENBERGER (1947), WILSON u. KARR (1951), WILSON (1954), HICKS (1953), sowie BRENT (1960), RUGH (1963), HICKS u. Mitarb. (1957), HICKS u. D'AMATO (1963) hauptsächlich Hirn-Mißbildungen wie Hydrocephalus auf, während nach einer Bestrahlung am 9.–10. Tag Augenmißbildungen überwiegen. MICHEL (1969), MICHEL u. FRITZ-NIGGLI (1969), FRITZ-NIGGLI u. MICHEL (1970) beobachteten ebenfalls nach der Bestrahlung von 9 tägigen Embryonen gehäuft schwere Störungen in der Entwicklung der Augen (Abb. 20, 21). Nach HICKS u. D'AMATO (1963) treten schwerere Augenmißbildungen nur nach Bestrahlung von Rattenembryonen bis zum Alter von 10 Tagen auf. Bestrahlte 11 tägige Rattenembryonen zeigen Störungen im Hirnstamm, Hydrocephalus, sowie Encephalocele.

Nach RUGH (1960) erzeugten 100 R bei Rattenembryonen am 9. Tag 90 % Augenmißbildungen, 45 % Hirnmißbildungen, in 27 % Mißbildungen der Aortabogen, 27 % Herzmißbildungen und 18 % Rückenmarkmißbildungen. Am 10. Tag sinken die Augenmißbildungen auf 75 %, hingegen steigen die Mißbildungen des Harntraktes von 5 auf 25 %. Am 11. bis 12. Tag werden Störungen der Skeletbildung sichtbar, ebenso Hydrocephalus. Während nach Rugh keine visceralen Anomalien auftreten, sieht Brent Nierenmißbildungen, fehlende Nieren, fehlende Gonaden usw. 13—14 Tage nach Befruchtung bestrahlte Individuen zeigen weitgehend Skelet-Anomalien und Mikrophthalmie. Hirnmißbildungen, Rosettenbildung in der Retina sind nach Rugh u. Hicks häufig.

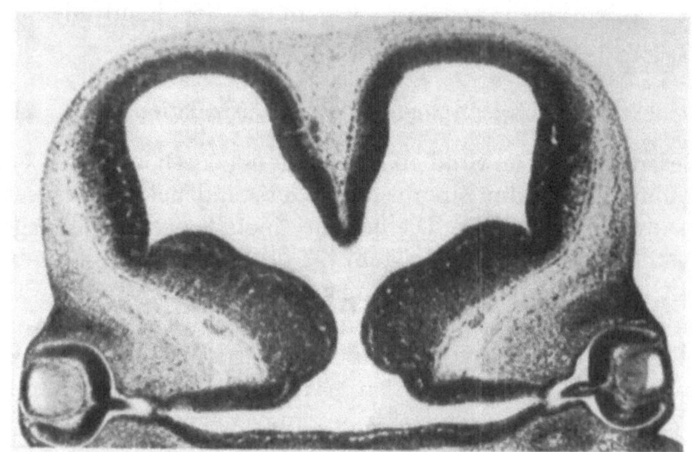

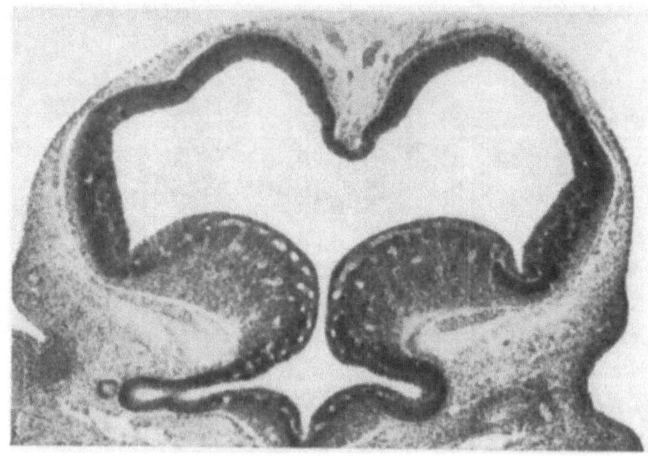

Abb. 21. Augenanomalien bei 13 tägigen Ratten-Feten nach Bestrahlung von 9 tägigen Embryonen mit 100 R (vorgängige Iodacetamidapplikation. 21 a unbestrahlte Kontrolle, 21 b Anophthalmie und Mikrophthalmie. (Michel, unveröffentlicht)

Für die Maus wird das gleiche Schädigungsmuster wie bei der Ratte beschrieben mit einer Anhäufung von Anomalien nach einer Bestrahlung der Embryonen in Organogenese (Russell u. Russell, 1950a, 1950b, 1954; Rugh, 1962c, 1963a, b, 1964). Kriegel u. Mitarb. (1962) fanden ebenfalls die folgenschwersten Mißbildungen nach der Bestrahlung der ersten Hälfte der Organbildungsperiode bei Mäusen. Während nach 300 R am 5. Tag nach Konzeption in 50 % Entwicklungsanomalien beobachtet wurden, stellte sich die gleiche Wirkung bereits mit 150 R ein, wenn 8 tägige Embryonen bestrahlt worden waren.

c) Fetalperiode

Nach einer Bestrahlung fetaler Stadien bleibt das zentrale Nervensystem weiterhin sensibel, wobei Hirndefekte wie Mikrocephalien, Mißbildungen des Corpus striatum, des

Corpus callosum und des Cerebellums vorwiegen. Nach HICKS (1953), COWEN u. GELLER (1960) treten bei im Alter von 15—17 Tagen bestrahlten Rattenfeten schwere Vorderhirndefekte auf, und nach Bestrahlung älterer Stadien häufen sich Cerebellum-Defekte (HICKS u. D'AMATO, 1963; COWEN u. GELLER, 1960).

Daneben treten Anomalien der Augen auf. So sind neben unregelmäßig ausgebildeten Linsen und Mißbildungen der Retina, sowie Rosettenbildung in der Retina, Katarakte häufige Folgen einer fetalen Bestrahlung.

Der Tod nach fetaler Bestrahlung tritt meistens nach Geburt in den ersten zwei Lebenswochen ein, und in seltenen Fällen und mit großen Strahlendosen abortieren die bestrahlten Feten (SCHINZ, 1923; KOSAKA, 1929a, b; DE NOBELE u. LAMS, 1925). Den postnatalen Todesfällen voran geht ein eigentliches Strahlensyndrom mit Anämie, Kachexie, Ikterus usw.

Bei den überlebenden in utero als Feten bestrahlten Säugetieren ist eine verminderte Sterilität festzustellen (HANSON, 1923; PARKES, 1927). Eine Bestrahlung von männlichen Ratten am 19. Tag ihrer Entwicklung mit 150 R führt zur Sterilität, während die Strahlenempfindlichkeit für die weibliche Keimzell-Linie etwas früher, nämlich am 15. Tag der Entwicklung den Höhepunkt erreicht (BEAUMONT, 1960; MANDL u. BEAUMONT, 1964). Oogonien und Oozyten in fetalen und neonatalen Affen erwiesen sich hingegen als strahlenresistenter als diejenigen von Nagetieren (BAKER u. BEAUMONT, 1967).

Werden (REINCKE, 1962) Rattenmütter am 18. Graviditätstag 265—280 R Totalkörperbestrahlung ausgesetzt, dann wird die neonatale Sterblichkeit bis zum 30. Tage nach Bestrahlung um beinahe 50 % erhöht. Die Tiere wurden termingerecht geboren, zeigten aber deutlich Veränderungen im Blutbild, die am 4.—8. Tag des Lebens am ausgeprägtesten sind. Lediglich für die Lymphozyten wurden unmittelbar nach der Geburt die niedrigsten Werte verzeichnet, gefolgt von einem baldigen Anstieg. Regenerative Vorgänge treten im Knochenmark bereits am 3. Lebenstag auf.

Nach diesen Befunden scheint es, als ob die überlebenden Jungtiere über eine Regenerationskraft verfügen würden, die derjenigen der Erwachsenen überlegen ist, da beispielsweise am 30. Lebenstag die Zahl der Erythrozyten über den Normalwerten steht.

d) Bestrahlungen neonataler Stadien

Nach REINCKE u. Mitarb. (1966, 1968a, b) zeigten unmittelbar nach der Geburt bestrahlte Ratten eine Dl 50 %/30 d von 212 R, die nach Bestrahlung viertägiger Säuglinge auf 348 R anstieg, um dann bis zur Entwöhnung gleich zu bleiben. Demnach tritt unmittelbar nach der Geburt eine vorübergehende größere Strahlensensibilität auf, die sich später etwas vermindert, um erst nach der Entwöhnung schlagartig zu sinken.

Es wurden keine signifikanten Unterschiede in der Strahlenreaktion männlicher und weiblicher Säuglinge festgestellt. Bei Mäusen zeigte sich hingegen nach LANGENDORFF u. LANGENDORFF (1966) sofort nach der Geburt eine hohe Strahlenresistenz, die dann wieder absinkt.

Sämtliche Gewebe, die sich noch in Entwicklung befinden, wie hauptsächlich das Skelet (s. z.B. HORVÁTH u. Mitarb., 1962), werden durch die Bestrahlung neonataler Stadien betroffen. Ebenso sind Katarakte und andere Augen-Anomalien häufig, während vom ZNS hauptsächlich das Cerebellum betroffen ist (HICKS, 1958; HICKS u. D'AMATO, 1963). Mit zunehmendem Alter treten Störungen auf, die beim Adulten anzutreffen sind (Beschreibung siehe HUG, 1959).

e) Zusammenfassung

Der Zeitpunkt des Entwicklungsstadiums, das bestrahlt wird, bestimmt Ausmaß und Art der Entwicklungsstörung (Tabelle 2, Abb. 18). In bezug auf den Entwicklungsstillstand, resp. Tod, nimmt die Resistenz mit fortschreitender Entwicklung zu. Die Blastogenese ist das empfindlichste Stadium (siehe auch Abb. 19), und während der Organogenese sinkt die Sensibilität, um in der Fetalperiode Werte zu erreichen, die denen der Adulten ähnlich sind. RUGH u. WOHLFROMM (1965) und MURPHREE u. PACE (1960) zeigen allerdings,

Tabelle 2. *Entwicklungsstadien und Entwicklungsstörungen*

	Stadien	Tod	Mißbildungen
	Blastogenese		
Maus	0–7,5 d	häufig	selten
Ratte	0–9 d		
Mensch	0–18 d		
	Organogenese		
Maus	7,5–13 d		
Ratte	9 d–14,5 d	weniger	häufig
Mensch	18 d–38 d	häufig	
	Fetalentwicklung		
Maus	13 d – Geburt		
Ratte	14,5 d – Geburt	selten	selten
Mensch	38 d – Geburt		

daß die niedrige Sterblichkeit nach fetaler Bestrahlung oft vorgetäuscht ist, wenn nur die Todesfälle in utero berücksichtigt werden. Verfolgt man die Todesfälle bei den Lebendgeborenen weiter, beispielsweise innerhalb der ersten 30 Tage, dann wird offensichtlich, daß die fetale Bestrahlung oft zu einem Entwicklungsstillstand und frühzeitigem Tod nach Geburt führt. So verursachen 220 R bei 12—16 tägigen Rattenfeten über 75 % neonatale Todesfälle.

Mißbildungen, Anomalien, Strahlenmodifikationen treten gehäuft nach Bestrahlung von Stadien während der Organogenese auf, wobei bestimmte Schädigungen Sensibilitätsmaxima aufweisen. Die Untersuchungen mit anderen Wirbeltieren zeigten ähnliche Abhängigkeiten der Schädigung vom Bestrahlungsalter, so die Experimente mit Hühner-Embryonen (Clapp, 1964, 1965; Rugh, 1960; Zusammenfassung Wendt, 1965), wobei aber hier die besonderen Umstände der Entwicklung die Vergleiche komplizieren. Wendt (1964) und Wendt u. Zöller (1965) glauben, daß bei Hühner-Embryonen indirekte Strahlenwirkungen vorwiegen, indem durch Bestrahlung erzeugte Ernährungsschwierigkeiten der embryonalen Zellen ausschlaggebend für die Schädigung seien. Übrigens haben Brent u. McLaughlin (1960) auch bei Ratten einen sogenannten indirekten Strahleneffekt festgestellt, wenn sie trächtige Ratten mit und ohne Abschirmung der neuntägigen Embryonen bestrahlten. Eine alleinige Bestrahlung des Thorax und des Kopfes mit 1400 R führte bis zu 40 % zu fetalen Todesfällen. Mißbildungen stellten sich aber keine ein, da anscheinend die Strahlenkrankheit der Mutter das embryonale Wachstum nicht modifiziert, sondern lediglich die Letalität erhöht.

2. Einige strahleninduzierte Entwicklungsstörungen bei Säugetieren

a) Zentrales Nervensystem

Neuroblasten und sich differenzierende Nervenzellen scheinen besonders strahlensensibel zu sein. Sowohl ihre Struktur, ihre Fähigkeit, ein Organ zu bilden, als auch ihre Funktionen werden beeinträchtigt.

α) *Makroskopisch und mikroskopisch faßbare Änderungen*

Während nach Rugh u. Grupp (1959a) bei menschlichen Geburten spontan Exencephalien mit einer Häufigkeit von $^1/_{4000}$, Anencephalien von $^1/_{1000}$ auftreten, wurden nach Bestrahlung von 7,5 tägigen Mäuse-Embryonen mit 50 R in 4 % der Fälle Exencephalien erzeugt, nach Bestrahlung von 0,5 tägigen Mäusen mit 15 R zu 0,7 % und nach Bestrahlung von 1,5 tägigen mit 15 R in 2,3 % (siehe auch Rugh u. Grupp, 1959b).

Je nach Versuchsanordnung (Dosis-Leistung, Dosis-Höhe, Intervall zwischen Bestrahlung und Beobachtung) werden Zusammenhänge zwischen Bestrahlungsalter und Art der Mißbildung erkennbar (Abb. 22).

Allgemein gilt bei der Ratte, daß schwerste Störungen, wie Anencephalie, nach Bestrahlung von Stadien zu Beginn der Organogenese (9—11 tägige Embryonen) auftreten, während bestrahlte Feten schwere Rückenmarkanomalien, Mikrocephalie, Störungen des Vorderhirns, der Hirn-Rinde, aufweisen können, die mit zunehmendem Bestrahlungsalter zum Teil abnehmen.

Hingegen treten Retina- und Cerebellumdefekte gehäuft mit zunehmendem Fetalalter auf, um sogar nach Bestrahlung neonataler Stadien ein Häufigkeitsmaximum zu erreichen (HICKS, 1954, 1957, 1958; HICKS u. D'AMATO, 1963; COWEN u. GELLER, 1960).

SCHJEIDE u. Mitarb. (1962) beobachteten nach lokaler Kopfbestrahlung 2 tägiger Rattensäuglinge mit 750 R gehäuft Cerebellumdefekte, ebenso LANDOLT (noch nicht ver-

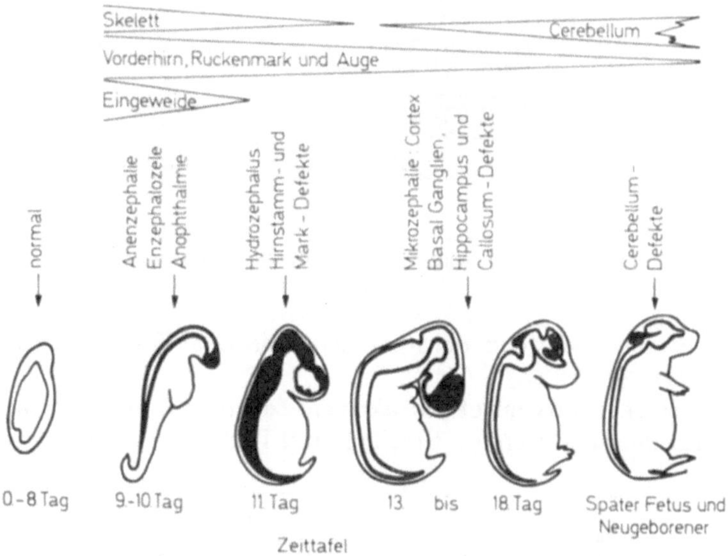

Abb. 22. Mißbildungen (hauptsächlich des zentralen Nervensystems in Abhängigkeit vom Bestrahlungsalter. (Nach HICKS, 1954)

öffentlicht), (Abb. 23). Bei zweitägigen Ratten erzeugte eine Teilbestrahlung des Kopfes (MOSIER u. JANSONS, 1970) mit 600 R neben einer allgemeinen Wachstumshemmung eine Reduktion der Hirngröße und hauptsächlich des Cerebellums.

Für Mäuse-Embryonen und Feten gelten ähnliche Abhängigkeiten der Defekte vom Entwicklungsalter (z. B. DEKABAN, 1969).

Nach HICKS (1954, 1958), HICKS u. Mitarb. (1959), HICKS u. D'AMATO (1963) ist für die Strahlenschädigung des ZNS hauptsächlich die besondere Strahlensensibilität primitiver Neuroblasten verantwortlich, die mit 30—40 R zerstört werden können. Dabei sind (HICKS u. D'AMATO, 1963) nicht nur die mitotisch aktiven Stadien sensibel, sondern postmitotische Stadien, die aus der proliferativen Zone auswandern und vor der Differenzierung stehen.

Die Hauptursache der Schädigung dürfte im Zellverlust, also in einem Ausfall von Organbezirken bestehen. Für die Cerebellum- und Cortex-Defekte verantwortlich ist vermutlich der Verlust jener postmitotischen Zellen, für die kein Nachschub mehr geleistet werden kann, da die mitotische Aktivität mit zunehmendem Alter versiegt. Selbst 20—30 R beeinflussen bereits die Entwicklung der Neuronen in Cerebellum und Cortex.

17*

Nach D'Agostino u. Brizzee (1966) manifestiert sich der Strahlenschaden in einer sofortigen und unspezifischen Pyknose der Zelle (Bestrahlung 13 tägiger Rattenfeten mit 130 R). 2 Tage (nach Hicks, 1958) sofort nach Bestrahlung lassen sich Erholungserscheinungen in Form von Rosettenbildung erkennen. Rosettenbildung tritt übrigens auch nach

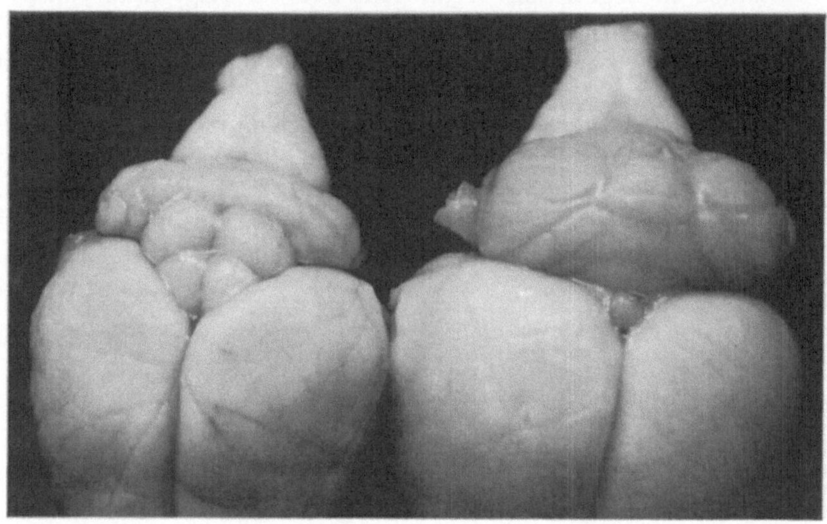

Abb. 23. Cerebellumdefekte in 35 tägigen Tieren nach lokaler Bestrahlung von 24–36 stündigen Ratten mit 750 R, links: bestrahlt, rechts: unbestrahlt. (Nach Landolt, in Publ.)

Bestrahlung von Stadien während der Organogenese auf (Hicks, 1953, 1957; Michel, 1969/1970), (Abb. 24).

Die Rosetten bestehen aus mitotisch aktiven Zellen, die um ein Lumen angeordnet sind und eine spezifische Reaktion auf Strahlen und Radiomimetica darstellen, die nur im

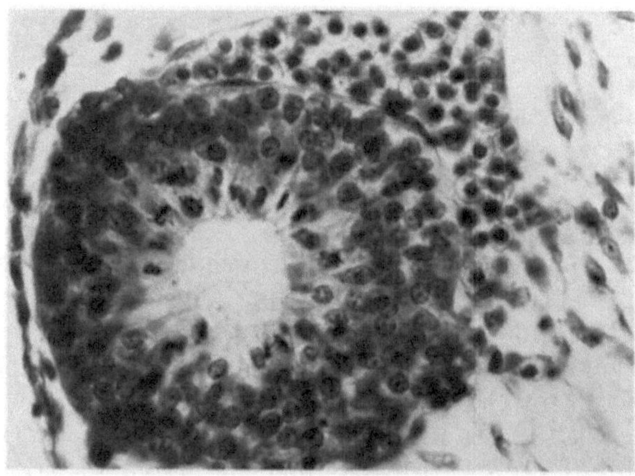

Abb. 24. Rosettenbildung in 13 tägigen Feten nach Bestrahlung von 9 tägigen Rattenembryonen mit 100 R. Von Wilson u. Mitarb. (1952) als embryonale Tumoren gedeutet. (Aus Michel, 1969/1970)

Nervensystem anzutreffen ist. Vermutlich sind es regenerierende Zellkomplexe, die den Zellschwund ausgleichen und vielleicht auch im Dienste des Abbaus nekrotischer Bezirke stehen. Früher (Wilson u. Mitarb., 1952) wurden sie als Tumoren beschrieben.

Stets wird nach der Bestrahlung eine Hemmung der mitotischen Aktivität der Nervenzellen beobachtet; allerdings sind abgesehen von Grossmann (1955) bei Xenopus-Larven und Hicks u. D'Amato (1966) bei Maus-Embryonen wenige systematische Untersuchungen durchgeführt worden. Nach D'Agostino u. Brizzee (1966) nimmt die mitotische Aktivität in mit 130 R bestrahltem fetalem Gehirn nach 50 min deutlich ab, um nach 100 min wieder den Normalwert zu erreichen. Vermehrt sind zudem (Fritz-Niggli u. Michel, 1970; Michel, 1969/1970) Chromosomenanomalien wie Brückenbildung bei Zellen in Anaphase (Abb. 25), die übrigens auch bei unbestrahlten Keimen in geringem Maße anzutreffen sind.

Elektronenoptische Untersuchungen (Roizin u. Mitarb., 1962; D'Agostino u. Brizzee, 1966) ergaben keine Besonderheiten, abgesehen vom Auftreten von Zelltrümmern sowie hie und da veränderten Mitochondrien.

Werden bestrahlte Neuroblasten von Amphibien (Amblystoma punctatum) in eine gesunde Umgebung verpflanzt, erholen sich die bestrahlten Zellen nicht mehr (Rugh u. van Dyke, 1964).

Diese Untersuchungen bestätigen frühere Befunde an Strahlenchimären und parabiotischen Amphibien (Fritz-Niggli, 1958b).

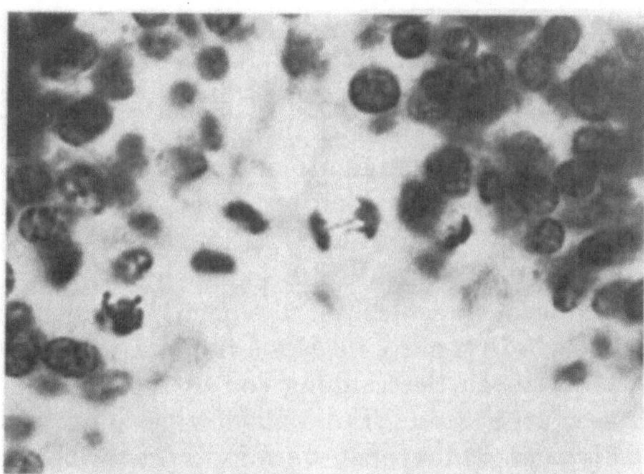

Abb. 25. Chromosomenanomalie (Brückenbildung) nach Bestrahlung von 9 tägigen Rattenembryonen mit 50 R und Iodacetamidvorbehandlung. (Aus Fritz-Niggli u. Michel, 1970)

β) *Biochemische Änderungen und Funktionsstörungen*

Einige Untersuchungen befassen sich mit allgemeinen Stoffwechselstörungen des bestrahlten embryonalen, fetalen und neonatalen ZNS. Wegner (1965, 1969), Wegner u. Mecking (1969) wiesen nach einer Bestrahlung von 9 Tage alten Embryonen mit 150 R eine Störung des DNS-Stoffwechsels im Gehirn nach, die sich 24 Std nach der Bestrahlung normalisierte. Ein erneuter Abfall 2 und 3 Tage nach Bestrahlung hing offensichtlich mit dem verspäteten Schluß des Neuralrohrs zusammen. Wurden 11- und 14 tägige Embryonen bestrahlt, war die Störung des DNS-Stoffwechsels weniger ausgeprägt, jedoch die mitotische Aktivität stark gehemmt. Eine Lokalbestrahlung des Kopfes von 8—30 tägigen Ratten mit 100—1 500 R setzt nach de Vellis u. Schjeide (1968), de Vellis u. Mitarb. (1967) die Bildung von Glycerol-Phosphat-Dehydrogenase im Hirnstamm und den Hirnhemisphären herab. Dieser Effekt wurde nicht mehr beobachtet, wenn die Tiere im Alter von 40 Tagen bestrahlt wurden. Die Hemmung war dosisabhängig und zeigte keine Recovery-Phänomene. Eine lokale Kopf-Bestrahlung 2 tägiger Ratten mit 750 R hatte eine Erniedrigung des Eiweißgehaltes des Hirnstamms zur Folge. Dieser Effekt war deutlich im Alter von 8 Tagen, während im Alter von 12 Tagen der Lipid- und Proteolipid-Gehalt gesenkt war. Bis zum Alter von 57 Tagen zeigte sich kein Anschein einer Erholung. Mit der gleichen Dosis konnte auch eine Hemmung der Bildung und der spezifischen Aktivität verschiedener Enzyme wie der Glycerol-Phosphat-Dehydrogenase und der Isocitrat-

Dehydrogenase in den cerebralen Hemisphären und dem Hirnstamm nachgewiesen werden. Die Untersuchungen deuten darauf hin, daß Störungen im Enzymmuster verantwortlich sind für gewisse ZNS-Schäden, so könnte die beobachtete Hemmung der Myelinisierung (Schjeide u. Mitarb., 1967) durch die Blockierung der Synthese von Phospholipiden zustande kommen. Die Störung des Protein-Musters wird nach de Vellis u. Schjeide (1969) auf der Transcriptionsstufe verursacht.

Die biochemischen Strahleneffekte lassen vermuten, daß auch das funktionelle Geschehen in hirnbestrahlten Säugetieren gestört sein könnte. Es existieren etliche Untersuchungen vornehmlich mit Ratten auf diesem Gebiete, die sich zum Teil widersprechen. Diese Widersprüche lassen sich dadurch erklären, daß eine Prüfung der Funktion des Hirns bei Nagetieren nicht einfach ist.

Nach Piontkowski u. Semagin (1963) zeigten adulte Ratten, die während ihrer Entwicklung in utero vom nullten bis zwanzigsten Tag täglich mit 1 R bestrahlt worden waren, neben der Reduktion des Hirngewichtes und Cortex-Dicke, Störungen der nervösen Aktivität, so wogen die bestrahlten Hirne 2,384 ± 0,046 g gegenüber 2,568 ± 0,017 g der unbestrahlten Hirne, wobei Anpassungsschwierigkeiten zu vermerken waren. Verhaltungsstörungen wurden auch von Yamazaki u. Mitarb. (1962) nach Bestrahlung von $^1/_2$—15tägigen neugeborenen Ratten beobachtet, wobei sich die 1. postnatale Woche als die sensibelste erwies.

Nach einer Bestrahlung von 10-, 14- und 18tägigen Rattenfeten mit 150 R (Graham u. Mitarb., 1959) war das Lernvermögen deutlich eingeschränkt. So antworteten nichtbestrahlte Tiere in 80 % korrekt auf einen Lichttest nach 9tägiger Belehrung, während als 10- und 18tägige Feten bestrahlte Tiere einen Tag länger brauchten. Gleicherweise beobachteten Kaplan (1962a, b), daß sich in utero lediglich mit 25 und 50 R vorbestrahlte 2,5-, 6,5- und 6,7tägige Embryonen schlechter in einem Labyrinth zurechtfinden konnten; für 1,5tägige Embryonen wurde sogar eine Dosis minima von 15 R gefunden.

Die Stärke der Motorik ist nach Bestrahlung von 10- und 15tägigen Ratten in utero mit 50 R und 100 R herabgesetzt, ebenso ist die allgemeine motorische Aktivität nach Bestrahlung von 5- und 10tägigen Embryonen vermindert, aber bei bestrahlten 15- und 20-tägigen Feten erhöht (Werboff u. Mitarb., 1961, 1962, 1964).

Stark vom Entwicklungsstadium und Geschlecht abhängig ist nach den gleichen Autoren die Beeinflussung des lokomotorischen Lernvermögens; so scheinen Frühstadien auf die Bestrahlung mit einer verbesserten Leistung zu antworten, hingegen Fetalstadien und besonders 15tägige Feten mit einer Verschlechterung. Übereinstimmend beobachteten Walker u. Furchtgott (1970) eine Herabsetzung der Lernfähigkeit nach Bestrahlung 16tägiger Rattenfeten mit 100 und 200 R, während 50 R ohne Effekt blieb.

Neugeborene 1tägige Mäuse (Manosevitz u. Rostkovski, 1966) zeigen im Gegensatz zu 1tägigen Ratten (Furchtgott u. Echols, 1958) eine erhöhte allgemeine motorische Aktivität (Bestrahlung mit 300 R). Genetische Unterschiede zwischen und innerhalb der Arten scheinen eine große Rolle zu spielen (Nash u. Mitarb., 1970).

Verschiedentlich wurde auch die Krampfbereitschaft von Mäusen und Ratten auf verschiedene Streß untersucht. So führt (Miller, 1962) bereits 1 R oder eine chronische Exposition von Geburt bis 30 Tage mit einer totalen Dosis von 0,14 R zu einem Anstieg der Krampfbereitschaft von Mäusen. Wenn 23—30tägige Mäuse 350 Millirad pro Tag ausgesetzt wurden, dann stellte sich eine erhöhte Empfindlichkeit auf verschiedene Streßfaktoren bei einer totalen Dosis von 1,5—2 R heraus. Cooke (1963), Cooke u. Mitarb. (1964) bestätigten diese Befunde bei Ratten für eine Totaldosis von 20 R (2 R pro Tag während der ersten 10 Tage der Entwicklung). Werboff u. Mitarb. (1961) beobachteten eine übersteigerte zentralnervöse Antwort auf Streß (Lärm) nach Bestrahlung 15tägiger Ratten-Feten mit 100 R, hingegen eine Abnahme der Empfindlichkeit, wenn am 5. und 10. Tag der Entwicklung bestrahlt wurde.

Verschiedene Entwicklungsstörungen könnten in einer Schädigung von Hirnfunktionen beruhen, so allgemeine Wachstumshemmung, Fertilitätsstörungen, Verminderung der

Paarungsaktivität etc. Eine Bestrahlung mit 50—150 R beginnend mit dem 10. und 14. Lebenstag führte bei männlichen Ratten (FURCHTGOTT u. Mitarb., 1959) zu einer herabgesetzten Paarungsaktivität, ebenso eine einmalige Bestrahlung 18—20tägiger Feten mit 150 R (HUPP u. Mitarb., 1960).

Nach einer lokalen Kopfbestrahlung 2tägiger Ratten tritt eine allgemeine Hemmung des Körperwachstums auf, neben einer verminderten Fertilität. Anscheinend verursacht nicht die Strahlenschädigung der Hypophyse (MOSIER u. JANSONS, 1970) diese allgemeine Wachstumsstörung, sondern bilaterale Strahlenschädigungen von Strukturen im Hypothalamus-Gebiet.

Von Interesse sind Studien von SAVKOVIĆ (1969), der nach lokaler Kopfbestrahlung 2tägiger Ratten mit 600 R eine Verminderung der Fertilität von 95 % auf 40% beobachtete. Er glaubt die Änderung mit einer Beeinflussung der Sekretion von Gonadotropin zu deuten, schließt aber eine Wirkung von Radiotoxinen nicht aus.

b) Augenmißbildungen

Mißbildungen des Auges sind ein außerordentlich häufiger und augenfälliger Strahlenschaden. Bereits geringe Strahlenmengen (WILSON, 1954; FRITZ-NIGGLI u. MICHEL, 1969; MICHEL u. FRITZ-NIGGLI, 1969; MICHEL, 1969/1970) nämlich $12^1/_2$ und 25 R führen bei bestrahlten 9tägigen Rattenembryonen zu Entwicklungsstörungen der Augen. Die sensible Periode für Augenschädigungen ist die Organogenese. So weisen nach HICKS (1954), JOB u. Mitarb. (1935) bestrahlte 9—13tägige Rattenembryonen am häufigsten Augenanomalien auf. Wird das Entwicklungsstadium kurz vor der Bildung der Augenmulde (für die Ratte

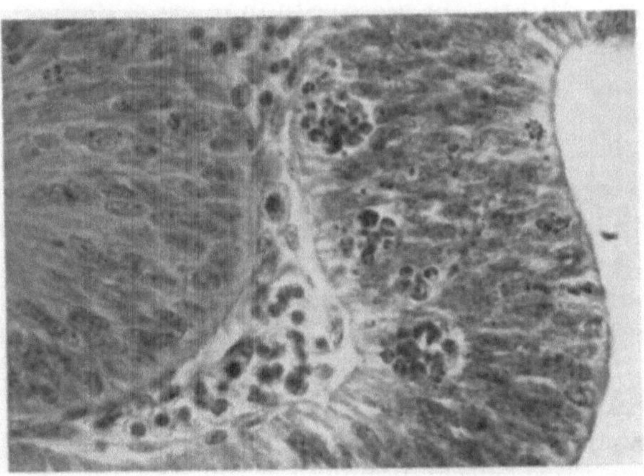

Abb. 26. Nekrosen in der Retina von 13tägigen Rattenfeten nach Bestrahlung als 9tägige Embryonen mit 100 R. (MICHEL, unveröffentlicht)

9 Tage nach Befruchtung) bis zur Organisation des tiefen Augenbechers bestrahlt, sind schwerwiegende Augenstörungen wie Mikrophthalmie und Synophthalmie, Anophthalmie (Abb. 20, 21, 26) die Folge.

Nach der Augenblasenbildung bestrahlte Stadien weisen Unterentwicklung, wie Mikrophthalmien (HICKS, 1954) auf. Nach Bestrahlung 11tägiger Ratten-Embryonen wurden persistierende Colobome, z.B. der Chorioides gefunden. Bei Mäuse-Embryonen (RUSSELL u. RUSSELL, 1954) treten Colobome nur nach Bestrahlung $8^1/_2$—$9^1/_2$tägiger Embryonen auf, so daß dort die sensible Periode mit dem Schluß des Augenspaltes beendet wäre.

In einer eingehenden Studie beschreiben HICKS u. D'AMATO (1963) den möglichen Mechanismus der strahlenbedingten Augenmißbildungen. Strahlensensibel sind nach ihnen Mesenchymzellen zwischen Ektoderm und Augenblase und zwar hauptsächlich Zellen, die sich zu differenzieren beginnen (in postmitotischer Phase), ferner Zellen in G_2-Phase und Prophase. Der Zellverlust kann vor dem 10. d der Entwicklung (Ratte) nicht mehr kompensiert werden, und Mikrophthalmien, Anophthalmien, Synophthalmien und morphologische Störungen der Retina sind die Folge. So sah Michel (1969/1970) keinen Unterschied im Ausmaß der Augendefekte nach der Bestrahlung 9tägiger Rattenfeten, wenn die Tiere 4 oder 28 Tage nach Bestrahlung untersucht wurden. Spätere Stadien vermögen den Strahlenschaden zu kompensieren oder sind a priori weniger anfällig.

Kriegel u. Shibata (1964) bestätigen, daß grobe Augenmißbildungen nur dann erwartet werden können, wenn die Bestrahlung während des Wachstums der Augenblase bis zur Differenzierung des Auges erfolgt, wobei als kritische Entwicklungsphase bei der Maus der 8. und 9. Entwicklungstag angegeben wird. Nach ihnen trägt die mangelnde Koordination der Blasteme die hauptsächliche Schuld an der Entwicklungsstörung.

Die größten morphologischen Änderungen stellen sich nach der Bestrahlung sensibler Stadien mit kleinen Strahlenmengen in der Retina ein (siehe auch Shively u. Mitarb., 1969).

Nach Bestrahlung späterer Stadien dominieren Linsentrübungen, aber auch Retinadefekte. Nach Rugh u. Skaredoff (1965) ist die fetale Retina extrem strahlenempfindlich und erst kurz nach der Geburt nimmt ihre Strahlenresistenz zu. Im Zusammenhang mit einer Restitution sind Rosettenbildungen häufig.

An einem großen Versuchsmaterial mit gegen 15000 Mäusen wurde die Katarakt-Bildung von Rugh u. Mitarb. (1964a) untersucht. Sonderbarerweise erwies sich das Stadium unmittelbar nach der Befruchtung für männliche und weibliche Tiere als das strahlenempfindlichste, indem 60 % der Augen von Mäusen, die mit 100 R sofort nach der Befruchtung bestrahlt worden waren, Katarakte aufwiesen und zwar auf beiden Augen. Als Dosis minima nehmen Rugh u. Mitarb. für dieses Stadium etwa 10 R an, wobei sich die männlichen Mäuse als etwas strahlenempfindlicher erwiesen.

c) Skeletanomalien

Augenfällig ist ein anderer Strahlenschaden sich entwickelnder Wirbeltiere, nämlich Anomalien der Skeletbildung, die sich in einer Wachstumshemmung oder einer eigentlichen Mißbildung äußern können (Abb. 27). Naturgemäß werden sie auch induziert, wenn neugeborene und kindliche Individuen bestrahlt werden. Ausführliche Untersuchungen sind an Mäusen durchgeführt worden (Warkany u. Schraffenberger, 1947; Russell u. Russell, 1950a, b, 1954; Hicks, 1954; Rugh u. Mitarb., 1964b; Murakami u. Mitarb., 1963; Murakami u. Kameyama, 1964).

Skeletanomalien wurden auch als Kriterium für die Bestimmung einer Schwellendosis der embryonalen Strahlenschädigung gewählt. So untersuchte Jacobsen (1965, 1966, 1969) das Sternum und die Hals-Wirbelsäule sowie Extremitäten von Mäusen, die geringen Strahlenmengen ausgesetzt worden waren. Bereits mit 5 R konnten signifikante Unterschiede gegenüber der Kontrolle festgestellt werden, so nach Bestrahlung von 8tägigen Embryonen bei 2279 untersuchten Tieren in 0,3 % Individuen Sternumdefekte (Kontrolle 0,19 %) und 0,63 % Wirbelsäule-Defekte gegenüber 0,45 % der Kontrolle. Von Ohzu (1965) wurde in 1,1 % (Kontrolle 0 %) Polydaktylie des Hinterfußes und 31,4 % (Kontrolle 13,9 %) des Vorderfußes festgestellt, wenn die Embryonen im Alter von $1/_2$ Tagen mit 5 R bestrahlt worden waren. Die Entstehung bestimmter Skelet-Anomalien ist ausgesprochen stadienabhängig.

So fällt das sensible Stadium für Gliedmaßendefekte mit der Bildung der Beinknospen zusammen. Bei der Maus treten Schädelmißbildungen hauptsächlich ein, wenn $6^1/_2$—$8^1/_2$ Tage nach Befruchtung bestrahlt wird. Bei der Ratte hingegen dauert diese Sensibilitätsperiode etwas länger, nämlich 9—14 Tage nach Befruchtung. Palatum fissum findet sich bei der Ratte gehäuft nach Bestrahlung von 14—15tägigen Embryonen, also zu Beginn der Fetalentwicklung, tritt aber auch nach Bestrahlung früherer Stadien auf. Auffällig sind Rippenanomalien nach Bestrahlung von 9—15tägigen Embryonen der Ratte, sowie von $6^1/_2$—$9^1/_2$tägigen Mäusen. Während OHZU (1965) bereits nach einer Bestrahlung unmittelbar nach Befruchtung Vor- und Hinterfußdefekte beobachtete, sahen RUSSELL u. RUSSELL (1954) diese Extremitätendefekte nur nach Bestrahlung von $11^1/_2$—$13^1/_2$-tägigen Mäuse-Embryonen. Schwanzdefekte sind nach RUSSELL u. RUSSELL bei der Bestrahlung von mindestens $9^1/_2$tägigen Mäuse-Embryonen zu erwarten, während die sensible Periode bei den Ratten nach WARKANY u. SCHRAFFENBERGER (1947) sich über die Zeit von 9—14 Tagen erstreckt.

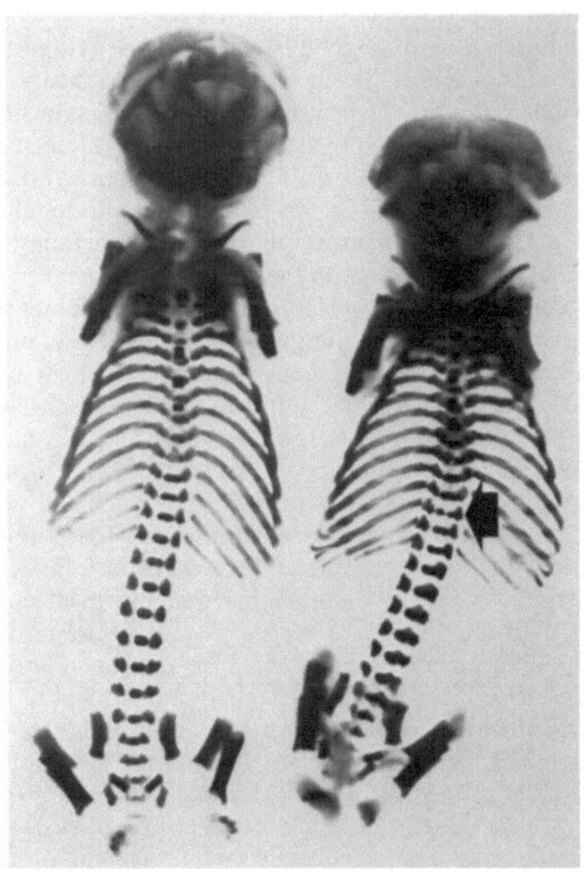

Abb. 27. Subtile Skelet-Anomalie nach Bestrahlung eines 11 tägigen Rattenembryos mit 50 R; statt eines ventralen Knochenkerns finden sich zwei getrennte (Pfeil) am 21. Tag der Entwicklung, links unbestrahlter Embryo (Färbung des Skelets mit Alizarinrot S). (MICHEL, unveröffentlicht)

Nach KNOPP u. TRAUTMANN (1962) ist das strahlenempfindlichste Stadium der Maus in bezug auf die Schwanzwirbelsäule der 13. Lebenstag. 200 R hemmten die Wachstumsgeschwindigkeit des Schwanzskeletes, wobei sich durch eine anscheinend elektive Störung einzelne Antimere der Sklerotome zusätzlich als Bestrahlungsfolge eine Blockwirbelbildung mit Knickschwanz einstellte. Weitere strahlenbedingte Anomalien sind:

Reduktion der Zahl der Wirbel durch einen Ausfall der Ossifizierung oder durch eine Verschmelzung der Wirbelkörper-Anlagen. Eine Verschmelzung von Ossifikationszentren innerhalb der einzelnen Wirbel, Störungen der Histogenese, Verzögerung in der Ossifikationsgeschwindigkeit usw. verursachen verschiedenste Anomalien der Wirbel wie u.a. auch Spina bifida.

d) Gonaden

Die Strahlenempfindlichkeit der sich in Entwicklung befindenden Gonaden ist verhältnismäßig wenig untersucht worden. Dabei wurde hauptsächlich die Funktionstüchtigkeit der adulten Gonaden von in utero bestrahlten Tiere analysiert und nur in wenigen Fällen histologische Untersuchungen angestellt (Übersichten Mandl, 1964; Schnetter u. Mitarb., 1968).

Die Reproduktionsfähigkeit kann durch die Bestrahlung sich entwickelnder Lebewesen, resp. Gonaden beeinflußt werden, indem die Fekundität, d.h. die Produktion der Gameten und die Fertilität, d.h. die Fähigkeit lebensfähige Nachkommen zu produzieren, gestört wird. Meist wird die Fertilität untersucht, die aber von so vielen Faktoren bestimmt wird, daß eine Kausalanalyse kaum möglich ist. Die Zahl der Gameten, ihre Befruchtungsfähigkeit kann direkt oder indirekt durch dominante Letalfaktoren verändert sein. Die Wanderung der Keimzellen und ihre Befruchtungsfähigkeit lassen sich durch Beeinflussung des ganzen Genitalsystems, selbst des physischen Gehabens (Paarungsunfähigkeit) ändern und auch eine Autopsie der Mutter mit Zählung der corpora lutea im Vergleich zu den Feten gibt keine genaue Auskunft über die Strahlenempfindlichkeit der Keimzellen in den sich entwickelnden Gonaden, da präimplantative Todesfälle (z.B. durch dominante Letalfaktoren verursacht) der Beobachtung entgehen.

Ebenso sollte die Fertilität der Nagetiere über Monate hinaus untersucht werden, da beispielsweise nach einer Bestrahlung junger weiblicher Tiere mit 25 R in den ersten Würfen (Mole, 1959) keine Beeinflussung bemerkbar ist, die aber in den weiteren Würfen mit einer Reduktion der Fertilität auf 50 % drastisch wird (auch bei adulten konnten wir diese Hemmung der Fertilität durch 25 R beobachten (Fritz-Niggli u. Michel, in Publ.).

Nach einer eingehenden Untersuchung von Murphree u. Pace (1960) zeigte sich sowohl in bezug auf die Durchschnittszahl der Feten als auch der corpora lutea ein deutlicher Effekt der Bestrahlung 18tägiger Ratten-Feten mit 150 R, nämlich 11 ± 3 corpora lutea bei den bestrahlten Weibchen gegenüber 13 ± 2 corpora lutea bei den unbestrahlten und eine Durchschnittszahl von 9 ± 3 Feten bei den bestrahlten Weibchen (gegenüber 12 ± 2 der Kontrolle). Wurden 18- und 20tägige männliche Feten in utero mit 150 R bestrahlt, dann war eine vollkommene Sterilität die Folge, wobei allerdings nicht entschieden werden konnte, ob diese Sterilität nicht auf einer mangelnden Kopulationsfähigkeit beruhte. Die Gewichtsabnahme des Testes der bestrahlten Männchen gegenüber der Kontrolle war signifikant, $0{,}5 \pm 0{,}05$ g beispielsweise im Alter von 66 d nach Bestrahlung am 20. Entwicklungstag gegenüber $3{,}3 \pm 0{,}21$ g der unbestrahlten Tiere. Nach Beaumont (1960), Beaumont u. Mandl (1962), Mandl u. Beaumont (1964) liegt das Maximum der Strahlenempfindlichkeit für die weibliche Keimzelle etwas früher, nämlich am 15.—16. Tag der Entwicklung gegenüber der männlichen Ratte am 19. Tag p.c. Das Ovar von neugeborenen Mäusen zeigt interessanterweise in der Zeitspanne von Geburt bis zu 4 Wochen extreme Schwankungen in der Strahlensensibilität (Rugh u. Wohlfromm, 1964). Während 30 R die Fertilität exponierter Neugeborener nicht beeinträchtigte, war die Zahl trächtiger Weibchen signifikant herabgesetzt, wenn sie als ein- bis dreiwöchige Tiere bestrahlt worden waren.

Entsprechend histologischen Untersuchungen sind die Oogonien der Neugeborenen strahlenresistent, währenddem die Oozyten vornehmlich beim Übergang vom primären zum sekundären Stadium strahlensensibel sind. Die Frühstadien der Keimzellen wurden von Schnetter u. Mitarb. (1968) untersucht, indem weibliche Mäuse am 3., 5., 6. und 7. Tag ihrer Entwicklung mit 150 R bestrahlt und am 9. und 10. Entwicklungstag analysiert wurden. Anhand ihres besonders hohen Gehaltes an alkalischer Phosphatase ließen sich die Urgeschlechtszellen auch in frühen Stadien in der hintern Darmregion des Embryos sicherstellen. Bei der Maus werden sie $7^1/_4$ Tage nach der Befruchtung erkennbar und beginnen vom $8^1/_2$. Tag an ihre aktive Wanderung und mitotische Aktivität, um in die Keimwülste einzuwandern.

Interessanterweise scheinen die Vorläufer der Urgeschlechtszellen in bis zu 7 tägigen Embryonen einer Bestrahlung mit 150 R gegenüber relativ strahlenresistent zu sein. Erst 6—12 h vor dem Beginn ihrer Differenzierung zu wandernden typischen Urgeschlechtszellen werden sie strahlenempfindlich, und ihre Zahl kann auf weniger als $^1/_3$ des Kontrollwertes vermindert sein. Die adulten weiblichen Tiere werden nicht steril, so daß diese sensible Periode am 7. Tag bisher kaum erkannt worden ist. Männliche Mäuse hingegen sind nach Bestrahlung mit 200 R am 7. Tag ihrer Entwicklung vermindert fertil (RUSSELL u. Mitarb., 1960). Ein zweites Empfindlichkeitsmaximum tritt bei den Männchen am Ende der Wanderungsphase der Urgeschlechtszellen auf, bei den Weibchen vor der Prophase der Meiose. Erneut steigt bei den Männchen die Strahlensensibilität am Ende der Vermehrungsphase, bei den Weibchen vor dem Eintritt in das Dictyotän-Stadium kurz nach der Geburt. Nach MINTZ (1958, 1959, 1960) führt eine fraktionierte Bestrahlung von 8—12-tägigen weiblichen Mäuse-Embryonen in utero (total 400 R) zu ihrer fast vollständigen Sterilisation. Einige Feten zeigen überhaupt keine Keimzellen mehr und nachträgliche in vitro-Kulturen deuteten auf keine Erholung evtl. überlebender Zellen. Ebenso führte dieselbe Behandlung bei männlichen Embryonen zu einer erheblichen Verminderung der Keimzellen. Die wenigen überlebenden Keimzellen entwickelten sich nicht mehr zu Typ A-Spermatogonien.

Interessanterweise sind die embryonalen und fetalen Gonaden von Mäusen und Ratten etwa gleich strahlenempfindlich, währenddem sich in der Sensibilität adulter Gonaden Art-Unterschiede zeigen. Ebenso scheinen übrigens sich entwickelnde Gonaden von Nagetieren extrem strahlensensibel zu sein; so konnten ERICKSON u. Mitarb. (1963) nach Bestrahlung von 45—90 tägigen fetalen Gonaden des männlichen Schweines selbst mit einer Dosis von 400 R keine vollkommene Sterilität erreichen (Untersuchung 154 Tage post partum). Noch strahlenresistenter sind die primordialen Keimzellen im 2 monatigen Rhesusaffen. Selbst mit 1 000 R und mehr trat keine vollkommene Sterilisierung ein (BAKER u. BEAUMONT, 1967). Die Minimaldosis für eine vollkommene Sterilisation wird auf 2 000 R geschätzt, also um ein Mehrfaches größer als bei den Nagetieren. Nach BAKER (1969) reagieren bei niedrigen Dosen in vitro bestrahlte Oozyten von Ratten und Affen gleich wie in vivo. Um die Zahl der Oozyten auf 50—70 % zu reduzieren, sind bei den Ratten 148 R nötig, beim Affen 5 000 R. Bei höheren Dosen allerdings sind die in vitro-Bestrahlten resistenter als in vivo. Die Untersuchungen der Strahlenempfindlichkeit von in vitro bestrahlten fetalen menschlichen Gonaden ergab eine hohe Strahlenresistenz von Oogonien und Oozyten, die noch höher liegt als diejenige von Rhesus-Affen. BAKER hält die menschlichen Oozyten und Oogonien für die strahlenresistentesten Keimzellen überhaupt.

In den neugeborenen Rhesus-Affen ist eine Dosis von 1 800 R notwendig, um innerhalb 2 Wochen 80—100 % der primordialen Oozyten zu eliminieren, während für die neugeborene 5 tägige Ratte 100 R genügen. Die Resistenz der primordialen Oozyten steigt etwa um das Dreifache an zwischen Geburt und Maturität.

Es liegen nur wenige systematische Untersuchungen über die Wirkung kleiner Strahlenmengen und kontinuierliche kleinere Strahlenbelastungen vor. RUSSELL u. Mitarb. (1960) fanden bei männlichen Mäusen, die im Alter von 0,5—14,5 Tagen kontinuierlich mit 8,9 mR/min bestrahlt worden waren, keine verminderte Fertilität. Im Gegensatz dazu zitierte LANGENDORFF (1969), daß eine Bestrahlung wiederum männlicher Mäuse mit 8 mR/min (allerdings über die ganze Gestationszeit hinweg) 5 Monate nach der Geburt zur Sterilität führte, die durch histologische Untersuchung festgestellt wurde. Mit einer Dosisleistung von 4 mR/min ebenfalls während der ganzen Entwicklungsperiode traten hingegen keine Änderungen auf, während eine Bestrahlung mit 16 mR/min 10 Tage lang eine vollkommene Sterilität von Anfang an bewirkte.

Anscheinend sind die weiblichen Keimzellen in embryonalen und fetalen Gonaden einer Erholung weniger zugänglich als in adulten. So zeigte eine Bestrahlung mit einer Totaldosis von 20 R/d die gleiche Wirkung, ob sie kurz- oder langzeitig 14 mR/min oder 42 R/min (Faktor 3000) verabreicht wurde (LANGENDORFF, 1969).

Im Gegensatz dazu können sich die primären Oozyten bei den geschlechtsreifen Tieren erholen, indem dort die kontinuierliche Bestrahlung 4mal weniger wirksam ist als die fraktionierte konzentrierte.

Über Gefährdung durch Radionuklide existieren kaum Untersuchungen. Injektionen von 20 μCi 90 Sr i.v. (11 und 16 Tage nach der Befruchtung) reduzierten z.B. die Zahl der Oozyten (Typ I—III) auf 50 %, wobei der schädigende Effekt am deutlichsten wurde, wenn 16 tägige Individuen betroffen wurden (Nilsson u. Henricson, 1969).

e) Weitere Anomalien

Alle übrigen Gewebe und Organe können nach Bestrahlung ihrer Blasteme oder auch im Zustand der Differenzierung durch die ionisierenden Strahlen erheblich geschädigt werden. Herzmißbildungen und Gefäßmißbildungen stellen sich hauptsächlich nach Bestrahlung von 9 tägigen Ratten-Embryonen (Wilson u. Mitarb., 1953) ein. Mit 100 R ereignen sich in 24 % der Fälle Mißbildungen der Aortabögen und des Herzens.

130 rad 14,1 MeV-Neutronen (Okamoto u. Mitarb. 1969) auf 8 tägige Ratten-Embryonen erzeugten in 85 % der Feten Mißbildungen des Herzens und der großen Gefäße. Elektronen-optisch wurden große Lysosome in den Myokard-Zellen beobachtet, die für den Zelltod verantwortlich gemacht werden. Nach Bestrahlung von Hühnchen-Embryonen wurden innerhalb 2—3 h nach einer letalen Strahlendosis Schädigungen der Mikrozirkulation, gesteigerte Permeabilität und Degeneration der Gefäßwände gesehen (Stearner u. Mitarb., 1969). Die gleichen Autoren nehmen an, daß die Gefäß-Schädigung im zentralen Nervensystem nach Bestrahlung neugeborener Ratten mit 600 R und 1000 R für den Tod innerhalb 48 h verantwortlich ist.

Nach einer Bestrahlung von 6 tägigen Mäuse-Embryonen wurde Herzvorfall beobachtet, während Defekte im Urogenitalsystem durch eine Bestrahlung früher Stadien der Organogenese ausgelöst werden. $9^1/_2$ Tage nach Befruchtung differenziert sich bei der Ratte das embryonale Mesoderm, das Niere und Ureter bilden wird. Der Wolffsche Gang wird $10^1/_4$ Tage nach Befruchtung angelegt und mündet $12^1/_2$ Tage nach Befruchtung in die Kloake. Störungen wie Nierenfusion und Unterentwicklung der Niere erscheinen deshalb vornehmlich bei Ratten-Embryonen, die zu Beginn der Mesoderm-Entwicklung bestrahlt wurden.

Bei der Maus hingegen treten nach Russell u. Russell (1954) Mißbildungen im Urogenitalsystem erst nach Bestrahlung späterer Stadien auf. Sobald der Wolffsche Gang in die Kloake einmündet, wird die Topographie der Nieren durch die Bestrahlung kaum mehr gestört. Nach Frilley u. Raynaud (1946) führt eine Bestrahlung der Nierenanlagen mit hohen Strahlendosen (24 000 R) zu einer beinahe vollkommenen Zerstörung des Gewebes.

Strahlenempfindlich sind die Blasteme der Leber bei der Ratte (Wilson u. Mitarb., 1953) am 10. Tage nach der Befruchtung, indem mit 100 R gegen 30 % der bestrahlten Tiere Leberschädigungen aufwiesen. Die sensible Phase fällt genau mit der Blastembildung zusammen. Auch die fetale Leber bleibt strahlensensibel, und zwar zeigte sich bei der Maus nach einer Lokalbestrahlung der Leberregion 13- bis 18 tägiger Feten ein Empfindlichkeitsmaximum für die Leberzellen am 13. Entwicklungstag mit einer ausgeprägten Dosis-Abhängigkeit (240 R, 580 R, 960 R). Nach dem 15. Tag wird die Leber resistent.

Das hämatopoietische Gewebe hingegen der Leber wird am meisten nach Bestrahlung 14 tägiger Stadien gestört. Interessanterweise ist das hämatopoietische System der fetalen Leber weniger empfindlich als die blutbildenden Zellen des Adulten (Duplan, 1963), die sich auch später von der Strahlenschädigung erholen. Nach einer Ganzkörperbestrahlung ist das fetale hämatopoietische System strahlensensibel am 15. Entwicklungstag (Hazzard u. Budd, 1969).

Neben spezifischen Änderungen treten postnatal nach Bestrahlung der sich entwickelnden Säugetiere verschiedene allgemeine Störungen auf, wie Lebensverkürzung, allgemeiner Entwicklungsrückstand, erhöhte Anfälligkeit gegenüber Krankheiten. So war z.B. nach

MURPHREE u. PACE (1960) die neonatale Todesrate nach Bestrahlung 15—18 tägiger Rattenfeten mit 110 R (60 Co) signifikant erhöht, wobei sich die meisten Todesfälle am 7. Tag ereigneten. Auch subtilere Schädigungen können nach Bestrahlung in utero eintreten, so wurde eine erhebliche Zunahme der Karies-Anfälligkeit nach Bestrahlung 10 tägiger Rattenembryonen mit 150 R (ERSHOFF u. BAVETTA, 1958) gefunden.

3. Strahlenschädigung des menschlichen Embryos und Fetus

Nachdem bereits VON KLOT (1911) von einer Unterbrechung der Schwangerschaft des Menschen mit Röntgenstrahlen berichtet, prägte SCHINZ(1923) den Begriff des Röntgenaborts. Vermutlich die erste Mißbildung am Menschen beobachtete FRIEDRICH (1910), weitere Beobachtungen stammen von ASCHENHEIM (1920) über eine schwere Strahlenschädigung eines Kindes, das im 3. bis 6. Lebensmonat in utero wegen einer therapeutischen Bestrahlung der Mutter geschädigt wurde, nämlich Mikrocephalie mit verkümmertem Opticus und Linsentrübung, ferner sahen BASIC u. WEBER (1956) eine ausgesprochene Wachstumshemmung an einem Kind, das als zweimonatiger Fetus im Mutterleib bestrahlt worden war. Stets wird als auffälligster Schaden Mikrocephalie geschildert, wenn Entwick-

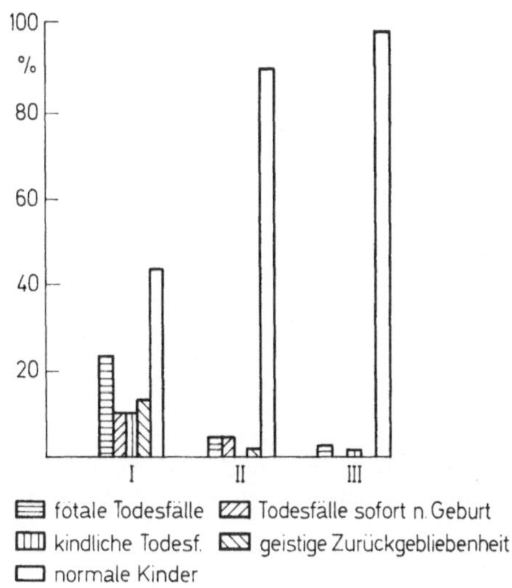

Abb. 28. Sterblichkeit von Embryonen, Feten und Kindern, die in utero der Strahlung der Atombombenexplosion von Nagasaki ausgesetzt waren. I = Mütter innerhalb 0–2000 m mit größeren äußerlichen Strahlenschäden, II = Mütter innerhalb 0–2000 m ohne größere Strahlenschäden, III = Mütter innerhalb 4000–5000 m. (Nach YAMAZAKI u. Mitarb., 1954)

lungsstadien jünger als 5 Monate bestrahlt worden waren. Da diese Angaben meistens aus den Anfängen der Strahlentherapie stammen, kann die genaue Strahlenmenge nicht mehr ermittelt werden. Aus neuerer Zeit existieren hauptsächlich die Untersuchungen über die Überlebenden der Atombomben-Explosionen von Nagasaki und Hiroshima. So wurden (YAMAZAKI u. Mitarb., 1954) die Kinder von total 98 Frauen untersucht, welche während der Explosion innerhalb von 2000 m vom Hypozentrum entfernt und zu dieser Zeit schwanger waren. Die Mütter wurden unterteilt in Frauen, die starke Anzeichen von Strahlenschädigung zeigten, wie Epilation, Petechien (Purpura) (I), und solche, die Anzeichen einer Strahlenschädigung aufgewiesen hatten, nämlich Fieber, Übelkeit, Diarrhoe (II). Als Vergleichsgruppe wurden Mütter gewählt, die 4000–5000 m vom Hypozentrum entfernt waren. Dabei wurden nur Areale ohne größeren nachträglichen Fall-out von radioaktivem Material berücksichtigt. Die Gesamtsterblichkeit der Kinder von Müttern mit Strahlenschädigungen betrug 43 % gegenüber 9 % von Müttern ohne äußere Strahlenschädigungen und 6 % der Kontrollgruppe (Abb. 28). Besonders die fetalen Todesfälle

überwiegen bei den Müttern mit Strahlenschädigungen gegenüber den Kindern von Müttern
ohne sichtbare Strahlenschäden, und ebenso zeigten sich unter den 16 überlebenden Kindern
der Mütter mit Strahlenschädigungen 4 verschiedene Grade von geistiger Zurückgebliebenheit. Sowohl in der Größe als auch im Gewicht blieben die meisten Kinder der Bestrahlten
hinter der Norm zurück.

Nach einer Untersuchung an 205 japanischen Kindern im Alter von $4^1/_2$ Jahren (Plummer, 1952), die im ersten Trimester ihres Lebens in utero der Atombomben-Bestrahlung
ausgesetzt waren, wiesen von 11 Kindern der Mütter, die sich zur Zeit ihrer Schwangerschaft innerhalb 1250 m vom Hypozentrum entfernt befanden, deren 7 ausgesprochene Mikrocephalien mit Schwachsinn auf. Unter den 205 Kindern traten insgesamt 24
Anomalien auf (Augenanomalien, Pigmentstörungen), wobei Mikrocephalien die häufigste Erscheinung waren. Übereinstimmend stellte Miller (1956) fest, daß 33 Kinder (die
in utero der Atombombenstrahlung von Hiroshima ausgesetzt waren (24 im Alter von
7—15 Wochen) einen kleineren Kopfumfang aufwiesen. 15 dieser 33 Untersuchten zeigten

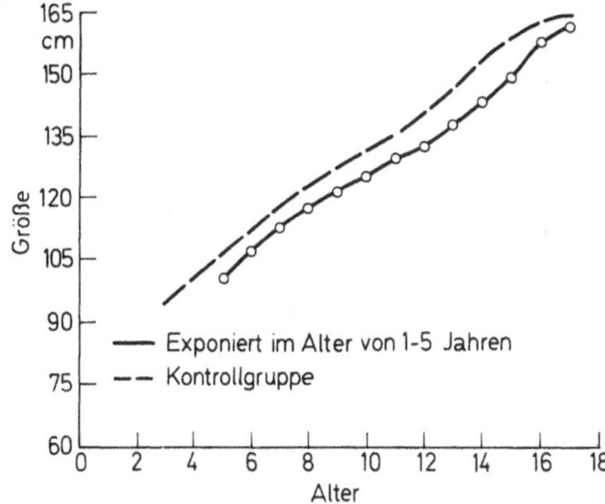

Abb. 29. Wirkung der Fallout-Bestrahlung auf das Wachstum der Kinder auf der Rongelap-Insel. Durch unglückliche Umstände wurden nach einem Atombombentest 1954 Einwohner der Marshall-Inseln einer Fallout-Bestrahlung ausgesetzt. (Nach Sutow u. Conard, 1969)

geistige Zurückgebliebenheit und zwar in Abhängigkeit von der Distanz vom Hypozentrum
und dem Alter während der Bestrahlung. Kinder, die 1954 auf der Rongelap-Insel (Marshall-Inseln) einer Fallout-Bestrahlung während einem Atombomben-Test-Programm ausgesetzt waren, zeigten eine geringe Wachstumshemmung (Abb. 29) und Schilddrüsen-Anomalien (Knötchen), (Sutow u. Conard, 1969). Die externe Totalkörperbestrahlung
wird auf 175 rad geschätzt, die totale Dosis (incl. absorbierte Radionuklide) auf die
Schilddrüse auf etwa 700—1400 rad.

Ob eine röntgendiagnostische Belastung der Mutter den Embryo oder Fetus im Mutterleib bereits morphologisch schädigen könnte, ist noch nicht geklärt.

In einer Studie an 3024 Kindern, von denen 1008 in utero mit 1,5—3 rad bestrahlt
worden waren (Griem u. Mitarb., 1969), konnten weder eine Zunahme von Mißbildungen
noch von Leukämie (siehe nächstes Kapitel) beobachtet werden, lediglich eine unerwartet
hohe Häufigkeit von Hämangiomen.

Nach Lejeune u. Mitarb. (1960) wurden unter 1101 in utero durch röntgendiagnostische Untersuchung der Mutter bestrahlte Kinder später in 1,4 % hyperchromatische Stellen
in der Iris gefunden, gegenüber 0,2 % der Kontrolle (total 7092 Fälle). Diese Beobachtungen wurden von Cheeseman u. Walby (1963) nicht vollumfänglich bestätigt, die wohl
Differenzen in der gleichen Richtung (1,2 % bei den Bestrahlten und 0,8 % bei den Unbestrahlten) fanden, aber den Unterschied für zufällig halten.

4. Induktion von Neoplasmen

Bestrahltes kindliches und embryonales Gewebe zeigt zum Teil eine erhöhte Bereitschaft zur malignen Entartung. Während tierexperimentell kaum Daten vorliegen, liegen mehrere statistische Untersuchungen über die Gefährdung des Menschen vor.

a) Schilddrüsencarcinom

(Übersicht. *UN-Bericht*, 1962, 1964, 1966; STEWART, 1969). Eine Bestrahlung der Kopf- und Nackenregion während der Kindheit (hauptsächlich wegen Hypertrophie des Thymus, der Tonsillen und Lymphknoten), fördert die Entstehung von Schilddrüsen-Tumoren (Tabelle 3).

So berichteten DUFFY u. FITZGERALD (1950), daß von 28 Patienten mit Schilddrüsencarcinomen deren 10 zwischen dem 4. und 16. Monat ihres Lebens einer Thymusbestrahlung unterworfen worden waren. Ebenfalls 50 % von 22 jugendlichen Schilddrüsencarcinom-Patienten hatten nach RAVENTOS u. Mitarb. (1962) eine Strahlen-Vorgeschichte. SIMPSON u. HEMPELMANN (1955) stellten ebenfalls eine signifikante Erhöhung der Fälle mit Schilddrüsencarcinomen und Adenomen in thymus-vorbestrahlten Kindern fest. Nach

Tabelle 3. *Schilddrüsen-Krebs nach therapeutischer Bestrahlung.*
(Aus UN-Report 1964)

Autor	Alter bei Bestrahlung	Mann × a	durchschnittl. Exposition (R)	Fälle	Fälle x 10^{-6}/a	Risikoschätzung auf 10^{-6}/a/R
CONTI u. Mitarb. (1960)	Kinder	21896	168	0	0	0,0 (0,0–1,1)
HANFORD u. Mitarb. (1962)	Kinder/Adulte	5711	900	8	1400	1,6 (0,7–3,1)
LATOURETTE u. HODGES (1959)	Kinder	15130	214	1	66	0,3 (0,01–1,7)
PIFER u. Mitarb., *Series I* (1963)	Kinder	26843	329	8	298	0,9 (0,4–1,8)
PIFER u. Mitarb., *Series II* (1963)	Kinder	11000	126	1	91	0,7 (0,01–4,0)
SAENGER u. Mitarb. (1960)	Kinder	24871	330	11	442	1,3 (0,9–2,3)
SIMPSON u. HEMPELMANN (1957)	Kinder	18829	520	10	531	1,0 (0,5–1,9)

CLARK (1955) waren von 15 Kindern mit Schilddrüsencarcinomen im Alter von 15 Jahren und darunter sämtliche im frühen Kindesalter mit 200—725 R (Dosis in Luft gemessen) bestrahlt. Dabei verstrich durchschnittlich zwischen Bestrahlung und Diagnose des Carcinoms 6,9 a.

Nach WILSON u. ASPER (1960) hatten von unter 17 jährigen Schilddrüsenkrebs-Patienten (s. auch WILSON u. Mitarb., 1958) deren 72 % eine Strahlenvorgeschichte. Allerdings scheint die Feldgröße eine Rolle zu spielen, da bei einer weiteren Untersuchung von CONTI u. Mitarb. (1960) nach einer Bestrahlung der Thymus-Region mit einem Feld von 4 × 4 cm unter bestrahlten 1564 Kindern keine Carcinome auftraten.

In einer prospektiven Studie an 1644 Patienten (SAENGER u. Mitarb., 1960), die im Alter unter 16 Jahren wegen benigner Leiden mit weniger als 50—5 000 R in der Kopf-, Brust- und Nackenregion bestrahlt worden waren, wurden 11 Fälle von Schilddrüsenkrebsen festgestellt, gegenüber 0,12 Fällen, die normalerweise erwartet worden wären. Die ebenfalls prospektive Übersicht von PIFER u. Mitarb. (1963) zeigte, daß durch therapeutische Bestrahlung des Thymus bei Kindern Schilddrüsenkrebs induziert wurde. Die Gefährdung war höher, wenn die Kinder eine anteriore und posteriore Behandlung als nur eine anteriore erfuhren.

Nach Winship u. Rosvoll (1961 a, b) hatten 80 % von 286 Schilddrüsenkrebs-Patienten als Säuglinge oder als Kind eine therapeutische Bestrahlung des Kopfes oder des Nackens erhalten, wobei die Strahlendosen zwischen 180—6000 R (Durchschnitt: 600 R) variierten und das Intervall zwischen Bestrahlung und Diagnose des Krebs durchschnittlich 8,6 a betrug. Wenn sich auch in vereinzelten Arbeiten (z.B. Uhlmann, 1956; Garland, 1961) besonders nach Bestrahlung mit kleinen Dosen keine erhöhte Krebsanfälligkeit Vorbestrahlter nachweisen ließ, sprechen doch die Mehrzahl der zum Teil extensiven Studien für einen kausalen Zusammenhang der Entstehung von Schilddrüsentumoren mit einer Bestrahlung im Säuglings- und Kindesalter. Die Erhöhung des Risikos an Schilddrüsenkrebs zu erkranken wird pro R auf 0,5—1,5 Fälle pro 10^6 pro Jahr geschätzt (*UN-Bericht*, 1964; siehe auch Tabelle 3), wobei stets berücksichtigt werden muß, daß sämtliche Risikoschätzungen von Studien mit Dosen über 100 R und mehr stammen. Für das ganze Leben haben Beach u. Dolphin (1962) ein Risiko von 35 Fällen pro 10^6 pro rad geschätzt (Latenzzeit 6,9—8,6 Jahre). Neuere Schätzungen (*UN-Bericht*, 1966) sprechen von 10—20 Fällen pro Million pro R. Neben Schilddrüsencarcinomen können auch noch andere Tumoren auftreten. So hatten nach Takahashi u. Mitarb. (1966) 906 Patienten mit Krebs des Pharynx, Larynx, Zungenwurzel etc. (Schilddrüsencarcinome ausgeschlossen) 11, also 1,21 % eine Strahlenvorgeschichte im kindlichen Alter, verglichen mit 0,45 % bei den Patienten ohne Vorgeschichte (relatives Risiko von 2,7).

Osteochondrome scheinen ebenfalls (Pifer u. Mitarb., 1963) nach kindlicher Bestrahlung häufiger (relatives Risiko 7,5) aufzutreten als bei unbestrahlten Kindern.

b) Leukämie nach therapeutischer Bestrahlung von Kindern und Säuglingen

Eine Reihe von Analysen (Zusfassg. s. *UN-Bericht*, 1962, 1964) befaßt sich mit dem Auftreten von Leukämie, nach einer Bestrahlung in der Kindheit hauptsächlich wegen Thymusvergrößerung. Nach Simpson u. Hempelmann (1957), Hempelmann (1960), Hempelmann u. Mitarb. (1967) stellte sich vermehrt Leukämie ein. Pifer u. Mitarb. (1963) und Toyooka u. Mitarb. (1963 a, b) fanden nach einer mittleren Dosis von 329 R eine Vermehrung der Leukämiefälle um das 6fache. Hingegen wurde mit einer niedrigeren mittleren Dosis von 126 R keine signifikante Vermehrung der Leukämiefälle mehr gefunden. Ebenso beobachteten Conti u. Mitarb. (1960) nach einer Thymusbestrahlung mit kleinem Feld (150 R; 4 × 4 cm) keine Vermehrung der Leukämiefälle. Die Induktion von Leukämie im kindlichen Alter scheint demnach streng dosisabhängig zu sein.

c) Leukämie bei Kindern nach einer Bestrahlung in utero
(strahlendiagnostische Untersuchung der Mutter)

In bezug auf die Induktion der Strahlenleukämie scheinen Embryonen und Feten die sensibelsten Stadien darzustellen. Diese Feststellung machten bereits 1956 Stewart u. Mitarb., indem sie in einer retrospektiven Analyse von an Leukämie erkrankten Kindern beobachteten, daß die Erkrankten zu einem größeren Prozentsatz eine Strahlen-Vorgeschichte in utero aufwiesen als gesunde Kinder. Dabei wurden nur diagnostische Untersuchungen der Mutter mit Strahlen berücksichtigt. Das relative Risiko (Stewart, 1961), durch die Vorbestrahlung an Leukämie zu erkranken, wurde mit 1,83 berechnet. In der Folge wurden etliche Analysen unternommen (Tabelle 4).

Während Court-Brown u. Mitarb. (1960) in einer extensiven prospektiven Untersuchung bei 39166 lebend geborenen Kindern von Müttern, welche während ihrer Schwangerschaft zwischen 1945 und 1956 diagnostisch untersucht worden waren, keine Erhöhung des Leukämiebefalls gegenüber Unbestrahlten fanden, konnte MacMahon (1962) in einer prospektiven Bevölkerungsstudie über 734243 Kinder eine signifikante Erhöhung der Leukämie-Sterblichkeit durch eine Bestrahlung der Kinder in utero nachweisen. Nach Berücksichtigung verschiedenster Variablen, wie Alter der Mutter, Geburtsordnung, errechnete MacMahon eine um etwa 40% höhere Leukämie-Mortalität der Kinder, die eine Strahlenvorgeschichte aufwiesen. Bei der Verwertung aller Ergebnisse der statistischen Untersuchungen (Tabelle 4) stellt sich ebenfalls ein durchschnittlicher Risikofaktor von 1,4 heraus. Das heißt nichts anderes, als daß die geringe Strahlenbelastung einer diagnostischen Untersuchung der Mutter von ca. 1—5 R, die Wahrscheinlichkeit, an Leukämie zu erkranken, erhöht. Stewart nimmt an, daß die frühen Entwicklungsstadien des ersten Trimesters am gefährdetsten sind. Es treten Lymphosarkome, Reticulosen und

Tabelle 4. *Relatives Leukämie-Risiko in retrospectiven Studien an Kindern, die an Leukämie nach diagnostischer Bestrahlung in utero gestorben sind.* (Nach UN-Report 14, 1964)

Autor	Alter (in Jahren) beim Tod	Datum der Todesfälle	% der Mütter mit abdominaler Strahlenbelastung während der Schwangerschaft		Relatives Risiko (95% Vertrauensgrenze in Klammer)
			Fälle Leukämie	Kontrollen	
Stewart (1961)	< 10	1953—55	96/780 (12,3%)	117/1,638 (7,1%)	1,8 (2,4—1,4)
Ford u. Mitarb. (1959)	< 10	1951—55	20/70 (28,6%)	48/247 (19,4%)	1,7 (2,9—0,8)
Kaplan (1958)	?	1955—56	37/150 (24,7%)	24/150 (16,0%)	1,7 (3,7—1,0)
Kaplan (1958)	?	1955—56	34/125 (27,2%)	27/125 (21,6%)	1,4 (2,5—0,7)
Polhemus u. Koch (1959)	?	1950—57	72/251 (28,7%)	58/251 (23,1%)	1,3 (2,0—0,9)
Kjeldsberg (1957)	?	1946—56	5/55 (9,1%)	8/55 (14,5%)	0,6 (2,0—0,2)
Murray u. Mitarb. (1959)	< 20	1940—57	3/65 (4,6%)	3/65 (4,6%)	1,0 (12,0—0,6)
Murray u. Mitarb. (1959)	< 20	1940—57	3/65 (4,6%)	7/93 (7,5%)	0,6 (2,4—0,1)
Murray u. Mitarb. (1959)	< 20	1940—57	3/65 (4,6%)	2/82 (2,4%)	1,9 (40,0—1,1)

akute lymphatische Leukämien auf. Im Gegensatz also zum Erwachsenen dominiert bei der kindlichen Strahlenleukämie nicht der myeloische Typ. Dabei kann das Intervall zwischen Noxe (Bestrahlung) und Erkennbarkeit kürzer als 2 Jahre und länger als 10 Jahre sein (Stewart, 1969).

Der beste Beweis für die Existenz eines erhöhten Risikos durch kleinste Strahlenmengen an Leukämie zu erkranken, ist die Tatsache, daß die radiogenen Leukämien (nach in utero-Bestrahlung) eine andere Altersverteilung (Abb. 30) aufweisen als nicht radiogene Tumore (Stewart, 1969). Ebenso wird durch die Bestrahlung in utero die Wahrscheinlichkeit, an Knochentumoren (Knochensarkom), zu erkranken, mit einem Risikofaktor von 1,5 erhöht.

d) Zusammenfassung

Zusammenfassend kann gesagt werden, daß in bezug auf alle Leukämien der menschliche Embryo 2—5mal gefährdeter ist als der Adulte. Im übrigen hat nach Stewart u. Kneale (1968) die Gefährdung des Kindes in utero bereits durch verbesserte röntgendiagnostische Untersuchungen (mit geringerer Strahlenbelastung) abgenommen. So stellt sich auch bei Griem u. Mitarb. (1969) nach einer Studie an 3024 Kindern, von denen 1008 in utero 1,5 bis 3 rad ausgesetzt waren, kein erhöhtes Risiko, an Leukämie zu erkranken, heraus, hingegen eine erhöhte Häufigkeit von Hämangiomen.

Der sich entwickelnde Mensch ist auch in bezug auf die Induktion von Knochensarkomen sensibler als der Adulte. Studien über das Auftreten von Knochensarkomen
nach Injektion von 224 Radium (ThX) in 217 Jugendliche und 708 Adulte (Behandlung von
Tuberkulose, Spondylitis ankylopoetica und andere Krankheiten) zeigen für die Jugendlichen eine Häufigkeit der Tumoren in 1,5 % pro 100 rad, für Adulte 0,9 % pro 100 rad
(Spiess u. Mays, 1970).

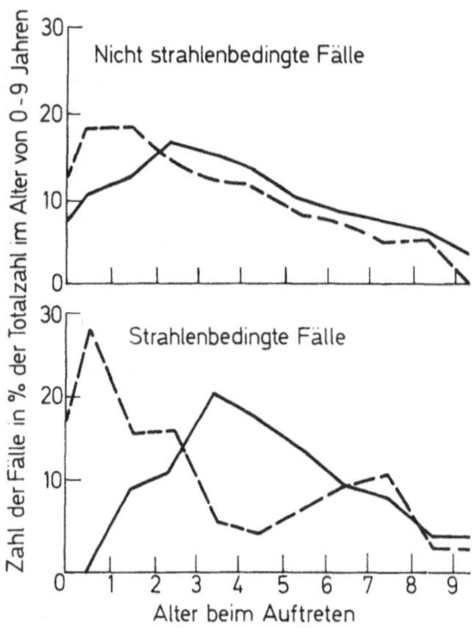

Abb. 30. Alter des Auftretens für nicht radiogene und radiogene hämatopoietische Neoplasmen und solide
Tumoren bei 0–9 jährigen Kindern. (Nach Stewart, 1969)

5. Radionuklide und Entwicklungsstörungen

Grundsätzlich stellen sich für Entwicklungsstörungen, die durch Strahlen von zer-
fallenden Radionukliden erzeugt werden, qualitativ keine neuen Probleme. Sie seien deshalb nur kurz erwähnt. Hingegen sind Aufnahme und biologische Halbwertszeit gewisser
Radionuklide bei sich entwickelnden Lebewesen wesentlich von derjenigen im Adulten
verschieden. Die potentielle Gefährdung kann größer oder kleiner sein. Im Zusammenhang
mit den ausgedehnten Untersuchungen über die radioaktive künstliche Verseuchung unserer Umwelt sind auch die besonderen Probleme des Embryo, Fetus und Kind untersucht
worden (Daten in UN-Bericht 1962, 1964, 1966; Kriegel u. Langendorff, 1964;
Radiation Biology of the Fetal and Juvenile Mammal, edit. by Sikov and Mahlum, 1969).
Die Strahlenmengen, die auf Embryonen und Feten im Mutterleib einwirken, variieren in
Abhängigkeit vom Entwicklungsalter und hauptsächlich den Veränderungen des plazen-
taren Durchganges (Transport: Mutter—Kind). Lamm-Feten im Mutterleib nehmen am
meisten ^{45}Ca, ^{65}Zn, ^{35}S auf, wenn die Radionuklide der Mutter im 3. Trimester der
Gravidität verabreicht werden (Abb. 31). Die größte Menge der Radionuklide wird vom
mütterlichen Körper aufgenommen, so beim Schwein 95 % von ^{65}Zn, 91 % von ^{35}S
(Hansard, 1969). Die Feten nehmen etwas mehr ^{45}Ca auf (80 % Inkorporation im mütterlichen Körper). Es wird vermutet, daß die Retention in der Plazenta den Austausch
Mutter—Kind reguliert. Besonders interessiert die Aufnahme von radioaktivem Jod in
Embryo und Fetus, das vielfältig zu diagnostischen Untersuchungen herangezogen wird.
Nach Czerniak u. Mitarb. (1969) ist beim menschlichen Fetus bis zum Alter von 4,5 Monaten eine geringe Jodaufnahme nach Applikation von ^{131}J an die Mutter zu verzeichnen,
hingegen eine 2,6 mal größere Aufnahme in der Schilddrüse des sechsmonatigen Fetus als
in der Mutter.

Von Meerschweinchen (NELSON u. Mitarb., 1969) wird ebenfalls 131 Jod mit zunehmendem Entwicklungsalter vermehrt aufgenommen (Abb. 32), wobei das Aufnahmemuster sich nach dem 25. Entwicklungstag dem des Adulten angleicht. Applikation von ^{131}J während der Organogenese (15 μ Ci/d während 6 Tagen) führte zu Änderungen im prä-

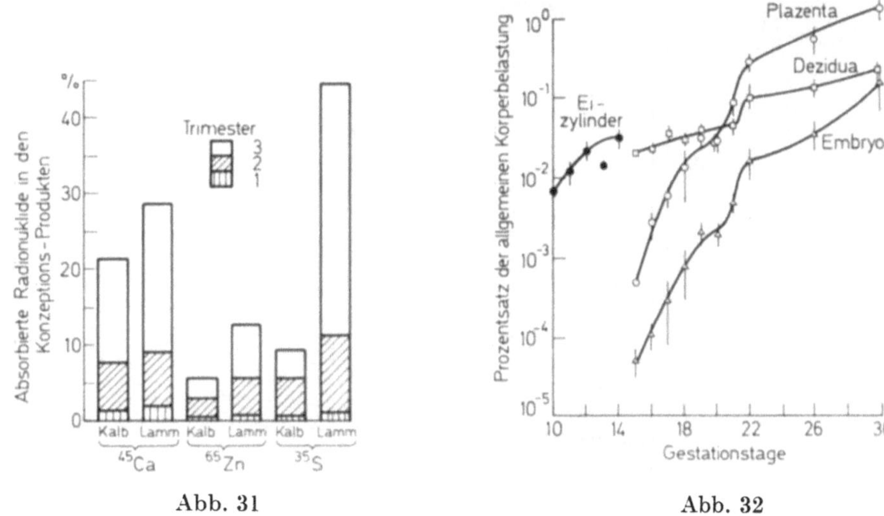

Abb. 31   Abb. 32

Abb. 31. Aufnahme von Radionukliden während der 3 Trimester der Entwicklung in utero beim Lamm und Kalb. (Nach HANSARD, 1969)

Abb. 32. 131 Jod-Aufnahme vom embryonalen Gewebe und der mütterlichen Decidua, 24 h nach einer oralen Applikation von 100 μ Ci. (Nach NELSON u. Mitarb., 1969)

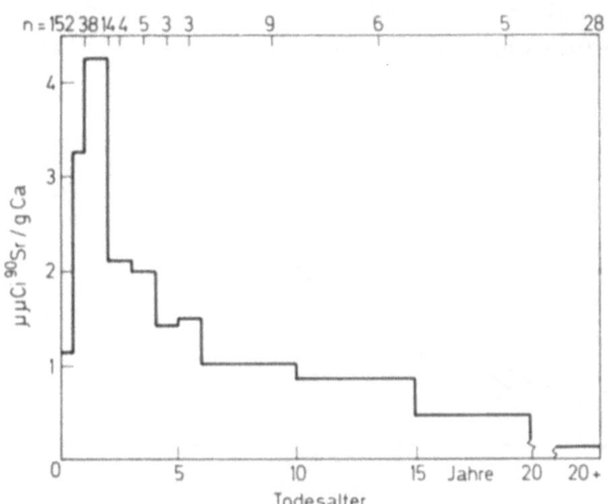

Abb. 33. Konzentration von 90 Strontium in menschlichen Knochen im United Kingdom 1959 in Abhängigkeit vom Todesalter. n = Zahl der Untersuchungen. (Nach Report of UN, 1962)

natalen Körpergewicht und Mißbildungen der Retina. Nach der Geburt werden besonders knochensuchende Radionuklide von Neugeborenen und Kindern in vermehrtem Maße inkorporiert. Das Verhältnis zwischen der Retention von 90 Strontium und Calcium ist größer bei Kindern als beim Erwachsenen (STRAUB u. Mitarb., 1964). Die Aufnahme ist altersabhängig (Abb. 33). Interessant sind die Beobachtungen von IINUMA u. Mitarb. (1969)

über die 137 Caesium-Aufnahme bei Säuglingen. Mit Kuhmilch ernährte Säuglinge und Kinder wiesen eine größere Strahlenbelastung auf als Erwachsene, während Feten und brustgenährte Kinder weniger 137 Caesium aufnahmen als Erwachsene (Abb. 34).

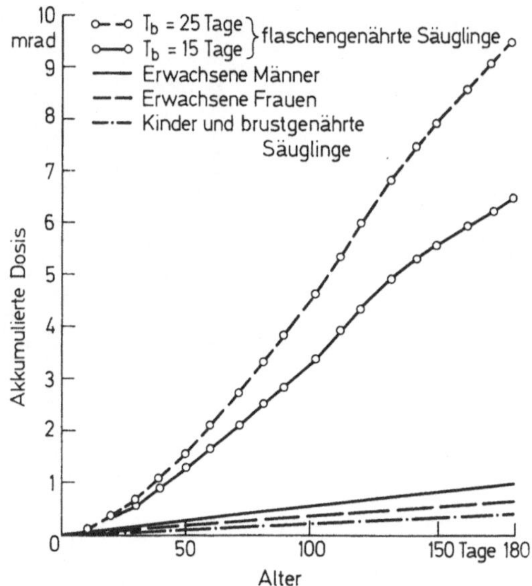

Abb. 34. Vergleich der akkumulierten Dosis von 137 Caesium in mrad zwischen flaschen- und brustgenährten Kindern und Erwachsenen. (Nach Iinuma u. Mitarb., 1969)

In verschiedenen Experimenten mit Tieren wurden Mißbildungen und Todesfälle bei Embryonen und Feten nach der Applikation von ^{32}P, ^{89}Sr in relativ hohen Dosen beobachtet.

Während eine Applikation von 1,6 μCi/g/d 3H-Thymidin an Ratten während dem 9.—22. Tag der Gravidität ohne Effekt war, zeigten sich mit höheren Dosen (3,2; 4,8 und 6,4

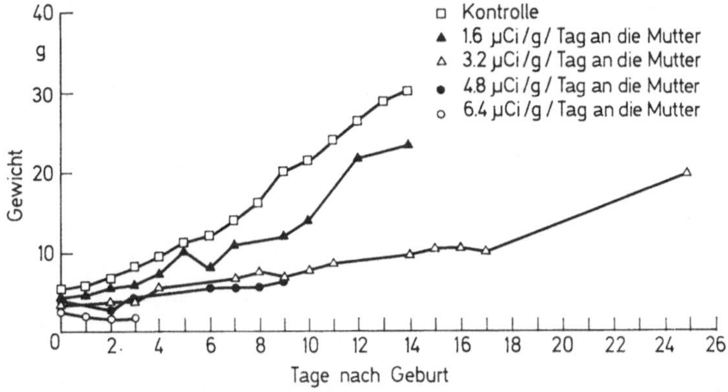

Abb. 35. Gewichtsänderung bei neugeborenen Ratten nach Applikation von 1,6 μ Ci/g/d–6,4 μ Ci/g/d ^{3}H-Thymidin an die Mutter vom 9.—22. Gestationstag. (Nach Fliedner u. Mitarb., 1969)

μCi/g/d) ein Anstieg der Totgeburten, eine Störung im Wachstum und in der Entwicklung der blutbildenden Gewebe (Fliedner u. Mitarb., 1969). Schwere Mißbildungen traten nach 8,0 μCi/g/d ein (Abb. 35).

Für eine bessere Schätzung der Gefährdung des werdenden Menschen durch Inkorporierung kleiner Mengen von Radionukliden werden noch eingehende Untersuchungen notwendig sein.

6. Abhängigkeit der embryonalen Strahlenschädigung von physikalischen (LET, Intensität, Fraktionierung) und physiologischen Parametern (Milieufaktoren)

Wie andere strahlenbiologische Effekte ist auch die embryonale Strahlenschädigung bei Wirbeltieren keine Konstante, sondern hängt von verschiedenen physikalischen und physiologischen Parametern ab.

a) Strahlenqualität und LET (linear energy transfer)

Die meisten schlüssigen Untersuchungen sind an Drosophila-Embryonen und Puppenstadien durchgeführt worden, während bei Wirbeltieren Experimente mit Hühner-Embryonen vorwiegen, die zum Teil eine Abhängigkeit der Wirkung vom LET zeigten. COOPER u. Mitarb. (1962) verglichen die Wirkung von ultraharten 20 MeV-Elektronen mit derjenigen von 250 keV-Photonen auf 12 Tage alte Hühner-Embryonen (RBE von 0,82). Cobalt 60-Gammastrahlen sind (LOKEN u. Mitarb., 1960) etwas weniger wirksam (RBE von 0,82) als 220 keV-Photonen. HUMPHREY u. SINCLAIR (1962) fanden für Cobalt-60-Gammastrahlen gegenüber 200 keV-Gammastrahlen eine RBE von 0,92, ferner von 0,93 im Vergleich von 22 MeV-Photonen gegenüber 200 keV-Photonen, währenddem sich die biologische Wirksamkeit von 22 MeV-Photonen nicht von derjenigen der Cobalt 60-Strahlen unterschied.

Wenn der LET-Wert außerordendlich hoch ist, wie z. B. für schwere Ionen, ist es möglich, daß der embryonale Schaden qualitativ und quantitativ verändert wird. Dies gilt besonders für Störungen, die auf multifaktoriellen oder multizellulären Ereignissen beruhen. Das heißt der Schaden wird durch das gleichzeitige Zusammenwirken mehrerer Schädigungen bewirkt, wie z. B. der Ausfall einer Mehrzahl benachbarter Zellen. Die Strahlung würde gleichsam „Löcher" in die embryonalen Systeme schießen. Tatsächlich konnten TODD u. Mitarb. (1972) an Mais-Keimlingen mit 3,9 GeV-Stickstoff-Ionen für bestimmte Schädigungen eine RBE von 1000 errechnen und neuartige Anomalien feststellen.

b) Abhängigkeit der Wirkung von Verdünnung und Applikation (einmalige Bestrahlung und Fraktionierung)

Gerade in bezug auf die besondere Gefährlichkeit des embryonalen Strahlenschadens interessiert die Frage, ob eine verdünnte chronische Bestrahlung, wie sie sich beispielsweise durch eine geringe Erhöhung des Strahlenpegels in der Umwelt des heutigen Menschen einstellen könnte, gleich wirkt wie eine konzentrierte einmalige Bestrahlung.

Die meisten Untersuchungen gerade mit niedrigen Dosen, zur Bestimmung eines Schwellenwertes, sind mit einmaliger und konzentrierter Bestrahlung gemacht worden. Neben diesen praktischen Überlegungen interessiert das Problem auch in bezug auf die Genese des embryonalen Strahlenschadens. Das Erholungsvermögen der Zelle kann durch Fraktionierungs- und Verdünnungs-Experimente abgeschätzt werden. Da der embryonale Strahleneffekt aber ebenfalls stark vom Alter des bestrahlten Stadiums abhängt, sagt ein Verdünnungs- oder Fraktionierungseffekt kaum etwas Endgültiges über den Mechanismus der Strahlenschädigung, resp. über die Möglichkeit der Erholung aus. So kann ja die einmalige Dosis auf ein strahlensensibles Stadium einwirken, währenddem die fraktionierte auch Stadien bestrahlt, welche nicht mehr empfindlich sind oder umgekehrt. AUERBACH (1956) stellte fest, daß nach einer Bestrahlung von $9^1/_2$ tägigen Mäuse-Embryonen mit einer einmaligen Applikation von 300 R sowohl weniger schwere Mißbildungen des Skelets, als auch der Augen (Colobom) auftraten, als wenn die Dosis in 3mal à 100 R mit einem Intervall von 30 min appliziert wurde (80 R/min sowohl für die einmalige als auch für die fraktionierte Bestrahlung, 250 keV-Photonen). Die Kurz-Intervall-Fraktionierung erweist sich als die gefährlichere.

Wird die Dosis hingegen über einen längeren Zeitraum auf Mäuse verdünnt oder fraktioniert verabreicht (Russell u. Mitarb., 1960), dann sind bei einer Totaldosis von 200 R die verdünnte und die fraktionierte Bestrahlung weniger wirksam (Abb. 36). Allerdings wurde für die kontinuierliche verdünnte Bestrahlung (0,0086 R/min) eine andere Strahlenqualität, nämlich γ-Strahlen einer 137 Cäsiumquelle gewählt wie für die einmalige Be-

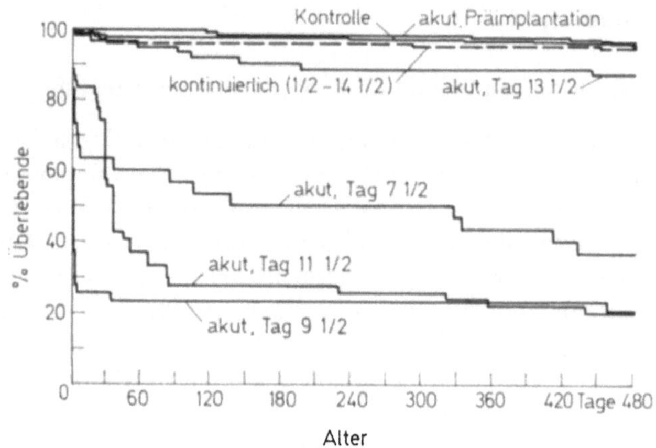

Abb. 36. Postnatale Überlebenszeit von Mäusen (am 486. Tag nach Geburt) die akut (83 R/min) und chronisch (0,0086 R/min) bestrahlt worden waren. Ganzkörperbestrahlung, Totaldosis = 200 R für akute Bestrahlung (250 keV) und 171 R für chronische Bestrahlung mit ^{137}Cs. (Nach Russell u. Mitarb., 1960)

strahlung und auch dort wurde eine „schützende" Wirkung der Fraktionierung gefunden.

Erstreckt sich die fraktionierte Bestrahlung über die ganze Tragzeit der Maus (Dosisleistung 45 R/min, 150 keV-Photonen, Bestrahlung einmal täglich mit 2,5 R—80 R), (Kriegel u. Langendorff, 1964), dann wurde erst bei einer Dosis von 20 R/d eine geringe

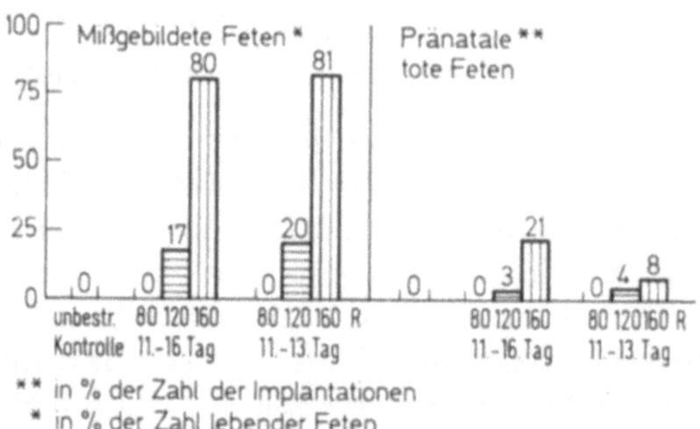

Abb. 37. Mißgebildete Feten und pränatale Todesfälle bei Mäusen nach fraktionierter Totalkörperbestrahlung (180 keV, 90 R/min) während 11–16 d nach Konzeption. (Nach Kriegel u. Reinhardt, 1969)

Zunahme der Mißbildungs- und Resorptionsrate, sowie eine Gewichtsverminderung der Feten beobachtet. Die Fraktionierung scheint hier wiederum schützend zu wirken. Interessanterweise ist ein plötzlicher Anstieg der fetalen Todesfälle nach 60 R/d zu beobachten, wobei Fehlbildungen und Resorption ab 20 R/d zunehmen. Nach Ansicht von Kriegel u. Langendorff wird durch die fortgesetzte Bestrahlung der Embryo in der Blastogenese latent geschädigt (siehe auch Kriegel 1965).

Keine Strahlenschäden (Abb. 37) bei 18 tägigen Mäuse-Feten traten nach einer fraktionierten Bestrahlung mit 80 R/d (180 keV, 90 R/min) am 11.—16. Tag, am 11.—13. Tag und am 14.—16. Tag der Entwicklung auf (KRIEGEL u. REINHARDT, 1969). Erst wenn 120 und 160 R/d verabreicht wurden und nur, wenn die Bestrahlung während der Zeit 11—16 d oder 11—13 d nach Befruchtung erfolgte, stellten sich Mißbildungen, wie anomale Schwänze, Extremitätenanomalien ein.

Nach einer kontinuierlichen Bestrahlung durch Inkorporierung von radioaktiv markiertem Thymidin wurden erst nach einer täglichen Gabe von 8,0 μ Ci/g/d an Ratten (vom 9.—22. Trächtigkeitstag) Mißbildungen beobachtet, während eine reversible Hemmung in der Entwicklung des hämatopoetischen Systems bereits nach 3,2 μCi/g/d einsetzte (FLIEDNER u. Mitarb., 1969).

Die Untersuchung 18tägiger Mäuse-Feten (KONERMANN, 1968a und b), die während der gesamten Entwicklung einer täglichen Bestrahlung von 5 R, 10 R, 20 R, 40 R, 60 R und 80 R (148 R/min, 150 keV-Photonen) ausgesetzt waren, ergab wiederum, daß eine Fraktionierung über eine längere Entwicklungszeit in kleinen Tagesraten gegeben weniger schadet, als wenn die entsprechende Gesamtdosis mit höheren Einzeldosen in kurzer Zeit gegeben wurden. 5 R pro Tag führten zu keinen makroskopisch erkennbaren Schäden. 10 R/d hingegen erhöhten die Resorptionsraten, wenn während der ganzen Entwicklungsdauer oder während der Organogenese bestrahlt wurde, währenddem eine Bestrahlung der Blastogenese und Fetalperiode ohne Wirkung blieb. Mit 20 R/d erhöhte sich lediglich nach der Bestrahlung der Blastogenese-Stadien die Letalität.

Bei Bestrahlung der Fetalperiode allein blieb auch eine Erhöhung der Tagesdosis auf 80 R ohne Wirkung, ebenso wenn die Keime bereits während der Blastogenese (KONERMANN, 1970) vorbestrahlt und einer Gesamtdosis von 400 R ausgesetzt waren. Wesentlich scheint allerdings das strahlenfreie Intervall zwischen Erstbestrahlung während der Blastogenese und der Zweitbestrahlung während der Fetalperiode zu sein, da nach einer Vorbestrahlung während der Organogenese die bestrahlten Feten strahlengeschädigt sind (hauptsächlich Gewichtsverminderung). Für eine verdünnte Bestrahlung mit Cobalt-60 von 10 R bis 119 R/d stellte sich stets eine geringere Mißbildungsrate heraus als nach einer konzentrierten (KONERMANN, 1969). Auch bei Ratten-Feten wurde nach einer Fraktionierung von 150 R in 3 Einzeldosen (50 R/min) mit einem Intervall von 9 h (JACOBS u. BRIZZEE, 1966) eine geringere Wirkung der fraktionierten Bestrahlung festgestellt. Beobachtet wurden ein Tag nach Bestrahlung Mißbildung des Gehirns (Pyknosen, Rosettenbildung). Nach der fraktionierten Bestrahlung von 14tägigen Feten wurde keine Rosettenbildung und von 17tägigen Feten überhaupt keine Strahlenschädigung festgestellt.

Eine Fraktionierung von 150 R in 3—9 Fraktionen während 12 Std schädigten bei 13tägigen Ratten-Feten die Hirnzellen weniger als eine einmalige Bestrahlung oder eine zweimalige mit einem Intervall von 3 h (BRIZZEE u. Mitarb., 1966).

Eine Verringerung des Strahleneffektes nach chronischer, verdünnter oder fraktionierter Bestrahlung wurde von LANGENDORFF (1963) besonders bei Adulten auch für das Auftreten von Spätschäden beobachtet. Sowohl Veränderung des Blutbildes, Leukämie-Induktion, Tumorwachstum, Lebensverkürzung, Fertilitätsstörungen werden bei chronischer Strahlenbelastung nur bei relativ hohen Gesamtstrahlenmengen beobachtet.

Dieser Schutzeffekt der verdünnten, fraktionierten Bestrahlung kann als Ausdruck der Erholungsfähigkeit der bestrahlten Zellen gedeutet werden. Ferner wäre es möglich, daß sich embryonale und fetale Strahlenschäden erst dann manifestieren, wenn ein gewisses Maß an hemmender oder tötender Wirkung erreicht wird. Nur ein Ausfall einer bestimmten Zahl Zellen würde zur embryonalen Schädigung führen (s. Diskussion „Analyse des embryonalen Schadens" und LET-Effekt, Seite 277, 286).

Für größere Säugetiere dürfte allerdings das letzte Wort nicht gesprochen sein, indem MURPHREE u. GRAVES (1969) beispielsweise bei einem Vergleich (allerdings mit kleinen Zahlen) von 1 R/min- und 47 R/min-60 Co-Bestrahlung auf 23tägige Lämmchen in utero mehr Mißbildungen bei der verdünnten Applikation und einer Totaldosis von 188 R beobachteten.

c) Milieufaktoren

Genau wie bei den Wirbellosen (siehe Seite 240) dürften Änderungen des intra- und extrazellulären Milieus vor, während und nach der Bestrahlung die Entwicklungsstörungen von Wirbeltieren beeinflussen. Die wenigen Untersuchungen bestätigen diese Ansicht. Bei 6tägigen Hühnerembryonen wurde der sogenannte indirekte Strahleneffekt (Wendt, 1964) durch Thyroxinvorbehandlung verstärkt, durch Methylenblau vermindert.

Eine Schutzwirkung von subletalen Vorbestrahlungen mit 375 R auf eine Zweitbestrahlung mit 725 R nach 20—25 h schützt Hühner-Embryonen 100%ig vor dem Strahlentod (Wendt, 1970) vermutlich mit einer Aktivierung unspezifischer zellulärer Abwehrreaktionen. Ebenfalls bei Hühnerembryonen wurde mit einer Verfütterung von Zink ein Schutzeffekt erzielt (Clapp u. Kienholz, 1966). 15—18tägige Rattenfeten wurden durch

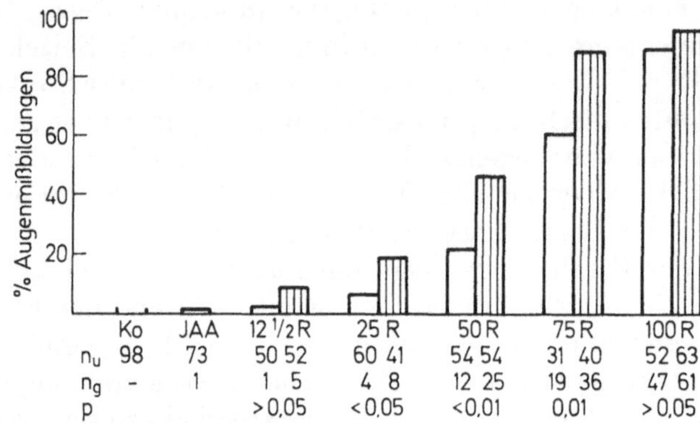

Abb. 38. Sensibilisierung der Strahlenschäden bei 9 tägigen Rattenembryonen mit Iodacetamid. Befunde 4 Tage nach Bestrahlung. Leere Säulen: Alleinige Bestrahlung, schraffierte Säulen: Bestrahlung und Vorbehandlung mit Iodacetamid, i.p. 0,925 mg/kg Körpergewicht 1 h vor Bestr.); nu = Anzahl der untersuchten Feten, ng = Anzahl der geschädigten Feten. (Aus Michel, 1969/70)

eine Behandlung mit Mercaptoaethylamin vor Bestrahlung mit 300 R vor dem Strahlentod geschützt (Maisin u. Mitarb., 1955). Junge Mäuse im Alter von 10—60 Tagen ließen sich ebenfalls mit einer Injektion von 50 mg/kg Serotonin 5 min vor Bestrahlung mit einer Dosis letalis 50 %/30 d schützen, währenddem die Wirkung des Strahlenschutzstoffes bei eintägigen Tieren am geringsten war (Langendorff u. Langendorff, 1966).

Von großem Interesse für die Beurteilung der Strahlengefährdung des Menschen ist die Frage, ob an und für sich nicht teratogene Substanzen, vornehmlich Pharmaka, die Wirkung kleiner Dosen sensibilisieren. Tatsächlich verdoppelt eine Applikation von Jodazetamid i.p. (0,925 mg/kg Körpergewicht) eine Stunde vor Bestrahlung 9tägiger Ratten-Embryonen die Zahl der Mißbildungen (Fritz-Niggli u. Michel, 1970; Michel u. Fritz-Niggli, 1969; Michel, 1969/1970). So stieg die Zahl der in der Kopfregion geschädigten 14tägigen Feten durch Applikation von Jodazetamid vor Bestrahlung mit 12,5 R von 5 auf 9,6 % nach 25 R von 8,3 auf 24,4 % (Abb. 38). Eine noch größere Sensibilisierung wurde durch eine einmalige Applikation von Antibiotica (Ledermycin) erreicht (Fritz-Niggli u. Michel, 1971). Es ist wahrscheinlich, daß diese sensibilisierenden Substanzen hauptsächlich das Repairsystem blockieren.

IV. Dosis minima

Die Schätzung oder Bestimmung der Dosis minima, die zu einer Entwicklungsstörung führt, stellen für die Beurteilung der Strahlengefährdung des Menschen ein äußerst wichtiges Problem dar. Verständlicherweise sind wir bei den Schätzungen zumeist auf Experimente an Ratten und Mäusen angewiesen.

Im Tierexperiment werden fast ausschließlich auffällige, morphologisch faßbare Veränderungen erfaßt und dann auch nur größere Abweichungen. Subtile Stoffwechseländerungen und geringe Abweichungen in der Morphologie und der Leistung einzelner Organe entgehen der Beobachtung. Vereinzelte Untersuchungen mit besonderen Methoden, die sich mit der Aktivität des ZNS befassen, zeigen bereits nach einer geringen Strahlenbelastung Funktionsstörungen.

Die meisten Experimente sind mit einer einmaligen, konzentrierten Bestrahlung des ganzen Körpers des Muttertieres durchgeführt worden (abgesehen von der lokalen Bestrahlung des Embryos durch WILSON u. KARR (1951), WILSON u. Mitarb. (1952), WILSON u. Mitarb. (1953), BRENT (1960).

Wie aus Tabelle 5 hervorgeht, variieren die Minimaldosen nach Autor, Kriterium und Bestrahlungsalter (s. auch Übersicht LANGENDORFF, 1969). Unterschiedliche Versuchsanordnungen können das Ergebnis verändern.

Nach JACOBSEN (1969) sind sogar zwischen „Winter"- und „Sommer"-Experimenten bedeutende Unterschiede möglich. So sind 8tägige Mäuse-Embryonen, die mit 5, 20 und 100 R (175 keV, 59 R/min) während des Winters bestrahlt wurden, eindeutig strahlenempfindlicher als im Sommer. Auch die Wurfgröße, der Zustand der Mutter, die Ernährung der Neugeborenen etc. könnte die Schädigungsrate beeinflussen.

Eindeutig steht fest, daß sowohl bei der Ratte als auch bei der Maus und einer Bestrahlung von strahlensensiblen Stadien mit 5 R Mißbildungen und Entwicklungsstillstand erzielt werden. Bei der Bestrahlung von *Ratten*-Embryonen während der Organogenese treten nach 30—50 R mit Sicherheit erhöhte Letalität, Augen- und Hirnanomalien auf (JOB u. Mitarb., 1935; HICKS u. Mitarb., 1957). Mit 25 R (WILSON u. KARR, 1950, 1951; WILSON, 1954) lassen sich Augenmißbildungen, sowie Neubildungen (Rosetten) in der Kopfregion nachweisen und mit 12,5 R treten besonders in Kombination mit dem Strahlensensibilisator Jodazetamid Augen- und Kopfanomalien auf (FRITZ-NIGGLI u. MICHEL, 1970). Dosen unter 10 R führen nach Bestrahlung fetaler Stadien (D'AMATO u. HICKS, 1965) zu Anomalien der Neuronen und 25 R (HICKS u. D'AMATO, 1963) zu Reduktion des Hirngewichtes und zu anomalem Wachstum der Neuronen in Cerebellum und Cortex. Auch eine Bestrahlung der Blastogenese-Stadien mit 5—25 R (BRENT, 1960) führt zu Wachstumshemmung.

Bei der *Maus* stellen sich nach Bestrahlung der Embryonen in Organogenese mit 5 R Skelet-Anomalien und Entwicklungsstillstand (JACOBSEN, 1965) ein. Empfindlich sind die Stadien vor den ersten Furchungen oder während der ersten Furchung, indem 5 R nicht nur Entwicklungsstillstand, sondern auch Exencephalien (RUGH u. GRUPP, 1959a) und Polydaktylien (OHZU, 1965) erzeugen. Mit Dosen etwas höher als 10 R kann Katarakt induziert werden. Verschiedene Autoren (s. Tabelle 5) verzeichnen sowohl bei der Ratte als auch bei der Maus sowohl nach verdünnter als auch nach konzentrierter einmaliger Bestrahlung bei Totaldosen von 20—25 R eine erhöhte Krampfbereitschaft auf audiogene Reize. MILLER (1962) glaubt sogar nach chronischer verdünnter Gammabestrahlung eine Dosis minima von 0,14 rad beobachten zu können. Mit 25 R scheint die Lernfähigkeit von 400tägigen Rattenembryonen (KAPLAN, 1962a), die im Alter von 2,5 Tagen bestrahlt worden waren, eingeschränkt zu sein, während 15 R auf 1,5tägige Embryonen im Alter von 90 d die Lernfähigkeit herabsetzen (KAPLAN, 1962b).

Soweit die Schwellendosen für strahleninduzierte Entwicklungsstörungen bei der Ratte und der Maus. Es besteht kein Grund zur Annahme, daß sich der menschliche Embryo im Mutterleib anders verhält als die Nagetier-Embryonen. Während für den Menschen keine schlüssigen Angaben über die kleinsten Dosen für Mißbildungen und Entwicklungsstillstand zu finden sind, läßt sich hingegen klar erkennen, daß der menschliche Embryo im Mutterleib in bezug auf Krebsgefährdung äußerst strahlensensibel ist. Im Anschluß an die Arbeiten von STEWART u. Mitarb. (1956, 1958) zeigten verschiedene statistische Untersuchungen, daß eine diagnostische Untersuchung der Mutter bereits das keimende Lebewesen schädigen kann. Nach einer ICRP-Publikation (1969) verfaßt vom Committee

Tabelle 5. *Dosis minima für Entwicklungsstörungen*

	Bestrahltes Stadium	Bestrahlungsdaten	Dosis minima	Kriterium	Autor
Ratte	8 d, 9 d	112 keV, 36 R/min	36–40 R	Hirn, Auge	Job u. Mitarb. (1935)
	9 d	85 keV (12,5 R/min)	25 R	Wachstumshemmung	Wilson u. Karr (1951)
	9 d	85 keV (12,5 R/min)	25 R	Rosettenbildung Kopfregion	Wilson u. Mitarb. (1952)
	9 d	85 keV (25 R/min)	50 R	Resorption	Wilson u. Mitarb. (1953)
	9 d	85 keV (12,5 R/min)	25 R	Mikrophthalmie Anophthalmie	Wilson (1954)
	8 d	85 keV (12,5 R/min)	12,5 R	Wachstumshemmung	Wilson (1954)
	vom 9. d an	250 keV	30–40 R	Zerstörung der Neuroblasten	Hicks (1952) Hicks u. Mitarb. (1957)
	18 d und 2–3 Wochen nach Geburt	250 keV (50–70 R/min)	25 R	Anomales Wachstum (Neuronen von Hirn-Cortex, Cerebellum)	Hicks u. D'Amato (1963)
	18 d	250 keV (60 R/min)	< 10 R	Anomalien der Neuronen Reflexe	D'Amato u. Hicks (1965)
	Neugeborene	250 keV (60 R/min)	10 R		
	0–20 d	1 rad/d schnelle Neutronen	20 R		
	0–8 d	?	5–25 R	Wachstumshemmung	Brent (1960)
	9 d	200 keV (36,5 R/min)	12,5 R	Augen- und Hirnanomalie (verstärkt durch Jodazetamid)	Fritz-Niggli u. Michel (1970) Michel (1969/70)
	Bestrahltes Stadium	**Bestrahlungsdaten**	**Dosis minima**	**Kriterium**	**Autor**
Maus	0–6 d	250 keV (80 R/min)	25 R	Reduktion der Wurfgröße	Russell u. Russell (1954)
	7,5 d; 8,5 d	250 keV (80 R/min)	25 R	Skeletanomalien	Russell (1955, 1957)
	8 d	200 keV (14 R/min)	25 R	Anomalien des ZNS	Murakami u. Kameyama (1958)
	0,5 d	184 keV (15 R/min)	5 R	Resorption	Rugh u. Grupp (1959a)
	2-Zellstadium	184 keV (50 R/min)	10 R	Exencephalien	Rugh (1963b)
	0,0–0,5 d	184 keV (50 R/min)	etwas höher als 10 R	Katarakt	Rugh u. Mitarb. (1964a)

Bestrahltes Stadium	Bestrahlungsdaten	Dosis minima	Kriterium	Autor
0,5 d } 1,5 d }	160 keV (24,5 R/min)	{ 5 R { 5 R	Polydaktylie	OHZU (1965)
7,5 d	175 keV (67 R/min)	5 R	Letalität Letalität	JACOBSEN (1965)
7,5 d	175 keV (67 R/min)	5 R	Hydroamnion Skeletanomalien	JACOBSEN (1966)

	Bestrahltes Stadium	Bestrahlungsdaten	Dosis minima	Kriterium	Autor
Ratte	15–20 d	250 keV (9,4 R/min)	25 R	Krampfbereitschaft (vorbehandelt mit Metrazol)	WERBOFF u. Mitarb. (1961, 1962)
	1,5 d	180 keV (15 R/min)	15 R	Lernfähigkeit als 90 d Ratten (Lashley Maze)	KAPLAN (1962b)
	2,5 d	180 keV (25 R/min)	25 R	als 400 d-Ratten	KAPLAN (1962a)
	0–20 d	1 R/d	20 R	Nervöse Aktivität Reduktion des Hirngewichtes und der frontalen Rinde	PIONTKOVSKY u. SEMAGIN (1963)
	0–10 d	γ-Strahlen (^{60}Co) 2 R/d : 23 h/24 h Tag	20 R	Audiogene Krampfbereitschaft	COOKE (1963) COOKE u. Mitarb. (1964)
	postnatal 0–30 d	γ-Strahlen (^{60}Co) 0,0048 rad/d	0,14 rad	Audiogene Krämpfe	MILLER (1962)
	postnatal 23–30 d	γ-Strahlen (^{60}Co) 0,35 rad/d	1,5–2 rad	Audiogene Krämpfe	MILLER (1962)
	6 d, 11 d, 16 d	γ-Strahlen (^{60}Co) 2,4 R/min	> 10 R	Audiogene Krämpfe	TACKER u. FURCHTGOTT (1962)
Mensch	hauptsächlich 0–90 d	Strahlendiagnostische Belastung der Mutter	1–5 R	Leukämie	STEWART u. Mitarb. (1956) MACMAHON (1958)

of the International Commission on Radiological Protection, ist diese Tatsache heute unbestritten. Nicht nur die Wahrscheinlichkeit, an Leukämie zu erkranken, ist nach einer Bestrahlung in utero erhöht, sondern auch für andere Krebsarten besteht eine erhöhte Bereitschaft. Die Dosen, die während einer ausgiebigen diagnostischen Untersuchung der Mutter den Keim belasten, betragen etwa 1—5 R.

Zusammenfassend stellen wir fest, daß im Stadium der Blastogenese Dosen von 5—15 R die Entwicklung ändern können, und zwar nicht nur im Sinne eines Entwicklungsstillstandes, sondern auch einer Anomalie des Neugeborenen. Ebenso kann während der Organogenese eine einmalige Bestrahlung von 5 R Skeletmißbildungen und Entwicklungshemmungen erzeugen und eine Dosis von 12,5 R in Kombination mit einem Strahlensensibilisator führt mit Sicherheit zu Augen- und Hirnschädigungen. Nicht nur embryonale Zellen, sondern auch fetale sind strahlensensibel, so sind Neuronen nach 25 R mißgebildet und gleicherweise treten Linsentrübungen auf. Bis Beweise vorliegen, daß die Embryonen von Nagetieren besonders strahlenempfindlich sind und sich in ihrer Strahlenreaktion nicht mit derjenigen menschlicher Embryonen vergleichen lassen, müssen wir annehmen, daß auch für den sich entwickelnden Menschen gleiche Minimaldosen existieren.

Es wäre übrigens durchaus möglich, daß viele subtile Änderungen, die aber für den Betroffenen sehr unangenehm sein könnten, bereits mit noch niedrigeren Dosen induziert werden. Es sei deshalb noch einmal mit allem Nachdruck die Forderung von Russell (1955) unterstützt, daß eine Frau im fortpflanzungsfähigen Alter nur dann strahlendiagnostisch untersucht werden sollte, wenn mit Sicherheit noch keine Befruchtung vorliegt, d.h. also in den ersten Tagen des Zyklus (lebensbedrohende Zustände natürlich ausgeschlossen). Bei vorliegender Schwangerschaft sollten röntgendiagnostische Untersuchungen nur im äußersten Notfall durchgeführt werden. Es ist durchaus möglich, daß an und für sich nicht teratogene Pharmaka und Chemikalien den Strahleneffekt noch verstärken können.

Experimente mit Jodazetamid und Antibiotika deuten in diese Richtung.

V. Mechanismen der strahlenbedingten
Entwicklungsstörungen

Das komplexe Geschehen der Entwicklungsvorgänge erschwert die Analyse der strahlenbedingten Störungen und gestattet nur bruchstückweise einen Einblick in den Schädigungsablauf. Ionisierende Strahlen vermögen vieles. Sie können Zellen in der mitotischen Aktivität stören, sie können die Entstehung und die Leistung von Biomolekülen ändern, Hemmstoffe vernichten oder produzieren; sie können Zellen subletal und letal schädigen, Zellbezirke ausschalten, Gestaltungsbewegungen beeinflussen oder mit subtilen Änderungen von Membranen, Funktion und Struktur ändern. Da gerade zeitliche und räumliche Koordination verschiedenster Vorgänge für die richtige Heranbildung der Individuen unabdingbare Voraussetzung sind, bieten sich den ionisierenden Strahlen zahlreichste Angriffspunkte. Dieser extremen Verletzlichkeit des Embryos steht seine große Erholungsfähigkeit, sein Regulationsvermögen entgegen. Das erwachsene Individuum hingegen läßt sich nur in bestimmten Bezirken beeinflussen, kann aber Schäden schlecht reparieren. Zwischen Embryonen und Adulten sind in bezug auf Regulationsvermögen und Sensibilität Feten und Kinder einzureihen.

Strahlensensibilität und Reparaturvermögen bestimmen das Ausmaß der strahlenbedingten Entwicklungsstörung.

Da sich diese beiden Faktoren während der Entwicklung ändern und für jedes Organ und jeden Zelltyp verschieden sind, muß Art und Ausmaß des Strahlenschadens in strenger Abhängigkeit der Entwicklungsphase stehen.

1. Einige Möglichkeiten der „primären" Strahlenwirkung

In Abb. 39 sind schematisch einige Angriffspunkte der ionisierenden Strahlen während der Differenzierung eines Organs dargestellt. Der histologischen Differenzierung geht voran (oder ist mit ihr verknüpft) die zytologische. Aus der neutralen prädifferenzierten, omnipotenten Zelle bilden sich einhergehend mit Transcriptionsprozessen protodifferenzierte Zellen mit eingeschränkter (aber modellierbarer) Potenz. Diese pluripotenten Zellen können sog. Blasteme bilden und sich dann zu in Form und Funktion spezialisierten Zellen heranbilden. Translationsprozesse — Membrandifferenzierung stehen makromolekular im Vordergrund.

Gewisse Stadien sind empfindlich auf extrazelluläre Faktoren, und interzelluläre Kommunikationen sind oft wichtigste Voraussetzung der Entwicklung. Dabei spielen neben der Bildung und Aktivität von Effektoren und Repressoren auch degenerative Prozesse eine bestimmte Rolle (siehe z. B. FORSBERG u. KAELLEN, 1968).

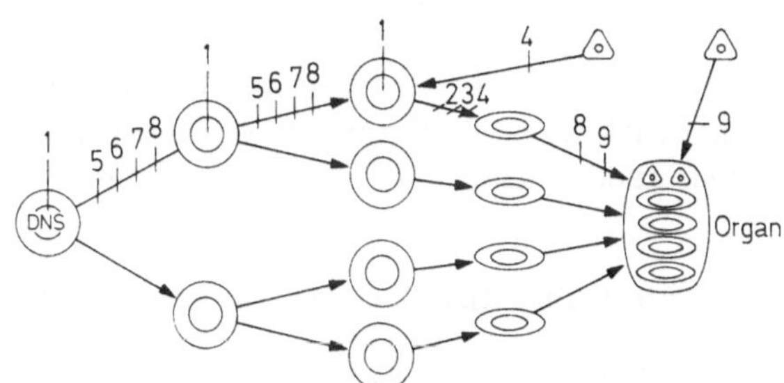

Abb. 39. Bildung eines Organs aus omnipotenten Stammzellen (rund) zu spezialisierten, differenzierten Zellen. 2 Typen von adulten, differenzierten Zellen (ovale und dreieckige) sind an der Bildung des adulten Organs beteiligt. Eingezeichnet sind einige mögliche Interventionen ionisierender Strahlen, die zu Entwicklungsstörungen führen. 1 = DNS mutiert, 2 = DNS → m RNS gestört, Transcription gestört, 3 = r RNS → Proteinsynthese, Translation gestört, 4 = Membranschädigungen, 5 = Hemmung und Stop der mitotischen Aktivität, 6 = Zelltod, 7 = Hemmung oder Induktion von Repressoren, 8 = Interzelluläre Kommunikationsstörungen, 9 = Wanderung gehemmt

An der Bildung des funktionstüchtigen Organs sind verschiedene Zelltypen beteiligt, wobei Bewegungsvorgänge (Zellwanderung etc.) zur endgültigen Struktur beitragen.

Verschiedene bereits bekannte biologische Strahlenwirkungen können nun in dieses komplexe Geschehen eingreifen.

In Abb. 39 sind einige der wichtigsten dargestellt, nämlich:

1. Mutation, falsche Geninformation
2. Störung der Bildung der m RNS (Transcriptionshemmung)
3. Bildung der r RNS, Eiweiß-Synthese (Translation gestört)
4. Membranschädigungen
5. Hemmung und Stop der mitotischen Aktivität
6. Zelltod
7. Hemmung oder Induktion von Repressoren
8. Interzelluläre Kommunikationsstörung
9. Hemmung von Zellwanderung

Die embryonale Schädigung kann durch singuläre oder multiple Ereignisse, die sich auf physikalisch-chemischer oder zellulärer Ebene abspielen, induziert werden.

Durch diese Strahleneffekte (zu denen sich noch etliche andere gesellen mögen) kann die endgültige Heranbildung eines adulten Phänotyp in den verschiedensten Phasen gestört werden, und in den meisten Fällen wird ein Zusammenwirken etlicher Faktoren die

Schädigung verursachen. Von einigen Strahlenbiologen wird allerdings des öfteren eine einzige Strahlenschädigung in den Vordergrund gesetzt, so z. B. die somatische Mutation, die für fast alle Mißbildungen verantwortlich gemacht wird. Daß somatische Mutationen Zellbezirke und Organe ändern und mißbilden, ist eine Tatsache, die sich besonders gut bei Mosaik-Lebewesen wie Drosophila ablesen läßt.

Aber auch bei der Maus (Russell u. Major, 1957) ließen sich nach der Bestrahlung von 10tägigen Embryonen, die heterozygot für 4 Fellfarbgene waren, Mosaik-Flecken im Fell nachweisen, die vermutlich auf rezessive somatische Mutationen in den prospektiven Pigmentzellen zurückgingen. Lejeune u. Mitarb. (1960) stellten bei in utero bestrahlten Kindern ein gehäuftes Auftreten von heterochromatischen Bezirken in der Iris fest, die sie auf somatische Mutationen zurückführten.

Nicht nur dominante Mutationen oder rezessive Mutationen in heterozygoten Genotypen können Organe und Zellbezirke phänotypisch ändern, sondern auch das Auftreten von somatischem Crossing over in heterozygoten Zellen. Die Größe des veränderten Bezirks hängt mit dem Alter der bestrahlten Stammzellen zusammen, je früher die Bestrahlung in der Entwicklung, um so größer das Areal.

Während in bestimmten Fällen Mutationen direkte Ursache einer Anomalie sein können, dürften allgemeine Entwicklungsschädigungen durch komplexes Geschehen verursacht werden, an denen sich auch Mutationsereignisse beteiligen können.

2. Erholungs- und Reparationsprozesse

Intrazelluläres Repairvermögen und Milieufaktoren, die eine Erholung begünstigen, spielen auch bei der strahlenbedingten Entwicklungsstörung eine entscheidende Rolle. Zudem sind besonders frühe Entwicklungsstadien fähig, Zellverluste zu kompensieren, Lücken zu schließen, indem die verschonten Zellen in vermehrter Proliferation den Verlust wettmachen. Dieses Regulationsvermögen zeichnet besonders die Zellen in der Blastogenese aus, aber auch spätere Stadien sind zur Kompensation fähig. Daß solche Repara-

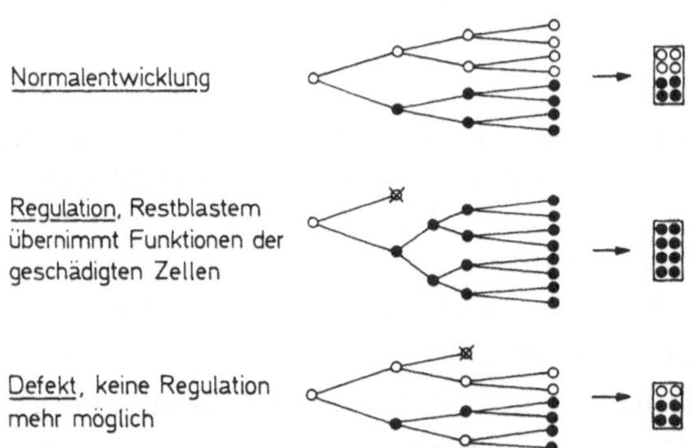

Abb. 40. Bedeutung der Reparatur von Blastem-Schäden durch proliferative Prozesse

turmechanismen stattfinden, beweisen u. a. die Mehrfachbildungen nach verschiedenen Noxen. In diesen Fällen wird sogar überkompensiert (Abb. 40).

Bei Drosophila lassen sich mit Hilfe der Induktion von somatischen Crossing over proliferative Reparationsprozesse direkt nachweisen (Schweizer, 1972). Bestrahlung von verschiedenaltrigen Genitalimaginalscheiben zeigen für die Mißbildung bestimmter Strukturen (Borstenausfälle) ein Sensibilitätsmaximum später Stadien (in 92stündigen Larven), während eine Bestrahlung jüngerer Stadien (in 68 h-Larven) kaum zu Schädigungen und sogar zu Mehrfachbildungen führte. Durch die Bestrahlung wird gleichzeitig somatisches Crossing over induziert, das sich in besonders markierten heterozygoten Zellen manifestiert, so daß der Anteil von einzelnen bestrahlten Zellen an der Bildung bestimmter Strukturen sich ablesen läßt.

Wird nun in einem bestrahlten jugendlichen Blastem, das Restblastem in vermehrter Proliferation den Schaden aufregulieren, dann wird die Nachkommenzahl der überlebenden Zelle gegenüber der Norm vermehrt sein. Eine Urzelle (markiert durch die Induktion des

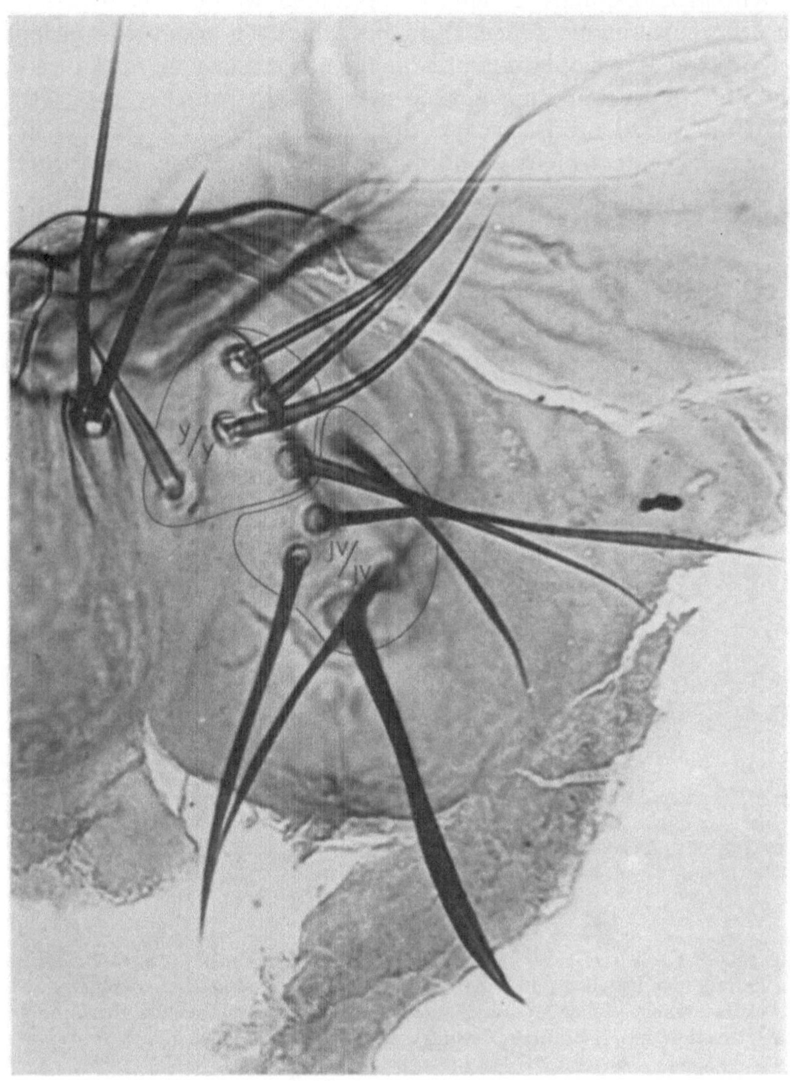

Abb. 41. Strahleninduzierte somatische Crossing over bei Drosophila melanogaster. Genetische Konstitution der bestrahlten somatischen Zellen = y + / + jv; y (yellow) = gelbe Borsten, jv (javelin) = Speerborsten. Durch Bestrahlung der für y und jv heterozygoten Zellen ereignet sich somatisches Crossing over und Zwillingsflecke mit yy- und jvjv-Genotyp. Die Borsten des homozygoten y/y sind gelb, des andern Flecks jv/jv und speerförmig, Bestrahlung 72stündiger Larven mit 4000 R. Rücktransplantation in 48stündigen Larven. (Nach SCHWEIZER, 1972)

somatischen Crossing overs) wird einen größeren Zellkomplex bilden. Tatsächlich entstanden aus bestrahlten Genitalscheiben in 68 h-Larven große Mosaikflecken, deren Größe mit zunehmender Dosis zunahmen (Abb. 41, 42).

Dabei dürfte die induzierte Reduktion des embryonalen Gewebes (Massenreduktion) die mitotische Aktivität der Überlebenden stimulieren, wie dies beim embryonalen Lungengewebe der Maus ALESCIO u. DI MICHELE (1968) nachweisen konnten.

3. Strahlensensibilität und Strahlenresistenz

Zusammenfassend kann ausgesagt werden, daß die Strahlenempfindlichkeit, resp. die Strahlenresistenz verschiedener Entwicklungs-Phasen und die besonderen Schädigungsmuster von mehreren Faktoren abhängig sind. Strahlenresistent sind Strukturen, die biochemisch die genaktive Phase abgeschlossen haben, wobei unter Genaktivität DNS-abhängige primäre makromolekulare Ereignisse verstanden werden. Die drastisch zunehmende Resistenz sich differenzierender Zellen kann u. a. dadurch gedeutet werden, daß biochemische Vorgänge automatisch ablaufen und die Geninformationen resp. ihre Folgeprodukte in genügender Zahl zur Verwendung vorliegen.

Ferner hängt die Strahlenresistenz von der mitotischen Aktivität der Zellen und Zellkomplexe ab. Ganz besonders wichtig sind die sog. kritischen Teilungen, die z. B. die Phase

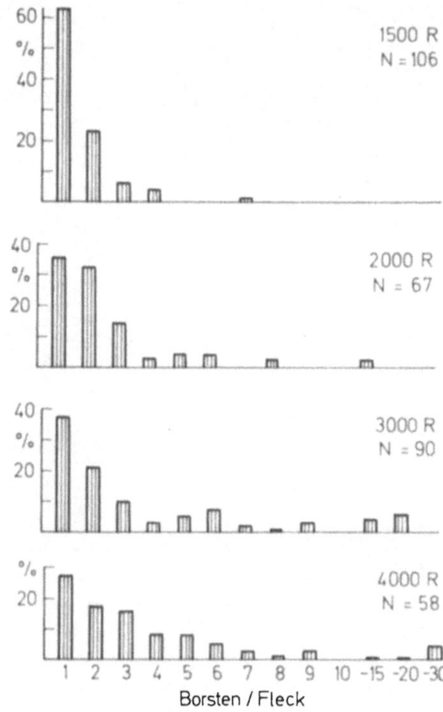

Abb. 42. Abhängigkeit der Größe der Mosaike von der Dosis nach Bestrahlung von 48 stündigen Larven mit 1 500–4000 R. Markierung der Urzellen mit Hilfe des induzierten somatischen Crossing over. Mit zunehmender Dosis nimmt die Häufigkeit großer Mosaik-Bezirke zu, d.h. das Restblastem übernimmt in proliferativer Reparatur Funktion und Enddifferenzierung der geschädigten Zellen. (Nach Schweizer 1972)

der endgültigen Differenzierung unmittelbar einleiten. Vor der kritischen Teilung kann ein embryonales System sehr verletzlich, nach der Teilung resistent sein. Stillstand von Bewegungen, Abschluß von Zellwanderungen führen ebenfalls zu Strahlenresistenz, zusammen mit einer Unabhängigkeit von interzellulärer Kommunikation. Konsolidierung von Membranen dürfte ebenfalls Strahlenresistenz bedeuten.

Daneben aber bestimmen inter- und intrazelluläre Erholungsmechanismen die Strahlenresistenz und vor allem führt die Fähigkeit zu proliferativen Reparationsprozessen zu einer „Pseudo"-Strahlenresistenz, indem der induzierte Zellverlust durch Überlebende kompensiert wird. Je entfernter eine noch nicht differenzierte Zelle von der letzten kritischen Teilung steht, um so größer wird die Möglichkeit einer Kompensation. Bei Drosophila zeigten Rücktransplantationen älterer strahlengeschädigter Blasteme in jugendlicheren Stadien, daß tatsächlich Schäden durch die künstlich verlängerte Entwicklungsdauer kompensiert werden.

Es wird offenkundlich, daß die strahlenbedingten Entwicklungsstörungen zum größten Teil durch das Zusammenwirken vieler Faktoren bedingt werden. Ein Modell der Strahlenwirkung aufzustellen, wie es Hug u. Kellerer (1966) vornehmlich für zelluläre Effekte getan hatten, dürfte vorläufig auf größte Schwierigkeiten stoßen. Nur einige wenige Störungen lassen sich von primären Absorptionsereignissen ableiten.

Verschiedene in diesem Beitrag erwähnte Arbeiten sind dank der Unterstützung des Schweiz. Nationalfonds und der Hartmann-Müller-Stiftung durchgeführt worden, denen wir an dieser Stelle bestens danken.

Literatur

Alescio, T., di Michele, M.: Relationship of epithelial growth to mitotic rate in mouse embryonic lung developing in vitro. J. Embryol. exp. Morph. **19**, 227–237 (1968).

Ammon, J.: Zur Frage der Wirkungsweise einer radonhaltigen Atmosphäre auf embryonale Stadien von Drosophila melanogaster. Biophysik **2**, 29–41 (1964).

Aschenheim, E.: Schädigung einer menschlichen Frucht durch Röntgenstrahlen. Strahlentherapie **11**, 789–795 (1920).

Auerbach, R.: Effects of single and fractionated doses of x-rays on mouse embryos. Nature **177**, 574 (1956).

Baker, T. G.: The sensitivity of rat, monkey, and human oocytes to x-radiation in organ culture. Radiation biology of the fetal and juvenile mammal. Eds.: Sikov, M. R., Mahlum, D. D. Oak Ridge: USAEC 955–961, 1969.

— Beaumont, H. M.: Radiosensitivity of oogonia and oocytes in the foetal and neonatal monkey. Nature **214**, 981–983 (1967).

Bar, Boulle: zit. nach Job. et al. 1935: Amer. J. Anat. **56**, 97–117 (1935).

Basic, M., Weber, D.: Damage to the intrauterine fetus by roentgen rays. Strahlentherapie **99**, 628–634 (1956).

Beach, S. A., Dolphin, G. W.: A study of the relationship between X-ray dose delivered to the thyroids of children and the subsequent development of malignant tumours. Physics in Med. and Biol. **6**, 583–598 (1962).

Beaumont, H. M.: Changes in the radiosensitivity of the testis during foetal development. Int. J. Radiat. Biol. **2**, 247–256 (1960).

— Mandl, Anita, M.: A quantitative and cytological study of oogonia and oocytesin the foetal and neonatal rat. Proceedings of the Royal Society **155** (Series B), 557–579 (1962).

Bergonié, J., Tribondeau, L.: Action des rayons x sur le testicule. Arch. Elect. méd. **14**, 779, 823, 874, 911 (1906).

Bohn, G.: Influence des rayons du radium sur les animaux en voie de croissance. C. R. Acad. Sci. (Paris) **136**, 1012–1013 (1903).

Brent, R. L.: The effect of irradiation on the mammalian fetus. Endocrinology (Clinial Obstetrics and Gynecology) H/H, Fetal Physiology and Distress. Ed. Greenblatt, R. B., Montgomery, Th. L., 928–950, 1960.

Brent, R. L., McLaughlin, M. M.: The indirect effect of irradiation on embryonic development. I. Irradiation of the mother while shielding the embryonic site. Amer. J. Dis. Child. **100**, 94–102 (1960).

Brizzee, K. R., Jacobs, L. A., Bench, C. J.: Effects of fractionated x-irradiation of fetal cerebral hemisphere. Radiat. Res. **27**, 509–510 (1966).

Brunst, V. V.: Effects of ionizing radiation on the development of amphibians. The Quarterly Review of Biology **40**, 1–68 (1965).

Burckhard, G.: Über den Einfluß der Röntgenstrahlen auf den tierischen Organismus, insbesondere auf die Gravidität. Volkmanns klin. Vortr. **404** (Gyn. 150), 469–480 (1905).

Butler, E. G.: The effects of radium and x-rays on embryonic development. Biol. effects radiat. **1**, 389–410 (1936).

Cheeseman, E. A., Walby, A. L.: Intra-uterine irradiation and iris heterochromia. Ann. Hum. Genet. Lond. **27**, 23–29 (1963).

Clapp, N. K.: 50 LD (24 hours) observations in the chick embryo after exposure to x-rays. Radiat. Res. **22**, 457–462 (1964).

— Histopathologic changes in the kidney of the chick embryo following x-irradiation. Radiat. Res. **25**, 180 (1965).

— Kienholz, E. W.: Radioprotection in chick embryos from hens fed zinc. Radiat. Res. Abstr. **27**, 511 (1966).

Clark, D. E.: Association of irradiation with cancer of the thyroid in children and adolescents. J.A.M.A. **159**, 1007–1009 (1955).

Conti, E. A., Patton, G. D., Conti, J. E., Hempelmann, L. H.: Present health of children given x-ray treatment to the anterior mediastinum in infancy. Radiology **74**, 386–391 (1960).

Cooke, J. P.: Low-level chronic gamma irradiation as a factor in audiogenic seizures of mice. Radiat. Res. **20**, 298–302 (1963).

— Brown, S. O., Krise, G. M.: Prenatal chronic gamma irradiation and audiogenic seizures in rats. Experimental Neurology **9**, 243–248 (1964).

Cooper, G. W., van Dyke, J. G., Nickson, J. J., Laughlin, J. S.: The relative biological efficiency of 20-mev electrons and 25 o-ekvp x-rays as measured in the 12-day-old chick embryo. Radiat. Res. **16**, 686–691 (1962).

Court-Brown, W. M., Doll, R., Hill, A. B.: Incidence of leukaemia after exposure to diagnostic radiation in utero. Brit. Med. J. **11**, 1539–1545 (1960).

Cowen, D., Geller, L. M.: Long-term phatological effects of prenatal x-irradiation on the central nervous system of the rat. J. Neuropath. Exp. Neurol. **19**, 488–527 (1960).

Crowther, J. A.: An analysis of some observations on the action of x-rays on drosophila eggs. Brit. J. Radiol. **23**, 292 (1927).

Czerniak, P., Soferman, N., Chajchik, S.: Development of a thyrotoxic fetus in the uterus of an euthyroid mother. Radiation biology of the fetal and juvenile mammal. Eds.: Sikov, M. R., Mahlum, D. D. Oak Ridge: USAEC 63–71, 1969.

D'Agostino, A. N., Brizzee, K. R.: Radiation necrosis and repair in rat fetal cerebral hemisphere. Arch. Neurol. **15**, 615–628 (1966).

D'Amato, C. J., Hicks, S. P.: Effects of low levels of ionizing radiation on the developing cerebral cortex of the rat. Neurology (Minneapolis) **15**, 1104–1116 (1965).

Dekaban, A. S.: Effects of x-radiation on mouse fetus during gestation emphasis on distribution of cerebral lesions, part II. J. nucl. Med. **10**, 68–77 (1969).

de Nobele et Lams: Action des rayons Roentgen sur l'évolution de la grossesse et le développement du foetus. Bull. Acad. roy. Méd. Belg. **5**, 66–82 (1925). Deutsch: Strahlentherapie 25, 702–707 (1927).

de Vellis, J., Schjeide, O. A.: Time-dependence of the effect of x-irradiation on the formation of glycerol phosphate dehydrogenase and other dehydrogenases in the developing rat brain. Biochem. J. **107**, 259 (1968).

— — Effects of ionizing radiation on the biochemical differentiation of the rat brain. Radiation biology of the fetal and juvenile mammal. Eds.: Sikov, M. R., Mahlum, D. D. Oak Ridge: USAEC 857–875, 1969.

— — Clemente, C. D.: Protein synthesis and enzymic patterns in the developing brain following head x-irradiation of newborn rats. J. of Neurochemistry **14**, 499–511 (1967).

Dolphin, G. W., Beach, S. A.: The relationship between radiation dose delivered to the thyroids of children and the subsequent development of malignant tumours. Health Physics **9**, 1385–1390 (1963).

Duffy, B., Fitzgerald, P. J.: Thyroid cancer in childhood and adolescence: a report on 28 cases. Cancer **3**, 1018–1032 (1950).

Duplan, J. F.: Effet de l'irradiation x sur la fonction hémopoiétique du foie foetal de la souris. Nouv. Rev. franc. Hémat. **3**, 121–132 (1963).

Dyer, N. C., Brill, A. B.: Fetal radiation dose from mate nally administered 59 Fe and 131 I. Radiation biology of the fetal and juvenile mammal. Eds.: Sikov, M. R., Mahlum, D. D. Oak Ridge: USAEC 73–88, 1969.

Erickson, B. H., Murphree, R. L., Andrews, J. F.: Effects of prenatal gamma irradiation on the germ cells of the male pig. Radiat. Res. **20**, 640–648 (1963).

Ershoff, B. H., Bavetta, L. A.: Potentiating effects of prenatal x-irradiation on dental caries in the rat. Proc. Soc. exp. Biol. and Med. **97**, 202–205 (1958).

Fellner, O. O., Neumann, F.: Der Einfluß der Röntgenstrahlen auf die Eierstöcke trächtiger Kaninchen und auf die Trächtigkeit. Z. Heilk. **28**, 162–202 (1907).

Finsinger, F. X.: Abtötungs- und Mutationsraten nach Röntgenbestrahlung frisch abgelegter Drosophila-Eier in verschiedenen Sauerstoffkonzentrationen. Promotionsarbeit. Zürich: Leemann AG 1964.

Fliedner, T. M., Haas, R. J., Bohne, F., Harriss, E. B.: Radiation effects produced in pregnant rats and their offspring by continuous infusion of tritiated Thymidine. Radiation biology of the fetal and juvenile mammal. Eds.: Sikov, M. R., Mahlum, D. D. Oak Ridge: USAEC 263–282, 1969.

Ford, D. D., Paterson, J. C. S., Trueting, W. L.: Fetal exposure to diagnostic x-rays and leukemia and other malignant diseases in childhood. J. nat. Cancer Inst. **22**, 1093–1104 (1959).

Forsberg, J. G., Kaellen, B.: Cell death during embryogenesis. Rev. roum. d'Embryologie et de Cytologie, Série d'Embryol. **5**, 91–102 (1968).

Försterling, K.: Wachstumsstörungen infolge von Röntgenisierung. Verh. dtsch. Röntgenges. **3**, 126–128 (1907).

Friedrich, O.: Histologische Untersuchung eines intrauterin mit Röntgenstrahlen bestrahlten menschlichen Fötus. Z. Röntgenk. **12**, 404–412 (1910).

Frilley, M., Raynaud, A.: Destruction des ébauches des reins des embryons de souris âgés de 14 jours, par irradiation in utero, au moyen des rayons x. C. R. Soc. Biol. (Paris) **140**, 962–964 (1946).

Fritz-Niggli, Hedi: Erste biologische Versuche mit dem 31 MeV-Betatron. Arch. Klaus-Stift. Vererb.-Forsch. **26**, 454–459 (1951).

— Biologische Analyse der Strahlenschädigung von Drosophila-Eiern durch 180 kV-Röntgenstrahlen und ultraharte 31 MeV-Strahlen. Naturwissenschaften **39**, 485–486 (1952a).

— Quantitative und qualitative Analyse der Röntgenschädigung im Drosophila-Versuch. Fortschr. Röntgenstr. **76**, 218–254 (1952b).

— Biologische Versuche mit dem 31 MeV-Betatron. Fortschr. Röntgenstr. **80**, 28–38 (1954).

— Vergleichende Analyse der Strahlenschädigung von Drosophila-Eiern mit 180 keV und 31 MeV. Fortschr. Röntgenstr. **83**, 178–200 (1955).

— Die unterschiedliche biologische Wirkung von 30 MeV-Elektronen, 31 MeV-Röntgenstrahlen und 180 keV-Röntgenstrahlen. Betatron- und Telekobalttherapie, Internat. Symp. 1957, 113–130. Heidelberg: Springer 1958a.

— Strahlenchimären und Parabiose. Strahlentherapie **106**, 378–390 (1958b).

— Strahlenbiologie. Stuttgart: Georg Thieme 1959.

— Allgemeine Strahlenbiologie. Handbuch der allg. Pathologie Bd. 10. Heidelberg: Springer 1–126, 1960.

— Die Bedeutung des Repairsystems für die relative biologische Wirksamkeit von Strahlen verschiedener Qualität; eine Zwei-System-Theorie. Strahlentherapie **135/2**, 202–212 (1968).

— Diener, E., Schleuss, P.: Sauerstoffeffekt nach konventioneller Röntgen- und hochenergetischer

Elektronen-Bestrahlung bei einer Strahlenmodifikation (Phänokopie). Biophysik **1**, 51–59 (1963).

FRITZ-NIGGLI, HEDI, MICHEL, CH.: Chemical sensitization of the damaging effects on embryos produced by low radiation doses: the role of energy metabolism and immediate repair. Radiation Protection and Sensitization, Eds: MOROSON, H. L., QUINTILIANI, M. London: Taylor & Francis Ltd., 311–317, 1970.

— — Sensibilisierung der Strahlenschädigung von Rattenembryonen durch Demethylchlortetracyclin (Ledermycin). ATKE **18**, 105–108 (1971).

— SCHINZ,H.R.: Biologische Wirksamkeit von 30 MeV-Elektronen in Abhängigkeit von der Gewebetiefe und im Vergleich mit 180 keV- und 31 MeV-Photonen. Strahlentherapie **115**, 379–393 (1961).

— — Biologische Wirksamkeit von 30 meV-Elektronen in Abhängigkeit von der Gewebetiefe und im Vergleich mit 180 keV- und 31 MeV-Photonen. II. Letalitätstest an vierstündigen Drosophila-Embryonen. Strahlentherapie **118**, 503–517 (1962).

FURCHTGOTT, E., ECHOLS, M.: Activity and emotionality in pre- and neonatally x-irradiated rats. J. comp. physiol. Psychol. **51**, 541–545 (1958).

— MURPHREE, R. L., PACE, H. B., DEES, J. W.: Mating activity in fetally irradiated male swine and rats. Psychol. Rev. **5**, 545–548 (1959).

GARLAND, L. H.: Cancer of the thyroid and previous irradiation.Surg.Gynec.Obstet. **112**,564–566(1961).

GLASSER, O., MAUTZ, F. R.: Studies on the effect of Roentgen rays and gamma rays upon the eggs of Drosophila melanogaster. Amer. J. Roentgenol. **29**, 815 (1933).

GLOCKER, R.: Röntgen- und Radiumphysik für Mediziner. Stuttgart: Georg Thieme 1949.

GRAHAM, T. M., MARKS, A., ERSHOFF, B. H.: Effects of prenatal x-irradiation on discrimination learning in the rat. Proc. Soc. exp. Biol (N. Y.) **100**, 78–83 (1959).

GRIEM, M. L., MEWISSEN, D. J., MEIER, P., DOBBEN, G. D.: Analysis of the morbidity and mortality of children irradiated in fetal life (II). Radiation biology of the fetal and juvenile mammal, Eds.: SIKOV, M. R., MAHLUM, D. D. Oak Ridge: USAEC 651–659, 1969.

GROSSMANN, ANNEMARIE: Über die Wirkung der Röntgenstrahlen auf die gesamte Mitoseaktivität der Xenopuslarve nach verschiedenen Zeitabschnitten. Diss. Oncologia **8**, 259–272 (1955).

HADORN, E.: Letalfaktoren. Stuttgart: Georg Thieme 1955.

— Differenzierungsleistungen wiederholt fragmentierter Teilstücke männlicher Genitalscheiben von Drosophila melanogaster nach Kultur in vivo. Develop. Biol. **7**, 617–629 (1963).

— Konstanz, Wechsel und Typus der Determination und Differenzierung in Zellen aus männlichen Genitalscheiben von Drosophila melanogaster nach Dauerkultur in vivo. Develop. Biol. **13**, 424–509 (1966).

HAMILTON, W. J., BOYD, J. D., MOSSMAN, H. W.: Human embryology (prenatal development of form and function). Cambridge: W. Heffer & Sons Limited, 1962.

HANFORD, J. M., QUIMBY, E. H., FRANTZ, V. K.: Cancer arising many years after radiation therapy, incidence after irradiation of benign lesions in the neck. J. Am. Med. Assoc. **181**, 404–410 (1962).

HANSARD, S. L.: Transplacental movement and maternal-fetal organ accretion rates of selected radiominerals in gravid cattle, sheep, and swine. Radiation biology of the fetal and juvenile mammal, Eds:. SIKOV, M. R., MAHLUM, D. D. Oak Ridge: USAEC 9–23, 1969.

HANSON, F. B.: The effects of x-rays on the albino rat. Anat. Rec. **24**, 415 (1923).

HAVIN, E., OFTEDAL, P.: Radiation sensitivity of Drosophila embryos in relation to age, in air and in nitrogen. Int. J. Rad. Biol. **14**, 149–160 (1968).

HAZZARD, D. G., BUDD, R. A.: Effect of in utero x irradiation on the peripheral blood of the newborn rat. Radiation biology of the fetal and juvenile mammal, Eds.: SIKOV, M. R., MAHLUM, D. D. Oak Ridge: USAEC 357–364, 1969.

HEMPELMANN, L. H.: Epidemiological studies of leukemia in persons exposed to ionizing radiation. Cancer Res. **20**, 18–27 (1960).

— PIFER, J. W., BURKE, G. J., TERRY, R., AMES, W. R.: Neoplasms in persons treated with x-rays in infancy for thymic enlargement. J. nat. Cancer Inst. **38**, 317–341 (1967).

HENNEBERG, B.: Normentafel zur Entwicklungsgeschichte der Wanderratte. Normentafeln zur Entwicklungsgeschichte der Wirbeltiere. Jena: Verlag G. Fischer, Heft 15, 1–162 (1937).

HERTWIG, G.: Radiumbestrahlung unbefruchteter Froscheier und ihre Entwicklung nach Befruchtung mit normalem Samen. Arch. mikr. Anat. **77**, 165–209 (1911).

HERTWIG, O.: Die Radiumkrankheit tierischer Keimzellen. Ein Beitrag zur experimentellen Zeugungs- und Vererbungslehre. Arch. mikr. Anat. **77**, 1– 164 (1911).

HERTWIG, P.: Partielle Keimesschädigung durch Radium und Röntgenstrahlen. Handbuch der Vererbungswissenschaft Bd. 3. Berlin: Gebrüder nervous Bornträger, 1–48, 1927.

HICKS, S. P.: Some effects of ionizing radiation and metabolic inhibition on the developing mammalian nervous system. J. Pediat. **40**, 489–513 (1952).

— Developmental malformation produced by radiation. Amer. J. Roentgenol. **69**, 272–293 (1953).

— The effects of ionizing radiation, certain hormones, and radiomimetic drugs on the developing nervous system. J. cell. comp. Physiol. **43**, Suppl. 1, 151–178 (1954).

— Some aspects of developmental neurology: A review. Cancer Res. **17**, 251–265 (1957).

— Radiation as an experimental tool in mammalian developmental neurology. Physiol. Rev. **38**, 337–356 (1958).

— D'AMATO, C. J.: Effects of radiation on the developing embryo and fetus. Progr. in Gynecology **4**, 58–74 (1963).

— — Effects of ionizing radiation on mammalian development, Advances in Teratology Vol. I. London: Logos Press Ltd. 196–264, 1966.

— — LOWE, M. J.: The development of the mammalian nervous system: I. Malformations of the brain, especially the cerebral cortex, induced in rats by radiation, II. Some mechanism of the malformations of the cortex. J. comp. Neurol. **113**, 435–469 (1959).

Hicks, S. P., Brown, Barbara L., D'Amato, C. J.: Regeneration and malformation in the nervous system, eye, and mesenchyme of the mammalian embryo after radiation injury. Amer. J. Path. **33/1**, 459–481 (1957).

Horikawa, M., Sugahara, T.: Studies on the effects of Radiation on Living Cells in Tissue Culture: I. Radiosensitivity of various imaginal discs and organs in larvae of Drosophila melanogaster. Radiat. Res. **12**, 266–275 (1960).

Horváth, J., Horváth, F., Juhász, E., Urbányi, L.: Über die Strahlenschädigung wachsender Knochen. Strahlentherapie **118**, 462–478 (1962).

Hug, O.: Die akuten Allgemeinrekationen bei Ganz- und Teilkörperbestrahlung. Strahlenbiologie, Strahlentherapie, Nuklearmedizin und Krebsforschung, Ergebnisse 1952–1958, Eds.: Schinz, H. R., Holthusen, H., Langendorff, H., Rajewsky, B., Schubert, G., Stuttgart: G. Thieme, 581–662, 1959.

— Kellerer, A. M.: Stochastik der Strahlenwirkung. Berlin: Springer 1966.

Humphrey, R. M., Sinclair, W. K.: The relative biological effectiveness of 22-mevp x-rays cobalt-60 gamma rays, and 200-kvcp x-rays: VI. Determined by lethality in the 4-day chick embryo. Radiat. Res. **16**, 384–393 (1962).

Hupp, E. W., Brown, S. O., Austin, J. W.: Continuous and acute irradiation effects on developing animals. Radiation biology of the fetal and juvenile mammal. Eds.: Sikov, M. R., Mahlum, D. D. Oak Ridge: USAEC 589–600, 1969.

— Pace, H. B., Furchtgott, E., Murphree, R. L.: Effect of fetal irradiation on mating activity in male rats. Psychological Reports **7**, 289–294 (1960), Southern Universities Press 1960.

ICRP-PUBLICATION: Radiosensitivity and spatial distribution of dose. Radiation Protection **14**. London: Pergamon Press 1969.

Iinuma, T. A., Yashiro, S., Ishihara, T., Uchiyama, M., Nagai, T., Yamagata, N.: Estimation of internal dose in human fetus and newborn infants due to fallout cesium-137. Radiation biology of the fetal and juvenile mammal. Eds: Sikov, M. R., Mahlum, D. D. Oak Ridge: USAEC 105–116, 1969.

Jacobs, L. A., Brizzee, K. R.: Effects of total-body x-irradiation in single and fractionated doses on developing cerebral cortex in rat foetus. Nature **210**, 31–33 (1966).

Jacobsen, L.: Low-dose embryonic x-irradiation in mice and some seasonal effects in the perinatal period. Radiat. Res. **25**, 611–625 (1965).

— Radiation-induced effects in mouse foetuses. A preliminary report. Acta Radiol. Suppl. **254**, 82–86 (1966).

— Radiation-induced teratogenesis in relation to season and some features of reproduction biology. Radiation biology of the fetal and juvenile mammal. Eds.: Sikov, M. R., Mahlum, D. D. Oak Ridge: USAEC 229–242, 1969.

Job, T. T., Leibold, G. J., Fitzmaurice, H. A.: Biological effects of roentgen rays. Amer. J. Anat. **56**, 97–117 (1935).

Jüngling, O., Langendorff, H.: Biologische Ausdosierung von Radiumpräparaten. Strahlentherapie **48**, 174 (1933).

Kaplan, H. S.: An evaluation of the somatic and genetic hazards of the medical uses of radiation. Amer. J. Roentgenol. **80**, 696–706 (1958).

Kaplan, S. J.: Learning behavior of rats given low level x-irradiation in utero on various gestation days. Response of the nervous system to ionizing radiation. New York: Academic Press 645–657, 1962a.

Kaplan, S. J.: Behavioural manifestations of the deleterious effects of prenatal x-irradiation. Effects of ionizing radiation on the nervous system. Vienna: IAEA 225–243, 1962b.

Kjeldsberg, H.: Radioaktiv bestraling og leukemifrekvens hos barn. T. norske Laegenforen **77**, 1052–1053 (1957).

von Klot, B.: Die Unterbrechung der Schwangerschaft durch Röntgenstrahlen. Inaugural-Dissertation, München 1911.

Knopp, J., Trautmann, J.: Zur Frage der Fruchtschädigung durch ionisierende Strahlen. Beitrag zur formalen Genese von postnataler Knickschwanzbildung bei der in utero bestrahlten weißen Maus. Strahlentherapie **117**, 161–190 (1962).

Kohn, H. I., Kallman, R. F.: Relative biological efficiency of 1000-kvp and 250-kvcp x-rays: V. Determinations based on the LD_{50} of the 4-day-old chick embryo. Radiat. Res. **5**, 710–714 (1956).

Konermann, G.: Die Wirkung fraktionierter Röntgenbestrahlung zu den einzelnen Hauptphasen der Embryonalentwicklung der Maus. Teil I, Strahlentherapie **136**, 336–348 (1968a); Teil II, Strahlentherapie **136**, 484–495 (1968b).

— Die Keimesentwicklung der Maus nach Einwirkung kontinuierlicher Co 60-Gammabestrahlung während der Blastogenese, der Organogenese und der Fetalperiode. Strahlentherapie **137**, 451–466 (1969).

— Erholungsvorgänge bei Mäuseembryonen nach fraktionierter Röntgenbestrahlung. Strahlentherapie **139**, 73–83 (1970).

Kosaka, S.: Der Einfluß der Röntgenstrahlen auf die Feten: III. Mitteilung. Untersuchungen an weißen Ratten. Zbl. ges. Radiol. **6**, 538–539 (1929a). IV. Mitteilung. Untersuchungen an Meerschweinchen. Zbl. ges. Radiol. **6**, 777 (1929b).

Kriegel, H.: Embryonalschäden durch Strahlenbelastung mit kleinen Dosen. Strahlenschutz in Forschung und Praxis. Eds.: Melching, H. J., Frik, W., Keim, H., Ladner, H. A., **5**, 105–115, Freiburg i./Br.: Verlag Rombach 1965.

— Langendorff, H.: Die Wirkung einer fraktionierten Röntgenbestrahlung auf die Embryonalentwicklung der Maus. Strahlentherapie **123**, 429–437 (1964).

— — Shibata, K.: Die Beeinflussung der Embryonalentwicklung bei der Maus nach einer Röntgenbestrahlung. Strahlentherapie **119**, 349–370 (1962).

— Reinhardt, S.: Effect of a fractionated x-irradiation on the development of the mammalian fetus.

Radiation biology of the fetal and juvenile mammal. Eds.: SIKOV, M. R., MAHLUM, D. D. Oak Ridge: USAEC 251–262, 1969.

KRIEGEL, H., SHIBATA, K.: Histologische Untersuchungen über die Beeinflussung der Embryonalentwicklung bei der Maus nach Röntgenbestrahlung: I. Mitteilung. Frühembryonale Veränderungen und Beeinflussung der Augenentwicklung. Strahlentherapie **124**, 573–587 (1964).

LANGENDORFF, H.: Zur Induktion von Spätschäden bei chronischer äußerer Einwirkung kleiner Strahlendosen. Strahlentherapie **122**, 1–15 (1963).

— Die Wirkung kleiner Strahlendosen und Dosisleistungen auf die Embryonalentwicklung von Säugetieren. Strahlentherapie **138**, 181–185 (1969).

— LANGENDORFF, M.: Untersuchungen über einen biologischen Strahlenschutz. 68. Mitteilung: Strahlenempfindlichkeit und Schutzwirkung des Serotonins bei Mäusen verschiedener Altersstufen. Strahlentherapie **129**, 425–431 (1966).

— SOMMERMEYER, K.: Strahlenwirkung auf Drosophilaeier, I. Fundamenta Radiol. **4**, 196–209 (1939).

— — Strahlenwirkung auf Drosophilaeier, II. Strahlentherapie **67**, 110 (1940).

LATOURETTE, H. B., HODGES, F. J.: Incidence of neoplasia after irradiation of thymic region. Amer. J. Roentgenol. **82**, 667–677 (1959).

LEJEUNE, J., TURPIN, R., RETHORE, M. O., MAYER, M.: Résultats d'une première enquête sur les effets somatiques de l'irradiation foeto-embryonnaire in utero (cas particulier des hétérochromies iriennes). Rev. franç. études clin. et biol. **5**, 982–989 (1960).

LENGFELLNER, K.: Über Versuche von Einwirkung der Röntgenstrahlen auf Ovarien und den schwangeren Uterus von Meerschweinchen. Münchner med. Wschr. **53**, 2147–2148 (1906).

LOKEN, M. K., BEISANG, A. A., JOHNSON, E. A., MOSSER, D. G.: The relative biological effectiveness of cobalt-60 gamma rays and 220-kvp x-rays on the viability of chicken eggs. Radiat. Res. **12**, 202–209 (1960).

MAISIN, H., DUNJIC, A., MALDAGUE, P., MAISIN, J.: Au sujet de la protection des embryons irradiés in utero, par la mercaptoéthylamine. Comptes Rendus Soc. Biologie (Paris) **149**, 1687–1690 (1955).

MACMAHON, B.: Prenatal x-ray exposure and childhood cancer. J. nat. Cancer Inst. **28**, 1173–1191 (1962).

MANDL, ANITA M.: The radiosensitivity of germ cells. Biological Reviews **39**, 288–371 (1964).

— BEAUMONT, H. M.: The differential radiosensitivity of oogonia and oocytes at different developmental stages. Effects of ionizing radiation on the reproductive system. Eds.: CARLSON, W. D., GASSNER, F. X. New York: 311–321, 1964.

MANOSEVITZ, M., ROSTKOWSKI, J. R.: The effects of neonatal irradiation on postnatal activity and elimination. Radiat. Res. **28**, 701–707 (1966).

MATTER, B. E.: Schwefelwasserstoff-Radiomimetikum und Strahlenschutzstoff bei Drosophila-Eiern. Radiol. clin. biol. **36**, 299–307 (1968).

— Zur Ursache der unterschiedlichen Strahlenempfindlichkeit verschiedener Kernteilungsstadien in der frühen Furchung von Drosophila melanogaster. Mutat. Res. **10**, 567–582 (1970).

MEYER, G. F.: Die Funktionsstrukturen des Y-Chromosoms in den Spermatocytenkernen von Drosophila hydei, D. neohydei, D. repleta und einigen anderen Drosophila-Arten. Chromosoma **14**, 207–255 (1963).

— Experimental studies on spermiogenesis in Drosophila. Genetics (Suppl.) **61**, 1 (1969).

MICHEL, CHR.: Chemische Sensibilisierung von Strahlenschädigungen bei Rattenembryonen. Arch. Klaus-Stift. Vererb.-Forsch. **43/44** (1969/1970).

— FRITZ-NIGGLI, HEDI: Chemische Sensibilisierung der Strahlenschädigung bei Rattenembryonen. Experientia **25**, 1135–1136 (1970).

MILLER, D. S.: Effects of low level radiation on audiogenic convulsive seizures in mice. Response of the nervous system to ionizing radiation. New York: Academic Press 513–531, 1962.

MILLER, R. W.: Delayed effects occurring within the first decade after exposure of young individuals to the Hiroshima atomic bomb. Pediatrics **18**, 1 (1956).

MINTZ, BEATRICE: Irradiation of primordial germ cells in the mouse embryo. Anat. Rec. **130**, 341 (1958).

— Continuity of the female germ cell line from embryo to adult. Arch. Anat. micr. Morph. exp. T **48 bis**, 155–172 (1959).

— Embryological phases of mammalian gametogenesis. J. of Cellular and Comparative Physiology **56**, Suppl. 1, 31–47 (1960).

MOLE, R. H.: Impairment of fertility by whole-body irradiation of female mice. Int. J. Rad. Biol. **1**, 107–114 (1959).

MOSIER, H. D., JANSONS, REGINA, A.: Effect of x-irradiation of selected areas of the head of the newborn rat on growth. Radiat. Res. **43**, 92–104 (1970).

MÜLLER, J. H.: Vergleichende Untersuchungen über die Wirksamkeit von 200 kV-Röntgen- und -Gammastrahlen auf die Puppen von Drosophila melanogaster. I. Bestimmung des „äquivalenten Röntgenwertes" für Gammastrahlen. II. Untersuchung über die Summation von Röntgen- und Gammastrahlen. Strahlentherapie **64**, 633–654 (1939).

MURAKAMI, U., KAMEYAMA, Y.: Effects of low-dose x-radiation on the mouse embryo. A. M. A. J. Dis. Child **96**, 272–277 (1958).

— — Vertebral malformation in the mouse foetus caused by x-radiation of the mother during pregnancy. J. Embryol. exp. Morph. **12**, 841–850 (1964).

— — NOGAMI, H.: Malformation of the extremity in the mouse foetus caused by x-radiation of the mother during pregnancy. J. Embryol. exp. Morph. **11**, 549–569 (1963).

MURPHREE, R. L., GRAVES, R. B.: Effect of dose rate on prenatally irradiated lambs. Radiation biology of the fetal an juvenile mammal. Eds.: SIKOV, M. R., MAHLUM, D. D. Oak Ridge: USAEC 243–250, 1969.

— PACE, H. B.: The effects of prenatal radiation on postnatal development in rats. Radiat. Res. **12**, 495–504 (1960).

MURRAY, R., HECKEL, P., HEMPELMANN, L. H.: Leukemia in children exposed to ionizing radiation. New Engl. J. Med. **261**, 585–589 (1959).

Nash, D. J., Napoleon, A., Le Etta Sprackling: Neonatal irradiation and postnatal behavior in mice. Radiat. Res. **41**, 594–601 (1970).

Naville, B.: Die Beeinflussung des Borstenmusters der Drosophila melanogaster durch Röntgenstrahlen (180 keV und 31 MeV). Oncologia **8**, 55–67 (1955).

Nelson, N. S., Stara, J. F., Hoar, R. M.: Concentration, distribution, and effects of radioiodine in embryonic guinea pigs during early organogenesis. Radiation biology of the fetal and juvenile mammal. Eds.: Sikov, M. R., Mahlum, D. D. Oak Ridge: USAEC 45–62, 1969.

Newcombe, H. B., McGregor, J. F.: Heritable effects of radiation on body weight in rats. Genetics **52**, 851–860 (1965).

Nilsson, A., Henricson, B.: The effect of 90 Sr on the ovaries of the fetal mouse. Radiation biology of the fetal and juvenile mammal. Eds.: Sikov, M. R., Mahlum, D. D. Oak Ridge: USAEC 313–324, 1969.

Ohzu, E.: Effects of low-dose x-irradiation on early mouse embryos. Radiat. Res. **26**, 107–113 (1965).

Okamoto, N., Ikeda, T., Satow, Y.: Effects of 14.1 MeV fast-neutron irradiation on the cardiovascular system of the rat fetus. Radiation biology of the fetal and juvenile mammal. Eds.: Sikov, M. R., Mahlum, D. D. Oak Ridge: USAEC 325–340, 1969.

Packard, Ch.: The measurement of quantitative biological effects of x-rays. J. Cancer Res. **10**, 319–339 (1926).

Palmer, R. F., Watson, C. R., Beamer, J. L.: Radiation dose to fetuses of miniature swine ingesting 90 Sr. Radiation biology of the fetal and juvenile mammal. Eds.: Sikov, M. R., Mahlum, D. D. Oak Ridge: USAEC 89–96, 1969.

Parkes, A. S.: On the occurrence of the oestrous cycle after x-ray sterilisation, Part. II. Irradiation at or before birth. Proc. roy. Soc. B. **101**, 71–95 (1927).

Pifer, J. W., Toyooka, E. T., Murray, R. W., Ames, W. R., Hempelmann, L. H.: Neoplasms in children treated with x-rays for thymic enlargement, I. Neoplasms and mortality. J. Nat. Canc. Inst. **31**, 1339–1356 (1963).

Piontkovski, I. A., Semagin, V. N.: Higher nervous activity of adult rats prenatally irradiated with small doses of x-rays. J. of Comparative and Physiological Psychology **56**, 748–751 (1963).

Plummer, G.: Anomalies occurring in children exposed in utero to the atomic bomb in Hiroshima. Pediatrics **10**, 687–693 (1952).

Polhemus, D. W., Koch, R.: Leukemia and medical radiation. Pediatrics **23**, 453–461 (1959).

Raventos, A., Horn, R. C., Ravdin, I. S.: Carcinoma of the thyroid gland in youth: a second look ten years later. J. clin. Endocr. Metab. **22**, 886–891 (1962).

Raynaud, A.: Effets des rayons-x sur l'embryon et le foetus des mammifères. Radiobiology appliquée, Vol. 2. Paris: Gauthier-Villars, 513–581, 1966.

Reincke, Ursula: Auswirkungen einer pränatalen Röntgenganzbestrahlung auf die Hämatopoese junger Ratten. Strahlentherapie **118**, 570–580 (1962).

Reincke, Ursula, Goldmann, Ehrentraud, Mellmann, J., Jesdinsky, H. J.: Zur altersabhängigen Strahlenempfindlichkeit weißer Ratten. III. Mitteilung: Bestimmung der LD 50 (30) während der Säuglingszeit und im Wachstumsalter. Strahlentherapie **136**, 349–359 (1968 a).

— Mellmann, J., Rother, Mechthildis: Zur altersbedingten Strahlenempfindlichkeit weißer Ratten. I. Bestrahlungsanordnung und Bestimmung der Gewebedosis. Strahlentherapie **129**, 622–628 (1966).

— Rother, Mechthildis, Andris, R.: Zur altersabhängigen Strahlemempfindlichkeit weißer Ratten. II. Bestimmung der LD 50 (30) im späten Fötalalter und kurz nach der Geburt. Strahlentherapie **136**, 93–99 (1968 b).

Rivers, T. M., Warkany, J., Fraser, F. C., Wilson, J. G., Matson, D. D., McIntosh, R.: National foundation conference on congenital malformations. J. chron. Dis. **10**, 83–151 (1959).

Roizin, L., Rugh, R., Kaufman, M. A.: Neuropathologic investigations of the x-irradiated embryo rat brain. J. Neuropath. exp. Neurol. **21**, 219–243 (1962).

Rosenthal, H. L.: Accumulation of environmental 90 Sr in teeth of children. Radiation biology of the fetal and juvenile mammal. Eds.: Sikov, M. R., Mahlum, D. D. Oak Ridge: USAEC 163–171, 1969.

Rugh, R.: Vertebrate Radiobiology: Embryology. Annual Review of Nuclear Science, **3**, 271–302 (1953).

— Symposium on effects of radiation and other deleterious agents on embryonic development: effects of ionizing radiation on amphibian development. J. cell. comp. Physiol. **43**, 39–75 (1954).

— Vertebrate Radiobiology (Embryology). Ann. Rev. nuclear Sci. **9**, 493–522 (1959).

— General Biology: Gametes, the developing embryo, and cellular differentiations. mechanisms in Radiobiology, Vol. 2. Eds.: Errera, M., Forssberg, A. 1–94. New York: Academic Press, 1960.

— Low levels of x-irradiation and the early mammalian embryo. Am. J. Roentgenol. Rad. Therapy and Nuclear Med. **87**, 559–566 (1962 a).

— Neurological sequelae to low-level x-irradiation of the developing embryo. Effects of ionizing radiation of the nervous system. Wien: IAEA 207–224, 1962 b.

— Major radiobiological concepts and effects of ionizing radiations on the embryo and fetus. Response of the Nervous System to Ionizing Radiation. Eds.: Haley, T., Snider, R. S. New York: Academic Press 3–26, 1962 c.

— The impact of ionizing radiations on the embryo and fetus. American Journal of Roentgenology. Radium Therapy and Nuclear Medicine **89**, 182–190 (1963 a).

— Ionizing radiations and the mammalian embryo. Acta radiol. **1**, 101–113 (1963 b).

— Why Radiobiology? Radiology **82**, 917–920 (1964).

— Chairman's Remarks. Radiation biology of the fetal and juvenile mammal. Eds.: Sikov, M. R., Mahlum, D. D. Oak Ridge: USAEC 381–391, 1969.

Rugh, R., Duhamel, L., Chandler, A., Varma, A.: Cataract development after embryonic and fetal x-irradiation. Radiat. Res. **22**, 519–534 (1964a).

— — Osborne, A. W., Varma, A.: Persistent stunting following x-irradiation of the fetus. Amer. J. Anat. **115**, 185–198 (1964b).

— — Somogyi, C., Chandler, A., Cooper, W. R., Smith, R., Stanford, G.: Sequelae of the LD/50 x-ray exposure of the preimplantation mouse embryo: Days 0.0 to 5.0. Biological Bulletin **131**, 145–154 (1966).

— Grupp, Erika: Response of the very early mouse embryo to low levels of ionizing radiations. J. Exp. Zool. **141**, 571–587 (1959a).

— — Exencephalia following x-irradiation of the preimplantation mammalian embryo. J. Neuropath. exp. Neurol. **18**, 468–481 (1959b).

— Skaredoff, L.: Radiation and radiomimetic chlorambucil and the fetal retina. Arch. Ophtalmology **74**, 382–393 (1965).

— van Dyke, R. H.: The fate and effect of x-irradiated neuroblasts (presumptive neural ectoderm) in an normal environment. J. Exp. Zool. **157**, 197–216 (1964).

— Wohlfromm, M.: X-irradiation sterilization of the pre-mature female mouse. Atompraxis **10**, 511–518 (1964).

— — Prenatal x-irradiation and postnatal mortality. Radiat. Res. **26**, 493–506 (1965).

Russell, Liane Brauch: The effects of radiation on mammalian prenatal development. Radiation Biology, Vol. 1. High Energy Radiation. Ed. Hollaender. London: McGraw-Hill Book Comp., Inc., 861–918, 1954.

— Hazards to the embryo and fetus from ionizing radiation. Internat. Conf. A/CONF. 8/P/77, USA, 1955.

— Effects of low-dose x-rays on embryonic development. Proc. Soc. exp. Biol. and Med. **95**, 174–178 (1957).

— Badgett, Susan, K., Saylors, Clyde, L.: Comparison of the effects of acute, continuous, and fractionated irradiation during embryonic development. Immediate and Low Level Effects of Ionizing Radiations. Ed.: Buzzati-Traverso, A. A. London: Taylor & Francis Ltd., 343–359, 1960.

— Major, Mary H.: Radiation-induced presumed somatic mutations in the house mouse. Genetics **42**, 161–175 (1957).

— Russell, W. L.: The effects of radiation on the preimplantation stages of the mouse embryo. Anat. Record **108**, 521 (1950a).

— — Changes in the relative proportions of different axial skeletal types within inbred strains of mice brought about by x-irradiation at critical stages in embryonic development. Genetics **35**, 689 (1950b).

— — An analysis of the changing radiation response of the developing mouse embryo. J. cell. comp. Physiol. **43**, 103–147 (1954).

Rutter, W. J., Kemp, J. D., Bradshaw, W. S., Clark, W. R., Ronzio, R. A., Sanders, T. G.: Regulation of specific protein synthesis in cyto-differentiation. J. cell. Physiol. **72** (Suppl. 1), 1–18 (1968).

Saenger, E. L., Silverman, F. N., Sterling, T. D., et al.: Neoplasia following therapeutic irradiation for benign conditions in childhood. Radiology **74**, 889–904 (1960).

Savković, N. V.: Effect of local irradiation of the head of 2-day-old rats: morphological and functional disorders and genetic changes in their progeny. Radiation biology of the fetal and juvenile mammal. Eds.: Sikov, M. R., Mahlum, D. D. Oak Ridge: USAEC 453–474, 1969.

Schaper, A.: Experimentelle Untersuchungen über den Einfluß der Radiumstrahlen und der Radiumemanation auf embryonale und regenerative Entwicklungsvorgänge. Anat. Anz. **25**, 298–314, 326–337 (1904).

Schinz, H. R.: Der Röntgenabort. Strahlentherapie **15**, 146–181 (1923).

— Fritz-Niggli, Hedi: Die Wirkung der Röntgenstrahlen und des cancerogenen Stoffes „Styryl" auf die Embryonalentwicklung. Strahlentherapie **90**, 345–352 (1953).

Schjeide, O. A., De Vellis, J., San Lin, R. I.: Changes in myelin elaborated following irradiation. 15th annual meeting of the Radiation Res. Society, San Juan, Puerto Rico, 1967.

— Yamazaki, J. N., Clemente, C. D., Ragan, N., Simons, Sue: Biochemical effects of irradiation in the brain of the neonatal rat. Response of the Nervous System to Ionizing Radiation. Eds.: Haley, T. J., Snider, R. S. New York: Academic Press, 95–108, 1962.

Schleuss, P.: Einfluß einer Kältebehandlung nach Bestrahlung auf den Ausfall der seta dorso centralis anterior bei Drosophila melanogaster „Sevelen" und „Berlin-Inzucht". Strahlentherapie **123**, 139 (1964).

Schmidt, H. E.: Zur Frage der Schwangerschaftsunterbrechung durch Röntgenbestrahlung. Dtsch. med. Wschr. **35**, 1064–1065 (1909).

Schneider-Minder, Annemarie: Cytologische Untersuchung der Embryonalentwicklung von Drosophila melanogaster nach Röntgenbestrahlung in frühen Entwicklungsstadien. Int. J. Radiat. Biol. **11**, 1–20 (1966).

Schneider, E., Schraub, A., Sattler, E. L., Waldvogel, H.: Untersuchungen über die Alphastrahlen-Empfindlichkeit embryonaler Stadien von Drosophila melanogaster. Strahlentherapie **137**, 119–121 (1969).

Schnetter, M., Langendorff, H., Schwaier, Anita: Strahlenschäden bei Urgeschlechtszellen von Mäusen. Strahlentherapie **135**, 337–345 (1968).

Schweizer, P.: Strahleninduzierte Hemmung der Entwicklung des männlichen Genitalsystems bei Drosophila melanogaster. Radiol. clin. biol. (Basel) **36**, 292–298 (1967).

— Wirkung von Röntgenstrahlen auf die Entwicklung der männlichen Genitalprimordien von Drosophila. Strahlentherapie **137**, 749–759 (1969).

— Wirkung von Röntgenstrahlen auf die Entwicklung der männlichen Genitalprimordien von Drosophila melanogaster und Untersuchung von Erholungsvorgängen durch Zellklon-Analyse. Biophysik **8**, 158–188 (1972).

Shively, J. N., Phemister, R. D., Epling, G. P.:

Radiation-induced cellular and subcellular morphologic alterations in the developing and in the mature mammalian eye. Radiation biology of the fetal and juvenile mammal. Eds.: Sikov, M. R., Mahlum, D. D. Oak Ridge: USAEC 493–510, 1969.

Sievert, R., Forssberg, A.: The time factor in the biological action of x-rays. Acta Radiol. 12, 535–551 (1931).

Sikov, M. R., Lofstrom, J. E.: Sensitization and recovery phenomena after embryonic irradiation. The American Journal of Roentgenology. Radium Therapy and Nuclear Medicine 85, 145–151 (1961).

— Mahlum, D. D.: Radiation biology of the fetal and juvenile mammal. Oak Ridge: USAEC, 1969.

Simpson, C. L., Hempelmann, L. H.: The association of tumors and roentgen-ray treatment of thorax in infancy. Cancer 10, 42–56 (1957).

— — Fuller, L. M.: Neoplasia in children treated with x-rays in infancy for thymic enlargement. Radiology 64, 840–845 (1955).

Snell, G. D.: Biology of the laboratory mouse. New York: Dover Publications, Inc. 1941.

Spiess, H., Mays, C. W.: Bone cancers induced by 224 Ra Th X in children and adults. Health Physics 19, 713–729 (1970).

Stearner, S., Phyllis, Christian, Emily, J. B.: Early radiation injury to the microcirculation: relation to mortality. Radiation biology of the fetal and juvenile mammal. Eds.: Sikov, M. R., Mahlum, D. D. Oak Ridge: USAEC 341–356, 1969.

Stewart, A. M.: Aetiology of childhood malignancies. Congenitally determined leukaemias. Brit. Med. J. 1, 452–460 (1961).

— Radiogenic cancers of childhood. Radiation biology of the fetal and juvenile mammal. Eds.: Sikov, M. R., Mahlum, D. D. Oak Ridge: USAEC 681–692, 1969.

Stewart, Alice, Hewitt, D.: Leukaemia incidence in children in relation to radiation exposure in early life. Current topics in radiation research Vol. 1. Eds.: Ebert, M., Howard, Alma. North Holland Publ. Comp., 221–253, 1965.

— Kneale, G. W.: Changes in the cancer risk associated with obstetric radiography. The Lancet 1, 104–106 (1968).

— Webb, Josefine, Giles, D., Hewitt, D.: Malignant disease in childhood and diagnostic irradiation in utero. The Lancet II, 447 (Preliminary Report) 1956.

— Webb, J., Hewitt, D.: A survey of childhood malignancies. Brit. Med. J. 1, 1495–1508 (1958).

Straub, C. P., Kahn, B., Wellman, H. N., Telles, N. C., Seltzer, R. A.: Retention of radionuclides by infants. I. Study techniques and error evaluation. Assessment of radioactivity in man, Vol. 2. Vienna: IAEA 345–362, 1964.

Suter, K.: Biologische Wirksamkeit von 100 keV- und 200 keV-Röntgenstrahlen, geprüft an der Puppenletalität von Drosophila melanogaster. Diplomarbeit Universität Zürich 1967.

Sutow, W. W., Conard, R. A.: The effects of fallout radiation on marshallese children. Radiation Biology of the fetal and juvenile mammal. Eds.: Sikov, M. R., Mahlum, D. D. Oak Ridge: 661–673, 1969.

Tacker, R. S., Furchtgott, E.: Low-level gamma irradiation and audiogenic seizures. Radiat. Res. 17, 614–618 (1962).

Takahashi, S., Kitabataki, T., Wakabayashi et al.: a statistical study on human cancer induced by medical exposure. To be published in Nippon Acta Radiologica. From: UN-Report 1966.

Todd P., Schroy, C. B., Schimmerling, W., Vosburgh, K.: Cellular effects of heavy charged particles, Cospar meeting, 10–24 may 1972, Madrid.

Toussey, S.: In discussion of a paper by E. C. Titus. J. adv. Therapy 23, 640 (1905).

Toyooka, E. T., Pifer, J. W., Crump, S. L., Dutton, A. M., Hempelmann, L. H.: Neoplasms in children treated with x-rays for thymic enlargement. II. Tumor incidence as a function of radiation factors. J. nat. Cancer Inst. 31, 1357–1377 (1963a). v. e. UN-document A/AC. 82/G/L. 891/Add. 1.

— — Hempelmann, L. H.: Neoplasms in children treated with x-rays for thymic enlargement. III. Clinical description of cases. J. nat. Cancer Inst. 31, 1379–1405 (1963b). v. e. UN-document AC. 82/G/L. 891/Add. 2.

Trautmann, J., Kollath, J., Munscheck, H.: Strahlenschäden des Mäuse-Embryos in der Frühschwangerschaft (Resorptionen, Wurfgrößen, Gewichte, Hirnmißbildungen). Strahlentherapie 133, 585–593 (1967).

Uhlmann, E. M.: Cancer of the thyroid and irradiation. J.A.M.A. 161, 504–507 (1956).

Ulrich, H.: A convenient method of collecting large numbers of Drosophila eggs homogeneous in age. Drosophila Information Service 27, 124 (1953).

— Wuergler, F. E.: Oxygen effect in newly laid Drosophila eggs. Second International Congress of Radiation Research, p. 187 (Abstract), Harrogate (England), 1962.

UNITED NATIONS REPORT: Scientific Committee on the effects of Atomic Radiation, General Assembly, Official Records:
— 17. Session, Suppl. No. 16 (A/5216) UN, N. Y. 1962.
— 19. Session, Suppl. No. 14 (A/5814) UN, N.Y. 1964.
— 21. Session, Suppl. No. 14 (A/6314) UN, N.Y. 1966.

Walker, S., Furchtgott, E.: Effects of prenatal x-irradiation on the acquisition extinction and discrimination of a classically conditioned response. Radiat. Res. 42, 120–128 (1970).

Warkany, J., Schraffenberger, E.: Congenital malformations induced in rats by roentgen rays: Skeletal changes in offspring following a single irradiation of the mother. Amer. J. Roentgenol. 57, 455–463 (1947).

Wegner, G.: Autoradiographische Untersuchungen des embryonalen DNS-Stoffwechsels nach einmaliger Röntgenganzbestrahlung der Wistarratte am 11. Graviditätstag mit 150 R. Z. ges. exp. Med. 139, 798–809 (1965).

— Zum Entstehungsmechanismus strahleninduzierter Gehirnmißbildungen bei der Ratte (Autoradiographische Untersuchungen). Strahlentherapie 138, 496–505 (1969).

— Mecking, H.: Autoradiographische Untersuchungen der DNS-Neubildung in Gehirnanlagen nach einmaliger Röntgenbestrahlung später Embryonal- und Fetalstadien der Ratte. Z. ges. exp. Med. **149**, 2–12 (1969).

WENDT, E.: Der Einfluß von Thyroxin und Methylenblau auf die indirekte Strahlenwirkung bei Hühnerembryonen. Atompraxis **10**, 1–5 (1964).

— Untersuchungen über die Wirkung von Röntgenstrahlen auf den Hühnerembryo. Ber. der Kernforschungsanlage Jülich Nr. 313, 1965.

— Beobachtungen über die Verminderung der Strahlenempfindlichkeit durch subletale Vorbestrahlungen bei Hühnerembryonen. Strahlentherapie **139**, 372–378 (1970).

— ZÖLLER, W.: Weitere Versuche zur Analyse des Distanzeffektes bei bestrahlten Hühnerembryonen. Jahresbericht der Kernforschungsanlage Jülich p. 45, 1965.

WERBOFF, J., GOODMAN, I., HAVLENA, U., SIKOV, M. R.: Effects of prenatal x-irradiation on motor performance in the rat. J. Amer. physiol. **201**, 703–706 (1961).

— HAVLENA, J., SIKOV, M. R.: Effects of prenatal x-irradiation on activity, emotionality and maze-learning ability in the rat. Radiat. Res. **16**, 441–452 (1962).

— — — Effects of prenatal x-irradiation on the behavioral development of the albino rat. Response of the nervous system to ionizing radiation. Ed.: HALEY, T. J., SNIDER, R. S. London: J. &. A. Churchill Ltd., 632–638, 1964.

WIDERÖE, R.: Physik und Technik der Megavoltbestrahlung. Handbuch Strahlenbiologie, Strahlentherapie, Nuklearmedizin und Krebsforschung, Ergebnisse 1952–1958. Stuttgart: Thieme, 289–360, 1959.

WILSON, E. H., ASPER, S. P.: The role of x-ray therapy to the neck region in the production of thyroid cancer in young people. A report of 37 cases. A.M.A., Archives of Internal Medicine **105**, 244–251 (1960).

WILSON, G. M., KILPATRICK, R., ECKERT, H., CURRAN, R. C., JEPSON, R. P., BLOMFIELD, G. W., MILLER, H.: Thyroid neoplasms following irradiation. Brit. Med. J. **II**, 929–934 (1958).

WILSON, J. G.: Differentiation and the reaction of rat embryos to radiation. J. cell comp. Physiol. **43** (Suppl. 1), 11–37 (1954).

WILSON, J. G., BRENT, R. L., JORDAN, H. C.: Neoplasia induced in rat embryos by roentgen irradiation. Cancer Res. **12**, 222–228 (1952).

— JORDAN, H. C., BRENT, R. L.: Effects of irradiation on embryonic development. II. X-rays on the ninth day of gestation in the rat. Amer. J. Anat. **92**, 153–187 (1953).

— KARR, J. W.: Difference in the effects of x-irradiation in rat embryos of different ages. Anat. Rec. **106**, 259–260 (1950).

— — Effects of irradiation on embryonic development. I. X-rays on the 10 th day of gestation in the rat. Amer. J. Anat. **88**, 1–33 (1951).

WINSHIP, T., ROSVOLL, R. V.: Childhood thyroid carcinoma. Cancer **14**, 734–743 (1961a).

— — A study of thyroid cancer in children. Amer. J. Surg. **102**, 747–752 (1961b).

WÜRGLER, F. E.: Modification of x-ray induced embryonic mortality by different anoxia conditions before and during irradiation of uncleaved D. melanogaster eggs. Drosophila Information Service **35**, 102–103 (1961).

— Mutational and cellular effects: Dose effect relations II. a) Experimental analysis of a linear dose effect curve resulting from x-irradiation of Drosophila eggs. Second International Congress of Radiation Research (Abstract). Harrogate, 199, 1962.

— Induced mutations and lethality in Drosophila after x-irradiation of meiotic and post-meiotic stages of the egg. Effects of radiation on meiotic systems. Wien: IAEA 43–62, 1968.

YAMAZAKI, J. N., WRIGHT, ST. W., WRIGHT, PH. M.: A study of the outcome of pregnancy in women exposed to the atomic bomb blast in Nagasaki. J. Cell. comp. Physiol. **43** (Suppl. 1), 319–328 (1954).

— BENNETT, L. R., CLEMENTE, C. D.: Behavioral and histologic effects of head irradiation in newborn rats. Response of the nervous system to ionizing radiation. New York: Academic Press, 59–73, 1962.

ZIMMER, K. G.: Zur biophysikalischen Analyse des Vorgangs der Tötung von Drosophilaeiern durch Strahlung. Biol. Zbl. **60**, 287 (1940).

G. The radiation syndromes*

By

E. P. Cronkite** and T. M. Fliedner***

With 9 figures

I. Introduction

Until 1945 the question of radiation syndromes produced by exposure of the whole body or portions of the body to penetrating or poorly penetrating radiations was of little consequence except to the practising radiologist. Following the use of nuclear bombs in Japan, the entire world became vitally concerned with the effects of whole body exposure to penetrating gamma radiation. Later, with the development of the atomic energy industries and the application of nuclear energy in the production of electric power, injuries from exposure to combined gamma and neutrons were seen following criticality accidents in the processing of fissionable materials and in accidents involving nuclear reactors. There have been several deaths, and in the survivors the question of late effects of radiation constitutes important medical-legal problems. These are not trivial problems. The questions of monetary rewards for fractures, burns and other injuries are well established in the courts. The question of rewards for a statistical possibility of getting a disease at some future date remains unanswered.

On March 1, 1954, the world was again forcibly reminded of the hazards of radiation in the modern world when a fall-out accident occurred following the experimental detonation of a thermonuclear device. The exposure of numerous native Marshallese and American military personnel to fission products involved both exposure to penetrating gamma radiation and exposure to superficial beta radiation from the fissionable materials that were in contact with the skin.

Thus, in view of the contemporary possible exposures of human beings to harmful amounts of radiation, one can set up a general classification of radiation injuries to be covered in this chapter.

1. Classification

Radiation injuries can be divided into two general categories, early and late injuries. The early type results from brief, intense exposure; the late type either from exposure to large single doses, or from prolonged exposures of lower intensity. In this chapter the following will be considered.

---

* Research performed at the Brookhaven National Laboratory under contract with the United States Atomic Energy Commission and at the Institut für Hämatologie Freiburg under contract with the Gesellschaft für Strahlenforschung mbH and the European Atomic Energy Community (EURATOM).

** Medical Department, Brookhaven National Laboratory, Upton, L. I., N.Y., USA.

*** Abteilung für Klinische Physiologie, Zentrum für Klinische Grundlagenforschung, Universität Ulm, Ulm (Donau).

a) The early consequences of short-term exposure

α) *From penetrating radiation*

α_1) *Whole body exposure*

The acute illness produced by total body irradiation may occur in man from exposure to gamma and/or neutron radiation from a detonated atomic bomb, high gamma exposure from fall-out from atomic bombs, from accidents with radioactive materials, nuclear power sources, or in radiotherapy either for malignancy or as a means of depressing antibody response preparatory to organ transplantation.

β_1) *Partial body or markedly inhomogeneous exposures*

An acute illness may result from partial body exposure to penetrating radiations as is commonly seen in therapeutic radiation for cancer, and might again be seen following exposure in shielded criticality accidents and from radiation sources in radar devices.

β) *From poorly penetrating radiations*

In this situation acute injury of the skin or other body integuments may result from beta ray exposures of the skin as may occur in contact with fall-out radiation from military or experimental use of nuclear bombs or from accidents involving handling of radioactive materials. This injury is primarily limited to the surface of the skin.

b) Long-term exposure

α) Again, this must be sub-divided under injuries from penetrating radiation and those from poorly penetrating radiation. From penetrating radiation one may develop the following late effects: blood dyscrasias, namely leukemia; an increase in degenerative diseases; shortening of the life span; an increase in the incidence of cancer in general; retardation of growth and development in children; an increased incidence of cataracts; impaired fertility; and, of course, genetic effects in gererations yet unborn. In this chapter the question of leukemia, shortening of the life span, the question of thyroid cancer, and retardation of growth and development in children will be considered briefly.

β) Poorly penetrating radiation primarily produces injury of the skin, and this will be considered only in respect to exposure to fall-out or contact with radioactive materials.

γ) *Absorption of radioactive materials*

This will be considered only briefly and in the context of absorption of fall-out materials in the event nuclear warfare, laboratory radiation accidents and the results of past absorption of radium and mesothorium.

II. Historical

Although the early history is well known, certain humorous and tragic aspects serve well to introduce the subject. In the early days there was some little apprehension concerning the newly found and mysterious rays. Unfortunately, the early fears were largely absurd and misdirected. Since they are rather humorous in the light of our knowledge today, it is of interest to refresh one's memory. Scarcely anyone seemed to realize that there might be biological dangers. Instead, the public was treated to imbecilities. The Pall Mall Gazette considered X-rays revoltingly indecent. Punch poked fun at Roentgen and advised him to work on spooks. A New Jersey legislature later was concerned about the use of X-rays in opera glasses. In London X-ray proof underwear was offered for sale. Today the following from Punch, January 1896, is quite comic:

"We are sick of Roentgen rays. It is now said that Mr. ADDISON has discovered a substance — tungstate of calcium is its repulsive name — which is potential, whatever that means, to the said rays. The consequence of which is that you can see other people's bones with the naked eye — on the revolting indecency there is no need to dwell. It would be best to burn the works on these rays, execute the discoverer and whelm all calcium tungstate into the ocean. Let the fish contemplate each other's bones if they like, but not us."

> Oh roentgen, then the news is true
> And not a trick or idle rumor
> That bids us each beware of you
> And of your graveyard humor
> We do not want, like Dr. Swift
> To take our flesh off and to pose in
> Our bones, or show each little rift
> And joint for you to poke your nose in.

— From PUNCH, January 25, 1896.

Ill effects were usually blamed on such things as ultraviolet from the Crookes tubes, platinum particles, cathode rays, electrostatic discharges, heat and so forth. It was soon noted that erythema was frequently seen involving the hands, arms and faces of people working with X-ray apparatus, but it appeared that this was considered of scarcely any more importance than sunburn. Thus, before long a tragic list of disastrous consequences began to unroll and many of the early workers appeared as victims, often fatally injured.

One of the early reports of superficial radiation injury is that of Dr. KASSABIAN, who wrote of X-rays as an irritant in 1900 and described his own case: "About five months ago the fingers, knuckles and dorsum of the left hand exhibited a general erythematous condition. This continued about a month; the itching became intense, the skin became tough, glossy, edematous and yellow." His condition became worse, and in 1903, he again wrote, "In order to effect a cure I have used every remedial agent mentioned in all the textbooks — but nothing seemed any good." In 1908 an area of ulceration showed malignant changes. In 1909, in spite of amputation, there were axillary metastases and death soon followed. This story with minor variations could be told of many others indeed.

BOND, FLIEDNER and ARCHAMBEAU (1965) quote HOLTHUSEN (1959) as saying of the 336 early fatalities ascribed to radiation exposure, 251 died from cancer induced by repeated radiation exposure of the skin, and 56 others died from blood dyscrasias such as anemia or leukemia. Of course, in this chapter we are more concerned with the depressive effects of radiation upon the blood forming tissues and the sequelae of prompt bone marrow depression or aplasia. The harmful effects of whole body irradiation on animals were documented early in the excellent studies of HEINECKE (1903 to 1905). Radiation hemorrhage was described by FERNAU et al. in 1913. FABRICIUS-MOLLER observed the relationship of the hemorrhagic diathesis from X-ray exposure in guinea-pigs to the depressed platelet count. In his classical initial study in 1922 he demonstrated that shielding of one leg by lead prevented the depression in platelets and thus the bleeding. Later ALLEN et al. (1948) ascribed radiation hemorrhage to heparinemia. This has been subsequently refuted by JACKSON et al. (1952) and CRONKITE and BRECHER (1952). In subsequent studies CRONKITE et al. (1952) have demonstrated that the radiation hemorrhage can be prevented solely by platelet transfusions. The importance of infection in pancytopenic states has long been appreciated by clinicians. The specific importance of infection in radiation pancytopenia was emphasized by the studies of MILLER et al. (1951) in their classic studies on the incidence of bacteriemia in mice subjected to total body X-irradiation and the improved survival rate by the treatment if mice with antibiotics after exposure. The critical role of the bone marrow in the development of radiation injury was emphasized by a series of studies by JACOBSON et al. (1949—1950) in which it was shown that shielding of the spleen accelerated the regeneration of the bone marrow. Lorenz, Congdon and Uphoff (1952) demonstrated conclusively that transplantation of bone marrow would significantly increase the survival of irradiated animals. There followed a long period of time in which it was argued whether the beneficial effect of splenic shielding, injection of splenic and bone marrow cell suspensions was due to transplantation or a humoral stimulation of host cells. It is now clear that the beneficial effect is predominantly due to transplantation of hemopoietic stem cells. The huge literature on this subject has conclusively demonstrated the role of transplantation of the hemopoietic stem cells in protection against radiation injury. It is not clear when the hemopoietic effects of whole body irradiation were first observed in human beings. However, an early detailed report on the effects upon depression of the blood in human beings without blood dyscrasias by Roentgen ray therapy was published by Minot and Spurling in 1924. A classical review of the effects of radiation on normal tissues of man and animals covering the period prior to 1942 was published by Warren (1942).

The explosion of the nuclear bombs at Hiroshima and Nagasaki produced human radiation pancytopenia on a massive scale. Everything that had been observed in animals was abundantly observed in the Japanese. These observations are reported by Oughterson and Warren (1956). The potential hazardous effects of fall-out radiation were emphasized following the accidental exposure of a large number of human beings to fall-out radiation on March 1, 1954. The effects of radiation from fall-out in human beings is described by Cronkite, Bond and Dunham (1956).

Two other aspects of radiation injury are also of importance. First, there is the question of severe injury to the nervous system either by whole body irradiation or exposure of the head alone. This produces a rapidly fatal syndrome amply described by Gerstner. — This has subsequently been observed in part in human beings exposed to huge amounts of radiation in criticality accidents (Paxton et al., 1958). Another means by which animals can be killed is the acute intestinal radiation death that was initially described by Quastler et al. (1951).

III. Definitions of human exposure

A semantic problem exists. In the past various descriptive terms have been used to describe the types of exposure, such as acute, chronic, protracted, repetitive and continuous exposure, again sub-divided into various categories on the basis of the type of radiation, its energy or other specific characteristic. Much ambiguity existed in the use of the preceding approach. Exposure conditions should therefore be defined according to the method proposed by the United States National Academy of Sciences, National Research Council Sub-Committee on Hematologic Effects of Radiation. These are:

1. Short-term exposure

Short-term includes total body exposures to radiation over a short period of time (e. g. in nuclear warfare, nuclear reactor or accelerator accidents) and exposure of limited but substantial body areas when the radiation is delivered either as a single dose or fractionated over a few days or weeks (e. g. in therapeutic radiation, diagnostic radiology or tracer or therepeutic use of radioactive isotopes). In considering short-term exposure, a dose greater than 50 rads is defined arbitrarily as a high dose, less than 50 rads a low dose. These definitions are for prospective and retrospective classification and study of radiation effects.

2. Long-term exposure

Long-term exposure refers to continued or repeated exposure to radiation over long periods of time — months or years. The possibility of such exposure is greatest in certain occupational groups and in persons having body burdens of radioactive isotopes with relatively long, effective half-lives. X-ray examinations repeated frequently over a long time were also considered long-term exposure, as are exposures to cosmic radiation, naturally occurring radioactive isotopes, and world wide fall-out.

Although the total dose of radiation is important in long-term exposure, it is more useful and convenient to indicate the degree of exposure in terms of dose per unit of time, usually cumulative dose per week.

1. Minimal weekly dose is less than 100 millirads.
2. Low weekly dose is 100 to 1000 millirads.
3. High weekly dose is greater than 1000 millirads.

The minimal dose is less than the maximum permissible dose (MPD) recommended most recently by the International Commission on Radiological Protection and the National Committee on Radiation Protection and Measurements. The dividing line between low and high dose corresponds to the first MPD recommendations of these groups in effect between 1936 and 1948.

IV. Effect of physical factors on radiation response of mammals

Superficially it would appear unnecessary to discuss the role of physical factors upon the response of the whole body to irradiation. However, problems are involved which are significantly different from those encountered in radiation therapy. Clearly the preferable measure of the amount of radiation is the absorbed dose (rad). This unit, as is well-known, is completely independent of the energy and type radiation. However, the expression of biological effects from whole body exposure or large parts of the body in terms of the rad is not completely satisfactory. The distribution of dose in respect to time and space is also a major determinant of response. It is necessary to know whether the dose is essentially instanteneous, fractionated, short-term or long exposure, because distribution of dose with time also significantly influences the biological response. As will be pointed out later in this chapter, the response, recovery and resistance to subsequent doses of radiation is significantly altered by prior exposure to radiation. Further, the spatial distribution of the absorbed dose anatomically in depth within an organ significantly influences the biological response of the whole animal. The quality of the radiation is another meaningful parameter to be considered. High energy protons, alpha, beta, gamma, X-ray and neutrons, all have properties which may influence the quantitative response per unit of absorbed dose. Generally the relative biological effectiveness (RBE) per rad is a function of the linear energy transfer (LET). However, with very high proton energies and stripped nuclei, as may be encountered in space flight, one must also consider the possible influence of spalation. A problem to which there is no satisfactory solution is the anatomic inhomogeneities in the distribution of absorbed dose within the body. With most conditions of human exposure the relative homogeneity of absorbed dose will be the exception rather than the rule. It is fair to say that after accidental exposures true homogeneity in absorbed dose has never been seen. The problem on unpredictable inhomogeneity in dose raises an important practical difficulty in assessing the hazard of accidental exposure of man. The inhomogeneities simply cannot be described by any single meaningful value for the dose distribution received by the critical organs within the body, hence the biological response is the key to management, not a physical dose estimate.

Although exposure due to absorbed radioisotopes will rarely be observed, it does constitute a problem of difficult dosimetry. For practical purposes, it is almost impossible to measure directly the dose from internal emitters. Therefore, it is necessary to rely on calculations of the dose from estimations of the average concentration of the radioisotope involved and the biological half-life of the substance. From the preceding two, one can easily calculate the absorbed dose providing that there is uniformity in the deposition of the material within all of the organs involved. Since the distribution is always inhomogeneous, one can only estimate the average dose and rarely, if ever, is one able to determine at a microscopic anatomical level the range in dose from the minimum to the maximum, nor the influence of relatively uninjured tissues upon contiguous severely injured tissues.

The concept of the integral dose is very useful in radiotherapy. This refers to the total energy absorbed within the object. This unit of measurement of radiation is of very limited or no value considering the effects of radiation on the whole body of man or animals since it has been shown that gram roentgens or integral dose cannot be used to predict the degree of biological effect. This arises from the fact that the biological effect depends not only on the total dose absorbed, but also on the portion of the body receiving the dose, the relative homogeneity of the absorbed dose and, of most importance, the influence of non-irradiated or lesser irradiated hemopoietic tissue upon the recovery of the more heavily

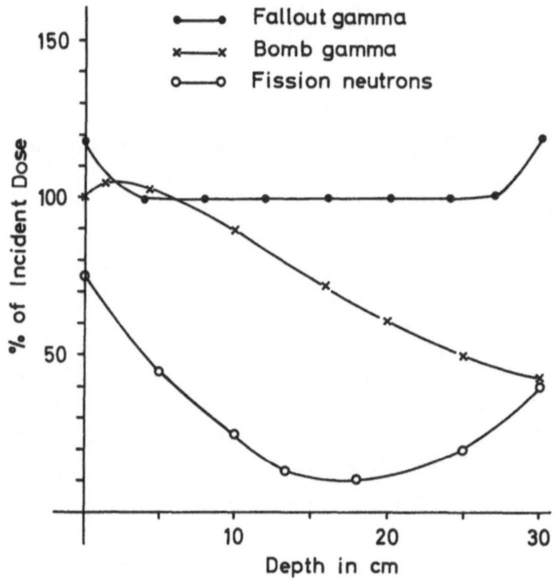

Fig. 1. Depth dose curves for three different types of radiation to which human being might be exposed

irradiated hemopoietic tissue. A very useful reference for a more technical and sophisticated discussion is the symposium on Physical Factors and their Modification of Biological Effects of Radiation (1964).

The relative biological effectiveness is analogous to the relative potency ratio for drugs in pharmacology. In radiation studies, a standard radiation, usually X-rays of prescribed characteristics, is used. The ratio of the dose in rads of X-rays to produce the same degree of biological effect to the dose of the test radiation is known as the RBE of the test radiation. When the targets are very small, one can obtain a precise estimate of the absorbed energy in each case and have a very scientific evaluation of the relative biological effectiveness. However, when one has larger targets, such as man, in a radiation field the problem is complicated by serious inhomogeneities in the distribution of absorbed dose. This is illustrated in Fig. 1. It will be noted that in the case of a diffuse field of gamma radiation coming from all directions at the individual, the surface dose is somewhat higher than the air dose due to back scatter, and the dose throughout the body is relatively uniform until the other side of the body is reached, at which point the dose again increases due to scatter and low energy components that are present. In the case of the penetrating initial bomb gamma radiation there is a very small increase in the absorbed dose in the first few centimetres, and then an attenuation with the unilateral irradiation, so that the exit dose is about 45 % of the entrance dose. In the case of fission neutrons, the first collision, absorbed dose at the surface is about 75 % of the incident dose. The absorbed dose is rapidly attenuated, reaching a low value of about 10 % of the entrance dose at 18 cm. Although the radiation is unidirectional, it is greater on the back surface of the body due to scattering from the air and entrance into the back side. These three examples of whole body exposure have three completely unique and different depth dose curves. Clearly, per rad of exposure there is a significantly different biological effect.

V. Qualitative and quantitative effects of radiation upon mammals

1. Dose mortality responses

Dose mortality responses have been used for decades to express the effect of radiation and to observe factors that modify the radiation response. All of the dose mortality curves have a characteristic sigmoidal appearance, as expressed in Fig. 2b. Generally, in respect to mammals most of the mortality is completed by 30 days and the mortality is scored at

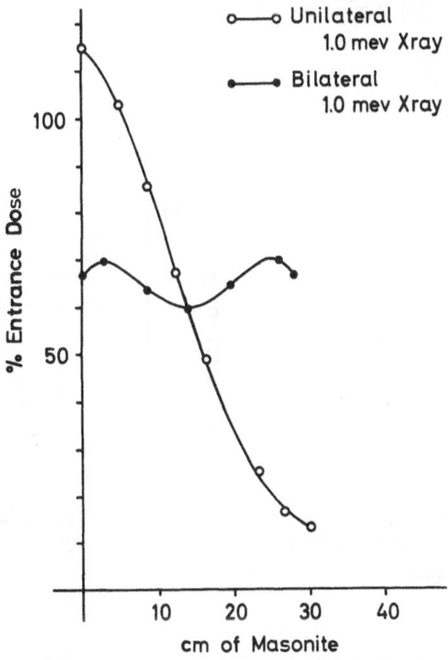

Fig. 2a. Depth dose curves for 1.0 MeV X-ray when all of the radiation is delivered to one side of the phantom and when half of the dose is delivered to both sides (bilateral)

this time. Note that the upper and lower portions of the curves are very poorly defined. It is theoretically impossible to ascertain the dose below which no individual would die or above which all individuals will die. However, these are in practice ascertained by exposure of large numbers of animals in the vicinity of zero and 100 % mortality. However, for comparative purposes the midpoint of the curve is used to characterize the entire dose response relationship. This dose is referred to as a median lethal dose, and is ordinarily abbreviated LD_{50}. It is a derived dose and does not mean that an individual animal exposed to this dose will necessarily live or die. It indicates only that in a very large population one can expect half of those exposed to die within the stated time. Usually with mammals the range in dose between no deaths and 100 % mortality is of the order of 200 to 400 rads. Theoretically the lower end of the curve approaches the abscissa asymptotically and does not cross it until zero dose. In actuality it crosses the abscissa at a relatively high dose, creating effectively a threshold dose for mortality. A very useful means of expressing the dose mortality is to plot it on probability paper, by which the sigmoidal curve is transformed into a line. Then one determines the slope of the curve and the LD_{50} to characterise the whole system.

a) Influence of depth dose pattern upon dose mortality

This problem has been studied by numerous investigators, and is illustrated from the work of Tullis *et al*. In Fig. 2a, the depth dose patterns of 2 MeV X-ray is plotted for a unilateral exposure and the depth dose pattern for bilateral exposure to the same total amount of radiation. In Fig. 2b the dose mortality curves for each type of exposure are

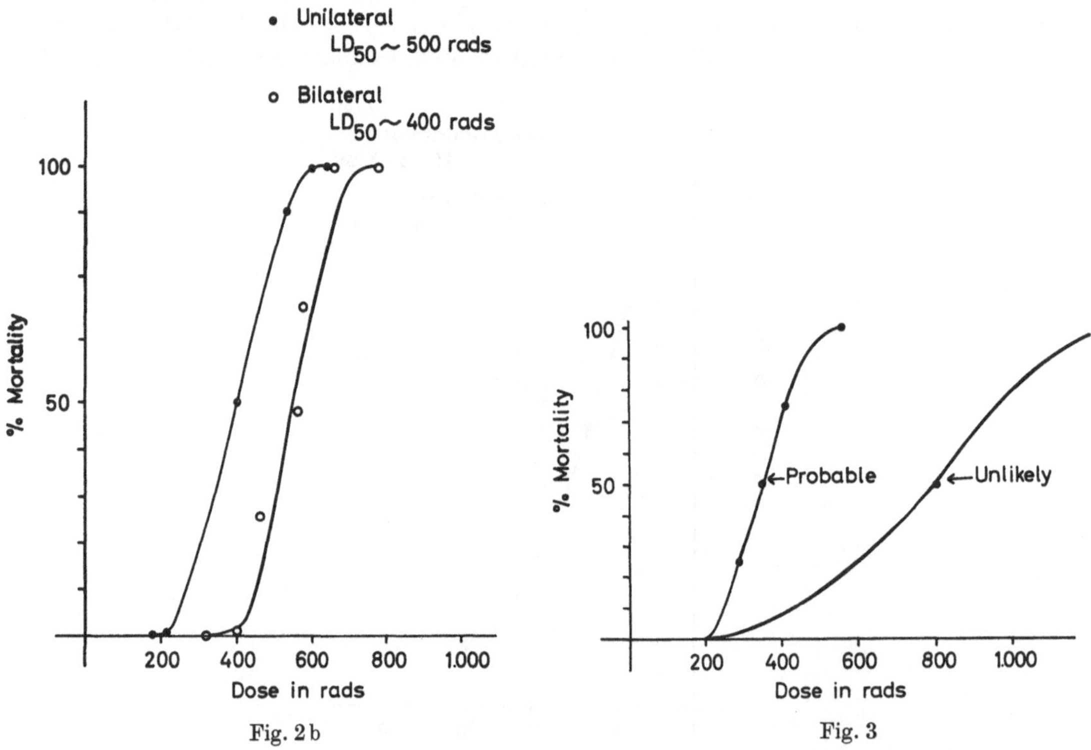

Fig. 2b. X-ray dose mortality curves in swine when the radiation is given unilaterally or bilaterally showing the different killing effect of the same amounts of radiation when given so that depth dose is different as in Fig. 2b

Fig. 3. Schematic presentation of dose mortality curves for man indicating the most likely human response and an unlikely response. See text for rationale

plotted. Note that the estimated LD_{50} for the unilateral exposure is 500 rads and for the bilateral exposure is 400 rads. Furthermore, with bilateral exposure animals commence to die at approximately 200 rads exposure, whereas with the unilateral exposure deaths were not observed until 400 rads. Similar studies using very low energy radiation have shown that one can go to many thousands rads of unilateral exposure without any acute mortality, although serious skin injury is produced.

Earlier in this chapter, Fig. 1, the depth dose curves for different types of radiation to which human beings might be exposed were plotted. Other types of accidents in which human beings may be involved are criticality accidents that consist of a combination of mixed gamma and neutrons, and here there are also inhomogeneities in the absorbed dose. However, the influence of the inhomogeneities in depth dose illustrates in Fig. 2a and b cannot be extrapolated for purposes of prediction to other types of exposure.

b) The median lethal dose for human beings

There are certain general facts that are pertinent to attempting to answer this vital problem. First, as shown by BOND and ROBERTSON (1957), all small mammals have a relatively high LD_{50} when expressed as mid-line absorbed dose, and all large mammals (swine, burros, dogs etc.) have a relatively low LD_{50}. The slopes of most dose mortality curves are roughly the same. In general the LD_{50} for large mammals is of the order of 250 rads for X-rays with uniform dose distribution, and that for small species is approximately double this value. Some investigators have considered primates to be more closely related to human beings. However, the LD_{50} of monkeys is similar to the small mammals rather than the large mammals. Large animals exposed under silimar geometric conditions have rather uniform dose mortality curves, perhaps partly because large animals, unlike small animals, provide their own constant maximum scatter of radiation. The experimental determination of LD_{50} is usually based on animals of a clearly defined genetic background, age and sex. In general females are a little more resistant to radiation than males. When one is concerned with human populations, one is dealing with a spectrum of ages, sex and races.

Knowledge about the LD_{50} for man is clearly needed, both for evaluation of radiation accidents and from the standpoint of planning possible whole body radiation therapy for specific purposes. CRONKITE and BOND (1960) have approached the problem of estimation of the LD_{50} for man in the absence of any therapy for the injury in the following manner. A large number of human beings were exposed to 175 rads of gamma radiation from fall-out. As illustrated in Fig. 1, the depth dose below 1 cm is quite uniform from this type of radiation. These individuals had a severe hematologic depression and were on the verge of developing purpura and had a severe granulocytopenia. From data on animals, it can be assumed that an increment of 50 to 100 rads probably would have placed these exposed human beings into the lethal dose range. One can therefore anchor the lower end of the dose mortality curve for man in the vicinity of 200 rads. The next assumption asserts that the slope of the dose mortality curve for large animals and for human beings will be almost the same. With the preceding two assertions one can draw a dose mortality curve through the lower anchor with the slope similar to that of dogs, and obtains an estimated LD_{50} of about 360 rads for man. This is illustrated in Fig. 3. Other human data are consistent with this estimate. One out of five of the Yugoslavs exposed to about 350 rads in a nuclear accident died. The hematologic response of the individuals exposed to approximately 300 rads in another criticality accident was significantly greater than that in the Marshallese. Some of these individuals developed purpura, and the depression in their granulocyte count was also greater than in the Marshallese. Furthermore, extensive studies on clinical radiation therapy exposing the entire body has resulted in a severe hematologic depression of individual with metastatic cancer after exposure to 200 rads, and an occasional death in these diseased individuals has been observed (MILLER *et al.*, 1957). The dose of radiation received by the Japanese in Hiroshima and Nagasaki is under continuing study by the joint Japanese-American Atomic Bomb Casualty Commission. With further refinements of their estimates, one may be able to ascertain the dose to a sufficient number of human beings to get a rather precise estimate of the human LD_{50} exposed to this type of radiation and given no therapy.

2. Cell renewal systems — the basis of understanding radiation effects in the mammal

A very sophisticated discussion of the role of disturbance in cellular kinetics of cell renewal systems as a basis for mammalian radiation lethality has been published by Bond, Fliedner and Archambeau (1965). For our purposes in this chapter only a brief summary of the different types of organ systems within the body and their characteristics are needed. Mammalian organs consist of three general types on the basis of cell production. First, there are those organs in which there is essentially no production of new cells from cessation of growth to death. Examples of this type are the brain, cardiac muscle, skeletal muscle and the collagenous tissues. Second, there is the class of organs in which there is the capa-

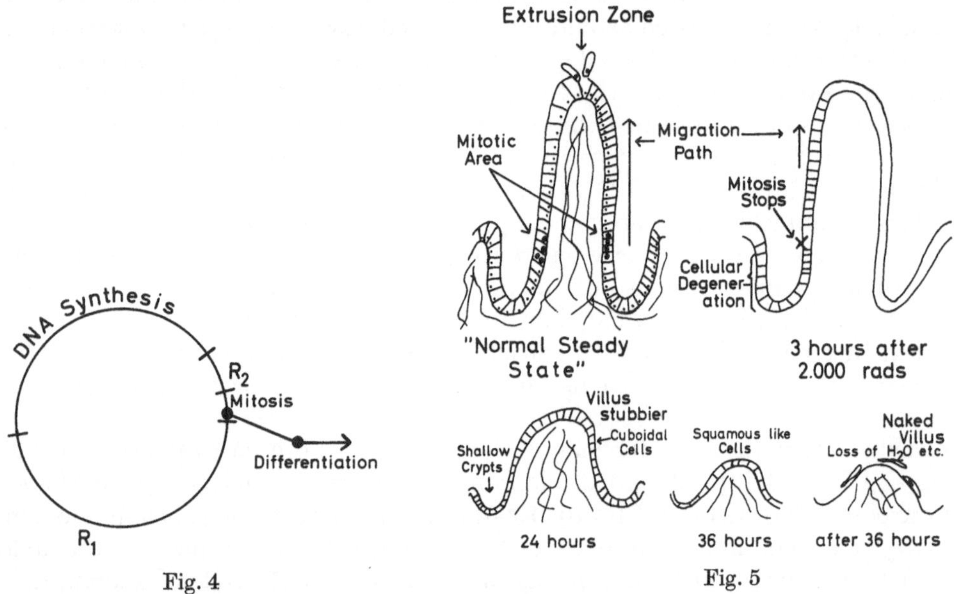

Fig. 4. Schematic of cell generative cycle indicating the different time phases between successive mitoses which have radiobiological significance

Fig. 5. Schematic presentation of cell renewal in the small intestinal epithelium and the effects of 2000 rads of radiation upon proliferation of bowel epithelium leading to the gastrointestinal syndrome

bility of repair following injury, such as the liver, fibrous tissue, periosteum and blood vessels. Normally there is practically no cell turnover in these tissues, but upon injury the remaining tissues delete can burst into cell proliferation and repair the loss of cells or the separation of the tissues. Third, there are those tissues which are in a steady state of cell proliferation, in which the production rate equals the death rate of cells. Examples of these tissues are the epithelium of gastrointestinal tract, the skin, and the hemopoietic tissues. Cell proliferation is maintained in each of these cell lines by "the stem cell" which has the properties of self-replication and differentiation to exogenous influences that direct it down specific cellular lines. The cell cycle for a stem cell is illustrated in Fig. 4. The cell cycle consists of the following periods commencing after mitosis. First there is a rest period (R_1) prior to the commencement of DNA synthesis or chromosomal replication. During the rest period, of course, other metabolic processes may be very active. During DNA synthesis the chromosomes are replicated to preserve the genetic code. Also during this time there is a substantial amount of RNA synthesis. Upon the completion of the replication of chromosomes there is another rest period termed R_2 prior to mitosis. When cells divide they can be assumed to be possessed of equal genetic capabilities. However, random influences impinge upon the stem cell pool and on an average induce half of the progeny to differentiate in order to maintain the steady state equilibrium of the stem cell pool and specific cell lines. One can measure the relative rate of cell proliferation by counting the number of mitotic figures, of cells that are in DNA synthesis, or by stopping mitosis at metaphase by stathokinetik agents such as colchicine, and observing the number of cells that accumulate in metaphase. For a more detailed description of the characteristics of cell renewal systems one is referred to BOND, FLIEDNER and ARCHAMBEAU (1965). The cell cycle is of particular importance in radiation effects, since the sensitivity of cells varies with the stage of the cell cycle. In general, cells are most sensitive to radiation during the mitotic, the late R_1 or early phases of DNA synthesis. In tissue culture after exposure to the same amount of radiation, 4 times the number of cells survive if exposed during late DNA synthesis, and most of the R_1 and R_2 periods as compared to exposure in synchronized cultures during the early DNA synthetic phases. Mitosis is also very sensitive, with about half as many cells surviving when exposed in mitosis as compared to late R_2 and early DNA synthesis. A simple cell renewal system for the gastrointestinal tract is illustrated in Fig. 5. Normally there is active proliferation of cells in the neck of the crypts of LIEBERKUHN. Cells migrate out the villus in an orderly fashion and are extruded at the tip. In the normal steady state it takes approximately 36 hours for cells to migrate to the tip of the villus.

Since the kinetics of cell proliferation in hemopoietic systems are described in considerable detail by BOND et al. (1965), only a pertinent summary will be presented herein.

a) Erythropoiesis

Stem cells are acted upon by erythropoietin to direct them down the erythropoietic pathway. The approximate generation time of erythropoietic precursors in the proliferating compartment is 24 hours in man. The total transit time from the stem cell to the reticulocyte is approximately 4 to 7 days. The mean life span of human red cells is 120 days. The steady state equilibrium is maintained by a feedback system that is sensitive to oxygen tension and perhaps the total mass of the red cells in the peripheral blood. Decreased oxygen tension increases the levels of erythropoietin which induces more stem cells down the erythropoietic pathway.

b) Granulocytopoiesis

Granulocytopoiesis is also reasonable well understood from the standpoint of the time involved in the flow of cells from the stem cell to the mature granulocyte in the peripheral blood (CRONKITE et al., 1960; FLIEDNER et al., 1965; CRONKITE and FLIEDNER, 1965). The factors that are responsible for the differentiation of stem cells into granulopoietic precursors are not known. The transit time for cells from the myeloblast to the first nondividing cell in man is about 6 days. The transit time through the maturing pool, that is from the metamyelocyte to the granulocyte, is 3 to 4 days. The total transit time from the stem cell to the mature granulocyte in the marrow is 9 to 10 days. Granulocytes disappear from the blood in a random fashion with a half-time of 6.6 hours (ATHENS et al., 1961). The random process is terminated by a senescent process at 30 hours (FLIEDNER et al., 1964).

c) Platelets

These are produced by the megakaryocytic system. The total transit time from the most immature megakaryocyte in the marrow to platelets in the peripheral blood has been described as lying between 4 and 10 days (man, CRONKITE et al., 1961; rat, EBBE and STOHLMAN, 1965). The life span in the peripheral blood of man is of the order of 10 days (LEEKSMA et al., 1956). Platelets are lost from the blood by a random process, and also have a finite life span that terminates the random loss.

d) Lymphopoietic tissues

The lymphocyte producing organs constitute a unique system. The lymphocytes may conveniently be divided into two classes on the basis of their size (Sipe *et al.*, 1966). The smaller class with volumes of 150 to 350 cubic microns is further sub-divided into two classes on the basis of life span. One is very short-lived and, at least in animal experiments, presumably is thymic in origin (Everett *et al.*, 1965). The other has a much longer life span, with some cells living in excess of a year (Robinson *et al.*, 1965). The larger lymphocytes have a relatively short life span measured in hours to a few days. A fraction of the small blood lymphocytes have a unique migration pathway from the blood through the postcapillary venules at the medullary cortical junction (Gowans *et al.*, 1963).

These cells migrate through this venule into the substance of the lymph node, and then recycle out through the efferent lymph and into the blood. This recycling accounts for a very large fraction of the lymphocytic output of the lymphatic ducts. Since lymphocytes have these widely varying life spans and migration patterns but are not unique in respect to morphology, it is difficult to study the kinetics of these cells adequately and separately with available techniques.

e) Bone marrow

The bone marrow is the site of the formation of red cells, granulocytes and platelets. Normally in man all myelopoiesis takes place within the cavities of bones. Thus it is contained within rigid walls which do not permit volume changes. The hemopoietic bone marrow is composed principally of three cell renewal systems: erythropoietic, granulopoietic and thrombopoietic. The parameters of cell proliferation for these have been listed earlier. All three cell renewal systems are distributed throughout the extra-sinusoidal marrow spaces. Normally one never sees erythroblasts outside the marrow parenchyma. In addition, it is rare to see granulocytic cells more immature than the band in the peripheral circulation. It is possible that the mature granulocyte spends some of its life span outside the blood vessels. However, there is no clear-cut evidence for re-entry of ganulocytes into the blood vessels. There is no question that lymphocytes spend a substantial fraction of their life span outside the blood vessels as described under the recycling of lymphocytes earlier. The vascular structure of the bone marrow has been studied extensively. It is a closed system with a series of unique arteries and veins connected by a very fragile sinusoidal system which receives blood from the arterial capillaries and from which blood empties into the venous side (Fliedner *et al.*, 1956). It is believed that cells enter the blood stream through the sinusoidal endothelium.

3. General cytological and histological effects of radiation on tissue

Radiation can produce immediate cellular death, suppression of the motility of cells, suppression of reproduction of cells, the induction of anomalies of cellular division, a retardation of growth and, in the germ cells, mutations. Whether mutations occur also in somatic cells maintaining the cellular renewal systems is open to question. What is observed microscopically in mammalian tissues following exposure to radiation is a function of the time after irradiation, the dose of radiation, and the tissue involved. The sequence of microscopic effects in the so-called radiosensitive tissues (those tissues that are continually renewing themselves) is different from that observed in the radioresistant tissues (tissues, the cells of which are rarely replaced if at all from the time of birth, or after cessation of growth).

There is nothing specific about the observable microscopic effects of radiation. There is no special type of necrobiosis. The cells degenerate according to the manner of the particular cellular type or tissue. The picture associated with cellular death in histopathology has been described as coagulative necrosis, liquefactive necrosis, granular degeneration, and cloudy parenchymatous degeneration. These phenomena are observed after irradiation. In a general sense, the more radioresistant types of tissues, for example, skeletal muscle, osseous, adipose, and glandular tissue, when exposed to sufficient amounts of radiation, undergo coagulative necrosis. It takes very large amounts of radiation to produce these changes. Although the cells themselves are still recognized, they undergo necrosis characterized by poor staining, disappearance of cellular detail, homogeneous appearing cytoplasm and disintegration of the nuclei. If the doses of radiation are sufficiently high, the necrosis will be visible in a matter of hours. The injured tissue may be absorbed very slowly following localized irradiation of radioresistant tissues. Following whole body irradiation with these large doses, survival time is very short, and there is not sufficient time for the whole sequence to unravel.

a) Central nervous system

Insight into the fact that there are a series of different modes of death following whole body irradiation arose from the fact that there are different survival times as a function of increasing dose of radiation. This is illustrated in Fig. 6. In the dose range of 200 to about 1 000 R, the mean survival time varies somewhat but is in the vicinity of 10 to

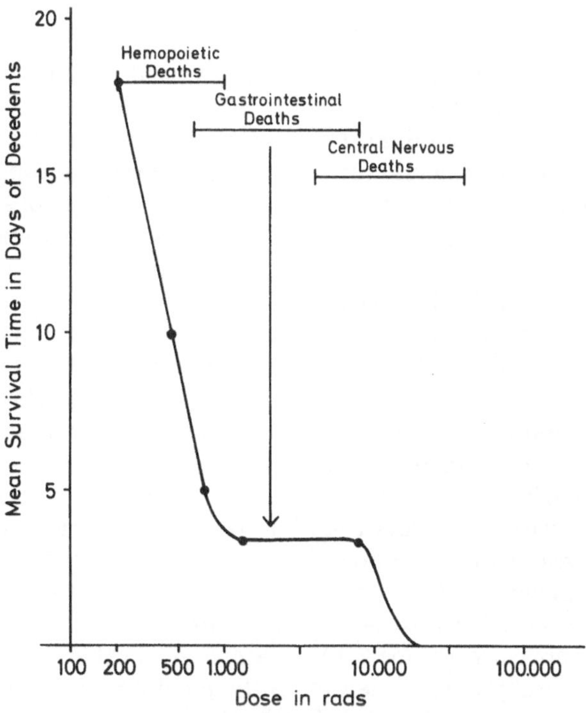

Fig. 6. Generalized curve for mean survival time of decedents as a function of the dose. Position of the curve varies with the species. Note overlapping in deaths from various modes and the plateau for gastrointestinal deaths

15 days depending upon the species. As the dose of radiation is increased over 1 000 rad, a stable survival time of about 3 to 4 days is seen, which corresponds to the gastrointestinal syndrome to be described later. This plateau in survival time is constant to roughly 5—7 000 R, with considerable variation between species. Again, the survival time commences to decrease, and with doses in excess of 10 000 rad given in a short period of time, the survival time is of the order of 24 hours. As the dose is increased further, the survival time progressively becomes shorter, and animals die under the beam. The survival time

versus dose has been published for mice by Cronkite (1951). As the survival time falls below 3 to 4 days, central nervous system symptomatology and severe injury of the central nervous system may be observed histologically. The central nervous system syndrome, when induced by whole body irradiation or irradiation of the head alone with uniform deposition of energy, is uniformly fatal in a short period of time. Only a brief summary will be presented. Details of the pathology and symptomatology are available from Gerstner (1958), van Cleave (1962) and Krayevskii (1965).

α) *The symptomatology of the CNS syndrome*

With extremely high doses of irradiation given at exceedingly high dose rates, respiratory difficulty commences, there may be a short period of agitation followed by marked apathy and death in a short period of time. When the radiation is given at slower dose rates, there may be a period of agitation followed by apathy, disorientation, disturbed equilibrium, ataxia, diarrhea, vomiting, opisthotonus, prostration, convulsions followed by coma and death. There is considerable variability in the sequence and the intensity of the various symptoms. In addition, there are also species differences. Part of the gastrointestinal symptomatology is due to irradiation of the gastrointestinal tract, but a portion is also due to direct injury of the head, since it can be produced by head irradiation alone.

Human symptomatology that has been observed will be described later.

β) *Histopathological changes in the central nervous system*

One of the characteristic phenomena is the perivascular and parenchymatous granulocytic infiltration of the meninges, chorioid plexuses and brain. These inflammatory infiltrations are composed predominantly of granulocytes and occur within a very few hours and later are replaced by mononuclear cells and later macrophages. If the survival is more than 4 to 5 hours, vasculitis is a constant finding. This consists of a perivascular granulocytic infiltration which involves all layers of the blood vessels, and may extend into the surrounding tissue. Veins and arteries of all sizes are equally involved. All parts of the cerebrum are involved. There are varying degrees of intensities, with the spinal cord and cerebellum apparently having less involvement. The intensity of the infiltration is biphasic, with peaks at 8 and 48 hours (Vogel *et al.*, 1958). Edema becomes prominent. Hyperchromatic granule cells of the cerebellum and pyknosis of these cells are characteristic, dose-dependent finding following whole body and head irradiation. The hyperchromatism of these cells is uniform throughout the cerebellum of the monkey. Changes in these cells appear as early as two hours, and are maximal at 24 hours.

In a general sense, with doses less than 500 rads to the brain, very little is seen. Of course, in the late stages of the hemopoietic syndrome, when there is a severe depression in the platelets and a generalized purpura, hemorrhage may be seen in the meninges and the substance of the brain. With doses in excess of 1000 rads, one sees distinct effects upon the brain that increase with dose. There are considerable differences in species sensitivity. There is no generally agreed view as to the most sensitive cells in the brain. Some pathologists are inclined to consider the oligodendroglia as most sensitive. The permeability of the blood brain barrier is disturbed. Trypan blue injected intravenously stains the brain. In summary, then, diffuse edema of the brain may be seen with perivascular infiltration of leukocytes. The acute inflammatory response, the degeneration of neurons and local hemorrhage may result in prompt death of the animals. If they survive the first day or so, later liquefaction and necrosis of the white substance of the brain may become prominent. Since there is no cellular turnover in the nervous system, all effects are due either to the inflammatory response and edema, or direct injury and necrosis of neurons.

When the irradiation is inhomogeneous in its deposition within the brain, as occurred in the Lockport incident (Howland *et al.*, 1961), there may be substantial nervous system symptomatology and direct physical evidence of cerebellar and cerebral injury, but prolonged survival, as will be described later in this chapter.

In marked contrast, apparently, to all of the other species, the burro develops severe nervous system symptomatology, and dies frequently from damage to the nervous system from doses of radiation below 1 000 rads (THOMAS and BROWN, 1961). There is no explanation as yet why this mammalian species has such a sensitive nervous system.

b) Gastrointestinal system

In the sub-lethal range, less than 200 rads, there is a diminution in the mitotic index of the small bowel (WILLIAMS *et al.*, 1958) and a depression in the weight of the bowel that is dose-dependent (CONARD *et al.*, 1956). A slight amount of pyknosis and karyorrhexis in the crypts of LIEBERKUHN, and an occasional bizarre mitotic figure may be seen. Recovery takes place promptly. The mitotic index returns to normal in a matter of a few days, and there may be an actual overshoot in both the mitotic index and the weight of the bowel.

In the mid-lethal dose range for mammals, effects are similar to those with sub-lethal doses of radiation, except that the depression in the mitosis is greater, the duration of the depression in the mitotic index is longer, and the decrease in the weight of the bowel is greater. The return to a normal histologic appearance takes somewhat longer. There is also an overshoot in both the mitotic index and the weight upon recovery (QUASTLER, 1956).

In the mid-lethal dose range, there are certain changes that take place later in the bowel that bear no direct relationship to the early injury. There are sequelae of the generalized effects of depression of bone marrow function and the resulting pancytopenia. About 10—20 days after exposure, a tendency to bleed becomes prevalent, due to the marked thrombocytopenia. There may be numerous petechial hemorrhages scattered throughout the mucosa of the bowel. In some areas there may be more extensive hemorrhage that will dissect the mucosa of the bowel from the underlying muscularis, and may even act as a site of commencement of intussusception, a point that has considerable clinical importance. If the animal survives the general effects of the depression of bone marrow function, the gastrointestinal tract will completely recover. In both the sub-lethal and mid-lethal range there is relatively little that can be observed with regard to the histologic changes in the stomach and the colon. When the doses of radiation are increased to the "supra-lethal" range, there are considerable differences in species sensitivity, with the rat being more sensitive than most mammalian species. In the general vicinity of 1 000 to 3 000 rads, the effect on the gastrointestinal tract is quite striking. There is complete cessation of mitosis in the crypts of LIEBERKUHN. With doses up to 1 600 rads this is temporary. However, if, as will be described later, animals are kept alive by appropriate therapy, regeneration will occur if the dose of radiation is not in excess of about 1 600 rads. The cells in the crypts undergo typical pyknosis, karyorrhexis and bizarre large cells with peculiar nucleoli make their appearance. As the production of new cells diminishes and ceases completely, the cells on the villi continue to migrate out to the extrusion zone at the tip of the villus. Thus, as cells are lost from the extrusion zone, the total number of cells covering the villi decreases. As the cells continue to move out, mature and become extruded into the lumen of the bowel, the epithelium changes from columnar to cuboid to squamous. When the last few stretched out squamous appearing cells are sloughed off into the bowel, generally around the third to the fourth day in rodents, the bare villi are left exposed. The preceding are shown schematically in Fig. 5. At this time there is a serious loss of plasma into the bowel, and death occurs promptly within a few hours from this massive loss of fluid and electrolytes unless antishock therapy is instituted, particularly with plasma, fluids and electrolytes. Animals can be saved when the vascular beds collapse if death is prevented by heroic fluid therapy (CONARD *et al.*, 1956). A striking series of events have been shown to take place in the small bowel after approximately 1 200 rads of gamma radiation. Therapy prevents death from the gut injury. Between the 4th and 6th days regeneration commences

(Brecher *et al.*, 1958). Mixed between the bizarre abnormal cells are numerous hyperchromatic cells with much mitotic activity. The crypts are reconstituted, and cells again begin to migrate out on to the villi and reconstitute the normal appearance of the bowel by the tenth to the twelfth day after exposure. The sequence of the degenerative effects on the bowel is shown in Fig. 5. Whether the recovery is abortive as in the case of hemopoiesis is not established.

As recovery in the small bowel occurs, a similar sequence of degenerative events takes place in the stomach of treated dogs, as seen earlier in the small bowel. Through the sixth day the stomach mucosa appears normal. However, there then appears an obvious necrosis of the cells in the necks of the gastric glands followed by a desquamation of epithelium from the mucous surface of the stomach in a way comparable to that described before for the small intestinal tract. These observations demonstrate the essential role of time in addition to dose of radiation in any discussion of relative radiosensitivity. Even under conditions in which the dose to the gastrointestinal tract is identical in all parts, the sequence of events takes place much more rapidly in the small intestine than in the stomach. Thus, any estimate of radiosensitivity based on observation after a single dose of radiation, or only at a single time after exposure, may be misleading.

c) The effect on lymph nodes, thymus and spleen

The magnitude of effect on these organs is a function of dose and time after exposure. Changes in the splenic and thymic weight of mice have been used practically to assay mixed gamma and neutron radiation. After the initial usual shoulder on the curve showing the relationship between the ratio of the control spleens to the irradiated spleen, the log of the ratio of irradiated spleen and thymus to normal spleen and thymus is linearly related to the dose of radiation. This has been a most useful biological dosimeter. Shortly after exposure of lymphatic tissue to even very small amounts of radiation down to the order of 25—50 rads, one can see a moderate amount of pyknosis and karyorrhexis in the lymphocytes during the first few hours after exposure. The nuclear debris is rapidly phagocytosed and disposed of. Mitosis returns and the lymph nodes, after small amounts of radiation, are reconstituted. Trowell (1946) has used the fraction of lymphocytes that are pyknotic as a dosimeter also. In the spleen and thymus one sees similar nuclear debris. After large doses of radiation, in the mid-lethal range, the destruction of the primary follicles of lymph nodes and spleen is quite striking and almost complete. Mitosis is essentially eradicated. By the third to the fifth day, at which time the maximum weight loss has taken place, the entire architecture of the lymph node is altered. The primary and secondary follicles have disappeared, the sinuses in the lymph nodes are distended with clear lymph, and there is an apparent increase in the number of plasma and stroma cells of the node due to the atrophy of the small lymphocytes normally present. As time goes on, there is a slow return to normal by an onset of mitosis and regeneration of the node. If the hemorrhagic phase of the whole body radiation syndrome commences, bleeding takes place peripherally in the tissues. The red cells are absorbed into the lymphatics and are in part phagocytosed by the reticulum cells of the sinuses as the bloody lymph flows past these phagocytic cells lining the sinuses. The lymph nodes become red very soon as a result of the concentration of red cells. At later time intervals the nodes become brown as the hemoglobin is destroyed.

In the thymus a similar sequence of events may be observed. The dense cortical portion of the thymus rapidly atrophies, and there may be reversal in the usual tinctorial appearance of the dense blue staining cortex and a lighter staining medulla. Upon regeneration the normal architecture returns. In the spleen the picture varies depending upon the species. In the mouse, and to a lesser extent the rat, the spleen normally has myelopoiesis in the red pulp in addition to lymphocyte production in the follicles and white pulp. One of the earliest observations is the inhibition of mitosis, followed by a depletion in erythropoiesis and myelopoiesis in the red pulp. Lastly, the megakaryocytes disappear by five to six days after exposure in the mid-lethal range. During this period of time there is an atrophy of the Malpighian follicles, so that practically nothing but the stroma cells and the central arteriole is still visible. If the animal enters the hemorrhagic phase of the disease, there is a marked erythro-phagacytosis as bleeding takes place into the spleen. Macrophages are active in clearing up the hemorrhagic areas. The minimum weight of the spleen usually is seen around the fourth day after exposure.

d) Bone marrow

In the bone marrow one can see, shortly after irradiation, pyknosis in the erythropoietic precursors. Pyknosis in other bone marrow cell lines is extremely rare. Mitosis is reduced, as shown by FLIEDNER *et al.* (1959). The mitotic index of human beings exposed to a nuclear accident has been shown to be significantly depressed by the fourth day after exposure. The significant finding is the progressive disappearance of parenchyma with minimal evidence of cell destruction. In the rigid bony container this is compensated by dilatation of the fragile sinusoids. These later rupture and intramedullary hemorrhage becomes prominent (FLIEDNER *et al.*, 1955). With the exception of the hemorrhage, most of the late atrophy can be explained on the basis that the differentiated, proliferating pools of all cell lines continue to differentiate and are finally extruded into the blood. Since the stem cell pool has a D_0 of about 95 rads, doses in the lethal range (200—600 rads) severely deplete this pool, and hence the replenishment of differentiated cell lines is drastically impaired until the stem cell pool recovers its size and is receptive to differentiating influences.

The preceding descriptions of the various tissues are predicated on homogeneous absorption of energy throughout the body. If some areas have had significant shielding, so that more stem cells survive, there may be a very rapid regeneration of more heavily irradiated areas of the hemopoietic tissues by migration, proliferation and differentiation of stem cells from the less severely injured areas.

e) Blood vessels and connective tissues

Radiation affects the capillaries, veins and arteries. The doses necessary to produce visible effects are large, usually greater than 1500 rads. There is a swelling of capillary endothelium. Bizarre forms of cells may appear. Changes usually take many days to weeks to appear. There is degeneration of the smooth muscle and connective tissue coats of the blood vessels, particularly arterioles. Endarteriitis and obliteration of vessels may be obvious, as are calcareous deposits at very late times. The vascular changes interfere with circulation and produce all of the sequelae of impaired circulation. In the kidneys typical nephrosclerosis may develop. All vascular changes take doses in excess of the minimum lethal dose for mammals and require many weeks to develop. There is a very extensive literature on these changes by WARREN (1942).

4. Blood counts

Observations on the concentration of blood cells in the peripheral blood reflect the injury to the production of new cells, the effect upon the life span in the peripheral blood, and any incrased death rate of cells within the peripheral blood. In a general sense then, if all new production of cells is eliminated, the decrease in the peripheral blood, providing there is no shortened life span, will reflect the normal life span and mode of loss from the peripheral blood. For example, the general case can be stated as follows. If produciton ceases, there is no reservoir of mature cells outside the blood, and if the loss from the blood is a random process, then the cells will disappear from the peripheral blood exponentially with time simply as the normal half-life of the item in the blood. If there is no random loss of the cell, and the other conditions listed above apply, then the disappearance from the peripheral blood will be a linear process. The relative radiation sensitivity of the stem cells has been determined by McCulloch *et al.* (1962). It has been shown that the D_0 is about 90 rads[1]. Accordingly, after doses in excess of 500 to 600 rads practically all new production from the stem cell level ceases until repletion of the stem cell compartment is complete and differentiation commences once again in each cell line. Actually at an LD_{50} it can be estimated from the dose effect curve that only about 1 of 500 stem cells would retain proliferative capabilities.

a) Effects upon erythrocytes

There is no significant effect upon erythrocytes in the peripheral blood until doses of many thousand rads are received. It has been shown in human beings by Schiffer *et al.* (1966) that human erythrocytes commence to have a shortened life span by the chromium labeling technique when doses in excess of 35000 rads are received. After doses in the lethal dose range (200—600 rads) are received by dogs, there is a shortened life span only during the hemorrhagic phase, and cells are subjected to an additional injury by circulating through the lymphatic spaces and lymph nodes. The normal human erythrocytes have a life span of 120 days. Thus, after doses of radiation that completely eliminate new red cell production, there would be a decrease in the red cell mass of about 0.83 % per day. After doses of radiation in the mid-lethal dose range, as has been observed many times in human accidents, the reticulocytes decrease to very low values or may, temporarily, disappear. During this period of time there is a slow decrease in the red cell mass. If hemorrhage occurs, due to thrombocytopenia, the decrease is accelerated. The status of erythropoiesis can be easily evaluated practically by counting the reticulocytes in the peripheral blood. The preceding is the sequence after homogeneous or near homogeneous exposure. After inhomogeneous exposure the sequence is different as will be described in a later section.

b) Granulocytes

Granulocytes are lost from the peripheral blood by a random process with a half-time of 6.6 hours. However, there is a large reservoir of mature granulocytes in the bone marrow in addition to the non-dividing pool of maturing granulocytes from the metamyelocyte through the band level that will continue to mature and be ultimately extruded into the peripheral blood. From the observations listed earlier on granulocytopoiesis, it has been shown that the transit time through the maturation pool (metamyelocytes to granulocytes) is about four days. There is no evidence that the non-dividing, maturing cells are significantly injured by radiation in the lethal dose range. Thus, if the proliferating granulocytic pool of cells were to be eradicated, maturation and entrance into the peripheral blood would continue. It would therefore take about four days before the last metamyelocytes formed just before radiation would be transformed into segmented neutrophils. With no further production, then, the granulocytes should commence to decrease in the peripheral blood between the fourth and fifth days with a half-time of close to seven hours. This has been observed, as will be illustrated later in the description of human cases.

Actually, one observes generally an initial granulocytosis. This is assumed to represent a mobilization of the marginal leukocytes in the peripheral blood, and perhaps also some mobilization of the medullary reservoir. It clearly is not due to an accelerated production of new cells.

After lower doses of radiation an initial granulocytosis is generally observed, followed by a more leisurely decrease in the granulocyte level, attaining in animals minimal values around the tenth to the fifteenth day. Around this time there may be then a temporary rise in the granulocytes that has been termed "the abortive rise".

---

1 D_0 is that dose which reduces the fraction surviving by 37% on the exponential part of the fraction surviving curve versus dose.

c) Platelets

In all mammalian species irrespective, apparently, of the dose of radiation, the platelets remain at normal level or perhaps increase moderately for four to five days after exposure. Thereafter the platelet counts diminish rapidly, and the depth to which they fall depends upon the dose of radiation. In all mammals, except man, the minimum platelet level is attained 8 to 10 days after exposure (CRONKITE and BRECHER, 1952). Below about the LD_{50} dose of radiation, the minimum level of platelets attained is dependent upon the dose of radiation (COHN and MILNE, 1956). Below 100 rads exposure there is a very minimal platelet depression. In human beings, after mid-lethal and lower doses of radiation, the minimal platelet levels are attained around 28 to 30 days after exposure (CRONKITE, BOND and DUNHAM, 1956). When reproduction of megakaryocytes is completely stopped, there is still an input of platelets into the blood for four to five days while the existing megakaryocytes continue to mature and produce platelets. Perhaps fewer platelets per megakaryocyte are produced (BOND, FLIEDNER and ARCHAMBEAU, 1965). As the megakaryocytes disappear from the bone marrow, there is then a disappearance of platelets from the peripheral blood, consistent with their life span and a random loss. It is not known at what level of exposure to radiation platelets are injured and disappear more rapidly.

5. Cytological effects of radiation on human bone marrow and peripheral blood

Pathologists have tended to say that study of the bone marrow and peripheral blood, except from the standpoint of changes in the concentration of cells and a relative hypoplasia, yields no useful information. In general, it is very useful to consider two types of morphologic injury that can be observed in the blood and the bone marrow. First are the phenomena seen in cells which are directly injured, and second are the abnormalities that occur as a result of abnormal mitoses. This has been studied extensively by FLIEDNER et al. (1961) in rats, and FLIEDNER et al. (1964) in accidentally irradiated human beings. In general, in the bone marrow the directly injured cells are for the most part red cell precursors. Direct injury is also very prevalent in the lymphocytic tissues. The effects seen are pyknosis, karyolysis and karyorrhexis. These phenomena are observed in cells before they have had a chance to enter mitosis after exposure to radiation. The mitotically connected cytologic abnormalities are observed later, after the irradiated cell has gone into or through mitosis. The directly injured cells are very rapidly removed from the bone marrow and other tissues, and this type of cell injury is not seen beyond the first few hours, or at most during the first day. Mitotically connected abnormalities reach their maximum incidence at approximately one day, but do no tdisappear from rat bone marrow until the third day and from human bone marrow until nine days or so. The characteristic types of abnormalities are chromatin dissociation with nuclear swelling, karyolysis, chromosome stickiness, chromosomal fragmentation, chromosomal bridges, tripolar or tretraploid mitosis, giant cells, binucleated cells, cytoplasmic chromatin clumps (karyomeres) and nuclear fragmentation. The preceding are illustrated by FLIEDNER et al. (1964).

In the peripheral blood abnormal myelocytic forms are seen, commencing about four days after exposure, and are present in the blood stream for about five to six days. The most prevalent is a giant neutrophil or metamyelocyte. In addition, one sees an occasional lymphocyte with a nuclear satellite. The latter may persist for very long periods of time (FLIEDNER et al., 1964).

Although animal studies have been performed, it is unfortunate that a systematic study of cytological abnormalities in human bone marrow and blood at various time intervals after exposure has not been made. It may be very rewarding to study systematically the appearance of cells in the blood and bone marrow during the period of the abortive rise. It would be of particular interest to determine the DNA content prior to and during the abortive rise.

After all obvious injuries to cells in blood and marrow have disappeared, one can still detect injury by culturing marrow or blood, and detect mitotic abnormalities (Bender and Gooch, 1962).

VI. Physiopathological effects

As a result of the destruction of tissue, the interference of mitosis in the ordinary renewal of many tissues described earlier, and the absorption of the products of destruction of the tissue (purines, pyrimidines, vasoactive peptides etc.), a sequence of events is observed that is reasonably well established. The symptomatology varies in intensity with the dose of radiation and, in the case of partial body irradiation, the area of the body exposed. The description of the physiophatological effects can be divided into four parts: vital signs, symtomatology, increased susceptibility to infection and the results of hemopoietic depression. The following are discussed in much greater detail by Ellinger.

1. The vital signs

The temperature remains constant following irradiation, except under two conditions. After massive doses of radiation, of the order of thousands of rads, there is general collapse and a rise and later fall in the body temperature. Also, after a few days, with doses in the mid-lethal range, there may be an increase in the temperature as a result of the development of infections. The pulse rate is variable, depending upon the dose of radiation and psychological factors. After the higher doses of radiation there is a tachycardia. The respiration is usually unchanged. After even moderate doses of radiation, there is a minor decrease in the blood pressure, presumably due to the release of histamine-like substances from the destruction of tissues. After massive doses of radiation, there is a precipitous fall of blood pressure. This may occur as a result of either irradiation of the abdomen alone or the head alone. The decrease in the blood pressure is precipitous, and a shock-like state develops which may be followed by death promptly unless heroic therapeutic measures of appropriate drug and fluid preplacement are instituted promptly. This is particularly well documented in the fatal radiation syndrome from an accidental nuclear excursion described by Karas and Stanbury (1965). This patient received a neutron dose of approximately 2200 rads and a gamma ray dose of 6600 rads for a total of 8800 rads, which is probably 10 to 20 times the mean lethal dose for a man. Within minutes after exposure the patient complained of severe abdominal cramps, headache, he vomited and was incontinent of diarrheal stool. Initially his blood pressure was elevated, as was the temperature. Within 4 hours the blood pressure was falling and the pulse rate was rising. From then until death about 48 hours after exposure, blood pressure as maintained only by continuous intravenous infusion of Levarterenol and methylprednisolone. In addition to the hypotension there was also moderate disorientation and difficulty with speech.

2. Symptomatology

Symptomatology, observed is definitely a function of the dose of radiation. In all mammals studied, after very large doses of radiation in excess of 5—6000 rads, there are signs and symptoms referable to the central nervous system that develop within minutes or hours. This symptom complex following massive doses of radiation to either the head or the whole body has been termed "the central nervous system syndrome". To date it has always been 100 % fatal when due to homogeneous absorption of radiation in the brain. The level of radiation that it takes to produce this very acute nervous system death in human beings is not established. The symptomatology of the nervous system syndrome is described in more detail under this title. After lower doses of radiation, the symptomatology may be very variable. Changes in pulse rate are closely related to physiological effects. Headache, irritability, anorexia, nausea and vomiting are variable. In the upper part of the lethal dose range these are quite prevalent. As the dose diminishes below the LD_{50}, the severity of all diminishes, and in the high sub-lethal range around 175—200 rads in human beings perhaps only a little nausea, transient vomiting and diarrhea will be observed.

3. Increased susceptibility to infection

This is a complex subject covered in detail by BOND, SILVERMAN and CRONKITE (1954) and summarized herein. One of the major causes of death is infection in all animals and in human beings. This was observed frequently after the nuclear bombing of Hiroshima and Nagasaki. The relationship of radiation injury to the various defenses against infection has been extensively studied. Defenses against infection can be divided into stationary and mobile forces. The stationary defenses are the surfaces of the body, the fixed phagocytic elements in the connective tissues, the connective tissues which react to local invasion, and the fixed macrophage elements in the various filters of the body (spleen, liver and lymph nodes). The mobile defenses are the circulating leukocytes and antibodies (natural and acquired) which can attack at the point of infection. Of great importance to the acquired antibody defenses is the ability to renew synthesis of specific antibodies on re-introduction of the antigen, or the so-called anamnestic response. Infection has been very well established as one of the lethal sequelae of whole body irradiation in the lethal and supra-lethal ranges, when the survival time is greater than 3 days (MILLER et al., 1951). However, death occurs also in irradiated germ-free animals, even though the survival time was prolonged by a moderate amount. This fact and other data discussed later shows that infection is not the only cause of death in the lethal range. It has been possible to control infection in irradiated animals with appropriate antibiotics (MILLER et al., 1951). If bacteria to which there is no known effective antibiotic invade, there is obviously no benefit. The bacteria that kill in irradiation injury frequently are the intestinal bacteria normally present. The normal physiology of intestinal bacteria is of interest. It is known that bacteria penetrate the normal intestinal wall, since one can culture orally introduced bacteria with distinctive color (S. marcescens) from mesenteric lymph nodes. In irradiated animals the organisms are able to pass through the mesenteric lymph nodes, and can be cultured from the spleen. The correlation of low granulocyte count with probability of death has been amply confirmed by many. However, the replacement of separated neutrophils in the dog (CRONKITE et al., 1954, 1955) did not increase the survival rate, it only modified the histological picture. However the application of granulocyte transfusions in granulopenic human beings with leukemia has been definitely beneficial (FREIREICH et al.). In addition to the granulopenia, irradiated leukocytes develop an impairment in their ability to phagocytize bacteria after irradiation. This does not develop immediately, but after a period of days, coinciding in time with the abortive rise. Thus, it is not clear whether this is due directly to an effect of radiation on the granulocyte or to the fact that cells remaining with time are progressively older and may be cytologically abnormal. In addition, the migratory ability of leukocytes in in vitro systems is impaired at the same time as phagocytosis. The opsonic and phagocytic indices are depressed. The bactericidal power of the blood is clearly decreased after exposure to radiation. The reticulo-endothelial system (RES) immediately after radiation has an intact capability to phagocytize injected bacteria. However, the reticulo-endothelial system is not able to kill the phagocytized bacteria, and they may break out into the blood stream at a later date, producing overwhelming bacterial sepsis, unless there has been a recovery of granulocytopoiesis. The reasons for the inability of the reticulo-endothelial system to kill the ingested bacteria are not known. However, the time of re-establishment of the bacteremia more or less parallels the depression in granulocytes and implies that there may be an interaction between the number of circulating granulocytes and the power of the fixed macrophages in the reticulo-endothelial system to kill ingested bacteria. In addition to the general diminution in the bactericidal power of the serum from irradiated animals, there is apparently a bona fide diminution in the properdin concentration of irradiated serum at the time when animals are most susceptible to infection. The experimental background for the preceding is reviewed (Bond et al., 1954; Bond and Cronkite, 1957). In summary then:

The increased susceptibility to infection in irradiated mammals is reasonably well understood. In most species, infection is a dominant cause of death in the lethal range. Obliteration of infection by means of the germ-free state does not eliminate death from other causes, primarily hemorrhagic phenomena. Protection by the mucosa of the normal bowel is relative, since bacteria can penetrate the normal bowel. The stationary defenses are altered. Changes in the morphological appearance and in the permeability of the connective tissues and skin following irradiation are known. The importance of these changes in defense against infection are not known. The ability of fixed reticuloendothelial cells to phagocytose bacteria appears to be relatively normal following whole body irradation, but the ability to retain and kill ingested bacteria appears to be impaired. Granulocytes are diminished in number, and evidence that they are functionally deficient is accumulating. New antibody production and in particular the secondary response for acquired antibody production are drastically inhibited. Lastly, the titer of natural antibodies (properdin) is reduced. Thus, there is little wonder that irradiated animals in the lethal range are exquisitely sensitive to the development of infection, even by the commensal organisms usually living in harmony on the surfaces of the body and within the gut.

4. Defects in hemostasis

Bleeding is a result of numerous facets, and the causes depend upon the dose of radiation and the time after exposure. After very high doses of radiation of many thousands of rads, there is apparently sufficient injury and disturbance to the capillary beds that result particularly in the gastrointestinal tract in stasis, apparent thrombosis and local bleeding of varying degrees. After very high levels of radiation, similarly one may also see capillary bleeding in cerebral blood vessels. After doses of radiation in the range of 200 to 1000 rads, a very definite tendency to bleed develops, providing that the animals live sufficiently long. Historically, the most critical observations on the pathogenesis of bleeding were made by Fabricius-Möller, who correlated plateled levels with bleeding and noted that lead shielding of a leg during irradiation prevented later bleeding and the thrombopenia was much less marked. The French workers, in particular Lacassagne et al., emphasized the probable importance of thrombocytopenia in the development of the bleeding tendency. Allen et al. claimed that heparinemia was a major cause of bleeding in addition to the thrombocytopenia in irradiated dogs, and that the thrombopenia actually sensitizes to heparin. Of the latter there is no doubt. Unfortunately, the concept of increased amounts of circulating heparin was readily accepted, probably because positive treatment by antiheparin agents, such as protamine or toluidine blue would neutralize the heparin and thus, in part at least, control the bleeding. Unfortunately, heparinemia has subsequently been proved not to be a cause of bleeding, and the anti-heparin agents of no value in treatment of radiation hemorrhage (Jackson et al., 1952). The defects in hemostasis that lead to bleeding are well documented. A progressive thrombopenia develops that is time- and dose-dependent. The thrombopenia leads to a quantitative deficiency in clot retraction, prothrombin utilization and capillary integrity. Lastly, at very low platelet levels with virtually no prothrombin conversion, the whole blood clotting time becomes remarkably prolonged. The bleeding tendency may take many forms, from merely a microscopic diapedesis of red cells into the connective tissue with absorption of the red cells into the lymphatics and their concentration in the filtering apparatus of lymph nodes. This very mild bleeding tendency may escalate to diffuse macroscopic purpura. When infectious processes become prominent, there may be ulcerations into small blood vessels with severe local bleeding that may result in exsanguination and death of the subject. Trauma and sepsis also increase the bleeding tendency.

The most direct evidence on the role of the platelet has been the proof that platelet transfusion will prevent bleeding or stop bleeding that has already commenced (CRONKITE *et al.*, 1954). It is of particular pertinence that the platelets must be viable and circulate in order to control the bleeding tendency. Lyophilized or frozen platelets are of no value in controlling the bleeding tendency (JACKSON *et al.*, 1957; FLIEDNER *et al.*, 1957). The platelet level at which bleeding may occur spontaneously has been studied by LAMERTON *et al.* in rats. At platelet levels above 40000 per cubic millimetre, bleeding and anemia did not occur. In human beings exposed to fall-out with platelets as low as 35000 per mm³, bleeding was not observed except for menorrhagia (CRONKITE, BOND and DUNHAM, 1956). As mentioned earlier, there is a significant difference in the rate at which platelets fall in man and in other mammals.

VII. Radiation syndrome due to short-term exposure to penetrating radiation

The following condensed summary on syndromes is based on reports of human radiation injury (BRUCER; CRONKITE, BOND, DUNHAM, 1956; GERSKOVA and BAISOGOLOV; HASTERLIK and MARINELLI; HEMPELMANN *et al.*; HOWLAND *et al.*; INGRAM *et al.*; LE ROY; MATHÉ *et al.*; OUGHTERSEN and WARREN; PENDIC; ROSSI *et al.*; SHIPMAN *et al.*; KARAS and STANBURY). It is highly unlikely that one will see human radiation injury in which there is a very uniform deposition of energy throughout the entire body following criticality and laboratory accidents. However, exposure of human beings in fall-out fields will result in quite uniform deposition of energy throughout the body one cm below the surface. It is useful pedagogically to describe a hierarchy of death related to dose and time after exposure to radiation, in which there is a relatively uniform whole body, short-term high dose exposure. The relation of survival time to dose was considered earlier. Modes of death have been established by experimentation with reasonable degrees of homogeneity of exposure particularly in the smaller mammals. The studies are believed to be particularly pertinent because they implicate various organ systems. Furthermore, the same syndrome can be produced by regional exposure of the implicated organ systems. For example, after very high doses of radiation delivered either to the head or the whole body, a characteristic syndrome is observed that has been termed "the central nervous system syndrome" because of marked symptoms of brain dysfunction that are consistent with neurologic damage. When radiation is delivered to the abdomen alone or to the whole body in the range of roughly 700 to 3000 rads, a very characteristic symptomatology develops. The symptoms are related to the gastrointestinal tract, and thus have been termed "the gastrointestinal syndrome". In animals it is characterized by a stable survival time, particularly in mice and rats, of about 3 to 4 days. The survival time for other mammals varies somewhat but is also stable over a wide range of doses. After lower doses of radiation, in the range of 200 to 1000 rads, a mild, transient gastrointestinal syndrome occurs, and a typical hemopoietic syndrome develops, which is characterized by sequelae of pancytopenia due to aplasia of the bone marrow. In most mammals, the killing process of the hemopoietic syndrome is completed by 30 days. However, in contrast, in man the killing process is not completed until about 60 days after exposure. Even after apparent recovery, hidden radiation injury (somatic mutations?) may manifest itself later in the form of neoplasia, particularly leukemia, cataracts, shortened life span, etc.

1. The central nervous system syndrome

This syndrome has been very well described in monkeys by LANGHAM *et al.* in 1956. The full blown cerebral form seen in animals has not been observed in human beings.

It was not observed in Hiroshima or Nagasaki bacause persons who where close enough to the hypocenter to receive such high doses necessarily experienced lethal thermal burns or mechanical injuries as well, and thus were lost during the confusion of the first three post-attack days without examination and recording. However, nervous system symptoms were observed in a criticality accident at the Los Alamos scientific laboratory by Shipman (1961) and by Karas and Stanbury (1965). From animal observations, one can attempt to predict and describe for man the acute cerebral form of disease. Weakness, irritability, ataxia, disorientation, drowsiness, and listlessness, will develop rapidly and may be present immediately. This will proceed within a very short time to severe apathy, prostration and lethargy. There will be progressive loss of physical and mental activity. With very high doses, probably in excess of 8—10000 rads, there will probably be disorientation and unawareness of reality almost immediately. In addition, after exposure to these very high doses, a disturbance of the motor system can be anticipated. Seizures may occur either in the form of generalized muscle tremors or ataxic movements, with the likelihood of full-blown epileptoid convulsions of the grand-mal type. If individuals survive the convulsive phase, they will be prostrate, somnolent, and will expire within 2 to 3 days following exposure. Animal studies have shown clearly that progressive cerebral symptoms result from widespread inflammatory foci that begin to develop within one hour after irradiation. These non-bacterial, radiation-induced reactions simulate meningitis, encephalitis and vasculitis, and are soon associated with oedema of the brain.

2. The gastrointestinal syndrome

This syndrome can appropriately be divided into the non-fatal type that is observed in the mid-lethal and sub-lethal dose range. Here there is temporary anorexia, nausea, vomiting, and perhaps a little diarrhea. This subsides within a few hours to a day or so. In the mid-lethal range, gastrointestinal symptomatology may return during the period of time of marked infectious processes and hemorrhage. This phase in man occurs 4 to 6 weeks after exposure, and is primarily due to the ulceration and hemorrhage into the bowel rather than from the direct radiation injury to the mucosa of the gastrointestinal tract. This will be described in more detail under the hemopoietic syndrome. In the fatal form of gastrointestinal injury there are considerable differences in species sensitivity, with the rat being more sensitive, particularly in the younger ages, than other mammalian species. The histologic effects of high doses of radiation in the range of 1000 to 3000 rads has been described earlier. As discussed in an earlier part of the chapter, following doses of irradiation in excess of roughly 700 rads, the cells in the crypts undergo pyknosis, karyorrhexis, and mitosis ceases. With no new cell production the cells on the villi continue to migrate out to the extrusion zone and are lost at the tip of the villus. The total number of cells covering the villi decreases. Finally, there are many denuded, swollen, stubby villi from which a serious loss of plasma into the bowel commences. Although it is probably an over-simplification one tends to connect severe diarrhea, hemoconcentration and shock followed by death with the anatomical disturbances that are observed. This is clearly an over-simplification because it takes of the order of 2 to 3 days for the denudation to be significant, and with the higher doses of radiation there is a persistent vomiting and diarrhea apparently as result of autonomic disturbances having their origin within the emetic center of the brain and elsewhere in the nervous system. However, at least in dogs, when the dose of radiation does not exceed roughly 1500 rads, the bowel will recover histologically and symptoms subside when there is adequate plasma and fluid replacement to prevent the shock-like death from hemoconcentration and peripheral vascular collapse.

Clinically, the following sequence may be observed after doses in excess of 700 rad. Nausea occurs within a few minutes, and vomiting may be severe by 60 minutes after exposure. The vomiting may increase in frequency, and diarrhea may become severe. The initial symptomatology after lower doses may subside. However, after very high doses, the signs and symptoms are persistent and continue until death. In the event that the initial symptomatology subsides, there may be a period of 1 to 3 days during which there is a sense of relative well-being, following which, around the third to the eight day a grave deterioration will occur. Severe nausea, vomiting and diarrhea again develop, and death occurs promptly as a result of a tremendous loss of plasma into the gastrointestinal tract. This severe gastrointestinal syndrome and its pathologic effects were described by HEMPELMANN *et al.* (1952) in a patient fatally irradiated at one of the nuclear accidents at the Los Alamos scientific laboratory. A very severe form of the gastrointestinal syndrome was described by KARAS and STANBURY (1965) after a critical excursion. A very mild, transient, non-fatal form of the gastrointestinal syndrome was observed in the Marshallese natives exposed to sub-lethal doses of radiation from fallout (CRONKITE, BOND and DUNHAM, 1956). In the preceding discussion on the pathogenesis and symptomatology observed, emphasis has been placed upon the local injury to the gastrointestinal tract. This is clearly an important facet, but not the only facet of the problem. As alluded to earlier, there is clearly a component mediated through the central nervous system, resulting in autonomic stimulation of motility in the gastrointestinal tract. In addition, it has been shown that ligation of the bile duct in the irradiated rat or cannulation and diversion of the bile prevents diarrhea (SULLIVAN, 1962). The role of bile in producing diarrhea has been related to an action of the bile salts on the irradiated bowel epithelium, since the diarrhea occurs at a time when there are marked histological disturbances of the gastrointestinal epithelium, and when depression of the absorptive function of the intestine is maximal. Ordinarily, bile salts are primarily absorbed in the distal ileum. Thus, bile salts increase in concentration in the colon. It is possible — though not proved — that the increased concentration of bile salts in the colon may produce the diarrhea. Another contributing fact that may have some clinical importance is that, in some animals at least, there is a substantial loss of sodium in the urine at least in the rat (JACKSON *et al.*, 1958).

Infection probably also plays a role, at least in some species of mammals, in the gastrointestinal syndrome. This is most clearly brought out in the studies that show it takes approximately 1.6 times as much radiation to produce the five day deaths in germfree mice as it does in conventional animals (WILSON, 1963). In addition, antibiotics and bone marrow transplantation that delay or prevent infectious processes also favorably, decrease the mortability of the gastrointestinal syndrome. Although infection plays a role in the gastrointestinal syndrome and the resulting mortality in the dose range from roughly 600 to 1 200 rads after higher doses of radiation greater than 2000 rads antibiotics and bone marrow transplantation do not increase the survival rate. Death ensues from the combined neurological disturbance of the gastrointestinal tract and the severe injury to the mucosa that results in the severe diarrhea, loss of plasma, disturbances in electrolyte metabolism, vascular collapse and death.

3. Hemopoietic syndromes

The disturbances in hemopoiesis that lead to the clinical syndromes have been described earlier. In this section, the general phenomena which may be observed after exposure of human beings in the lethal dose range will be summarized. First, there may be some overlap with a transient disturbance due to influence on the nervous system and the gastrointestinal tract as described earlier. The basic cause of the hemopoietic syndromes is hypoplasia to aplasia of the bone marrow. The simplest forms are seen when there is uniform deposition of energy throughout the entire hemopoietic system. The time sequence will be significantly altered by partial body exposure or marked inhomogeneities. There are three facets to the hemopoietic syndrome. First to be observed are usually the infectious aspects that generally come on earlier and may be seen as early as the seventh day after exposure. The reasons for the increased susceptibility to infection have been enumerated in an earlier section. The infections may be due to any bacteria. Generally, the infections result from invasion of the epithelial surfaces of the body by the commensal organisms that normally live on the surface of the body. Of course, any traumatic injury, thermal burn, or burns due to superficial ulceration of the skin from beta burns produced by fall-out material in contact with the skin provide portals of entry for bacteria. In addition, hemorrhagic areas in the bowel may result in superficial ulceration and hence further portals of entry for bacteria. The infectious processes will be much more severe and develop more rapidly wth overwhelming sepsis and prompt death if true pathogens invade. In addition, sites of chronic infection in the urinary tract or latent tuberculous lesions may be reactivated. The granulocyte depression is primarily responsible for the increased susceptibility to infection. This occurs earlier than the thrombopenia which is responsible primarily for hemorrhage. One may therefore see fatal infection before significant hemorrhagic manifestations develop.

In man, as described earlier, hemorrhage is due primarily to thrombocytopenia. After doses up to the mid-lethal dose range it takes approximately 30 days for the platelets to reach the minimum levels. Until the platelets fall below roughly 25000 per mm³, no bleeding is observed. The bleeding has been manifested in some individuals as only a mild cutaneous purpura. Sometimes it is manifested as a very severe epistaxis. There may be severe bleeding into the lungs that causes death. Bleeding may also be prominent around the larynx and result in respiratory obstruction. Another severe complication of bleeding may be the induction of intussusception of the bowel by hematomata with the concomitant acute abdominal episode that necessitates abdominal exploration under very hazardous conditions. Fatal hemorrhages may also take place from bacterial ulcerations of the bowel, and result in exsanguination. In addition, one may rarely have a fatal cerebral or myocardial hemorrhage. In man, hemorrhagic manifestations are rarely seen prior to the fourth week, and subsided by the end of the sixth to the seventh week in the Japanese.

Anemia may also be a major problem. This develops much more slowly for reasons described earlier. With complete cessation of blood production one will have a decrease in the red cell mass of 0.83 % per day. When hemorrhage occurs, two factors contribute to the acceleration of the development of the anemia.

First is the overt loss of blood from the body, and second is the shortened life span of red cells that recycle from the tissues throught the lymphatics. In the presence of severe bacterial infection, there may also be a severe hemolytic component.

4. Clinical evaluation of human beings exposed to radiation

There has been a strong desire on the part of physicians considering human radiation injury to depend upon estimates of radiation exposure for evaluation of the severity of the injury. One of the major objectives of this entire chapter is to demonstrate that, although precise estimates of radiation dose and — more important — the distribution of dose within the body are important from the standpoint of later statistical evaluation of radiation hazards, dose per se is not really essential for the management of radiation injury. Accordingly, from a practical standpoint, many years ago a practical clinical classification of radiation injury was proposed by Cronkite (1951). Initially this classification was proposed as a means of assisting in the management of mass radiation casualties in the event of nuclear warfare. It is still useful from a clinical standpoint. This classification consists of three general categories: survival improbable, survival possible, and survival probable. More recently Fliedner (1964) has analysed all available hematologic data that has been collected on human radiation exposures, and presented the hematologic picture for the above three categories.

a) Survival improbable

Individuals in the survival improbable group will experience prompt-intractable nausea, vomiting and diarrhea. Unless, as discussed earlier, there is drastic fluid and plasma replacement to compensate for the loss of fluid into the gastrointestinal tract, these individuals will die within a matter of a few days. Even with fluid replacement, they will yet experience sequelae of bone marrow aplasia and pancytopenia, and probably have 100 % mortality at a later date. The blood pictures for individuals in this category are scanty. In Fig. 7 the sequence in the granulocytes, lymphocytes and platelets is plotted. Note that there was a striking initial granulocytosis present in two of the three cases shown, sometime between the first and the third day. All of the patients had very low granulocyte counts by the fifth day after exposure. Unfortunately, it was impossible to

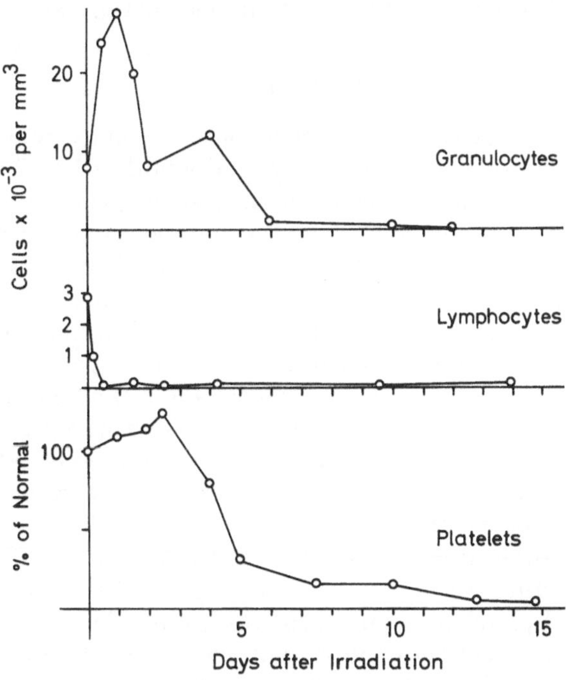

Fig. 7. Granulocyte, lymphocyte and platelet counts in survival improbable category. Curves idealized from
FLIEDNER (1964)

get blood counts in the Hiroshima casualties prior to the fifth day after exposure. However, in individuals dying in the first two weeks, the leukocyte counts between the fifth and the twelfth days were below 500 per mm³ (JACOBS *et al.*). The lymphocytes in these three cases had dropped to very low levels within hours after exposure. In one case, lymphocytes disappeared by 6 hours. Platelet counts were also very low by the eighth to the tenth day after exposure in the individuals in whom they were studied. Thus, with sufficiently high doses platelets diminish in human beings apparently as rapidly as they do in the other mammals. The cases which die within the first 3—4 days after irradiation have usually severe gastrointestinal symptomatology which is presumably due to a combination of central nervous system and gut injury. The relative importance of each varies with time after exposure. In the first few hours the gastrointestinal symptomatology is more likely central in origin and at later intervals the result of direct injury to the gut becomes more prominent. In addition, the most severe have been complicated by severe radiation injury to the cutaneous tissues. It is of interest in the patient presented by KARAS and STANBURY (1965) dying 49 hours after exposure, that lymphocytes had disappeared from the blood by 15 hours after exposure. During the period from exposure to death, the granulocyte count continually climbed until it reached almost 50 000,39 hours after exposure and 10 hours before death. This patient had severe gastrointestinal symptomatology until death. The patients observed by Hempelmann *et al.* (1957) and Oughtersen and Warren dying 7—16 days after exposure also had severe gut symptoms. At autopsy histopathologic examination of the bowel indicated a loss of the duodenal epithelium and complete erosion of the epithelium of ileum and jejunum. In the ulcerated portion of the jejunum, bacteria reportedly had invaded the intestinal wall. Thus, it appears, with the scanty information that is available, that the gastrointestinal syndrome reported in man may be accentuated by the granulocytic insufficiency and infection. Thus, prompt and continuous nausea, vomiting and diarrhea followed by virtual disappearance of neutrophils within 5 to 6 days, and a steady decline of platelets to low values by the 8th to the 10th day, are very poor prognostic signs. Survival in these cases must be considered improbable with all types of available therapy at the present time.

b) Survival possible

In general, the survival possible group will consist of individuals in whom the nausea and vomiting is relatively brief, subsiding within a period of 1 to 2 days, and followed by a period of well-being. These individuals will later suffer primarily from the hemopoietic syndrome. These are the patients who have a spontaneous statistical chance of survival that has been described by the classic sigmoid dose mortality curve. From data discussed earlier on the probable lethal dose for human beings, it has been postulated in the absence of therapy that the most likely human LD_{50} is in the vicinity of 360 rads. Patients in the survival possible group, after the subsidence of the initial symptoms, will show a typical series of changes developing in the peripheral blood, and ultimate granulocytopenia, thrombocytopenia and persistent lymphopenia. The patients on whom the blood picture in this category are based represent individuals who probably were exposed to relatively uniform whole body radiation in the range of 200 to 450 rads. There were marked variations in the circumstances of the exposure, the dose rate, radiation quality and energy, and a certain degree of additional complications were present. Despite these differences, a rather uniform hematological picture was observed. In Fig. 8, the probable sequence of leukocytes, lymphocytes and platelets is shown for this group. The graphs are redrawn, showing roughly the average response of the 17 individuals that Fliedner (1964) analysed in more detail. There is an initial granulocytosis occuring in most individuals within the first 2 to 4 days after exposure. Thereafter, there is a sharp decline which, if extrapolated, would reach zero values by 8 to 10 days. However, this decline is terminated by either a rebound or a plateau. The rebound or plateau lasts about 10 to 12 days. The preceding rise or plateau has been termed "the abortive rise". Around the 22nd day a final leukopenia commences. The granulocytes continue to decrease downwards, attaining the minimum values after about 34 days. A slow recovery in the granulocyte count commences after about the 36th day. However, in some patients this is a very slow process. In contrast, to the granulocyte count, the lymphocytes show a much less variable course. It is of interest and importance to note that the lymphocytes do not reach zero levels in any of the cases as in the category "survival improbable". Within 3 to 4 days the lymphocytes reach their minimum and remain at this level for at least 5 weeks. Thereafter the lymphocyte counts slowly recover, but may not reach normal values for weeks or many months.

In contrast to the patients in the "survival" improbable group, there is a much slower diminution in the platelet counts. The minimal values are not attained until about 28 to 39 days after exposure. Actually, there is a period during the first few days after exposure in which there is only a slight decrease or a constant platelet level. A thrombocytosis, as has been observed in animals, has not as yet been observed in the human beings. Actually, the sharp drop in platelet count does not commence until about 20 days. After the nadir is reached around the 30th day, a slow recovery commences with many weeks to return to normal.

Although extensive studies of the bone marrow have not been performed on human beings exposed in the survival possible category, it is believed that a useful procedure in this dose range is the serial determination of the mitotic index of the bone marrow. In normal individuals, the mitotic index of normal human bone marrow between the hours of 10.00 a.m. and 1.00 p.m. is approximately 9 per 100 cells (FLIEDNER *et al.*, 1959). In the casualties that occurred following exposure in the criticalty accident at Oak Ridge, the mitotic index was studied and found to be significantly decreased in the exposure of 50 to 200 rads. By the 4th day after exposure, in the more heavily exposed individuals,

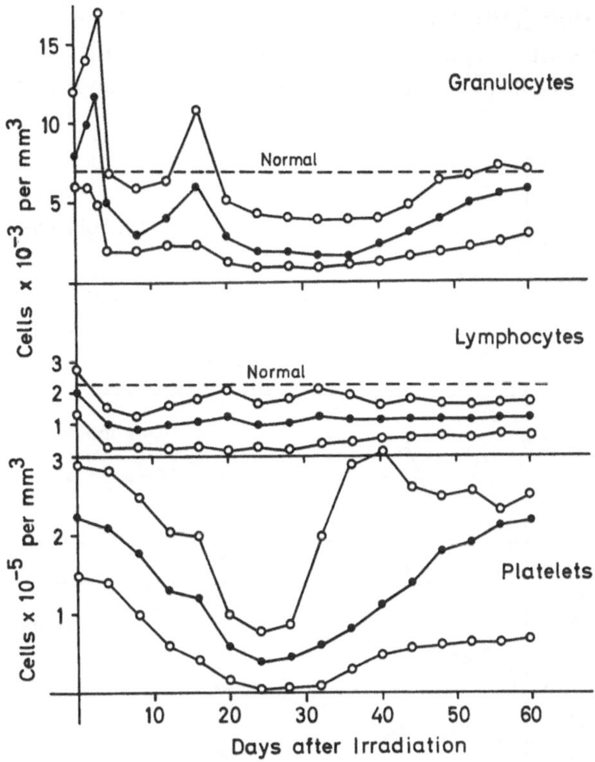

Fig. 8. Granulocyte, lymphocyte and platelet counts in patients in survival possible category. Open circle represent upper and lower limits of observed data and the solid points the mid trend. Curves idealized from FLIEDNER (1964)

the mitotic index reached almost zero. Furthermore, there was an apparent dose dependency in the depression. Thus, it is believed that the bone marrow aspirations performed promptly after an assumed exposure and at daily intervals for a period of one week would be most useful in detecting exposure to radiation in the 50 to 300 rads range. In addition to straightforward enumeration of the mitotic figures, qualitative changes are also evident. These changes consist of binucleated cells, mitotic bridges, fragments, stickiness and clumping of the chromosomes which can be quantitated. If a complete aplasia of the marrow has recurred, then examination of the marrow should be able to detect beginning regeneration, which is a most favorable prognostic sign.

A typical case of radiation injury in the survival possible category is summarized form OUGHTERSON and WARREN. A 25-year-old soldier was about 0.6 miles from the hypocenter in Hiroshima. He complained of malaise on the first day, but recovered. Between days 4 and 8 he worked on a drill field and marched 9.3 miles. Epilation began on day 8. On day 22, petechiae appeared. He was admitted to a hospital on day 26, with a sharp temperature rise on day 27, reaching 40.3° C on day 28, with subsequent gradual lysis. The petechiae began to clear on day 34, and the patient was discharged on day 59. Many other Japanese soldiers had malaise, nausea and vomiting on the first day of exposure. They recovered from the initial symptomatology, did hard physical work for 2 to 3 weeks and then developed purpura and severe infections. The mortality in this group was high.

c) Survival probable

This group consists of individuals who have had either no initial symptoms or mild or fleeting ones, disappearing within a few hours. Unless these individuals have sequelae of marrow depression, these patients will show no further subjective effects of irradiation, and obviously constitute no therapeutic problem. However, it is clear from many animal experimental studies that individuals in this category will be more susceptible to pathogenic organisms if present. Typical blood picture seen in this category is illustrated in Fig. 9. The granulocytes show an initial decrease during the first 8 days after exposure.

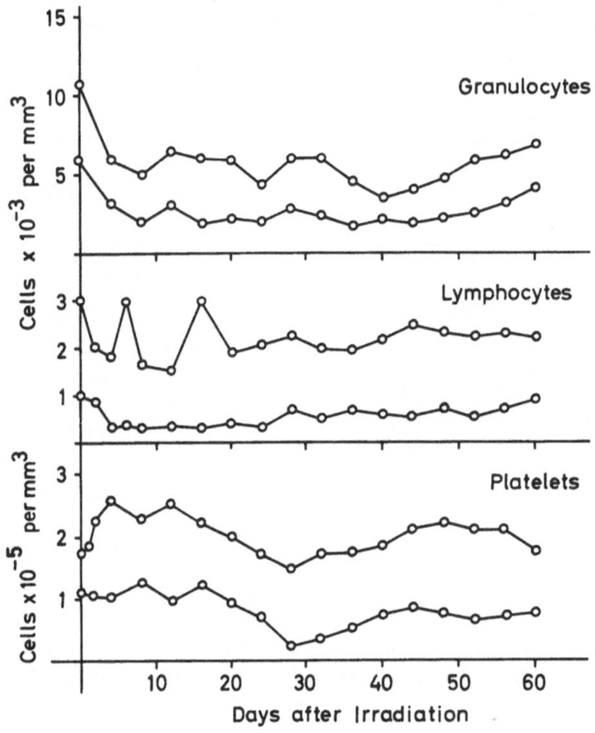

Fig. 9. Granulocyte, lymphocyte and platelet counts in survival probable category. Open circles represent highest and lowest values observed

However, they do not drop below 2000 per mm³. Thereafter, the declin elevels off and approaches a late minimum after about 40 days. During the first two weeks there is practically no change on the platelet counts. Thereafter, the platelet counts commence to fall and reach the minimal values around 28 days after exposure. Thereafter, there is a recovery in the platelet count which takes a matter of months.

The lymphocyte counts show a marked initial drop after exposure, the minimal values being attained within 2 to 3 days, with considerable variation from patient to patient. The depression remains constant for several weeks.

In general it has often been stated that the blood count has relatively little prognostic value. In respect to the lymphocyte, this is probably true, since doses up to about 300 rads produce almost a maximal depression in the lymphocytes, and further increase in dose, unless it is extremely high, do not depress this level further. However, the neutrophil count is extremely useful from a prognostic standpoint, as has been demonstrated in dogs, where there is a clear-cut difference in the rate of depression of the granulocyte count at 100 %, 80 %, and 10 % mortality respectively (CRONKITE and BRECHER, 1955). From the animal observations and the human observations summarized before, it can be seen that on clinical and laboratory grounds one can fairly well categorize patients into the relative degrees of radiation injury. This is clearly the first step in the management of radiation injury.

The preceding casualty sorting and general considerations about prognosis are relevant to therapy. In reality, one is confronted with the treatment of a patient who presents basically the same problems as the management of any other patient with pancytopenia. However, the irradiated patient presents the additional challenge that the aplastic state of the bone marrow may be reversible. Thus, if the patient can be carried through the critical period, he may recover, in contrast to the many cases of idiopathic or drug-induced bone marrow aplasia that are rarely reversible.

5. Influence of inhomogeneities of dose of radiation and partial body exposure

The first human radiation casualties from a criticality accident were characterized by marked inhomogeneities of the absorbed dose (HEMPELMANN et al., 1952). In some of the individuals, many thousands of rads were received by the hands with almost total destruction of the epithelium. The superficial skin over the abdomen and the face also received tremendous amounts of radiation, with the absorbed dose grading off towards the back and down to the legs that had some shielding. Very severe gastrointestinal injury was observed in two of the individuals. In the fatal cases, there was severe injury to the gastrointestinal tract, and marked necrosis of the skin of the hands and the face, with prominent oedema and erythema of the side of the body facing the criticality event. In addition, there was severe hemopoietic depression.

In the last criticality accident at Los Alamos scientific laboratory (SHIPMAN et al.), the dose to the head and the thorax was measured in thousands of roentgens. Immediately after exposure, the individual was disorientated, amnestic, and shortly thereafter went into collapse and was prevented from immediate death by extensive fluid and electrolyte replacement. He died within a short period of time, and at autopsy there was serious injury to the myocardium in addition to the central nervous system.

In the Lockport incident, a group of individuals had removed the lead shield from a Klystron tube that was not functioning properly. The device was emitting unfiltered 200 kV X-rays. The details of this incident are described by HOWLAND et al. (1961) and INGRAM et al. The dose distribution to the head of one individual showed marked inhomogeneities in the absorbed dose through the head. The initial neurologic symptoms were minimal, but later severe neurologic symptoms developed, demonstrating that neurologic injury per se is not necessarily fatal unless the absorbed dose is uniform throughout the head and greater than the minimum necessary to produce the neurologic syndrome. In the Lockport accident, vomiting was present initially and subsided in 4 patients out of 7 within the first day. Nausea was present in 5 of the patients and subsided more gradually, only after one week in the most seriously injured man. Headache was a serious problem in the Lockport incident. The type of pain experienced in the most heavily irradiated casualties, whose doses to the head were estimated to be about 1500 rads, was that of a deep pain located in the center of the head, unlike any headache experienced before. This is probably due to the relatively high inhomogeneous dose to the brain. In the more severe cases, small petechial showers and a few vesicular oral lesions were observed during the 4th week. The marked inhomogeneity and the component of the soft X-rays may have contributed to capillary injury in the Lockport cases. A clinical and hematologic course of the more severe Lockport patients that received of the order of 1500 rads to the head and 300 rads to the trunk differed significantly from syndromes described earlier. The symptomatology appeared to come in waves for weeks and months after exposure. These late reactions were preceded in one patient by transient erythema during the first 7 days, between days 13 and 19, and between days 24 and 29. However, on day 38, this patient became febrile, somnolent, and mentally depressed, with conjunctivitis, photophobia, and pain on movements of eyes. On day 44 another febrile attack was observed, with a new wave of somnolence and a moderate ataxia. With this, transient paresthesias of the right arm and left hand were present, and mild reflex changes were also noted. These neurological signs continued over a period of 12 days, the somnolence for 8 to 10 days. The neurological picture was compatible with diffuse involvement of the central nervous system. The Lockport cases are particularly confusing because of the sustained depression in the blood counts and the failure of the striking recovery around the 30th day in platelets observed in other human whole body injury. The reticulocytes showed a tendency to rise continually in both of the more severely exposed Lockport patients. This has not been observed in more uniform whole body exposure. The reasons for the discrepancies in the blood changes between more or less uniform whole body exposure and the X-irradiation to the trunk with a higher exposure of the head are not clear. From animal experiments in which partial body shielding produces a speedier recovery, one would expect inhomogeneous exposure such as in the Lockport incident to see more rapid recovery. Why erythropoiesis continued with a striking increase in the reticulocyte count from the very beginning with a continuous failure for a prolonged period of time in granulocytopoiesis and thrombocytopoiesis, is obscure. Clearly, much more information is needed on the influence of inhomogeneous exposure of human beings.

a) Partial body exposure

There is little direct information on human beings except from radiotherapy. There is considerable information on partial body exposure on animals, part of which will be summarized. Irradiation of the abdomen only produces gastrointestinal symptomatology. However, there are differences in survival time when the whole body is irradiated as compared to irradiation of the abdomen only, the exteriorized bowel or only a portion of the bowel. There is an extension of 2 to 3 days in survival time when only a portion of the abdomen or its contents are irradiated (Bond et al., 1950; Sullivan et al., 1959). In addition, there is also apparently a delay in the denudation of the epithelium of the irradiated bowel when only the abdomen or a portion of the bowel is irradiated. The longer survival time when the abdomen or the exteriorized bowel is irradiated is in part explained on the basis that a portion of the bowel is shielded, and thus fluid and electrolytes are better maintained. The increasing survival time with exposure of smaller segments of bowel is consistent with this concept. Selective irradiation of the oropharynx in the mouth has led to a syndrome described by Quastler et al. as "oral death".

Another source of information on the influence of partial body irradiation is derived from the aftermaths of excessive therapeutic radiation. This has been summarized by Cronkite (1966). The following is a condensation of the preceding reference. Large single doses in excess of 2000 rads or larger doses given over a longer period of time to the kidney will produce a radiation nephritis. Within a period of 6 to 13 months, or shorter in children, changes in renal function are observed. Chemical and cytological findings of nephritis are what one would expect. Hypertension and its sequelae follow.

Myopathy is produced by irradiation in single doses of around 1600 rads. Fractionation of the irradiation necessitates larger amounts of radiation. 5000 rads delivered over a 6 to 9 week period has resulted in severe inflammatory processes within muscles. Endarteriitis obliterans and the subsequent necrosis of muscle and connective tissue are characteristic.

Pneumonitis can be produced by single doses of roughly 2000 rads. The clinical symptoms are dyspnea, cough, pain and an increased temperature probably related to pneumonia. The clinical and pathologic severity is correlated with the volume and area of the lungs exposed.

Impaired bone growth and osteonecrosis. This has long been recognized as a concomitant of heavy reontgen therapy over growing bones in children. With fractionated doses it is due primarily to progressive vascular obliteration. Bone necrosis inevitably follows in due course. The bones of growing children are a particular problem. In the Marshallese only 175 rads to the whole body resultet in impaired skeletal growth in some of the children (CONARD et al., 1963).

6. Therapy of the acute radiation syndromes

Therapy of all diseases is based on proved clinical principles that apply to the treatment of signs and symptoms that are present in the course of the disorder. As mentioned earlier, the diagnosis of radiation injury and its clinical management are not dependent upon an accurate knowledge of the radiation doses received. As a matter of fact, it may be simpler to manage radiation injury without any initial knowledge of dosimetry, since all initial estimates so far have been greatly in excess of the ultimate established dose. This tendency for the physicist to over-estimate initially is understandable, but may be very disturbing to the physician responsible and the patient if he happens to know it (and he almost certainly will).

In general sense, then, one is confronted with the following problems. First, there is symptomatic relief of the central nervous system and gastrointestinal symptoms. Second, there may be severe pain and discomfort due to intestinal cramps. Third, there may be anxiety and a depression. Fourth, there are problems concerning fluid and electrolyte replacement and the maintenance of reasonable blood pressure and pulse. Fifth, there is the question of direct therapy or prevention of infectious complications, thrombopenic purpura and anemia. These general problems may occur to varying degrees in any of the major divisions of the radiation syndrome.

In respect to the central nervous system syndrome produced by very large amounts of radiation, there is little that one can do other than give sedation to control symptoms. In the case of the gastrointestinal syndrome, the intestinal hypermobility and vomiting that comes on early is probably related more to the nervous system than direct injury of the gastrointestinal tract. In all probability this can be controlled to a large extent by dithenhydramine in 100 mg doses given intramuscularly. Probably the most efficacious agent for pain and irritability is morphine in 12 mg subcutaneous doses. Since, as pointed out earlier, there is probably a synergism between the injury to the gastrointestinal tract and a rapidly developing granulocytopenia producing local infection of the bowel, one should consider the desirability of sterilization of the intestinal tract with Neomycin in 1 g doses every 4 hours orally. In the very severe cases of radiation injury, intravenous methylprednisolone and levarterenol may be of some help in maintaining an adequate blood pressure. In desperate cases of hypotension, one may try metaraminol and hypertensinogen.

However, it is highly probable that if the condition is so severe in the first few hours after irradiation that the preceding type of therapy is needed for the combination of neurological and gastrointestinal symptomatology, no therapy will increase the probability of survival. However, it is mandatory to keep the patient comfortable and treat each symptom complex irrespective of the prognosis. The management of the hemopoietic syndrome involves prevention of infection, treatment of infection when it occurs, prevention of bleeding and its control if it occurs, and prevention of anemia by appropriate transfusion, and considering the possibility of marrow transplantation to restore hemopoietic function.

a) Definite therapeutic outline and guiding principles

α) The cardinal therapeutic principle is to do nothing without a clear-cur clinical indication. Except for the severe forms of radiation injury as discussed earlier, there is no urgency. However, if there is a question of neutron exposure, a sample of blood for determination of the activation of sodium must be obtained immediately. From the latter, an estimate of the thermal neutron dose can be made. Whole body counter measurement of induced radioactive sodium is better.

β) A history and physical examination is particularly pertinent, and must be detailed with special reference to detecting the possibility of prior chronic infections of any type. It is highly desirable to obtain immediately any earlier hospital records of the patient.

γ) Inform responsible medical, administrative, health physics and legal authorities promptly. In dealing with radiation accidents, one obviously is primarily concerned immediately with the welfare of the patient, but because of the great public interest in the problem one cannot avoid inquiries from the press and diverse curiously interested people and agencies.

δ) Hospitalize the individuals as rapidly as reasonable until the degree of exposure has been ascertained.

ε) Follow closely the peripheral granulocyte, lymphocyte, platelet counts and hematocrits. Blood counts should be performed at daily intervals for one week and thereafter 3 times a week for at least 4 weeks. Then, the interval for blood study should be determined on the basis of the prior sequence. A bone marrow aspiration is essential as soon as possible after exposure, and at 1, 2 and 4 days after irradiation. Thereafter, a marrow aspiration should be performed 1 to 2 times a week, in order to observe for the possibility of spontaneous regeneration. With these studies and the general clinical appearance, one can determine the survival category in which an individual should be placed by the 4th or 5th day, utilizing the principles described earlier in this chapter.

ζ) Weigh daily and record fluid intake and output with intermittent electrolyte studies on the blood.

η) Institute the highest quality of nursing care. Particular attention should be paid to oral and skin hygiene. Portals of entry for bacteria are frequently the oral mucosa, abrasions of the skin, or around the anogenital area. Strict asepsis is mandatory with all procedures involving a cutaneous puncture.

ϑ) If it is believed that the short-term exposure has been in excess of 200 rads, or if the patients conform to the survival possible group, reverse isolation should be instituted promptly in order to prevent to introduction of pathogens into the patient's environment. Perform throat and nasal cultures on the staff. Staphylococcal carriers should not be permitted to participate in the care of irradiated individuals.

ι) In addition to the regular recording of vital signs, blood pressure and pulse should be watched carefully in the event that there are serious gastrointestinal symptoms. In particular, pay attention to the fluid and electrolyte balance, and correct as necessary with the appropriate solutions or plasma.

$\varkappa$) If signs of infection develop, such as a sudden spike in fever, or the development of ulcerations when the leukocyte count is below 1500 per mm^3, give antibiotics in large doses. Antibiotics are rarely indicated prophylactically. It is recommended that antibiotic doses be 3 times those that are ordinarily used. If the temperature is not controlled with the antibiotic employed, switch to another antibiotic. If the temperature rises again, switch to still another antibiotic. Of course, the choice of antibiotic will be determined in part by the bacterial cultures, but do not wait for the sensitivities to be determined, since the introduction of true pathogens may result in rapid, progressive overwhelming infection in the pancytopenic state. With commensal organisms, the infections do not progress as rapidly, but it takes time to get bacterial cultural confirmation of the infecting organism.

Use oral antifungal antibiotics when giving broad spectrum antibiotics. Sulfonamides have been used with success in pancyteopenias from other causes, and should always be given due consideration.

λ) Watch the platelet count carefully and observe the patient for signs of bleeding. Watch for the presence of hematuria, cutaneous petechiae or retinal bleeding. If there is any indication of bleeding give platelets in a single, whole blood transfusion until the hematocrit is at a reasonable level. Blood must be fresh (less than 4 hours old). When the hematocrit is elevated to satisfactory levels, give freshly separated platelets in a single transfusion in amounts equivalent to those found in approximately one third of the blood volume of the patient. Follow the patient closely, and retransfuse as indicated by the clinical picture. Generally speaking, platelet transfusions will not be necessary at more frequent intervals than 3 to 5 days. It is not necessary to maintain a normal platelet count. The probability of bleeding, with platelets in excess of 40000, is very rare indeed. In fact, bleeding is rarely observed until platelets fall below 25000 per mm³.

μ) In summary, when indicated, push antibiotic therapy vigorously to control infection and platelet transfusion to stop bleeding. Above all, try to prevent serious infection by reserve isolation and prevent gastrointestinal bleeding by bed rest and careful attention to the bowels, since fatal hemorrhage has been initial by straining at stool in the pancyto-penic state. Combined antibiotic and transfusion therapy has significantly increased the survival rate of dogs exposed up to an $LD_{95\text{-}100}$ dose of radiation by SORENSEN *et al.* (1960). At supralethal doses this regimen has been of no avail. One can anticipate that a similar regimen would be equally as effective in man exposed to biologically comparable doses of radiation. Many individuals have now survived after even fairly high doses of radiation without any therapy. Thus, unless signs of hemorrhage of infection, or extreme depression of peripheral blood counts appear, no treatment is needed. In the Marshallese exposed to high sub-lethal doses of radiation, in whom an epidemic of upper respiratory infections developed, practically no therapy was indicated or needed. In the 5 individuals exposed to neutron and gamma radiation in the industrial Y-12 accident at Oak Ridge, therapy, was limited to treatment of infection in a single individual who responded well. In these individuals, peripheral blood count depression was severe and in the Oak Ridge accident some loss of hair and some evidence of bleeding were also noted.

The use of antibiotics prophylactically has been recommended by others. However, it is felt that this is definitely contraindicated, for this may result in unnecessary development of resistant bacteria within the irradiated individual prior to the onset of infection, thus shortening the period of time over which the antibiotics may sustain life, and thereby also shortening the period of time during which spontaneous regeneration in the bone marrow may take place. However, with the overwhelming doses with a very severe gastrointestinal syndrome, consideration to the use of non-absorbable antibiotics to sterilize the intestine and prevent local infection accentuating the gastrointestinal syndrome should be given. Perhaps it is of academic interest, since individuals exposed to such doses of radiation probably have no statistical chance of survival any way.

If the dose of radiation is high, in excess of 500 rads, or if the individuals are deteriorat-ing with a very rapid decline in the granulocyte and the platelet counts, one of course must consider the possibility of attempting homologous bone marrow transplantation. The selection of patients for homotransplantation of bone marrow is very difficult. Certainly, if the dose of radiation has been proved without doubt to be definitely in excess of 600 rads (probability of spontaneous survival nil) one should consider homologous transplantation of bone marrow. However, one cannot be very enthusiastic about the probability of a successful homologous bone marrow transplantation for two significant reasons. First, in animals the dose of radiation must be very high in order to suppress immunity sufficiently for the foreign tissue to settle out and grow, and second, the number of cells required to protect animals is so large that a comparable amount could only be obtained from a single human donor by multiple aspiration which necessitates general anesthesia. However, situations may well arise in which one must give serious consideration to attempting transplantation of marrow. The biological background of marrow transplantation has been presented by Loutit and Micklem (1966).

The situation may be summarized somewhat as follows. Homologous bone marrow contains cells which have the capability of repopulating bone marrow and restoring immunological competence by donor cells. The former is desired and the latter is to be avoided. The establishment of immunological competence by donor cells permits these cells to launch a graft versus host disease (secondary disease or allogenic disease). The foreign, immunologically competent cells attack kidneys liver, lymph nodes, skin, and intestinal tract, producing severe symptomatology and death in a large fraction of treated animals. This has been shown by Mathé et al. to be formidable problem also in man. Following any attempted homotransplantation in man, one desires a temporary take of the hemopoietic tissue to save a life. It is hoped that this will be followed by a slow recovery of the host's immunologically competent system, which would then reject the transplanted bone marrow. In parallel with this, one wishes the host's bone marrow to recover. This has been apparently observed from time to time in experimental animals by chance alone. It is not clear as to how one can deliberately attain the desired result in man. For certain possible situations one should give serious thought to the preservation of bone marrow for autologous transfusion. It has been established by Alpen et al. and Thomas et al. that autologous transfusions significantly increase the survival rate of fatally irradiated dogs. Kurnick et al. have evidence that suggests preserved autologous marrow is of value in human beings with marrow depressed from extensive chemotherapy. Since marrow can be preserved satisfactorily one should consider the possible conditions where one might have greater probabilities of severe radiation injury and consider the desirability of preparing and preserving one's own marrow for possible future use. However, in this case one is confronted with the problem of submitting the individual to a small but definite hazard to life by general anesthesia in obtaining enough of his own marrow to the small but definite possibility of being involved in an accident at a later time and then needing the preserved marrow.

The entire problem is when and how to transplant bone marrow and obtain the desired results described above, or, in the event that a permanent take of the marrow is needed, to suppress secondary disease. There is no doubt that if one gets a permanent take of the transplanted marrow, the individuals would have died had the marrow not been transplanted. Now the question is how to suppress the secondary disease. These complicated problems do not have satisfactory answers at the present time, and one is referred to the World Health Organisation monograph on "Diagnosis and Treatment of Acute Radiation Injury" and "La Greffe des Cellules Hématopoiétiques Allogénique" for more details.

7. Prophylactic therapy

No-one will disagree that in any operation where hazard is involved, every possible precaution must be taken at the planning stage. Work with radiation is no exception, and the remarkable rarity of accidents in modern radiation work is a tribute to the planners in the nuclear energy industry of all countries. Much of the credit is due to the health physicists.

The first and necessary function of the health physicist is to advise and help his colleagues in other scientific and engineering disciplines to design, test and operate their various installations with safety. Clearly, the first time an assembly is operated is the most hazardous time. However, experience has clearly indicated that the hazards also continue because of natural capability of humans to err. Even in the case of often repeated successful operations, accidents do occur. This was demonstrated clearly in the Oak Ridge accident at Los Alamos accidents. Acordingly, one of the most important functions in prevention of accidents is the continuing enthusiastic vigilance of the health physicist and his colleagues. This clearly is an unpleasant police function, and one to which industrial psychologists should well give significant attention. There is no substitute for planning adequate protective measures and continuing enthusiastic vigilance on the part of those who must continually observe potentially hazardous operations to see that they remain safe in functioning.

The question of chemical protection against radiation has been intensively studied, both for a basic understanding of the mechanism of action of radiation, and with the hope that some practical prophylactic measure might be developed that could protect individuals operating in a radiation area. In fact, it has been shown that there are many agents which will increase resistance of animals to radiation by about a factor of 2. The two most effective procedures are the induction of severe hypoxia, and the administration of high concentrations of certain sulfhydro compounds. The former clearly is too hazardous in itself, and the second also has serious pharmacological effects, that prevents, at the present time, practical use of these agents. Of course, basic studies are continuing in this important field, but it is regrettable that nothing as yet of a practical nature has arisen that can be administered prior to exposure and will protect individuals against radiation.

VIII. Beta exposure of the skin from fall-out

This general problem has been covered in great detail by CONARD *et al.* The problem will only be summarized briefly here in. Generally it was considered that beta radiation from fission products would not constitute any hazard to human beings. However, in 1954 the importance of this hazard became apparent when widespread radiation lesions of the skin developed in a large group of people accidentally exposed to fall-out radiation in Marshall Islands following the experimental detonation of a large nuclear device. In addition to exposure of some 239 Marshallese people and 28 Americans, there were 23 Japanese fishermen exposed on the fishing boat. Up to this time some beta burns had been observed on the backs of animals near the atomic energy testing site. In addition, exposure of the hands of several individuals who had carelessly handled fission products, samples from a detonation, resulted in the development of severe lesions.

The lesions of the skin induced by fall-out are primarily due to the beta radiation from the fission products adhering to the particular fall-out material, and are therefore referred to as beta burns. Actually, in the fall-out accident, the radioactive material fell out of the sky, resembling small snow flakes. In this instance, the fall-out material consisted of calcium oxide from the incineration of the calcium carbonate of the coral islands. However, the chemical and physical make-up of fall-out will vary according to the type of terrain or soil over which the detonation occurs. All fall-out is particulate in nature, but the size and other characteristics of the particles will depend on the physical and chemical properties of the soil. The calcium oxide of the fall-out material in this accident partly dissolved in the perspiration of the skin and brought the adsorbed radioactive particles in very close contact.

The beta emitters of the fall-out material have a wide range of energies from a few kV to a few MeV. The depth of penetration is limited by the most energetic component. When in direct contact with the skin 50% of the most energetic component will be absorbed within 1 000 microns. Thus injury will be relatively superficial. However, severe burns necessitating skin grafting have been produced by accidental contamination of hands by fission products (KNOWLTON *et al.*).

During the first 24—48 hours after the fall-out descended on the Marshallese there was a varying degree of itching, burning and tingling of the skin along with lacrymation. How much of this was due to or accentuated by the calcium oxide and its caustic action on moist skin is not known. These symptoms subsided and for a period of about 2 weeks there were no symptoms or signs referable to the skin. At this time small highly pigmented macules appeared accompanied by intense itching and burning. These lesions were located on the exposed skin and were most commonly seen on the neck, face, cubital fossa, and feet. These coalesced into larger plaques and finally superficial desquamation of the epidermis occured. In a few instances there was severe edema, pain, and deeper ulceration on the dorsum of the feet and in one patient the back of the ears. All lesions ultimately healed. The ones in which there was deeper ulceration left residual scars and de-pigmented areas.

In addition to the skin lesions there were varying degrees of epilation. All hair regrew with normal color and texture. Treatment was limited to local antibiotic ointments and cleanliness when ulceration appeared.

The people who had beta burns have been carefully observed. To date, 16 years after the accident, no cases of cutaneous cancer have developed. Scars are present. Biopsies have shown mild typical late radiation effects in blood vessels and connective tissue however no trophic ulcers have developed. Perhaps radiation injury of the epithelium is an insufficient injury to produce epitheliomata and the secondary trophic disturbances due to ulceration and its sequelae are required to produce radiation induced cancer of the skin.

IX. Recovery from radiation injury and influence of prior whole body exposure on response to later exposure

In general the first order model for exponential recovery from radiation injury formulated by Blair in 1950 has been widely accepted and used to estimate hazards and residual injury at various times after prior exposure. The experimental basis for this model is the extensive study of the behaviour of mice previously exposed to radiation of various doses and later challenged to determine changes in the LD_{50}. As a result of accumulation of data on radiation effects on mammals in general and the accidental exposure of human beings to fall-out considerable doubt was thrown on the validity of the general application of the exponential recovery concept. Alpen (1966) began some years ago to systematically study the mortality and hematological response of a wide spectrum of mammals (mice to swine) after the first and subsequent exposures to radiation. First the LD_{50} for mammals falls into two categories one for small mammals (rat, mouse, hamster, and rabbit) with an LD_{50} of 889—941 rads and one for large mammals (dog, burro, goat, sheep and swine) with an LD_{50} of 251—376 rads. The monkey is midway between and the guinea pig has an LD_{50} of 255 rads rather than the 900 rads one might expect in a small animal.

The hematological responses in the early phases are relatively similar with some differences in the rapidity of the development of the reduced counts. There are striking differences in the recovery patterns which depend upon the species and not the dose of radiation.

When all species were studied for radiation recovery following the administration of $^2/_3$ of the LD_{50} it was found that only the mouse gave an exponential recovery following exposure. Even with the mouse there are significant deviations during the first few hours following the conditioning dose. The recovery patterns for the mammals are quoted from Alpen:

a) "a temporary delay in the commencement of the decrease in radiosensitivity termed the recovery plateau"

b) "a two component decrease in radiosensitivity made up of an early fast phase and a later slower phase"

c) "a recrudescence of radiosensitivity such that the animal is more radiosensitive following a period of early recovery"

d) "a period of radioresistance of 'over recovery' of varying duration and character".

None of the animals had all four of the characteristics listed above. Each species has its own unique pattern. The response pattern of man of course is not known but there is no cogent reason to believe that man is different from all other mammalian species. Accordingly these general principles should be incorporated into one's thinking when trying to evaluate repetitive whole body exposure of human beings.

References

ALLEN, J. G., JACOBSON, L. O., *et al.*: Heparinemia – an anticoagulant in the blood of dogs with hemorrhagic tendency after total body exposure to roentgen rays. J. Exp. Med. **87**, 71–85 (1948).
— ALPEN, E. A., BAUM, S. J.: Modification of X-radiation lethality by autologous marrow infusion in dogs. Blood **13**, 1168 (1958).
— The comparison of hematological responses and radiation recovery in several mammalian species. International Atomic Energy Agency Symposium on Effects of Radiation, Vienna 1966.
ATHENS, J. W., RAAB, S. O., HAAB, O. P., MAUER, A. M., ASHENBRUCKER, H., CARTWRIGHT, G. F., WINTROBE, M. M.: Leukokinetic Studies III. J. Clin. Inv. **40**, 159–164 (1961).
BENDER, M. A., GOOCH, P. C.: Persistent chromosome aberrations in irradiated human subjects. Rad. Res. **16**, 44 (1962).
BLAIR, H. A.: Recovery from radiation injury in mice and its effect on LD$_{50}$ for durations of exposure up to several weeks. USAEC Report UR-312, University of Rochester, Rochester, N.Y., 1954.
BOND, V. P., CRONKITE, E. P.: Effects of radiation on mammals. Ann. Rev. Physiol. **19**, 299–328 (1957).
— ROBERTSON, J. S.: Vertebrate radiobiology (lethal actions and associated effects). Ann. Rev. Nucl. Sci. **7**, 135–162 (1957).
— SILVERMAN, M., CRONKITE, E. P.: Pathogenesis and pathology of post-irradiation infection. Rad. Res. **1**, 389–400 (1954).
— FLIEDNER, T. M., ARCHAMBEAU, J. O.: Mammalian Radiation Lethality, A Disturbance in cellular Cinetics. — A. I. B. S. Monograph, Academic Press, New York and London, 1965.
— SWIFT, M. M., ALLEN, A. C., FISHLER, M. C.: Sensitivity of abdomen of rat to x-rays. Amer. J. Physiol. **161**, 323–330 (1950).
BRECHER, G., CRONKITE, E. P., CONARD, R. A., SMITH, W. W.: Gastric lesions in experimental animals following single exposures to ionizing radiations. Amer. J. Path. **34**, 105–119 (1958).
BRUCER, M.: The acute radiation syndrome. A medical report on the Y-12 accident, June 16, 1958, USAEC Report ORINS, Oak Ridge, Tenn., 1959.
COHN, S. H., MILNE. W. L.: The effects of combined administration of 90 Sn and external radiation. U.S. Naval Radiological Defense Laboratory USNRDL-TR-89, San Francisco, Calif., 1956.
CONARD, R. A., CRONKITE, E. P., BOND, V. P.: Fall-Out Radiation: Effects on the Skin. Chapter 12. BEHRENS, C. F., KING, E. R.: Atomic Medicine. Baltimore, Md.: Williams and Wilkins, 1964.
— — BRECHER, G., STROME, C. P. A.: Experimental therapy of the gastrointestinal syndrome produced by lethal doses of ionizing radiation. J. Appl. Physiol. **9**, 227–233 (1956).
CONARD, R. A., MEYER, L. M., SUTOW, W. W., MOLONEY, W. C., CANNON, B., HICKING, A., RICKLON, E.: Medical survey of the Marshallese nine years after exposure to fall-out radiation. Brookhaven Natl. Lab. Report No. 7766, Upton, N.Y., 1963.
CRONKITE, E. P.: The diagnosis, prognosis and treatment of radiation injury produced by atomic bombs. Radiology **56**, 661–669 (1951).
— Radiation injury in man. Chapter 5 in: SCHWARTZ, E. E.: Biological Basis of Radiotherapy. Philadelphia: J. B. Lippincott, 1966.
— — BRECHER, G.: Defects in hemostasis produced by whole body irradiation. 5th Annual Conference on Blood Coagulation and Allied Subjects. New York: Trans. Josiah Macy Foundation, 1952.
— FLIEDNER, T. M.: Granulocytopoiesis. New Engl. J. Med. **270**, 1347–1352 (1964).
— BOND, V. P., FLIEDNER, T. M., KILLMANN, S. A.: The use of 3 H-thymidine in the study of hemopoietic cell proliferation. Ciba Foundation Symposium Hemopoiesis. London: Churchill and Co., 1960.
— BRECHER, G.: The protective effect of granulocytes in radiation injury. Ann. N.Y. Acad. Sci. **59**, 815–833 (1955).
— JACOBS, G., BRECHER, G., DILLARD, G. H. L.: The hemorrhagic phase of the acute radiation syndrome due to whole body exposure. Amer. J. Roentgenol. **67**, 796–803 (1952).
— BRECHER, G., WILBUR, K. M.: Development and use of a canine blood donor colony. I. Leukocyte and platelet transfusions in irradiation aplasia of the dog. Military Surgeon **111**, 359–365 (1954).
— BOND, V. P., DUNHAM, C. L.: Some effects of ionizing radiation on human beings. U.S. Government Printing Office, TID 5358, Washington, D. C., 1956.
— — Diagnosis of radiation injury. An analysis of the human lethal dose of radiation. U.S. Armed Forces Med. J. **11**, 249–260, 1960.
— — FLIEDNER, T. M., PAGLIA, D. A., ADAMIK, E. R.: Studies on the origin, production and destruction of platelets, pp. 595–609. Intern. Symp. Henry Ford Hospital, Detroit, Mich., 1961.
EBBE, S., STOHLMAN, JR., F.: Megakaryocytopoiesis in the rat. Blood **26**, 20–35 (1965).
ELLINGER, F.: Medical Radiation Biology. Springfield, Illinois: Charles C. Thomas, 1957.
EVERETT, N. B., COFFREY, R. W., RIEKE, W. O.: Recirculation of lymphocytes. Ann. N. Y. Acad. Sci. **113**, 887 (1964).

Fabricius-Moller, J.: Experimental studies of the hemorrhagic diathesis from x-ray sickness. Copenhagen: Levin and Munksgaard Forlag, 1922.

Fernau, Schramek, Zarzycki: Über die Wirkung von induzierter Radioaktivität. Wien. klin. Wschr. **26**, 94 (1913).

Fliedner, T. M., Sandkühler, S., Stodtmeister, R.: Die Knochenmarkstruktur bei Ratten nach Bestrahlung mit schnellen Elektronen. Z. Zellforsch. Mikroskop. Anat. **43**, 195–205 (1955).

— — — Research on the architecture of the vascular bed of the bone marrow. Z. Zellforsch. Mikroskop. Anat. **45**, 328–338 (1956).

— Sorenson, D. K., Bond, V. P., Cronkite, E. P., Jackson, D. P., Adamik, E.: Comparative effectiveness of fresh and lyophilized platelets in controlling irradiation hemorrhage. Proc. Soc. Exp. Biol. Med. **99**, 731–733 (1958).

— Cronkite, E. P., Bond, V. P., Rubini, J. R., Andrews, G.: The mitotic index of human bone marrow in healthy individuals and irradiated human beings. Acta Haemat. **22**, 65–68 (1959).

— Bond, V. P., Cronkite, E. P.: Structural cytological and autoradiographic changes in the bone marrow following total body irradiation. Amer. J. Pathol. **38**, 599–623 (1961).

— Andrews, G., Cronkite, E. P., Bond, V. P.: Early and late cytological effects of whole body irradiation on human bone marrow. Blood **23**, 471–487 (1964).

— Hämatologische Befunde beim akuten Strahlensyndrom. Strahlentherapie, Sonderbände 56, 1964.

— Cronkite, E. P., Robertson, J. S.: Granulocytopoiesis I. Senescence and random loss of neutrophilic granulocytes in human beings. Blood **24**, 402–414 (1964).

— — Killmann, S. A., Bond, V. P.: Granulocytopoiesis II. Emergence and pattern of labeling of neutrophilic granulocytes in human beings. Blood **24**, 683–700 (1964).

Freireich, E. J., Levin, R. H., Whang, J., Carbone, P. P., Bronson, W., Morse, E. E.: The function and fate of transfused leukocytes in leukopenic recipients. Ann. N. Y. Acad. Sci. **113**, 1081–1089 (1964).

Gerskova, A. K., Baisogolov, G. D.: Two cases of acute radiation disease in man. Proc. Intern. Conf. Peaceful Uses of Atomic Energy, United Nations. Geneva **3**, 35–44 (1956).

Gerstner, H. B.: Acute radiation syndrome in man. U.S. Armed Forces Med. J. **9**, 313–354 (1958).

Gowans, J. L.: The effect of continuous reinfusion of lymph and lymphocytes from the thoracic duct. Brit. J. Exp. Path. **38**, 67 (1957).

Hasterlik, R. J., Marinelli, L. D.: Physical dosimetry and clinical observations on four human beings involved in an accidental critical assembly excursion. Proc. Int. Conf. Peaceful Uses of Atomic Energy, United Nations, Geneva **2**, 25–34 (1955).

Heinecke, H.: Über die Einwirkung der Röntgenstrahlen auf Tiere. Münchner med. Wschr. **1**, 2090–2092 (1903).

Hempelmann, L. H., Lesco, H., Hoffmann, J. G.: The acute radiation syndrome; a study of nine cases and a review of the problem. Ann. Int. Med. **36**, 279–510 (1952).

Holthusen, H., Meyer, H., Molineux, W. M.: Ehrenbuch der Röntgenologen und Radiologen aller Nationen. Munich and Berlin: Verlag Urban und Schwarzenberg, 1959.

Howland, J. W., Ingram, M., Mermagen, H.: The Lockport incident. Accidental partial body exposure in: Diagnosis and Therapy of Acute Radiation Injury, pp. 11–26. World Health Organization, Geneva, 1961.

Ingram, M., Howland, J. W., Hansen, C. H.: Sequential manifestations of acute radiation injury versus "acute radiation syndrome" stereotype. Ann. N. Y. Acad. Sci. **114**, 356–367 (1964).

International Commission on Radiologic Protection. Pergamon Press, London, England. Health Physics **11**, 1–20 (1959).

Jackson, D. P., Cronkite, E. P., Le Roy, G. V., Halpern, B.: Further studies on the nature of the hemorrhagic phase of radiation injury. J. Lab. Clin. Med. **39**, 449–461 (1952).

Jackson, K. L., Rhodes, R., Entenman, C.: Electrolyte excretion in the rat after severe intestinal damage by x-irradiation. Rad. Res. **8**, 361–373 (1958).

Jacobs, G., Lynch, F. X., Cronkite, E. P., Bond, V. P.: Human radiation injury – a correlation of leukocyte depression with mortality in the Japanese exposed to the atomic bomb. Military Med. **128**, 732–739 (1963).

Jacobson, L. O., Marks, E. K., Gaston, E. O., Robson, J. J., Zirkle, R. E.: The role of the spleen in radiation injury. Proc. Soc. Exp. Biol. Med. **70**, 740–742 (1949).

— Recovery from radiation injury. Blood **6**, 769–770 (1951).

Jammet, H. P.: Treatment of victims of the zero energy reactor accident at Vinca. Diagnosis and Treatment of Radiation Injury. World Health Organization, Geneva, 1961.

Karas, J. S., Stanbury, J. B.: Fatal radiation syndrome from an accidental nuclear excursion. N. Eng. J. Med. **272**, 755–761 (1965).

Knowlton, N. P., Leifer, E., Hogness, J. R., Hempelmann, L. H., Blaney, L. A., Gill, D. C., Oakes, W., Shafer, C. L.: Beta ray burns of the skin. J.A.M.A. **141**, 239–246 (1949).

Krayevskii, N. A.: Studies on the Pathology of Radiation Disease. London: Pergamon Press, 1965.

Kurnick, N. B.: Autologous bone marrow in the treatment of severe iatrogenic myelo-suppression. Diagnosis and Treatment of Radiation Injury, World Health Organization, Geneva, 1961.

Lacassagne, A., Lattes, J., Lavedan, J.: Étude expérimentale des effets biologiques du polonium introduit dans l'arganesine. J. radiol. et electrol. **9**, 1–14 (1925).

Lamerton, L. F., Baxter, C. F.: An experimental study of radiation induced anemia with reference to shielding procedures and platelet changes. Brit. J. Radiol. **28**, 87–94 (1955).

Langham, W., Woodward, K. T., Rothermel, S. M., Harris, P. S., Lushbaugh, C. C., Storer, J. B.: Studies on the effect of rapidly delivered, massive doses of gamma rays on mammals. Rad. Res. **5**, 404–432 (1956).

LEEKSMA, C. H. W., COHEN, J. A.: Determination of life span of human platelets. J. Clin. Invest. **35**, 964–969 (1956).

LE ROY, G. V.: Hematology of Atomic Bomb Casualties. Arch. Internal Med. **86**, 691–710 (1950).

LORENZ, E., CONGDON, C., UPHOFF, D.: Modification of acute irradiation injury in mice and guinea pigs by bone marrow injections. Radiology **58**, 863 (1952).

MICKLEM, H. S., LOUTIT, J. F., FORD, C. E.: Tissue Grafting and Radiation. ABIS Monograph, Academic Press, New York and London, 1966.

MANNICK, J. A., LOCHTE, H. L., ASHLEY, C. A., THOMAS, E. D., FERREBEE, J. W.: Autografts of bone marrow in dogs after lethal total body radiation. Blood **15**, 255 (1960).

MATHÉ, G., JAMMET, H. P., PENDIC, B., SCHWARZENBERG, L., DUPLAN, J. F., MAUPIN, B., LATARJET, R., LAURIEN, M. J., KALIC, D., DJUKIC, L.: Transfusions et greffes de moelle osseuse homologue chez des humains irradiés à haute doses accidentalement. Rev. Franç. Études Clin. Biol. **4**, 226–238 (1959).

McCULLOCH, E. A., TILL, J. E.: The sensitivity of cells from normal mouse bone marrow to gamma radiation *in vitro* and *in vivo*. Radiat. Res. **16**, 822–832 (1962).

MILLER, C. P., HAMMOND, C. W., TOMPKINS, M.: The role of infection in radiation injury. J. Lab. Clin. Med. **38**, 331–343 (1951).

MILLER, L. S., FLETCHER, G. H., GERSTNER, H. B.: Systemic and clinical effects induced in 263 cancer patients by whole body x-ray with air doses of 15–200 r. School of Aviation Med. USAF Report No. 57–92, Brooks Air Force Base, San Antonio, Texas, U.S.A., 1957.

MINOT, G. R., SPURLING, R. G.: The effects on the blood of irradiation. Am. J. Med. Sci. **16**, 215–240 (1924).

National Committee on Radiation Protection and Measurements Permissible Dose Handbook 59, U.S. Government Printing Office, Washington, D. C., 1954.

National Academy of Sciences, National Research Council: Effect of ionizing radiation on the human hemopoietic system. Publication No. 875, Washington, D. C., 1961.

OUGHTERSEN, A. W., WARREN, S.: Medical Effects of the Atomic Bomb on Japan. New York: McGraw Hill Book Co., 1946.

PAXTON, H. C., BAKER, R. D., MARAMAN, W. J.: Nuclear critical accident at Los Alamos Scientific Laboratory. USAEC Report MS-2293, Los Alamos, New Mexico, 1959.

PENDIC, B.: The zero reactor accident at Vinca. Diagnosis and Treatment of Radiation Injury. World Health Organization, Geneva, 1961.

Physical Factors and Modification of Radiation Injury-Symposium. Ann. N.Y. Acad. Sci. **114**, 1–716 (1964).

QUASTLER, H., LANZL, E. F., KELLER, M. E., OSBORNE, J. W.: Acute intestinal radiation death. Studies on roentgen death in mice III. Amer. J. Physiol. **164**, 546–556 (1951).

QUASTLER, H., AUSTIN, M. K., MILLER, M.: Oral radiation death. Rad. Res. **5**, 338–353 (1956).

— The nature of intestinal radiation death. Rad. Res. **4**, 303–320 (1956).

ROBINSON, S. H., BRECHER, G., LOWRIE, I. S., HALEY, J. E.: Leukocyte labeling in rats during and after continuous 3 H-thymidine infusion in rats. Implications for lymphocyte longevity. Blood **26**, 281–296 (1965).

ROSSI, E., THORNGATE, A. H., LARSON, F. C.: Acute radiation syndrome caused by accidental exposure to cobalt 60. J. Lab. Clin. Med. **59**, 655–666 (1962).

SCHIFFER, L. M., ATKINS, H. L., CHANANA, A. D., CRONKITE, E. P., GREENBERG, M. L., JOHNSON, H. A., ROBERTSON, J. S., STRYCKMANS, P. A.: Extracorporeal irradiation of the blood in humans. Effects upon erythrocyte survival. Blood, **27**, pp. 831–843, 1966.

SHIPMAN, T. L.: A fatal radiation fatality resulting from massive over-exposure to neutrons and gamma rays. Diagnosis and Treatment of Radiation Injury, pp. 113–133, World Health Organization, Geneva, 1961.

SIPE, C. R., CHANANA, A. D., CRONKITE, E. P., JOEL, D., SCHIFFER, L. M.: Studies on lymphopoiesis. VII. Size distribution of bovine thoracic duct lymphocytes duct Proc. Soc. Exp. Biol. Med. **123**, 158–161, 1966.

SORENSEN, D. K., BOND, V. P., CRONKITE, E. P., PERMAN, V.: An effective therapeutic regimen for the hemopoietic phase of the acute radiation syndrome in dogs. Rad. Res. **13**, 669–685 (1960).

SULLIVAN, M. F.: Dependence of radiation diarrhea on the presence of bile in the intestine. Nature **195**, 1217–1218 (1962).

— MARKS, S., HACKETT, P. L., THOMPSON, R. C.: X-irradiation of the exterioriced or in situ intestine of the rat. Radiat. Res. **11**, 653–666 (1959).

TERASIMA, T., TOLMACH, L. J.: Variations in several responses of HeLa cells to x-irradiation during the division cycle. Biophysics. J. **3**, 11–33 (1963).

THOMAS, R. E., BROWN, D. G.: Response of burros to neutron — gamma radiation. Health Physics **6**, 19–26 (1961).

TULLIS, J. L., CHAMBERS, R. W., MORGAN, J. E.: Mortality in swine and dose distribution studies in phantoms exposed to supervoltage radiation. Amer. J. Roentgenol. **57**, 620–627 (1952).

VAN CLEAVE, C. D.: Irradiation and the Nervous System. New York: Rowman and Littlefield, 1962.

VOGEL, F. S., HOAK, C. G., SLOPER, J. C., HAYMAKER, W.: The induction of acute morphological changes in the central nervous system of monkeys by cobalt 60 irradiation. J. Neuropath. Exptl. Neurol. **17**, 138–150 (1958).

WARREN, S.: Effects of radiation on normal tissue. Arch. Path. **34**, 443, 562, 249, 917, 1070 (1942).

WILLIAMS, R. B., TOAL, J. N., WHITE, J., CARPENTER, H. M.: Effect of total body x-radiation on small bowel epithelium. I. Changes in rate of cell division. J. Natl. Cancer Inst. **21**, 17–48 (1958).

WILSON, B. R.: Survival studies of whole body x-irradiated germ-free mice. Rad. Res. **20**, 477–483 (1963).

H. Frequency of induction of malignancies in man by ionising radiation*

By

E. Eric Pochin

I. Introduction

The carcinogenic hazard of heavy exposure of tissues to ionising radiation was clearly recognized within a few years of the first use of roentgen-rays and of the discovery of radioactivity (FRIEBEN, 1902; PORTER and WHITE, 1907; ROWNTREE, 1908). Tumours were seen to develop in areas of skin which had been grossly damaged by irradiation, and the distribution of such tumours over the body surface did not correspond with the usual distribution of skin tumours occurring spontaneously.

It was soon appreciated that radiation was carcinogenic at high dose levels in other tissues than skin, and malignant changes were observed in many types of organ or body tissue following irradiation. Initially it was established that such tumours were detectable within a few years of irradiation. With wider experience, longer review of irradiated subjects, and fuller statistical analysis, it became clear that tumours might develop at many years after exposure, latencies of 20 or 30 years having been demonstrated as mean or median values in some groups of patients followed for prolonged periods (GOOLDEN, 1957; ANDREWS, 1957; RAVENTOS and WINSHIP, 1964). At first also, tumours were recognised as arising in tissues which by histological criteria were grossly damaged. It was later appreciated however that tumours might develop in irradiated tissues in which damage was not demonstrable histologically, so that the malignant change was not a simple consequence of tissue disorganisation at the microscopic level.

In a qualitative manner, therefore, a carcinogenic effect of radiation on many, or most, body tissues has long been known. Much more recently, attempts have been made to establish quantitatively the frequency with which malignant tumours develop following given absorbed doses in different body tissues (ICRP, 1966; UNSCEAR, 1964; POCHIN, 1970). This much more difficult type of enquiry, which is reviewed in the present chapter, has become necessary for two distinct reasons.

In the first place, while it has been readily demonstrable that irradiation at high doses may induce malignant tumours in various tissues, a lower frequency of induction by lower doses may only be detected, and discriminated from the normal tumour incidence that would occur in the absence of irradiation, by careful statistical analysis of the results of appropriate epidemiological surveys. The difficulty in detecting any carcinogenic effects of lower doses of radiation, and in studying the relationship between dose and frequency of effect, is the greater because of the long latencies for some tumours even after high doses. Moreover, the experience following radiotherapy has been a major source of information on radiation carcinogenesis and fewer data may be available for exposure to moderate than to high doses. The detection of carcinogenesis at the lower doses may be doubly difficult for this reason.

---

* This review is based upon analyses undertaken on behalf of the British Medical Research Council.

A second need for developing any possible quantitative estimates of the carcinogenic hazards of radiation, particularly at moderate dose levels, arises from the exposure of people to radiation in the course of their work, and the variety of ways in which such exposure may occur. It is clearly of the greatest importance to establish whether moderate or low doses are carcinogenic, and with what frequency if so, so that exposures may be controlled to levels at which any such risks are, at most, slight. The evaluation of exposures which should not be exceeded thus requires at least an approximate estimate of hazard, or of the maximum likely hazard. Moreover, when occupational exposure may result from ingestion or inhalation of radionuclides which become localised and remain in certain tissues selectively, some quantitative estimation of the carcinogenic effect of radiation is required for different organs or tissues, as well as for the body as a whole.

It is obvious that even approximate estimates of this type which are applicable quantitatively in man and are valid for low doses delivered at low dose rates, are at present difficult or impossible to obtain. Some data are available for the frequency with which tumours are induced in various tissues following moderately high doses of some hundreds of rads, delivered at high dose rates. The inference to the frequencies to be expected from lower doses and dose rates is, however, impossible to make with confidence, although these data may at least provide the basis for a maximum estimate of the hazard of lower doses, and may also allow some comparison between the sensitivity of different tissues. There are, indeed, extensive data yielding quantitative estimates of the sensitivity of different tissues in animals. The substantial variations in sensitivity for the same tissue in different species, and in different strains of the same species, however, make it impossible to derive any generally applicable values which could be applied to man, or even to arrange different types of tissue in order of sensitivity, and this information from animals will not therefore be reviewed in any detail. Nor will any account be given of the parallel problems, which are of equal importance to human radiation risk evaluation and of even greater present difficulty, of estimating the components of hazard arising from genetic and chromosomal changes, and from life shortening or other limitation due to non-malignant changes that may be induced by radiation.

II. Problems involved in epidemiological surveys

Certain difficulties are common to many of the relevant epidemiological surveys of the cancer incidence observed following radiotherapeutic or other exposure of certain tissues.

1. Estimation of control rate

Firstly, it is usually necessary, in estimating or detecting any excess of tumours following radiation, to calculate the number of such tumours to be expected normally in a population of the sex and age distribution concerned, on the basis of the frequency of tumours in the general population of the region in question. Where, however, the exposure has resulted from the treatment of a particular condition or group of conditions, the expected incidence of a malignancy may differ in these conditions from that in the population as a whole. A false estimate may thus be obtained of an excess incidence attributed to radiation unless a sufficient survey is possible and available of the tumour incidence in patients with these diseases but untreated, either by radiation or by any other possibly oncogenic agent. That such an error might occur, in particular where the tumour incidence following radiation is low, is suggested by the finding that, although the incidence of leukaemia following the radioiodine treatment of hyperthyroidism is not significantly higher than that following surgical treatment, the leukaemia incidence following either treatment in this condition is significantly higher than in the general population (SAENGER *et al.*, 1968).

Similarly, COURT-BROWN and DOLL (1965), in their review of tumours observed following radiotherapy of ankylosing spondylitis, have stressed the association of ulcerative colitis with ankylosing spondylitis, and of carcinoma of the colon with ulcerative colitis.

2. Latency

A second general difficulty in obtaining valid numerical estimates of carcinogenicity is that tumours may continue to be detected for long periods after irradiation. The reported mean latency and the observed distribution of latencies in different studies are affected by the lengths of follow-up of patients that have been achieved in the studies, and by the efficiency of ascertainment of tumours at long intervals after irradiation, as well as by the age distribution of the population at exposure, and so by the loss of late induced tumours owing to death from other causes. Some correction of different estimates could be achieved if data were available, and were generally applicable, of the cumulant curve of incidence with time for radiation induced tumours, from studies in which extensive follow-up had been made. Since, however, the time scale of such a curve is likely to be dependent upon the age of the subject at irradiation, as well as upon the type of tumour concerned, no accurate correction of data can be expected on this basis. Tentative corrections have however been attempted along these lines (DOLPHIN, 1968) and are obviously of considerable quantitative importance where mean periods of follow-up for the exposed populations are less than 20 years. If for example the median latency for detection of a radiation induced cancer of particular type in an adult were 20 years — and this may well be an underestimate, since mean latencies of over 20 years have been observed in some studies — then the final incidence would clearly be about twice that found in a group of subjects followed for only 20 years. With mean periods of follow-up of less than 20 years, considerable importance would attach, not only to the distribution of follow-up times around their mean value, but also to the shape of the curve relating incidence of diagnosable malignancies with time interval after exposure. Some data are available on this distribution of latencies for certain malignancies and ages at exposure — for example for thyroid cancer (RAVENTOS and WINSHIP, 1964) and for leukaemia in adults (JABLON and BELSKY, 1970) — but more information on this question would be of value if based on substantial numbers of irradiated subjects fully followed up for long periods.

The long latencies, and the low incidence of tumours likely to be induced after moderate exposures (of some hundreds of rads), necessarily imply that valid quantitative estimates for radiation carcinogenicity in different tissues or organs will only be obtainable for these dose levels if large numbers of the subjects exposed can be followed for several decades. This consideration immediately excludes most of the information obtainable from radiotherapy of malignant disease except where such treatment is commonly effective in controlling the original malignancy or is given prophylactically, for example after operation. Even in these circumstances, there may be difficulties in establishing with certainty whether a subsequent tumour is a recurrence of the original treated malignancy or is a new condition which may have been radiation-induced. For this reason, estimates that have been or can be drawn from radiotherapeutic experience are largely confined to the sequels of the treatment of benign conditions. Such treatment is, of course, limited in application and is becoming even more limited although it has, for the present purpose, the value that it may involve total therapeutic exposures of some hundreds of rads to the tissues concerned, rather than of the thousands of rads usually given for malignant disease. These moderate doses are more relevant to the problems of estimating radiation carcinogenesis, not only because they are nearer to the doses that may be sustained under conditions of occupational exposure, but also because they are less likely to be associated with extensive cell destruction, and so to a decreased estimate of the carcinogenic risk of cell irradiation. They may, however, involve very low incidences of induced malignancy. Any resulting estimates are therefore likely to be based upon small numbers of cases in excess of natural expectation, and their values will have large statistical uncertainty. For example, if the risk of carcinogenesis in a particular organ were 0.1 % per 100 rads, the follow-up of 500 patients in whom that organ had received 400 rads would yield 2 more malignancies than expected without radiation. Even if the natural incidence were trivial, the confidence limits of an estimate based on only 2 cases would be wide. The necessary imprecision of any such estimate may be of small importance when only an approximate estimate of, for example, occupational risk is required, and when other uncertainties in its application to the possible effects of lower doses and low dose rates are in any case considerable. Reference has already been made, however, to the uncertainty as to whether a particular tumour incidence is the same in the general population and in the condition for which radiotherapy is given. This question is of increased importance when the number of tumours observed only exceeds by 2 or 3 the number expected on the basis of incidence in the general population.

3. Dosimetry

A further problem arises when attempts are made to base estimates on the effects of prolonged internal irradiation, as from the incorporation of radium-226 in bone. In such cases, it is possible to estimate (although with numerous uncertainties) what total dose has been delivered to bone, or to the endosteal cells, by the time a sarcoma is detected. It is not possible, however, to state what proportion of this dose was responsible for initiating the process leading to the malignancy that finally became detectable, and what proportion is "wasted" radiation which did not influence this result. The long latencies that commonly follow the relatively brief periods of exposure in external radiotherapy, and that have followed the momentary exposures at Hiroshima and Nagasaki, suggest that much of the radiation delivered to bone cells by radium-226 should not be included in calculations of the absorbed doses responsible for observed incidences of subsequent malignancy.

4. Magnitude of dose

Despite these severe limitations on the types of experience upon which carcinogenic risk estimates can be based, and on the accuracy or validity of the estimates that can be derived from any series of exposures, there remain some instances in which approximate estimates can be made for various human tissues or organs. In addition, it is becoming possible to grade certain other tissues in a semi-quantitative way as being less sensitive to carcinogenesis than those in which an excess of tumours has been observed after an equal exposure. In each case, however, the estimates are ordinarily derived from situations in which the absorbed doses in the tissues concerned have been in the region of hundreds of rads, and are not therefore applicable without qualification to estimating the effects of lower doses. For this reason it seems appropriate to quote estimates in terms of the percentage of subjects developing a tumour in the relevant organ, in excess of expectation, per 100 rads to the organ. Such estimates result simply from dividing the excess number of tumours by the mean organ dose and by the number of subjects, and are not intended to imply that the excess would be proportional to the dose at different dose levels — a point on which evidence is rarely available; and still less that the frequency of tumours would remain proportional to the size of dose even at dose levels of a few rads. Such a figure, however, if combined with a reference to the period of follow-up in which the incidence was observed, or with some correction for the incidence to be expected ultimately, forms a convenient basis for estimating quantitatively the sensitivity of an organ or tissue to radiation carcinogenesis.

III. Estimated induction of malignancies

1. Leukaemia

The induction of leukaemia, in its acute and granulocytic forms, by radiation was first identified by the detection of an increased incidence of these forms in radiologists, as compared with that in other groups of medical specialists (DUBLIN and SPIEGELMAN, 1948). No numerical estimate of hazard is obtainable from these observations, however, since the radiation exposure was not ordinarily measured in the earlier radiologists in whom the excess incidence was observed; and amongst radiologists more recently, whose exposure has been recorded, no such excess has been detected (COURT-BROWN and DOLL, 1958).

Various estimates have, however, been made from other sources. The incidence of leukaemia amongst significantly irradiated survivors at Hiroshima and Nagasaki has been compared with that in other groups in these cities or elsewhere in Japan. An excess incidence developed within a short time after exposure, reached a maximum after about 6 years, and had fallen to about one quarter of this maximum rate at 20 years from exposure (JABLON and BELSKY, 1970). The estimation of an induction-rate is affected by some uncertainties as to dose, shielding of parts of the body, and the probable differences in effectiveness per rad of the gamma and neutron irradiations which occurred in different proportions at different ranges in the two cities. Nor are incidences from particular studies necessarily proportional to dose, even for exposures from 100 to 400 rads. (A suggestion has been made [POSTON *et al.*, 1970] that, if correction is made for a varying RBE of neutrons with dose, curves of incidence with estimated dose are obtained yielding frequencies, by 20 years, of about 0.2 % and 0.4 % per 100 rems for doses of 100 and 300 rems at Hiroshima, and about 0.1 % and 0.4 % for these levels at Nagasaki.)

On diagnoses made by 20 years from exposure (MAKI *et al.*, 1968), overall values of about 0.4 % per 100 rads may be derived (from ABCC's master sample; with a somewhat lower figure from the life span study). The continuation of some excess incidence shows that a final figure will be somewhat, but perhaps not greatly, higher: the estimate would be increased by a few per cent if the excess incidence were regarded as decreasing linearly with time, or by about one third if assumed to be decreasing exponentially. A final value in the region of 0.5 %/100 rads would thus seem likely on these data. It has also been indicated that a rather higher induction occurred if this exposure took place during childhood (BIZZEZERO *et al.*, 1967), the rate in childhood being about 1.8 times, and that in adolescence about 1.3 times, that for the adult. Some indication has also been obtained of higher rates for the elderly than for young adults (DOLL, 1962).

An additional indication that the sensitivity may be increased in the young has been obtained by examining the excess frequency of leukaemia occurring during the first 10 years of life of children irradiated in utero in the course of diagnostic pelvic radiography of the mother. The extensive survey by MacMAHON (1962) indicated an incidence of 47 cases in children so irradiated, as compared with 32.5 expected on the basis of unirradiated children. Since the study was retrospective, the dose to the foetus was not known, but was likely to have averaged between 1 and 5 rads, and probably about 2 rads. A mean dose of 2 rads would imply an induction rate of about 1.1 $\pm$ 0.45 % (SE)/100 rads, rather higher than the current estimates for induction in adults; and MacMAHON demonstrated that the rather variable results of other and somewhat smaller surveys were statistically consistent with this value. In reporting results of the continuance of his survey, however, he stated (MacMAHON, 1970) that the excess was of 94 observed cases as compared with 74.9 expected, now yielding an induction rate of 0.65 $\pm$ 0.35 % (SE)/100 rads on the same assumption of a 2 rad mean dose to the foetus. The present data thus appear consistent with, but not conclusive of, a somewhat increased sensitivity of the foetus as compared with the adult. It should be emphasised that even these estimates depend on an assumed dose. Insofar as the mean dose is rather unlikely to have been less than 2 rad, they are, however, unlikely to underestimate any difference in age sensitivity to leukaemia induction.

In patients treated for ankylosing spondylitis, the subsequent significant excess of leukaemia can be related to dose delivered to bone marrow. In this case, however, only part of the marrow will be irradiated in any course of treatment, and it is quite uncertain whether partial exposure of the marrow would be as leukaemogenic as uniform exposure at an equal mean dose. It is also uncertain whether the incidence of leukaemia in patients with ankylosing spondylitis, treated with the range of drugs ordinarily administered but not with radiation, is in fact equal to that in the general population at corresponding ages, although there is some evidence (DOLL, 1970) that any difference, if it exists, must be small, and unimportant in estimating the excess incidence after irradiation. For a follow-up period averaging 13 years, the total incidence of leukaemia and aplastic anaemia apparently attributable to radiation was of the order of 60 per 14,500 persons (COURT-BROWN and DOLL, 1965). For an average dose of 880 rads delivered to about 40 % of the marrow, this would yield a value of about 0.1 to 0.15 % per 100 rads "mean marrow dose". The survey suggested a small but continuing incidence after 15 years, and the late occurence of new cases after atomic bomb irradiation would suggest that the figure might finally rise to $1\frac{1}{2}$ or 2 times this value. In either case, the final estimate is somewhat lower than that from the Japanese cities.

DOLL and SMITH (1968) also reported 6 cases of leukaemia, with only 1.3 expected on a general population basis, amongst 2,068 patients followed for a mean period of $13\frac{1}{2}$ years after roentgen-ray induction of artificial menopause involving a "mean marrow dose" of about 135 rads. These data therefore yield a figure of 0.16 ± 0.09 (SE) % per 100 rads by 13 years, which might correspond with about 0.3 % per 100 rads finally. A further estimate from similar surveys was quoted by DOLL at the International Cancer Congress in 1970.

When phosphorus-32 has been used in the treatment of polycythemia vera, an increased incidence of leukaemia has been reported. This finding is, however, difficult to interpret since the disease, even when untreated by radiation, may terminate in acute leukaemia, and since a prolongation of life achieved by the treatment may preferentially increase this likelihood. Moreover, a clear dependence of the incidence upon splenic size suggests that factors other than radiation may be involved (CAMPBELL et al., 1970). The values that can be derived from these data are very variable, the series of MODAN and LILIENFIELD (1964) yielding a figure of 3.4 ± 0.8 % per 100 rads for an 8 year follow-up (if an absorbed dose to marrow of 12 rads per millicurie administered is assumed), that of CAMPBELL et al. (1970) giving 1.4 ± 0.5, with LAWRENCE et al. (1969) finding 2.7 ± 0.7, while HALNAN and RUSSELL (1965) found no excess.

In the treatment of inoperable thyroid adenocarcinoma with radio-iodine, it seems clear that leukaemia may be induced in a small percentage of patients so treated. An estimate of this leukaemogenesis was attempted in one series (POCHIN, 1969) of 200 patients giving a value of 1.2 ± 0.6 % (SE)/100 rads to blood. It should however be emphasised that, in studies of this sort, a particular series may become "self-selected" for analysis and publication purely because the incidence appeared to be high and therefore of interest. High results based on few cases — 4 in this instance — may therefore merely reflect the occurrence of random variation round a lower mean value, series with "negative" results not being reported.

In summary, therefore, the available quantitative data suggest that radiation leukaemogenesis in man, following mean absorbed doses of a few hundred rads to the marrow, may occur at a rate of about $\frac{1}{2}$ % or possibly up to 1 % per 100 rads. Size of dose, dose rate, uniformity of marrow irradiation and other factors may, however, affect any such figure in ways that cannot yet be defined.

2. Breast

The radiation induction of breast carcinoma was suspected by MacKenzie (1965) who reported an increased incidence of this condition following repeated fluoroscopies made in the course of artificial pneumothorax therapy of pulmonary tuberculosis. The condition occurred in 4.8 % of the 271 patients followed, an excess of about 4 % above rates for the general population. On the basis of recorded numbers of fluoroscopies and of probable rates and durations of exposure (with 150 exposures for 15 sec at 50 R per minute), the mean breast dose may have been in the region of 2,000 rad, giving a rate of 0.2 ± 0.07 %/100 rad, but the dose estimation is very tenuous and the author emphasises that exposures may have exceeded these estimates in number, duration and dose rate. More recently Myrden and Hiltz (1969) have observed a similar excess, breast carcinoma arising in 7.3 % of patients treated by pneumothorax, and occurring ordinarily on the same side as the pneumothorax, as compared with an incidence of about 1 % in tuberculous patients not so treated. The median estimated number of fluoroscopies in those developing breast cancer exceeded 176, but neither the numbers for the whole series nor the exposures involved were quoted.

Wanebo and others (1968a) reported a raised incidence of breast cancer in survivors of irradiation at Hiroshima and Nagasaki, 9 such tumours being observed between 1958 and 1966 with 3.7 expected, amongst 1,643 women examined under the Adult Health Survey, and estimated as having received over 90 rads. This excess rate of 0.32% would have a standard error of 0.18 %. If significant (and further observation was reported in 1970 (Jablon and Belsky, 1970) as having diminished the difference), the induction rate during the 9 years of review would in any case appear likely to be less than 0.15 % per 100 rads over the period.

A further suggestion, but of equal statistical uncertainty, for tumour induction in the breast appears in a review (Pochin, 1969) of patients treated for thyroid cancer. Apart from the increased occurrence of leukaemia referred to above, there was no increase in mortality, and no significant increase in incidence, of other malignancies (apart from that of the thyroid). Within the non-significant excess incidence, amounting to 2.9 ± 2.8 cases, were 4 breast cancers, compared with 0.9 expected. If this possible increase in morbidity is related to dose, on the tentative dosimetric basis of the iodide concentrations applicable to milk from a secreting breast, an induction rate of 0.05 ± 0.03%/100 rads is obtained, but the significance of this figure can be questioned on numerous grounds

There are thus indications of sensitivity of breast tissue, perhaps of the order of 0.1 %/100 rads.

3. Bone

Osteosarcomas of bone have for many years been observed following incorporation of radium 226 into the skeleton as a result of earlier work with luminising materials or for other reasons. The quantitative aspects of the extensive human data have been very fully examined (Evans, 1966; Hasterlik and Finkel, 1965), and afford a valuable basis for relating the activity retained in bone to the likelihood or improbability of tumours arising. There are, however, numerous difficulties in applying this information to any numerical relationship between absorbed dose and tumour incidence.

Firstly, the available measurements usually relate to the final retention in bone at many years after ingestion, and the initial dose rates, distributions and patterns of excretion are unknown. Secondly, it is uncertain what part of the total dose is relevant to tumour induction, or may have been delivered only after this process has been initiated. Thirdly, the efficacy of the predominant alpha radiation in inducing malignancy, relative to that of other radiations, is uncertain. And fourthly, the relevant dosimetry in any case depends upon the site or sites within bone at which the cells occur which are involved in the process of tumour induction. If, as seems probable (ICRP, 1968), the endosteal cells are predominantly responsible, the relevant dose is that corresponding to their situation rather than the mean dose throughout bone, and the distribution of the nuclide, particularly soon after ingestion, will be important.

The occurrence of osteosarcomas following the injection of radium-224 therapeutically may offer a clearer basis for estimating the sensitivity of bone cells, owing to the short half life of the nuclide (3.6 days, as compared with 1600 years for ^{226}Ra), although the problems remain of the relative biological effectiveness for alpha radiations and the site of the sensitive cells. On the basis of a careful analysis of available data, Spiess and Mays (1970) observed an induction rate corresponding to 0.7 % per 100 rads as mean bone dose in adults and 1.4 % in adolescents. Since the dose to endosteal cells was estimated as about 9 times the mean bone dose, the nuclide probably being located on or near bone surfaces during much of its period of decay, values of 0.08 and 0.16 %/100 rads to endosteal cells are obtained for adults and adolescents. If alpha radiations have a relative biological effectiveness of between 2 and 10 times that of roentgen, beta or gamma radiation, it is clear that the further reduction of these figures, say to between 0.01 and 0.04 %/100 rems for the adult for such other radiations, would indicate bone cells to be of low sensitivity to sarcoma induction.

It is of interest that the lowest mean dose to bone at which a sarcoma has appeared following ^{224}Ra is estimated as 90 rad, as compared to 1,200 rad from ^{226}Ra. If however the estimation is based upon dose to endosteal cells, the levels would be about 800 rads from ^{224}Ra owing to its high initial surface concentration, and 500 rads from ^{226}Ra due to its more general distribution. It may therefore prove to be the case that the extensive human experience from these two isotopes of radium is not discrepant, and that the low radiation sensitivity of bone cells to malignant change is more widely supported.

4. Mucous membranes

In each of the major studies of radium-226 toxicity (Evans, 1966; Hasterlik and Finkel, 1965), but not in that of radium-224 (Spiess and Mays, 1970), carcinomas of the mucous membrane of the cranial air sinuses, as well as osteosarcomas, have been observed in excess of expectation. It has been stated that the mucosal cells lie at distances from bone similar to those of the endosteal cells. The close proximity of endosteal cells to bone, mainly within 10 μm, and the presence, presumably, of such cells between mucosa and bone, however, make it uncertain whether doses to the two types of cells will be equal, particularly in view of the rapid fall-off with distance of the alpha dose rate from radium-226; and no quantitative histological studies appear to have been made on this point. The fact that the mucosal cells are likely to receive additional radiation from radon released during radium decay and retained in the air sinuses, but that the frequency of mucosal malignancies is nevertheless only about half that of osteosarcomas (Evans, 1966; Hasterlik and Finkel, 1965), suggests that mucosal cells may have an even lower sensitivity than endosteal cells. This cannot be asserted with confidence until more information is available on the dose to mucosal cells from radium in bone and from radon in the air spaces, relative to that to endosteal cells; and on the relative numbers of each type of cell "at risk" per unit surface area of bone. The position does, however, illustrate a way in which it may prove possible to establish the sensitivity of one cell type relative to that of another for which a numerical estimate is available.

5. Lung

The report of Wanebo and others (1968b) on the incidence of lung cancers in survivors of the atomic bombing of Hiroshima and Nagasaki suggests that a slight excess of such tumours occurred during the 17 years following exposure. Three numerical criteria are obtainable: from deaths from 1950 to 1966 amongst members of the life span study;

from the incidence during the same period in members of the adult health study; and from cases coming to autopsy between 1961 and 1965 from the life span study group. None of these yielded strongly positive or highly significant values (0.09 ± 0.04, 0.12 ± 0.08 and, approximately and for 5 years only, 0.06 ± 0.03 % per 100 rad) but the trend of the figures suggested a rate in the region of 0.1 % per 100 rads by 20 years, and so perhaps twice this ultimately. Extension of this study, however, is reported to have yielded lower values of doubtful significance.

It is, however, of interest that, amongst the tumours of tissues substantially irradiated during the treatment of ankylosing spondylitis (COURT-BROWN and DOLL, 1965), those of the bronchi accounted for about 45 % of the total excess (of deaths from cancer of heavily irradiated sites on the incomplete follow-up to January 1963), the excess numbers being about one sixth those for leukaemia, although of course the doses delivered to lung and bone marrow will not have been equal.

The occurrence of radiation carcinogenesis in lung tissue, leading particularly to "oat-cell" tumours (SACCOMANNO *et al.*, 1964), has been evident from uranium and other mining experience for many years and has been studied quantitatively in great detail by LUNDIN *et al.* (1969). This extensive experience on human radiation carcinogenesis does not, however, yet yield any clear estimate of sensitivity, since the mean dose to lung or bronchi of individual miners can be only very approximately derived from the air concentrations of radon measured intermittently at defined positions in the various mines; and the dose itself is likely to depend on the concentration of charged particulates in the air inhaled. If it is assumed that one month's exposure at 1 "working level" contributes about 12 rad to the bronchi, the mortality from lung cancer is found to occur at a rate, in excess of expectation, of about 0.02 %/100 rads for an average of 10 years exposure as based on deaths between 1950 and 1967 for white underground miners, or 0.04%/100 rads if based on 1964/1967-deaths after higher mean exposures but with fewer person years at risk. The rates per 100 rem would of course be even lower, according to the quality factor assumed for alpha radiation, but the short mean time of follow-up will involve a considerable underestimate of total risk.

Difficulties again arise in allowing for tumours that will occur after longer latency, and in discounting radiation exposure after tumours have been initiated. This evidence, therefore, cannot yield a valid estimate of sensitivity of lung or bronchial tissues, but suggests that this figure is not high, since, even if half the radiation dose were "wasted", and if a quarter of all tumours had developed within 10 years, both estimates would still be lower than 0.4%/100 rads and of course lower still per 100 rems. So many uncertainties are involved, particularly in linking mine samples with cell dose, that the estimation is perhaps of more value in demonstrating the type of information still needed than in indicating the value derived.

6. Gastro-intestinal tract

It is unfortunate that very little information is available on which to base any estimate of the sensitivity of gut tissues to radiation carcinogenesis, since these tissues — and specifically those of the lower colon — ordinarily receive the highest absorbed doses following ingestion of radionuclides particularly in forms having low aqueous solubility, and an estimate of their sensitivity is important for protection purposes.

BRINKLEY and HAYBITTLE (1969) observed 7 deaths from tumours of rectum and intestine, with only 1.5 expected, during a 15 to 25 (average 16) year follow-up of 277 patients given previous roentgen-ray treatment for induction of artificial menopause. With a 10×20 cm field from symphysis pubis to pelvic crest, and with a probable mean dose to gut within this field of about 800 rad (HAYBITTLE, personal communication) a value of 0.25 ± 0.12%/100 rads is obtained for irradiation of part of the gut. For the rectum alone, presumably fully in the field, with 3 observed cases and 0.5 expected, the estimate becomes very imprecise — 0.11 ± 0.07%/100 rad. Of the 4 intestinal cases, with 1.0

expected, 3 were regarded certainly, and the fourth probably, as from large intestine. If half the large intestine were in the field, the value for the whole large intestine would be 0.27 ± 0.18%/100 rads. These figures are thus subject to large statistical, apart from any other, imprecision and would merely suggest that (if half the small intestine were in the field and did not contribute tumours) the total value for all gut distal to the stomach may be of the order of 0.4 ± 0.2%/100 rads, but further data on this important point are needed.

In their survey of the sequels of radiotherapy for ankylosing spondylitis, Court-Brown and Doll (1965) hesitated to interpret the observed excess of deaths from cancers of colon (25 with 14.8 expected) in view of the association between ulcerative colitis both with spondylitis and with cancer of the colon. This excess was about one sixth that from leukaemia over the same period, or one twelfth if the risk of colon cancer were 36 % above normal in spondylitis, but the lower mean dose to gut than to marrow and the longer latencies of carcinoma induction compared with leukaemia would both tend to decrease the difference between estimates that might be derived for colon and for leukaemia.

An attempt was made (Dolphin and Eve, 1968) to derive a figure for stomach sensitivity from the results of this survey, but this value is again imprecise owing to inadequate information being available at present as to the mean dose to the stomach in the irradiated spondylitic patients. The excess of deaths from stomach cancer is, however, estimated with moderate precision from these data (Court-Brown and Doll, 1965) — the numbers on the complete follow-up to January 1960 having been 28 observed and 16.0 expected — with an excess of 12.0 ± 5.3 cases, and on the incomplete follow-up to January 1963, 38 observed and 23.6 expected, an excess of 14.4 ± 6.2 cases. An estimate of dose to stomach from the fields and exposures used should therefore yield a significant figure for gastric sensitivity, although still for periods of follow-up which are short compared with the likely median latency for such cancers.

7. Thyroid

An excess of thyroid cancers has been observed following the irradiation of the gland in infancy as treatment given for enlargement of the thymus or for other reasons. Certain estimates, combining a number of surveys with or without reported increases in incidence, yielded mean values of about 0.2%, 0.35 % and 0.4 % per 100 rads (UNSCEAR, 1964; Beach and Dolphin, 1967; Hempelmann et al., 1967) for 15 to 20 years follow-up, and of 0.15 % (Hanford et al., 1962; personal communication by Dr. Quimby of mean dose) for 12 years. With corrections for late tumour incidence, Dolphin's (1968) data give 1.0 %, and the closely studied "high risk subgroup C" of Hempelmann (1968) gives a value of 1.3 ± 0.4 %/100 rads. In 24 cases noted by Hempelmann, no deaths have occurred although the mean follow-up since irradiation is of about 25 years, but pulmonary metastases are present in 2 patients. As the average of all experience, and for expected incidence in prolonged follow-up, an incidence of between ½ and 1 % per 100 rads received in infancy seems likely, although the total for fatal thyroid malignancies seems unlikely to exceed 0.1 %/100 rads, since differentiated thyroid cancers of the type induced can commonly be treated radically by surgery or adequately by radioiodine, and are in any event of relatively low malignancy.

Several publications (Socolow et al., 1963; Sampson et al., 1969; Wood et al., 1969) have indicated an excess of thyroid cancers occurring in the irradiated populations of Hiroshima and Nagasaki. Wood et al. (1969) report data showing that, in the two cities combined and for estimated thyroid doses of 0 to 49, 50 to 199, and over 200 rads, the excess incidences in males, above a rate of 0.04 % in control populations, were 0.07, 0.21 and 0.37 % respectively. The corresponding incidences in females, above a control rate of 0.2 %, were 0.08, 0.48 and 0.71 %. If mean doses of 100 and 300 rads are assumed for the two higher dosage groups, the mean rates in these two groups would be about 0.35 and

0.2 %/100 rads. It is of interest that the mean rate in those irradiated at ages of 20 or over was about one third that when the age had been under 20, the mean rate for the whole population having been about half that for those irradiated at ages under 20. The figures quoted do not therefore appear inconsistent with those for irradiation in infancy.

Of the 51 tumours studied histologically, 42 were adenocarcinomas of papillary, follicular or mixed character, and 9 were "occult sclerosing" carcinomas, no anaplastic tumours having been seen. In a further study (SAMPSON et al., 1969) 536 thyroid tumours, mainly small "occult" papillary carcinomas, were found in the course of 3,067 autopsies in these cities, giving an incidence of 22.5 % in those exposed at over 50 rads as compared with 16 % in the unexposed, but the significance of a lesion of this type occurring in 16 % of unexposed subjects is very difficult to interpret clinically.

It is believed that irradiation of the gland from radioiodine, under usual conditions of distribution, rate and duration of dose delivery is less carcinogenic per rad than uniform external radiation of the gland at high dose rate for short duration. This appears to be supported by several lines of animal experimental (DONIACH, 1963) or indirect evidence, including the absence of any excess of thyroid cancers in some hundreds of thousands of thyrotoxic patients treated with radioiodine, but again no numerical comparison is available for the normal human thyroid. The Rongelap populations, irradiated accidentally by fallout, received high mean doses to the thyroids of the children, predominantly from radioiodines, with a high incidence of palpable nodularity of the gland with three malignancies recently reported (CONARD et al., 1970). Two of these have occurred in 42 subjects who were aged 10 or more at the time of exposure, and are likely to have received a mean thyroid dose of about 300 rads (corresponding to an incidence of 1.6 % per 100 rads in 15 years) and one occurred in 25 children who were under 10 when exposed with a mean dose of the order of 1000 rads (or 0.4 % per 100 rads). These data give no support to a higher sensitivity in early childhood unless the doses to children were, as suggested, higher than "optimal" for tumour induction. The total incidence, of 3 cases compared with 0.056 expected, would correspond to an induction rate of 0.8 ± 0.45 % per 100 rads and would not in itself support a lower carcinogenicity of internal as compared with external radiation of the gland.

8. Other tissues

The salivary glands of infants who were irradiated for thymic or other conditions are likely to have received mean doses of the same order as their thyroid glands, and the excess incidence of malignant tumours of the salivary glands has been about one sixth that for the thyroid (4 salivary tumours with 0.1 expected, compared with 24 of the thyroid and one expected [HEMPELMANN et al., 1967]). This comparison applies only for infancy, and for incidence not mortality, with assumptions as to equal dose and equally efficient ascertainment, and subject to differences in latency of tumour development. It would, however, suggest that salivary glands would have a sensitivity in the region of 0.1 to 0.2 %/100 rads, if that of the thyroid is of $\frac{1}{2}$ to 1 %/100 rads in infants.

It is of equal importance that no excess is noted of tumours arising from trachea, skin, oesophagus or other structures within the field of irradiation. As a general point, the negative findings for many tissues following reasonably uniform irradiation of a defined volume may be as valuable as the positive findings in other tissues irradiated, since these negative findings, and the confidence limits that apply to the observed zero or small incidence, may serve to give upper estimates for the sensitivity, or sensitivity per unit mass, of many tissues which are relatively insusceptible to malignant change following radiation. In studies where equal efficiency of ascertainment can be ensured for all tumours, even if they were not the primary object of the study, negative results may be of great value in defining protection criteria and should always be fully reported. It is of interest in this connection that GOOLDEN (1957) reported 12 carcinomas of the pharynx following thyroid irradiation for benign conditions, but no other malignancies. He noted reports of 20 pharyngeal cancers (18 carcinomas and 2 fibrosarcomas) as against 5 laryngeal carcinomas in previous published series.

Cells of the developing nervous system appeared to be susceptible to tumour induction in the results obtained by MacMahon (1962) following irradiation in utero, with a possibly significant excess of 19 observed over 12.0 expected, a rate of $0.45 \pm 0.28 \%/100$ rads if a 2 rad mean dose is assumed. This excess has not however been confirmed on further experience in this series (MacMahon, 1970).

Skin has been recognised as susceptible to tumour induction for 70 years, and it is perhaps surprising that no studies appear to be available on which an estimate of susceptibility can be based. The lack of reported skin tumours in other studies involving skin irradiation may indicate that the sensitivity is low. A typical radiotherapeutic field will however involve only about 1 or 2 % of the total skin surface and a substantial contribution of skin tumours to the total tumour incidence from a uniform whole body irradiation cannot be excluded. The long latency of many such tumours would also tend to reduce the numbers observed in limited series. Andrews (1957) has reviewed reports and experience of skin tumours following irradiation, and noted a mean latency of 27 years in 28 basal cell cancers, and 25 years in 19 squamous cell cancers apparently so induced. In a sequence of 13 patients treated for benign conditions with a mean dose of 630 R, 3 skin cancers developed in a period of follow-up of from 12 to 30 years. The analysis of larger studies of this type should yield a numerical value for tumour incidence per 100 rads and per unit area of skin, and would be of value, particularly in regard to protection criteria in situations with high skin beta radiation doses but little irradiation of the whole body from penetrating radiation. It is of interest in this connection that Andrews recorded a mortality of only 6 % for apparently radiation induced skin tumours followed for a mean period of 10 years from their diagnosis and treatment.

An apparent excess of lymphomas in Hiroshima was reported by Anderson and Ishida (1964), the numbers suggesting an induction rate about one tenth that for leukaemia at comparable times and distributed about equally between lymphadenoma and lymphosarcoma. If confirmed and extended, this type of information could yield a numerical estimate for lymphoid tissues, or certain lymphoid tissues, by comparison with that for leukaemia, subject to any relevant differences in latency between these conditions. Lewis (1963) noted an excess of deaths from multiple myeloma, of 5 observed against 1 expected, in radiologists. The corresponding excess of deaths from leukaemia was 8.

Ample quantitative data are available on induction of malignancies, including those of biliary and vascular epithelium in the liver, following the injection of Thorotrast and the hepatic concentration of insoluble particles of thorium dioxide (IAEA, 1968). Uncertainties about the appropriate alpha dosimetry from the aggregating and migrating particles in the liver, and as to any purely chemical carcinogenic effect of these particles, prevent the derivation of any useful measure of sensitivity for these tissues.

IV. Conclusions

It would be wrong to attach undue significance to the absolute values of the figures suggested above for the susceptibility to radiation carcinogenesis of the tissues discussed. Many of these values are subject to considerable statistical uncertainty and all of them are liable to a number of systematic errors due to incomplete ascertainment, insufficient length of follow-up, uncertainty about normal cancer incidences in various diseases, the significance of uniformity of radiation of the whole of a tissue, other injuries associated with atomic bomb radiation, drugs used as treatment of conditions for which radiotherapy is given, and chromosomal or other abnormalities correlating with the reasons for which the radiation was used. And, above all, the association of a given induction rate with a particular mean dose to the tissue concerned does not imply that the induction rate is proportional to the dose within the range of doses given, or independent of dose rate and fractionation of the dose, still less that the value derived for some hundreds of rads delivered at high dose rate can be used for estimating the effect of a few rads delivered at low dose rate, although it may serve for protection purposes as a maximum likely estimate of this effect. Nor can it be excluded that irradiation of one tissue may increase the likelihood of cancer in another tissue.

It is however of obvious importance for radiation protection purposes, particularly in regard to radionuclides which are locally concentrated in relation to certain tissues and cause selective irradiation of them, that the relative sensitivity of different types of tissue should be established, and approximate estimates obtained at least for the more sensitive of them. In this sense, the estimates discussed above may at least serve for defining the problem and illustrating the methods involved and the further information required, as well as for indicating which tissues appear on present evidence to be the most sensitive and which are less so. In quantitative terms, it appears as though several may have sensitivity in the region of 0.5 to 1 % per 100 rads, and some at 0.1 % or less. Figures of this magnitude appear reasonable in relation to the estimates obtained for the induction in experimental animals of tumours which probably have, in most cases, been selected for study because of the readiness with which they are induced by radiation in selected species or strains of animal (IAEA, 1969). Thus values per 100 rads (again, without presumption of proportionality of dose and effect) can be estimated as about 11% for mammary adenocarcinoma in rats from gamma radiation, and between 4 and 8 % for the highly non-linear yield of malignant renal tumours in rats following roentgen radiation. Small intestinal tumours in rats give values depending upon strain of rat, of about 0.5 %/100 R in SIMONSON, 0.75 % in AUGUST, and 2.5 % in HOLTZMAN rats. DONIACH (1970) has estimated the induction of thyroid carcinoma in rats by roentgen radiation at a rate of from 1 to 4 % per 100 rads.

A direct estimate of the total of all tumours induced by uniform whole body irradation has been attempted by comparing the excess number of cases of leukaemia in an irradiated population with the excess of all other malignancies, regardless of their tissue of origin. At present, however, the two available sources of such information appear to give widely discrepant ratios, and neither series has been followed for long enough to recognise all the malignancies likely to have been induced. Thus in the surveys of the irradiated populations of the Japanese cities, the excess numbers of cases of leukaemia and of fatal other malignancies appear to be about equal, for a follow-up of up to 20 years (MAKI *et al.*, 1968). On the other hand, the irradiated spondylitis have shown from 3 to 6 times (with a factor of 3.1 ± 1.1 on the complete follow-up data of COURT-BROWN and DOLL [1965], or 5.5 ± 1.4 on their incomplete follow-up data) as many other fatal malignancies as cases of leukaemia (ICRP, 1969), even though many body tissues will have received lower doses than those to the bone marrow. The excess of cancers of the colon in this group is quite inadequate to account for this discrepancy, even if these were all due to a partial correlation with ulcerative colitis. It is, however, impossible to exclude either that other cancers also had an increased incidence in ankylosing spondylitis, or that associated treatments of these patients had carcinogenic effects, although neither explanation is supported by direct evidence. By this approach therefore one can only state that, if leukaemia is induced at a rate of 0.5 % per 100 rads mean dose to the marrow, a dose of 100 rads to the whole body would, by 20 years, cause other malignancies in between 0.5 and 3 % of cases, with perhaps twice these rates ultimately, giving total incidences of fatal malignancies of between 1 and 7 % .This range does not appear inconsistent with the range of values discussed above for the individual tissues likely to be of higher sensitivity, given that the low fatality rate of thyroid and skin tumours would be likely to bring them into the lower part of this range. With a few tissues in the region of 0.5 to 1 %, a few more between 0.2 and 0.5 %, and a number with lower values, a total incidence of a few per cent per 100 rads would not appear unlikely.

Any present review of this subject, however, must be regarded as a challenge to further comprehensive and quantitative follow-up studies of groups of subjects in whom the body, or defined volumes of the body, have been irradiated, rather than as a schedule of estimated sensitivities on which reliance can yet be placed.

References

Andrews, P.: Rodent ulcers induced by X-rays and radium. Univ. of London Thesis for MD, 1957.

Anderson, R. E., Ishida, K.: Malignant lymphoma in survivors of the atomic bomb in Hiroshima. Ann. intern. Med. **61**, 853–862 (1964).

Bizzozero, O. J., Johnson, K. G., Ciocco, A., Kawasaki, S., Toyoda, S.: Radiation-related leukaemia in Hiroshima and Nagasaki, 1946–1964. Ann. intern. Med. **66**, 522–530 (1967).

Beach, S. A., Dolphin, G. W.: A study of the relationship between X-ray dose delivered to thyroids of children and the subsequent development of malignant tumours. Phys. med. Biol. **6**, 583–598 (1962).

Brinkley, D., Haybittle, J. L.: The late effects of artificial menopause by X-radiation. Br. J. Radiol. **42**, 519–521 (1969).

Campbell, A., Emery, E. W., Godlee, J. N., Prankerd, T. A. J.: Diagnosis and treatment of primary polycythaemia. Lancet **1**, 1074–1077 (1970).

Conard, R. A., Dobyns, B. M., Sutow, W. W.: Thyroid Neoplasia from Radioactive Fallout. J. Amer. med. Ass. **214**, 316–324 (1970).

Court-Brown, W. M., Doll, R.: Expectation of life and mortality from cancer among British radiologists. Br. med. J. **2**, 181–187 (1958).

— — Mortality from cancer and other causes after radiation therapy for ankylosing spondylitis. Br. med. J. **2**, 1327–1332 (1965).

Doll, R.: Age difference in susceptibility to carcinogenesis in man. Br. J. Radiol. **35**, 31–36 (1962).

— Cancer following therapeutic external irradiation. Paper delivered at 10th International Cancer Congress, Houston 1970. In course of publication.

— Smith, P. G.: The long term effects of X-irradiation in patients treated for metropathia haemorrhagica. Br. J. Radiol. **41**, 362–368 (1968).

Dolphin, G. W.: The risk of thyroid cancers following irradiation. Hlth. Phys. **15**, 219–228 (1968).

— Eve, I. S.: In: Gastrointestinal radiation injury, pp. 465–476. Ed.: Sullivan, M. F. Amsterdam: Exc. Med. Foundation, 1968.

Doniach, I.: Effects including carcinogenesis of 131 I and X-rays on the thyroid of experimental animals; a review. Hlth. Phys. **9**, 1357–1362 (1963).

— Experimental thyroidtumours. In: Tumours of the thyroid gland, pp. 73–99. Ed.: Sir David Smithers. Edinburgh & London: E. & S. Livingstone, 1970.

Dublin, L., Spiegelman, M.: Mortality of medical specialists, 1938–1942. J. Am. med. Ass. **137**, 1519–1524 (1948).

Evans, R. D.: The effect of skeletally deposited alpha ray emitters in man. Br. J. Radiol. **39**, 881–895 (1966).

Frieben, A.: Canceroid nach langdauernder Einwirkung von Röntgenstrahlen. Fortschr. Röntgenstr. **6**, 106 (1902).

Goolden, A. W. G.: Radiation Cancer: a review with special reference to radiation tumours in the pharynx, larynx and thyroid. Br. J. Radiol. **30**, 626–640 (1957).

Halnan, K. E., Russell, M. H.: Polycythemia Vera, comparison of survival and causes of death in patients managed with and without radiotherapy. Lancet **2**, 760–763 (1965).

Hanford, J. M., Quimby, E. H., Frantz, V. K.: Cancer arising many years after radiation therapy. J. Am. med. Ass. **181**. 404–410 (1962).

Hasterlik, R. H., Finkel, A. J.: Diseases of bone and joints associated with intoxication by radioactive substances principally radium. Med. Clins. N. Am. **49**, 285–296 (1965).

Hempelmann, L. H.: Risk of thyroid neoplasms after irradiation in childhood. Science **160**, 159–163 (1968).

— Pifer, J. F., Burke, G. J., Terry, R., Ames, W. R.: Neoplasms in persons treated in infancy with X-rays for thymic enlargement; report of the 3rd followup survey. J. natn. Cancer Inst. **38**, 317–341 (1967).

IAEA Techn. Report 106. The dosimetry and toxicity of thorotrast. Vienna 1968.

IAEA Report of Symposium, Athens 1969. Radiation Induced Cancer. IAEA, Vienna 1969.

International Commission on Radiological Protection, Publication 8. The evaluation of risks from radiation. Oxford: Pergamon Press 1966.
Publication 11. A review of the radiosensitivity of the tissues in bone. Oxford: Pergamon Press 1968.

— Publication 14. Radiosensitivity and spatial distribution of dose. Oxford: Pergamon Press 1969.

Jablon, S., Belsky, J. L.: Radiation induced cancer in atomic bomb survivors. Paper delivered at 10th International Cancer Congress, Houston 1970. In course of publication.

Lawrence, J. H., Winchell, H. S., Donald, W. G.: Leukaemia in Polycythemia Vera. Ann. intern. Med. **70**, 763–771 (1969).

Lewis, E. B.: Leukaemia, multiple myeloma and aplastic anaemia in American radiologists. Science **142**, 1492–1494 (1963).

LUNDIN, F. E., LLOYD, J. W., SMITH, E. M., ARCHER, V. E., HOLADAY, D. A.: Mortality of uranium miners in relation to radiation exposure, hardrock mining and cigarette smoking, 1950 through Sept. 1967. Hlth. Phys. **16**, 571–578 (1969).

MACKENZIE, I.: Breast cancer following multiple fluoroscopies. Br. J. Cancer **19**, 1–8 (1965).

MACMAHON, B.: Prenatal X-ray exposure and childhood cancer. J. nat. Cancer Inst. **28**, 1173–1191 (1962).

— Juvenile cancer associated with prenatal irradiation. Paper delivered at 10th International Cancer Congress, Houston 1970. In course of publication.

MAKI, H., ISHIMARU, T., KATO, H., WAKABAYASHI, T.: Carcinogenesis in atomic bomb survivors. Atomic Bomb Casualty Commission Technical Report 24–68 (1968).

MODAN, B., LILIENFELD, A. M.: Leukaemogenic effect of ionising radiation treatment in polycythemia. Lancet **2**, 439–441 (1964).

MYRDEN, J. A., HILTZ, J. E.: Breast cancer following multiple flouroscopies during artificial pneumothorax treatment of pulmonary tuberculosis. Can. med. Ass. J. **100**, 1032–1034 (1969).

POCHIN, E. E.: Long term hazards of radioiodine treatment of thyroid cancer. UICC Monograph Series, Vol. 12, Thyroid Cancer, pp. 293–304. Berlin: Springer-Verlag 1969.

— The development of the quantitative bases for radiation protection. Br. J. Radiol. **43**, 155–160 (1970).

PORTER, C. A., WHITE, C. J.: Multiple carcinomata following chronic X-ray dermatitis. Ann. Surg. **46**, 649–671 (1907).

POSTON, J.W., CHEKA, J. S., CHEN, W. L., FOX, W. F., HUBBELL, H. H., JACKSON, J. E., JONES, T. D., ROBINSON, E. M., SHINPAUGH, W. H., SNYDER, W. S., WAGNER, E. B.: Dosimetry for human exposures and radiobiology. ORNL-4584, UC-41 Hlth. & Safety, pp. 129–151, 1970.

RAVENTOS, A., WINSHIP, T.: The latent interval for thyroid cancer following irradiation. Radiology **83**, 501–508 (1964).

ROWNTREE, C. W.: Contribution to the study of X-ray carcinoma and the conditions which precede its onset. Archs. Middx. Hosp. **13**, 182–205 (1908).

SACCOMANNO, G., ARCHER, V. E., SAUNDERS, R. P., JAMES, L. A., BECKLER, P. A.: Lung cancer of uranium miners on the Colorado Plateau. Hlth. Phys. **10**, 1195–1201 (1964).

SAENGER, E. L., THOMA, G. E., TOMPKINS, E. A.: Incidence of leukaemia following treatment of hyperthyroidism. Preliminary report of the cooperative thyrotoxicosis therapy follow-up study. J. Am. med. Ass. **205**, 855–862 (1968).

SAMPSON, R. J., KEY, C. R., BUNCHER, C. R., IYIMA, S.: Thyroid carcinoma in Hiroshima and Nagasaki. J. Am. med. Ass. **209**, 65–70 (1969).

SOCOLOW, E. L., HASHIZUMA, A., NERIISHI, S., NIITANI, R.: Thyroid carcinoma in man after exposure to ionising radiation. New Engl. J. Med. **268**, 406–410 (1963).

SPIESS, H., MAYS, C. W.: Bone cancers induced by 224 Ra (Th X) in children and adults. Paper delivered at 10th International Cancer Congress, Houston 1970. Health Physics **19**, 713–729 (1970).

United Nations Scientific Committee on the Effects of Atomic Radiation. G. A. Off. Rec. 19th Session, Suppl. No. 14 (A/5814). United Nations, New York 1964.

WANEBO, C. K., JOHNSON, K. G., SATO, K., THORSLUND, T. W.: Breast cancer after exposure to the atomic bombings of Hiroshima and Nagasaki. New Engl. J. Med. **279**, 667–671 (1968a).

— — — — Lung cancer following atomic radiation. Am. rev. resp. Dis. **98**, 778–787 (1968b).

WOOD, J. W., TAMAGAKI, H., NERIISHI, S., SATO, T., SHELDON, W. F., ARCHER, P. G., HAMILTON, H. B., JOHNSON, K. G.: Thyroid carcinoma in atomic bomb survivors, Hiroshima and Nagasaki Am. J. Epidemiol. **89**, 4–14 (1969).

Sachverzeichnis

Bei gleicher Schreibweise in beiden Sprachen sind die Stichwörter nur einmal aufgeführt

Subject Index

Where English and German spelling of a word is identical, the German version is omitted

Aberrations, chromosomes, classification, *Aberrationen, Chromosomen, Klassifikation* 141
—, —, radiation induced, *Aberrationen, Chromosomen, strahleninduzierte* 127—180
aberration types, chromosomes, *Aberrationstypen, Chromosomen* 136—141
abortive cell division, *abortive Zellteilung* 68
— colonies, after irradiation, *abortive Kolonien, nach Bestrahlung* 70, 72
absorbed dose, induction of mammary neoplasms, *absorbierte Dosis, Induktion von Mamma-Tumoren* 32
— —, unit rad, *absorbierte Dosis, Einheit Rad* 1, 2
absorption events, dose-effect relation, *Absorptionsereignisse, Dosis-Wirkungsbeziehung* 26, 27
— —, size of sensitive region, *Absorptionsereignisse, Größe der sensiblen Region* 35
abnormalities, radiation induced, *Mißbildungen, strahleninduzierte* 253, 289
accidents, reactor, *Zwischenfälle, Reaktor* 307
achromatic gaps, chromosomes, *achromatische Lücken, Chromosomen* 139
actinomycin, blockade of mitosis, *Actinomycin, Blockierung der Mitose* 68
—, dose effect curve parameters, HeLa-cells, *Actinomycin, Dosiseffektkurvenparameter, HeLa-Zellen* 55
acute radiation syndrome, therapy, *akutes Strahlensyndrom, Behandlung* 331
alkylating agents, dose effect curves, *alkylierende Verbindungen, Dosiseffektkurven* 54
anemia, radiation syndrome, *Anämie, Strahlensyndrom* 324
anomalies, radiation induced, mouse, *Anomalien, strahleninduzierte, Maus* 252
anoxia, dose effect curves, *Anoxie, Dosiseffektkurven* 107
—, in-vitro experiments, *Anoxie, in-vitro-Versuche* 104
antibiotic drugs, effect upon "reproductive integrity", *Antibiotica, Wirkung auf die „reproduktive Integrität"* 47, 68
α-particles, cell inactivation, *α-Partikel, Zellinaktivierung* 15, 16, 17, 89
—, chromosomal aberrations, *α-Teilchen, Chromosomenaberrationen* 135
aplasia, bone marrow, radiation effect, *Aplasie, Knochenmark, Strahlenwirkung* 301
α-rays, different energy, radiation effect, *α-Strahlen, verschiedene Energie, Strahlenwirkung* 76
α-radiation, induction of malignancies, *α-Strahlung, Tumorinduktion* 347, 348
ascites tumour, dose effect curve parameters, *Ascites-Tumor, Dosiseffektkurvenparameter* 62, 64
— —, dose rate effect, *Ascites-Tumor, Dosisleistungseffekt* 82

autoradiography, proliferation kinetics, *Autoradiographie, Proliferationskinetik* 112
—, radiation induced mitotic delay, *Autoradiographie, strahleninduzierte Mitoseverzögerung* 66

babies, leukaemia, irradiation, *Säuglinge, Leukämie, Bestrahlung* 272
bacteria, inactivation dose, *Bakterien, Inaktivierungsdosis* 7, 8
bacteremia, radiation effect, *Bakteriämie, Strahlenwirkung* 319
basal cells, dose effect curve parameters, *Basalzellen, Dosiseffektkurvenparameter* 62
beta exposure, skin, fall out, *Beta-Exposition, Haut, Fall-out* 335
biochemical changes, radiation effect, *biochemische Änderungen, Strahlenwirkung* 261
biological dosimetry, *biologische Dosimetrie* 159, 165
biological dosimeter, spleen, thymus, *biologisches Dosimeter, Milz, Thymus* 314
blastogenesis, radiation induced death, *Blastogenese Strahlentod* 251
blood, cell renewal system, *Blut, Zellerneuerungssystem* 309
— counts, radiation effect, *Blutzellen, Strahlenwirkung* 315
— dyscrasias, radiation exposure, history, *Blutschäden, Strahlenexposition, Geschichtliches* 301
— vessels, radiation effect, *Blutgefäße, Strahlenwirkung* 315
bone, induction of malignancies by ionising radiation, *Knochen, Induktion maligner Tumoren durch ionisierende Strahlen* 346
— marrow, cell renewal, *Knochenmark, Zellerneuerung* 310
— —, depression, radiation exposure, *Knochenmark, Depression, Strahlenexposition* 301
— —, dose effect curves in vivo, *Knochenmark, Dosiseffektkurven in vivo* 60, 78
— —, hemopoietic syndromes, *Knochenmark, hämatopoetisches Syndrom* 323
— —, "oxygen enhancement ratio", *Knochenmark, „oxygen enhancement ratio"* 104
— —, radiation effect, *Knochenmark, Strahlenwirkung* 78, 315, 317
— —, tissue culture, dose effect curve parameters, *Knochenmark, Zellkultur, Dosiseffektkurvenparameter* 52, 62, 78
— —, transplantation, radiation protection, *Knochenmark, Transplantation, Strahlenschutz* 302
— — cells, reduction of extrapolation number, *Knochenmackzellen, Reduktion der Extrapolationsnummer* 79